Improve International Textbook of Small Animal Surgery

Improve International Textbook of Small Animal Surgery

Volume 1

Soft tissues

Edited by Hannes Bergmann

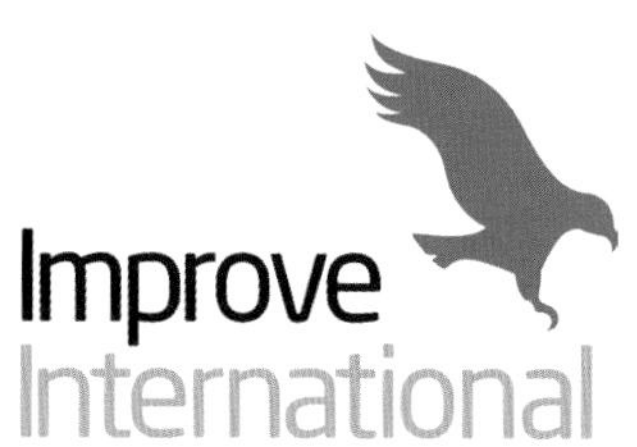

First published 2019

Published by
5M Publishing Ltd,
Benchmark House,
8 Smithy Wood Drive,
Sheffield, S35 1QN, UK
Tel: +44 (0) 1234 81 81 80
www.5mpublishing.com

A Catalogue record for this book is available from the British Library

ISBN 9781913352004

Book layout by Servis Filmsetting Ltd, Stockport, Cheshire
Printed by Replika Press Pvt Ltd, India
Photos by the authors unless otherwise indicated. The copyright of the photographs remains with the authors or person named in the credits.
Illustrations by Elaine Leggett

Contents

Contributors

Jonathan Bell, BVM&S, CertSAS, DipECVS, MRCVS, Swift Referrals

Kelly L. Bowlt-Blacklock, BVM&S, FHEA, DipECVS, MRCVS, Animal Health Trust

Guillaume Chanoit, DEDV, PhD, DipECVS, DipACVS, FHEA, MRCVS, Small Animal Referral Hospital Langford Vets, University of Bristol

Kate Forster, MAVetMB, CertSAS, DipECVS, MRCVS, Davies Veterinary Specialists

Ana Marquez, DVM, MACVSc, CertSAS, DipECVS, MRCVS, University of Edinburgh

Pieter Nelissen, DVM, CertSAS, DipECVS, MRCVS, Tierklinik Haar, Germany

Anna Nutt, BVM&S, MANZCVS, MRCVS, Small Animal Referral Hospital Langford Vets, University of Bristol

Donald Sheahan, BSc, BVSc, CertSAS, DipECVS, MRCVS, Dogwood Vets

Surgical asepsis and basic principles

1

Jonathan C. Bell

Chapter summary

1.1 Instrumentation and instrument handling

Key points

- The reader should be aware of the commonly used general surgical instruments that are available.
- An understanding of the correct handling and function of each instrument allows for efficient surgery and minimises tissue trauma.

Surgical instruments are the tools of our trade. It is important that the surgeon understands the intended function of each instrument and how to use the instrument properly to achieve that function. This chapter will describe the instruments contained within the author's standard surgical kit, along with additional commonly used instruments. It is not an exhaustive list of the available instruments, and different surgeons will have their own preferences regarding the instruments they use to make a standard surgical kit. It is the surgeon's responsibility to ensure they have the appropriate range of instruments available for their individual caseload. Poor quality or damaged instruments, or the use of instruments for an unintended purpose, can compromise the surgical procedure and increase the risk of complications.

1.1.1 Cutting instruments

Scalpel

The stainless steel scalpel has long since been held to be the gold-standard cutting instrument to which all other cutting instruments are compared. A correctly used scalpel blade creates the least traumatic incision. Skin incisions should be made full thickness with the blade perpendicular to the skin. The skin is stabilised by the non-dominant hand, being stretched perpendicular to the direction of the blade. A number 3 handle with a number 10 blade is most commonly used. Slide cutting gives the best control of length, depth and direction. Two grips are possible. The fingertip grip places the

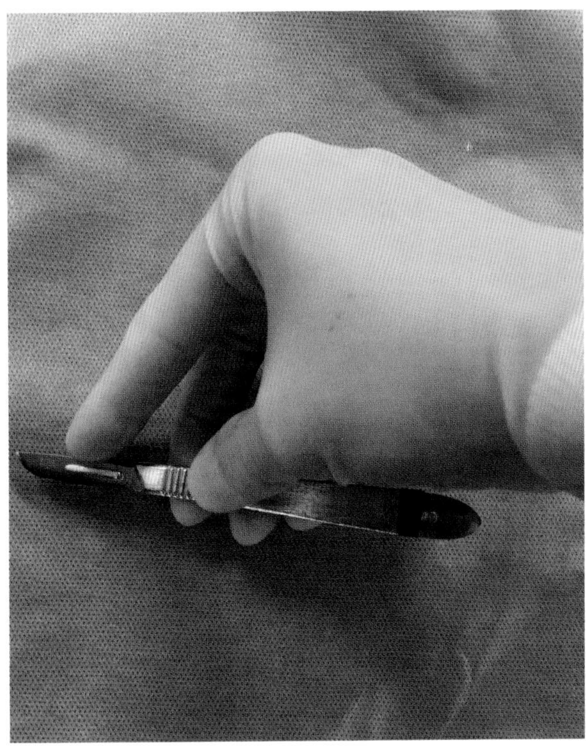

Fig. 1.1a Fingertip grip for holding a scalpel.

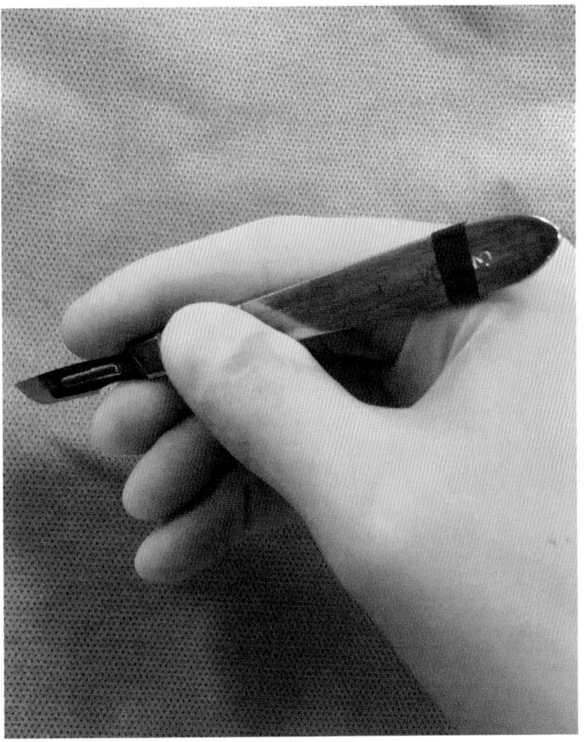

Fig. 1.1b Pencil grip for holding a scalpel.

length of the blade against the skin and is used for long incisions (Fig. 1.1a). The pencil grip increases precision and depth control and is used for shorter, delicate incisions (Fig. 1.1b). Press cutting and inverse press cutting are used to enter body cavities or fluid-filled organs, such as the linea alba or bladder.

Scissors

Scissors are articulated instruments which have the common features of ring handles, a shank of varying length, a box lock and blades of varying thickness and length. Blunt-tipped scissors are preferred to sharp-tipped scissors. Curved scissors improve visibility during dissection, but straight scissors offer a mechanical advantage. Metzenbaum scissors have thin, delicate tips and are used for most surgical dissections (Fig. 1.2a). Mayo scissors have longer, thicker blades and are used for cutting dense tissues (Fig. 1.2b). A dedicated pair of Mayo scissors should be kept in each kit to be used exclusively for cutting sutures and drapes. Long-length scissors are useful for dissection in deep cavities. It is useful to have available a selection of long instruments (needle holders, thumb forceps, Metzenbaum scissors and right-angled forceps) as a separate kit when performing such procedures.

The tripod grip gives the surgeon best control of the forces created when using scissors (Fig. 1.3). Closing forces cause the blades to come together. Shearing forces push the blades flat against each other during closing. Torque forces roll the leading edges of the blades inwards to touch each other.

Sharp dissection is accomplished by a standard double-blade cutting action (Fig. 1.4a). Only the tips are used in order to prevent crushing of tissues by the remainder of the blades. Push cutting is occasionally used to cut rapidly through less dense, areolar tissue (Fig. 1.4b). Blunt dissection is used to undermine skin edges or to break down loose connective tissue (Fig.

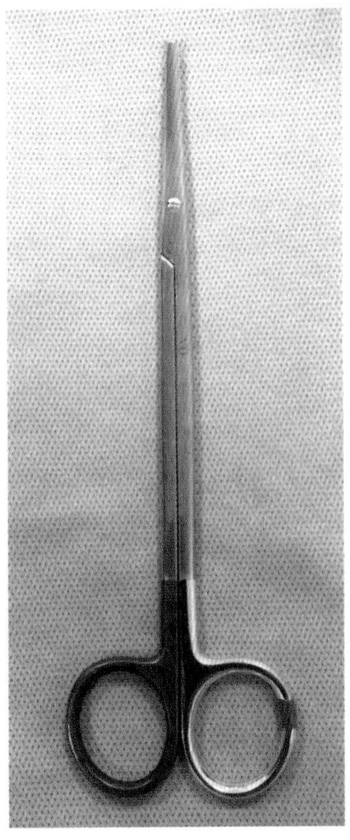

Fig. 1.2a Metzenbaum scissors.

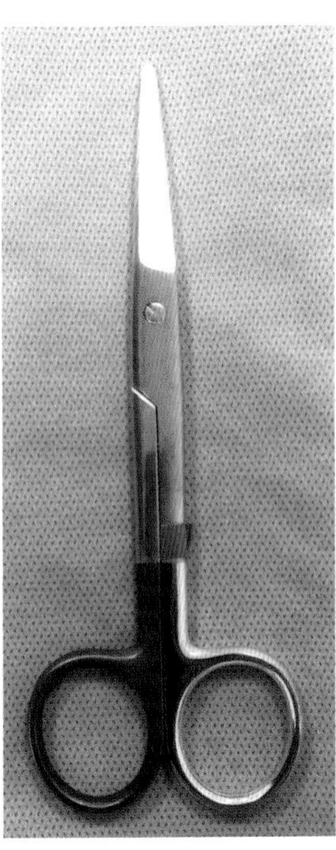

Fig. 1.2b Mayo scissors.

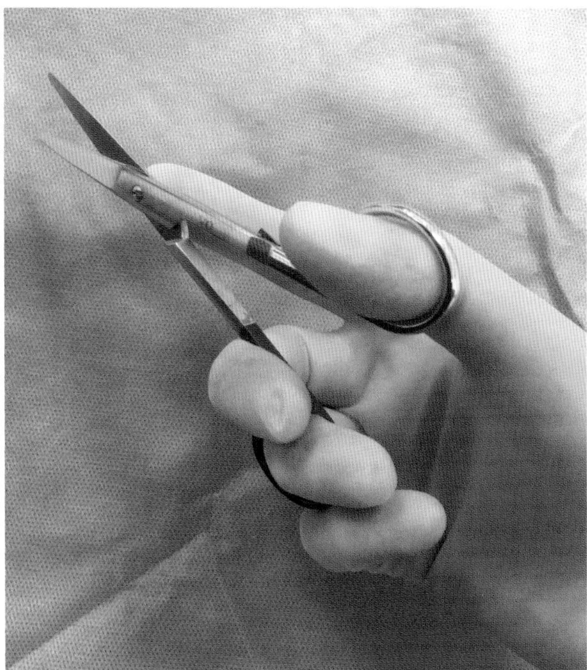

Fig. 1.3 Tripod grip for holding scissors.

1.4c). Again, only the tips are used to prevent tissue trauma. The tips are introduced under the skin, the blades opened, then withdrawn and then closed before reintroduction. Excessive blunt dissection should be avoided as this increases tissue trauma and dead space.

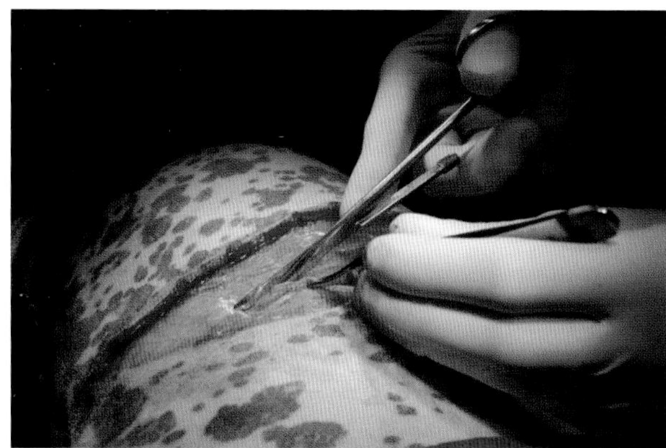

Fig. 1.4a Standard double-blade cutting.

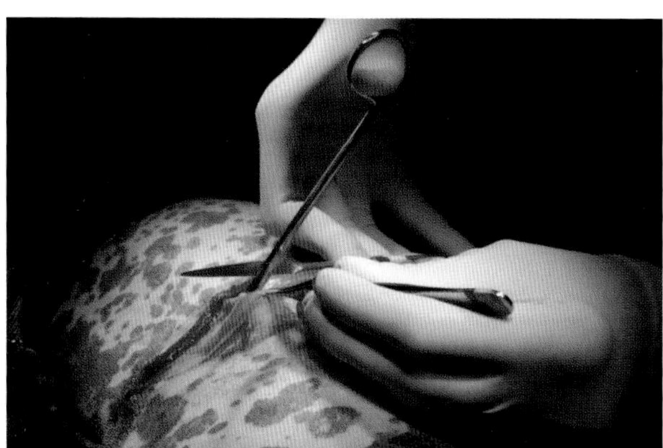

Fig. 1.4b Push cutting.

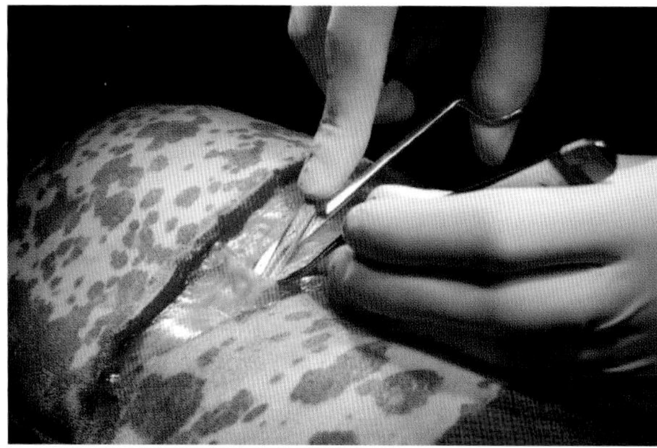

Fig. 1.4c Blunt dissection.

1.1.2 Grasping instruments

Needle-holders

Needle-holders are articulating instruments that, like scissors, have ring handles, a shank, a box lock, jaws and tips. In addition, a ratchet is usually present to allow the jaws to be locked. The jaws stabilise the needle and are usually straight. Tungsten carbide inserts are found in the better needle-holders and provide stability while protecting against suture damage. The Mayo–Hegar is the standard needle-holder (Fig. 1.5a); the Olsen–Hegar has a cutting blade built into the jaws (Fig. 1.5b). It is useful to have a pair of needle-holders with a long shank in a separate kit of long instruments.

Tripod, thenar, palmed and pencil grips are described. The tripod grip is most commonly used in general surgery. This grip allows easy grasping and release of the needle, as well as precise needle placement.

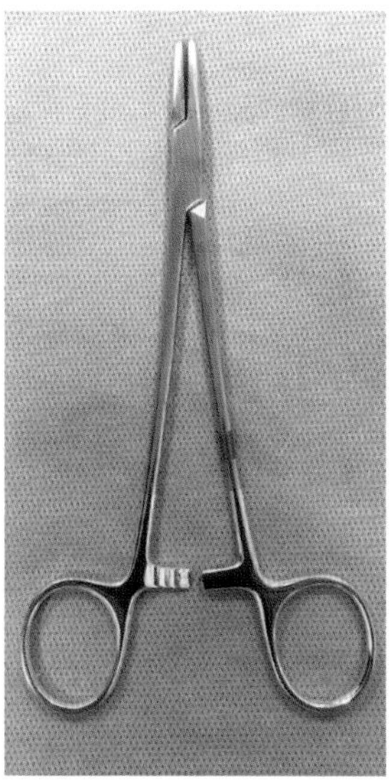

Fig. 1.5a Mayo–Hegar needle-holder.

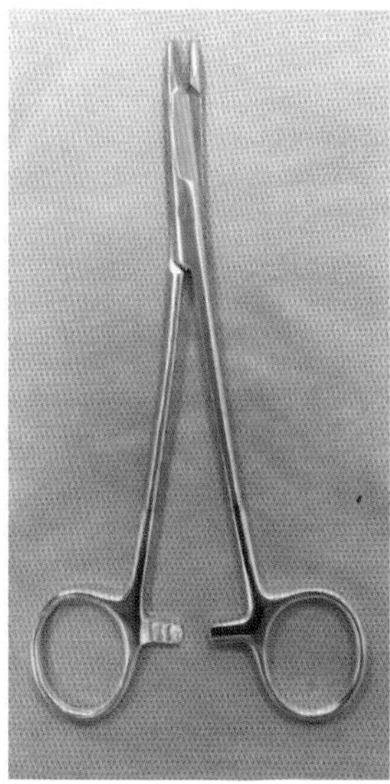

Fig. 1.5b Olsen–Hegar needle-holder.

Tissue forceps

Tissue forceps are used to grasp tissue and aid with dissection. They include crushing forceps, non-crushing forceps, haemostatic forceps, thumb forceps and towel clamps.

Crushing forceps are typically used to grasp tissue. These are articulating instruments with a ratchet lock next to the handle. The tips appose grasp tissue at right angles to the direction of pull. Allis forceps have serrated tips (Fig. 1.6a) while Babcock forceps have smooth tips (Fig. 1.6b). The former is used to grasp dense tissue and the latter to grasp more delicate visceral tissue. It is useful to have two of each in a standard surgical kit. These forceps cause tissue damage owing to crushing, and it is suggested that they are used only on tissue that is going to be excised. Right-angled forceps may or may not have a ratchet lock. These are used for dissecting around vessels to isolate them prior to ligation.

Non-crushing forceps are used to stabilise tissues without causing excessive tissue damage. Doyen intestinal forceps have slightly bowed jaws and fine longitudinal grooves (Fig. 1.7). The jaws may be straight or curved and come in a variety of lengths. They are used to occlude the bowel lumen during gastrointestinal procedures, preventing leakage of bowel contents. Other non-crushing forceps include vascular clamps (DeBakey and Cooley forceps) and partial-occlusion forceps such as Satinsky clamps.

Haemostatic forceps are used to grasp vessels or vascular pedicles, providing temporary or definitive haemostasis. These come in a variety of shank lengths and jaw sizes, and the tips may be straight or curved. The jaws are typically serrated. Halsted mosquito forceps are most commonly used (Fig. 1.8). The jaws of these forceps have transverse serrations along their length. These forceps are designed for

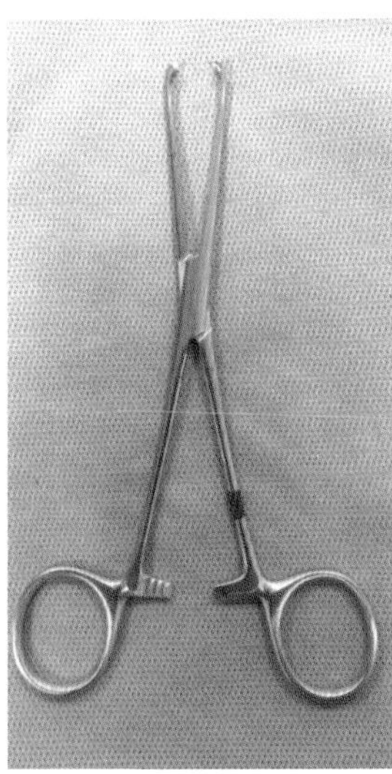

Fig. 1.6a Allis tissue forceps.

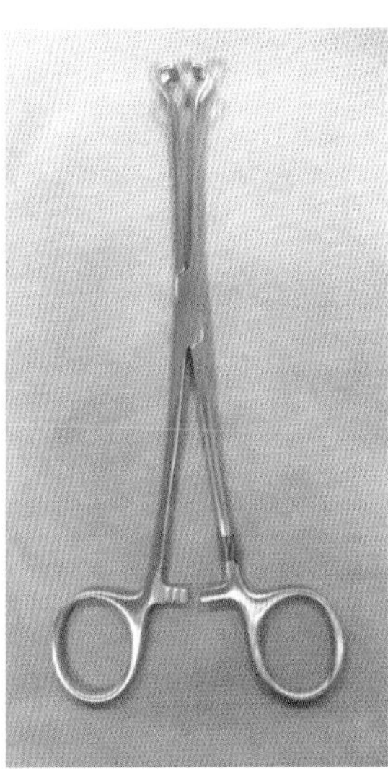

Fig. 1.6b Babcock tissue forceps.

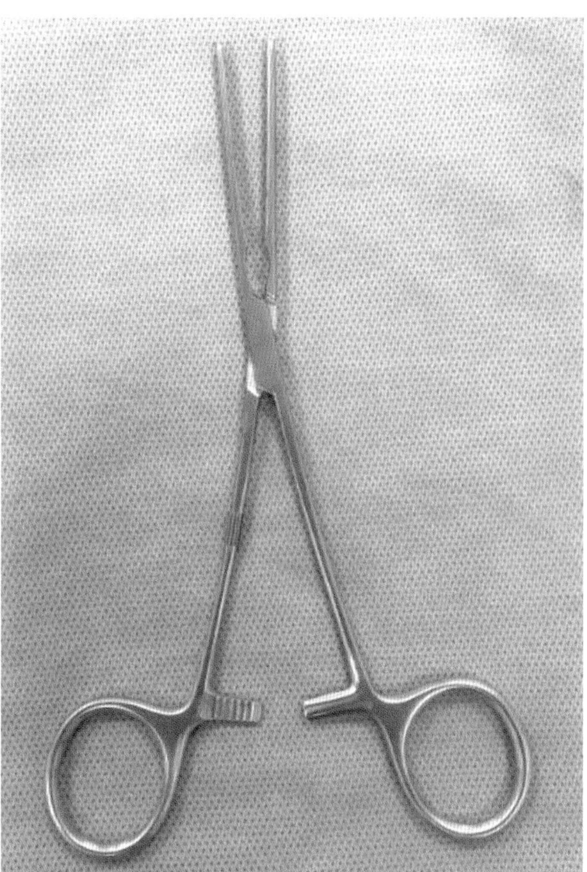

Fig. 1.7 Doyen intestinal forceps.

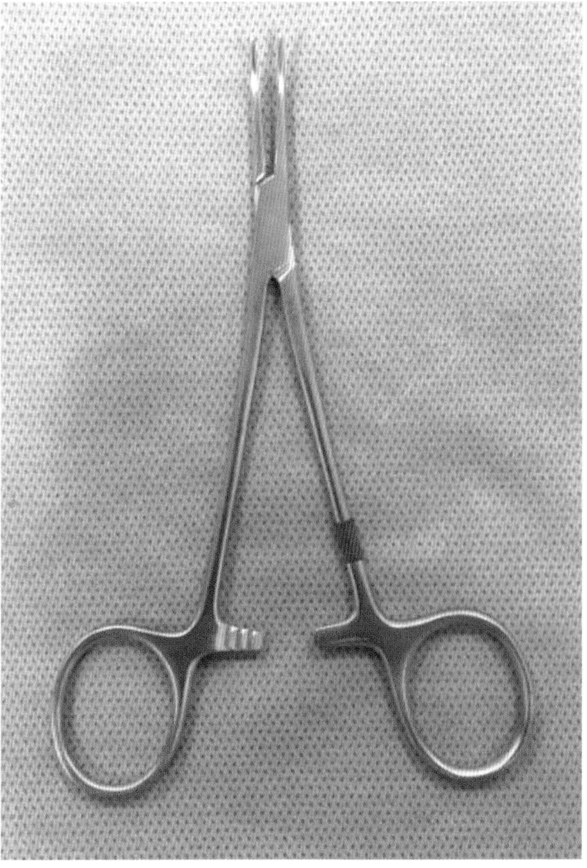

Fig. 1.8 Halsted mosquito forceps.

tip-clamping of small vessels. They can also be used for jaw-clamping of small vascular pedicles prior to ligature application. In the former application, the forceps are applied with the tips down; in the latter, they are applied with the tips up. A tripod grip is employed when applying the forceps. It is useful to have six to eight of these forceps in a standard surgical kit. Rochester–Carmalt forceps have longitudinal serrations and cross-hatched tips, and are used for jaw-clamping of larger pedicles.

Thumb forceps are used to stabilise tissue during dissection and suturing. The shafts are straight and serrated, to improve the surgeon's grip. These instruments are held between the thumb and index finger of the non-dominant hand (not between the thumb and fingers as would a philatelist). When not in use, they can be carried in the palm of the non-dominant hand, freeing up the thumb and index finger for suture manipulation and saving the surgeon from repeatedly putting them down and picking them up. For most dissection purposes, short, fine thumb forceps are indicated. Again, it is useful to have a selection of long thumb forceps in a separate long instrument kit. Brown–Adson forceps have two parallel rows of very fine teeth (Fig. 1.9a). Adson forceps (Fig. 1.9b) have tips with only two fine teeth, and may cause less crushing injury than Brown–Adson forceps. DeBakey forceps have long, thin tips with a ribbed configuration (Fig. 1.9c). These are used for handling delicate tissues within body cavities. Dressing forceps have tips with smooth serrations and are used for handling swabs (Fig. 1.9d). Their use on tissues is associated with crushing trauma owing to the increased force required to generate enough friction to hold the tissue.

Towel clamps have pointed tips designed to hold drapes and towels to the patient's skin. They are also used to secure tubing and cables. They may be penetrating or non-penetrating. The Backhaus has ringed handles and a ratchet lock, and is the most commonly used towel clamp (Fig. 1.10).

1.1.3 Retractors

Hand-held retractors

These are held by an assistant and provide short-term exposure of a focal area of the surgical field. Senn retractors are small, double-ended retractors, one end having three prongs and the other a right-angled blade (Fig. 1.11a). These are useful for retraction of superficial tissues. Army–Navy and Langenbeck retractors (Fig. 1.11b) have flat, right-angled blades (double- and single-ended, respectively) and are used for retracting

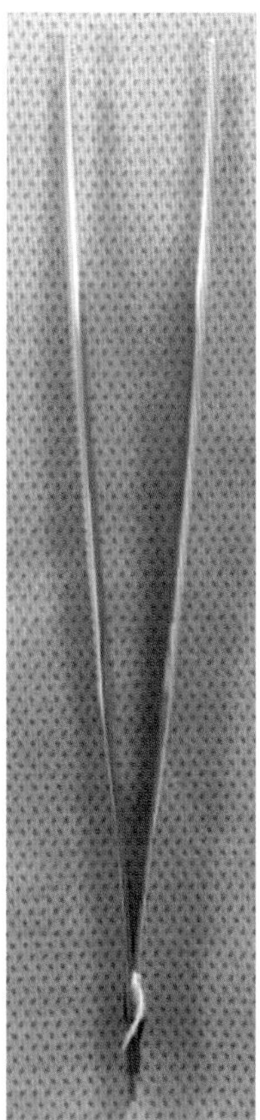

Fig. 1.9a Brown–Adson forceps.

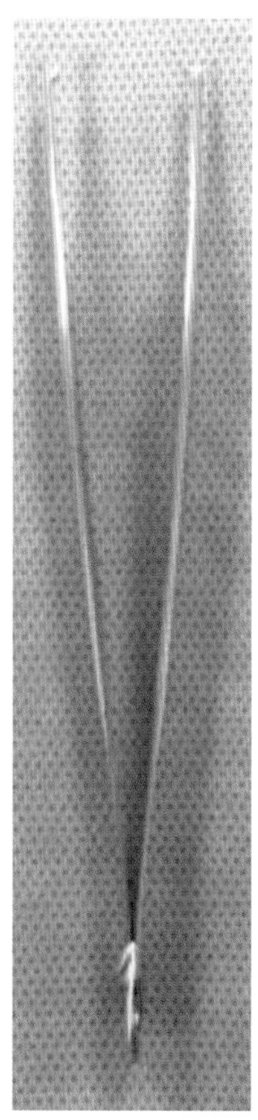

Fig. 1.9b Adson forceps.

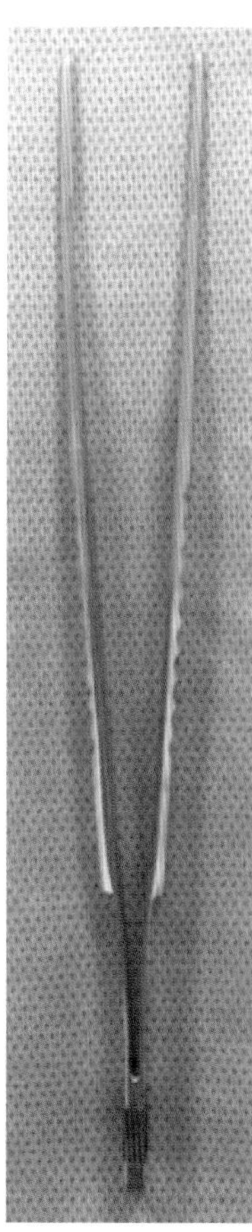

Fig. 1.9c DeBakey forceps.

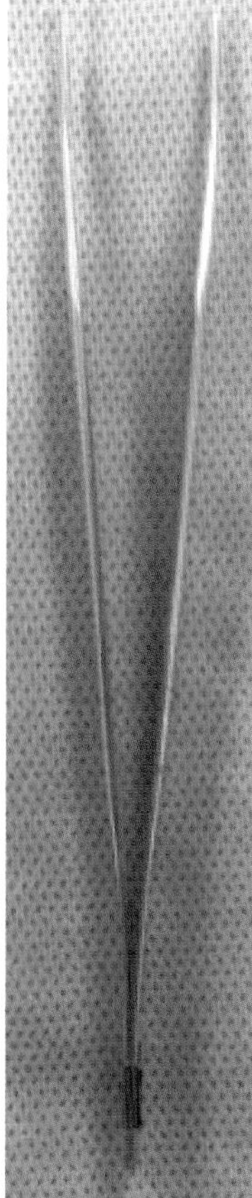

Fig. 1.9d Dressing forceps.

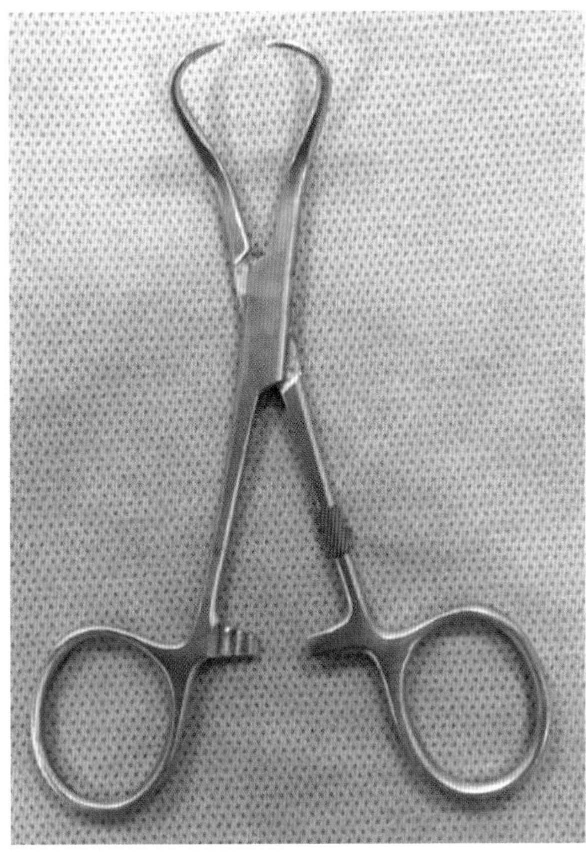

Fig. 1.10 Backhaus towel clamps.

deeper tissues and muscle bellies. Malleable retractors are flat and flexible; these come in different lengths and are used to retract within body cavities (Fig. 1.11c).

Self-retaining retractors

These provide long-term exposure of the whole surgical field. An assistant is not required to hold these retractors. Gelpi retractors have two arms, ring handles and a ratchet lock (Fig. 1.12). The arms vary in length and may be curved, straight or odd-legged; the tips may be sharp or smooth. These are ideal for retracting superficial tissues. Exposure is optimised when two Gelpi retractors are placed at right angles to each other. West, Weitlaner and Travis retractors have multiple prongs for more even tissue purchase and force distribution. Balfour retractors have two moveable arms mounted on parallel slide bars and are used for retraction of the abdominal wall during coeliotomy procedures (Fig. 1.13). The central blade that comes with these retractors is not used in veterinary patients. Finochietto retractors have two broad, outward-curved blades mounted on a ratcheted bar and are used for spreading the ribs or sternum during thoracotomy procedures (Fig. 1.14). With all self-retaining retractors, care must be taken to avoid tissue damage owing to excessive and prolonged pressure. Paediatric retractors are more appropriate to veterinary patients.

1.1.4 Suction tips

Suction is used to remove collections of fluid from the surgical field. It is also used to clear the surgical field when there is active haemorrhage prior to definitive haemostasis. Precise suctioning of small volumes of fluid is best achieved with a Frazier suction tip (Fig. 1.15a). Larger volumes of fluid are removed with a Yankauer tip (Fig. 1.15b) or a Poole tip (Fig. 1.15c). The Poole tip is ideally suited for suctioning fluid from body cavities. The outer fenestrated tube contains an inner pin-point suction tube and prevents occlusion by body tissues such as omentum.

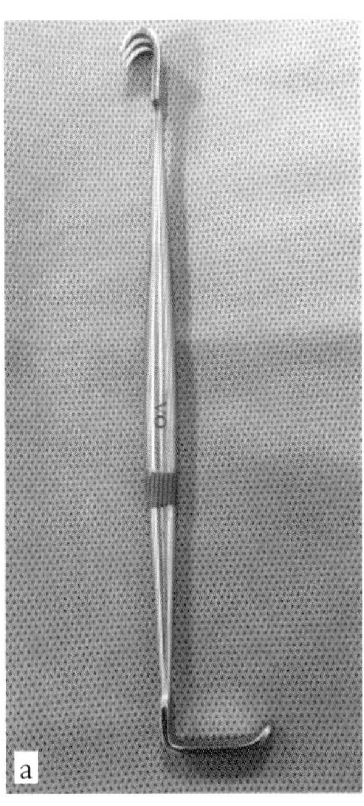

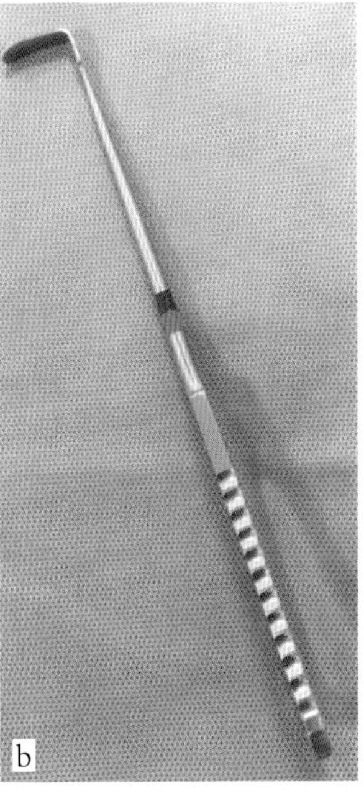

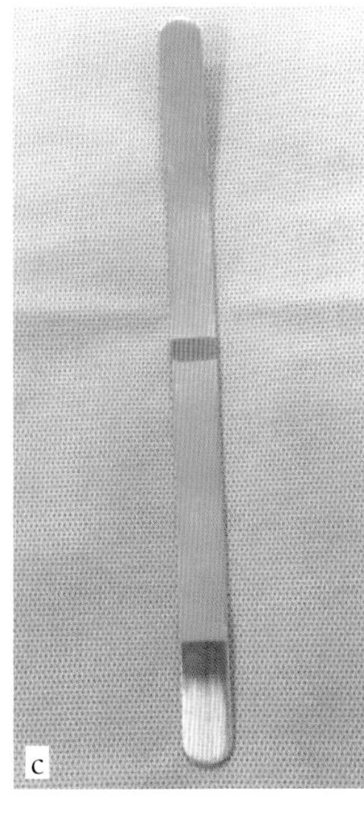

Fig. 1.11a Senn retractors.

Fig. 1.11b Langenbeck retractors.

Fig. 1.11c Malleable retractors.

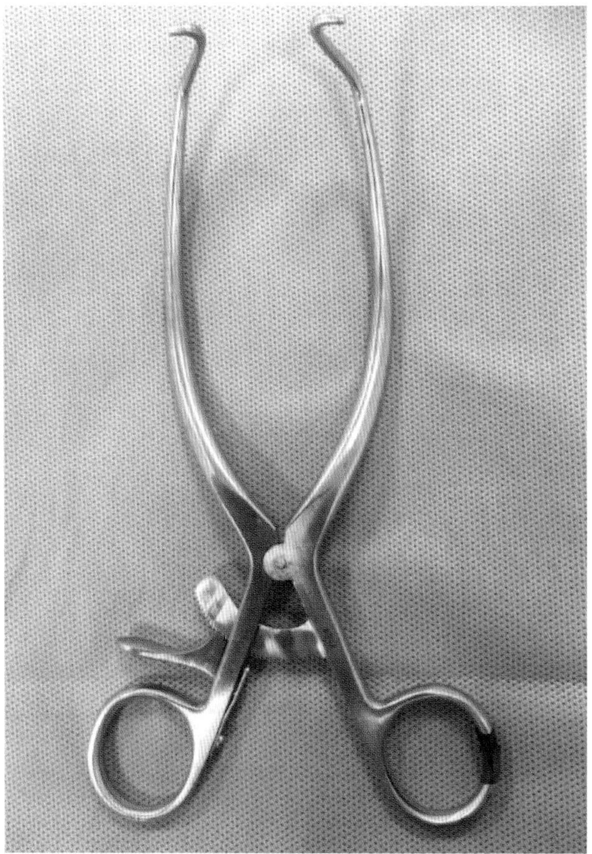

Fig. 1.12 Gelpi retractors.

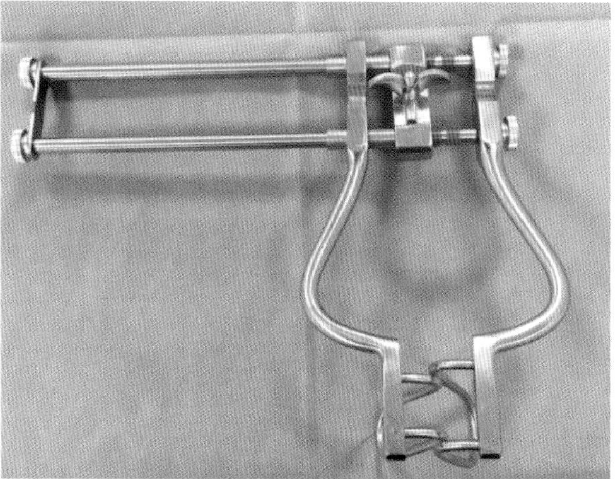

Fig. 1.13 Balfour retractors.

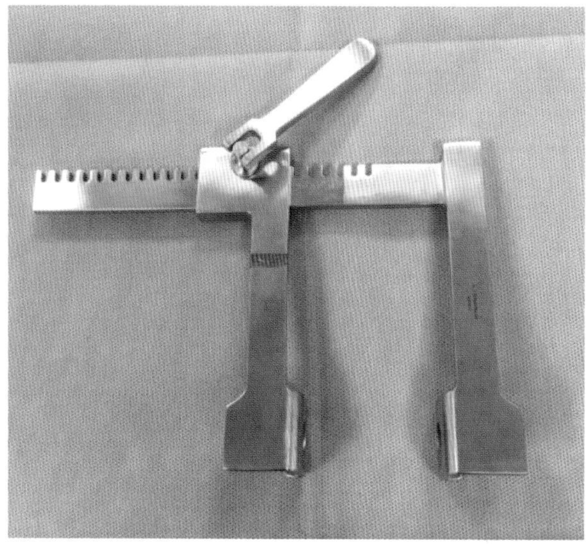

Fig. 1.14 Finochietto retractors.

1.1.5 Energy-based instruments

The use of energy-based tools in veterinary surgery is commonplace. These tools rely on electrons, photons and sound waves to transfer energy to tissue. Such tools can be relied upon to provide haemostasis and provide a bloodless incision, often resulting in decreased surgical times. Unfortunately, this gain in surgical expediency and haemostasis is at the expense of increased tissue damage compared with a conventional incision made by a scalpel blade (Dubiel et al., 2010; Meakin et al., 2017; Scott et al., 2017; Silverman et al., 2007).

Radiofrequency devices deliver a high-frequency alternating electrical current to tissues to generate heat energy, resulting in collagen denaturation and tissue shrinkage. The body's tissues have a high electrolyte content and are consequently an excellent conductor. Radiofrequency units may be monopolar or bipolar. With monopolar radiofrequency, the current is applied to the patient via a handpiece (the active electrode) (Fig. 1.16). This current passes back to the generator via an inactive return electrode attached to the patient; this return electrode (sometimes referred to as a grounding pad or dispersive pad) ensures that low-density current passes back to the radiofrequency generator (electrosurgical unit), preventing patient burns.

Monopolar units are used for dissection and haemostasis. A continuous, undamped waveform results purely in cutting while an intermittent or damped waveform results in haemostasis without cutting. Blending functions leads to varying degrees of cutting and coagulation. Radiofrequency energy achieves coagulation effectively by burning tissue. This can lead to charring and desiccation of tissue. High power settings and prolonged tissue contact can lead to injury to deeper tissues. If the ground plate is in contact with only a small area, there is a risk of thermal burns occurring at the site of the ground plate. Several studies have reported thermal damage to tissues and delayed wound healing following the use of monopolar electrocautery (Scott et al., 2017; Silverman et al., 2007). One study found that the use of monopolar radiofrequency did not result in additional tissue damage or delayed wound healing when used to create a coeliotomy incision (Meakin et al., 2017).

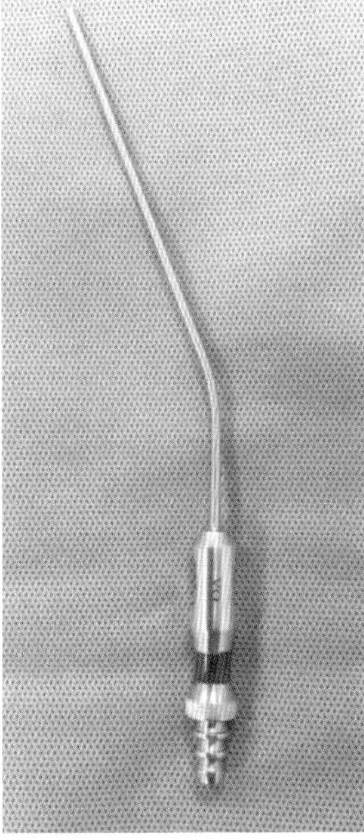

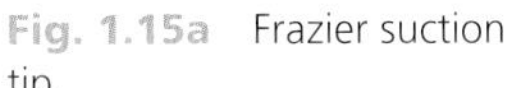

Fig. 1.15a Frazier suction tip.

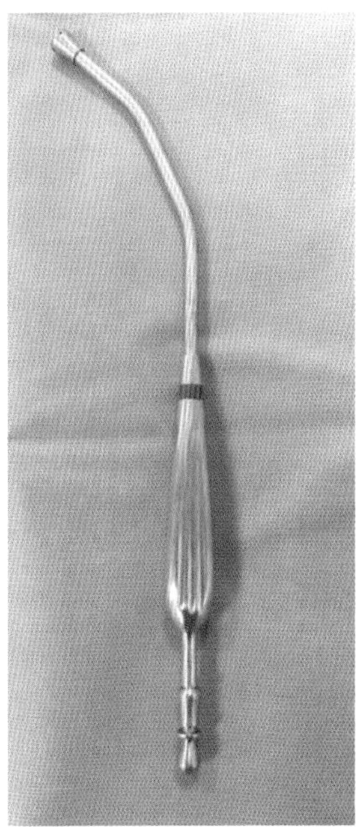

Fig. 1.15b Yankauer suction tip.

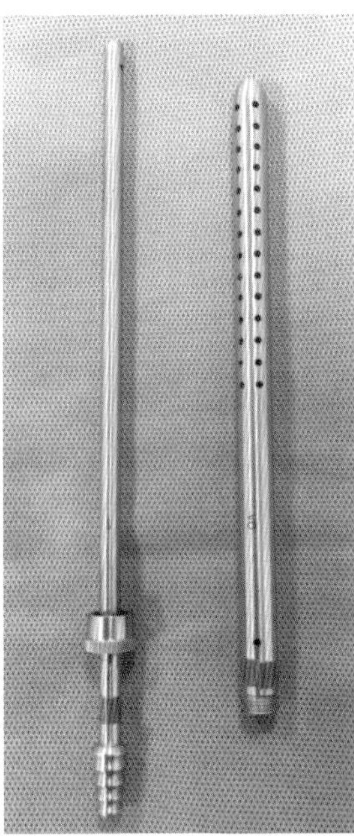

Fig. 1.15c Poole suction tip.

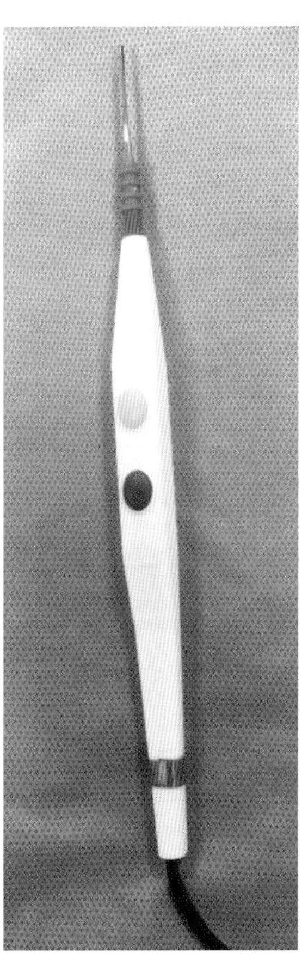

Fig. 1.16 Monopolar handpiece.

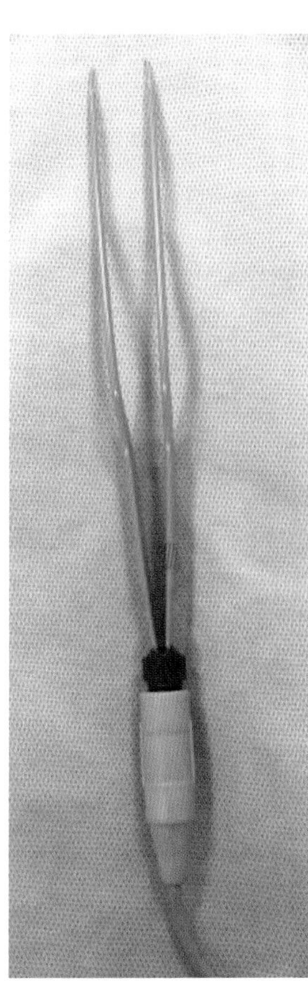

Fig. 1.17 Bipolar handpiece.

With bipolar radiofrequency, the handpiece is a pair of forceps containing the active electrode and the return electrode (Fig. 1.17). Current flows only through the tissue between the two electrodes, resulting in a more precise application of heat and less tissue damage. Unlike monopolar radiofrequency, which does not work well in liquid because of dispersion of the current, bipolar radiofrequency can be used in a wet surgical field.

Harmonic devices deliver ultrasound waves at 55.5 kHz. These ultrasonic vibrations generate heat and coagulate tissues. Scalpel and scissor tips can be used to deliver the energy to the tissues, simultaneously cutting and coagulating. These devices cut and coagulate at a lower temperature than radiofrequency devices and lasers owing to coaptive coagulation. This refers to the tamponade and sealing of vessels by a protein coagulum. This is in contrast to the obliterative coagulation of radiofrequency units, which occurs at much higher temperatures resulting in the burning of tissues. Coaptive coagulation minimises collateral tissue damage and prevents charring of tissue.

Surgical lasers have become increasingly popular in the veterinary field. There are two forms of photon emission: spontaneous and stimulated. With spontaneous emission, electrons are excited then return to their resting state, emitting photons in the process. The light produced consists of different wavelengths and is not in phase. With stimulated emission, the emitted photon is hit by second and subsequent photons. This photon-stimulated emission produces monochromatic light that is described as being coherent or in-phase. Coherent light interacts with the body's tissues to produce its effects. These differ depending on the wavelength of the light. Photochemical effects are chemical reactions induced directly by light. Photothermal effects are heat-related interactions such as ablation and coagulation. Photomechanical or photo-ionising effects lead to direct tissue destruction. Photo-ablation is associated with the direct breakage of molecular bonds. Photodynamic therapy is utilised in the treatment of some cancers. A chromophone is introduced into the diseased tissues. This absorbs laser light and converts it to heat or toxic oxygen radicals, thus destroying the tissue. Most medical lasers have a photothermal effect, that is they cut, cauterise, coagulate, vaporise or weld tissue. The amount of heat produced is determined by both laser- and tissue-related properties. This is intense and needs to be controlled by the handpiece. The depth of penetration of a surgical laser increases with increasing wavelength. Commonly used surgical lasers include argon, carbon dioxide, Nd:YAG, Ho:YAG and excimer. Lasers are damaging to the eyes and thus wavelength-specific protective goggles are required.

1.2 Sterilisation techniques, antiseptics and perioperative antibiotics

Key points

- Aseptic surgical technique pertains to a collection of mechanisms by which the surgeon strives to reduce the number of microorganisms present in the surgical wound, the overall aim being to reduce the incidence of surgical site infections.
- Sterilisation of surgical instruments and implants is commonplace in veterinary practice.
- The use of antiseptics to reduce the number of microbes on the patient's skin is also well established, and the antiseptic preparations commercially available are discussed.
- Despite an increased awareness in the veterinary profession of the importance of aseptic technique, surgical site infections remain a significant problem in surgery, resulting in patient morbidity and detrimental economic effects.
- The use of prophylactic perioperative antibiotics remains commonplace in the veterinary field, though there is increasing concern about the incidence of nosocomial and multidrug-resistant bacterial infections.

1.2.1 Sterilisation

Sterilisation is the destruction of all microorganisms on or in an object. Disinfection is anything less than sterilisation and may be high-, intermediate- or low-level depending on the range of microorganisms killed. In this context, microorganisms include bacteria, viruses, spores, fungi and prions. Critical items such as surgical instruments and implants, which enter a patient's body and pose a high risk of infection if contaminated, should be sterilised. Semi-critical items, which contact a patient's skin or mucous membranes, should be sterilised or subjected to a high-level disinfectant. Non-critical items, which contact a patient's skin only, can be disinfected.

All organic and inorganic debris must be removed prior to sterilisation. Failure to do so can lead to instrument damage (corrosion, rusting and damage to mechanisms) and inadequate sterilisation. Manual cleaning may be preferable for delicate instruments but is inferior to mechanical cleaning for general instruments. Enzymatic cleaners or detergents can help to remove organic debris. Surgical instruments should be completely submerged and rinsed prior to packaging. The use of abrasive brushes may damage surgical instruments. Mechanical cleaning is less efficient and possibly less hazardous to staff, though it is more expensive. Ultrasonic cleaning devices create minute gas bubbles that implode on contact with surgical instruments, creating a vacuum that removes particles and debris, a process called cavitation. On completion, dense particles fall to the bottom and finer soils rise to the surface; it is therefore important to rinse instruments.

Instruments should be dry before packing. Filtered medical-grade compressed air is the only approved method for drying instruments, though this modality is uncommonly used in veterinary practices. The ideal packaging material would be permeable to steam or gases, be resistant to heat and physical damage, have a long shelf-life, be durable and be an effective barrier to microorganisms. Paper/plastic pouches (Fig. 1.18a) and non-woven polypropylene (Fig. 1.18b) are commonly used in practice. Groups of instruments that are used for particular procedures – for example, thoracic surgical instruments – can be placed in a stainless steel box for convenience prior to wrapping and sterilisation. Ideally, instruments should be double-wrapped to reduce the risk of perforation and contamination.

Steam sterilisation is the most common method of sterilisation in veterinary practice. Steam kills microorganisms through coagulation and denaturation of proteins by moist heat. Water is a catalyst, hastening the process and allowing the use of lower temperatures. Heat is transferred by condensation and not simply by absorption. Steam sterilisers, or autoclaves, work under a balance of pressure, temperature and time. The pressure allows sterilisation to occur at a higher temperature than would otherwise be obtainable. Sterilisation times are temperature dependent, with 30 minutes at 121°C for a gravity-displacement autoclave and 4 minutes at 132°C for a pre-vacuum autoclave. Drying times are 15–30 minutes. Flash sterilisation is a process

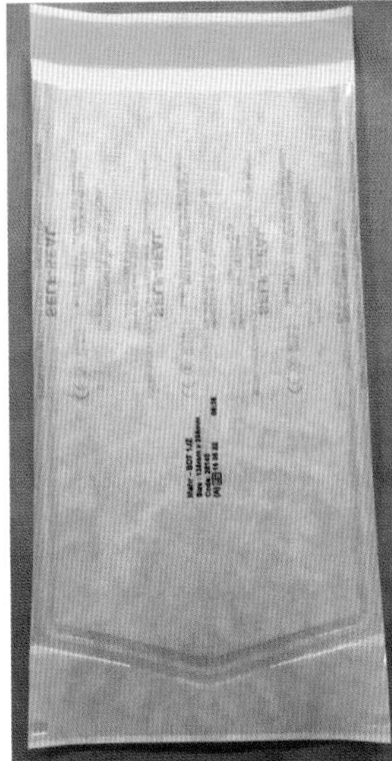

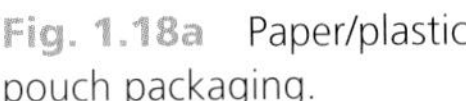

Fig. 1.18a Paper/plastic pouch packaging.

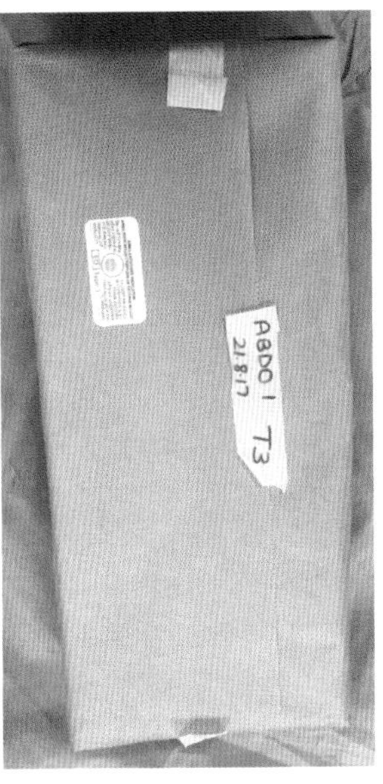

Fig. 1.18b Non-woven polypropylene packaging.

used to rapidly sterilise instruments for immediate use. This usually involves a higher temperature for a shorter time.

Gravity-displacement autoclaves introduce steam under pressure. Being lighter than air, steam rises and forces air out of a valve at the bottom of the unit. The coldest air is therefore always being forced out of the bottom of the unit and is used to measure the temperature of the autoclave, confirming that sterilisation conditions are being met. The efficacy of sterilisation depends on steam coming into contact with all items in the autoclave. Pre-vacuum autoclaves use a pump to remove air from the chamber prior to the introduction of steam, leading to a rapid and uniform distribution of steam.

Ethylene oxide is a colourless and odourless gas with a boiling point of 10.5 °C. It causes alkylation of proteins and nucleic acid, obstructing cell division and reproduction. It is mixed with carbon dioxide or hydrofluorocarbon to reduce its flammability. Instrument packs should be arranged loosely in the steriliser. Ethylene oxide doesn't penetrate glass and is adsorbed to rubber and plastic; this necessitates an aeration cycle before instruments are safe to handle. Sterilisation times are affected by concentration, temperature and humidity. Safety and environmental concerns make this method of sterilisation less popular.

Physical, chemical and biological indicators are used to monitor the efficacy of sterilisation. Physical indicators are monitors built into the steriliser and include printouts or graphs. Chemical indicators (Fig. 1.19) react to specific parameters that are critical to the sterilisation process, typically by a colour change. They confirm that the conditions of sterilisation have been met but not that the contents have been sterilised. Paper/plastic pouches have chemical indicators on their surface. It is common practice to place an additional chemical indicator strip inside the pouch amongst the instruments. Biological indicators consist of a culture of microorganisms that is evaluated after processing to determine its viability. *Geobacillus stearothermophilus* spores are used for steam sterilisation, and *Bacillus atrophaeus* spores are used for ethylene oxide sterilisation. These tests are more expensive and time consuming than chemical indicators, so are not suitable for day-to-day use, instead being used every 1–2 weeks as a failsafe to confirm the efficacy of chemical indicators.

Autoclaved instruments in double-layered paper/plastic pouches or non-woven polypropylene can be stored in closed cabinets for at least 96 weeks. The storage time for the same packaging following ethylene oxide sterilisation is around 100 days.

1.2.2 Antiseptics

Antiseptics are applied to living tissue to inhibit or kill microorganisms. Asepsis is the absence of micro-organisms on living tissue, a state which is never achieved. Aseptic technique, therefore, refers to the practices employed by the surgeon to keep the number of microorganisms within the surgical site to a minimum, the aim being to prevent surgical site infections. The ideal antiseptic should be effective against bacteria, fungi, viruses and spores. The immediate action of an antiseptic refers to the number of microorganisms killed or mechanically removed within the first 3 minutes of application. This is important as it equates to the time spent prepping the patient or, in the case of the surgeon, scrubbing up.

The persistent action refers to an antiseptic's ability

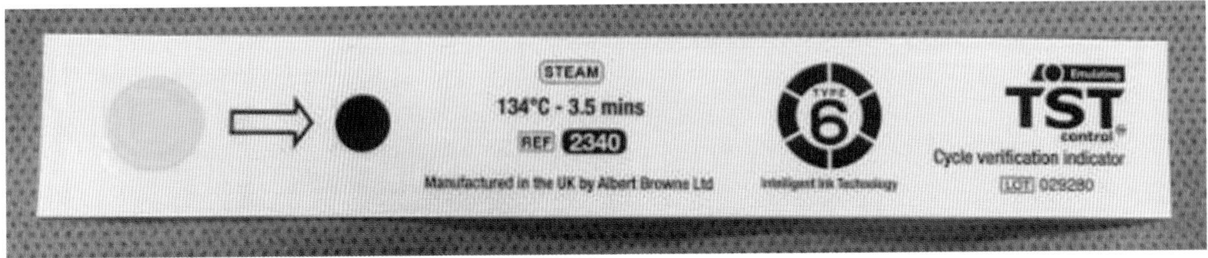

Fig. 1.19 A commonly used chemical indicator of sterilisation.

to prevent recolonisation of the skin within 6 hours of its application. This is also important as it corresponds to the time that the patient and surgeon are in theatre and the immediate post-surgical period, when the surgical wound is most vulnerable. This property is often now referred to as the sustained action. The residual action refers to a cumulative antimicrobial efficacy after repeated application of an antiseptic over at least 5 days. The importance of this is unknown.

Alcohols have traditionally been said to have a rapid bactericidal activity but a poorer activity against viruses and spores. This is related to the ethanol content of older preparations, which is around 60%. Preparations containing ethanol concentrations of over 80% have been shown to have greater efficacy against a wide range of fungi, viruses and spores, and are now commonly used as an alternative to traditional surgical hand-scrubbing preparations. Alcohols denature proteins, interfere with metabolism and cause lysis of cells. Their efficacy is reduced by the presence of organic debris, so this should be removed by washing prior to their application. Preparations containing over 80% ethanol have been shown to have a sustained action of up to 6 hours. They should not be applied to open wounds as they cause cell necrosis.

Iodophors contain iodine complexed to polyvinyl pyrrolidone. This high-molecular-weight carrier allows a slow, continuous release of free iodine, which is thought to reduce staining and toxicity. Povidone-iodine is the most commonly used iodophor. It is supplied as a 10% solution and the concentration of free iodine increases as it is diluted, reaching a maximum of 0.1%. The mechanism by which iodine exerts its antimicrobial effect is unknown, but involves interference with cell membrane protein synthesis. It is effective against a wide range of bacteria, fungi, viruses and spores. It has a rapid immediate action, but again this is reduced in the presence of organic debris. It has a sustained action of 4–6 hours. Contact dermatitis has been reported in almost 50% of animals. Care should be taken when applying iodine to open wounds, as higher concentrations are toxic to fibroblasts.

Chlorhexidine is a cationic bisbiguanide, and chlorhexidine gluconate is commonly used as a surgical scrub preparation. It has efficacy against a wide range of bacteria, but is variably effective against fungi and viruses. It is not effective against spores at room temperature. At low concentrations, chlorhexidine is bacteriostatic, interfering with the cell membrane and causing leakage of contents. At higher concentrations it is bactericidal, causing coagulation of cell contents. The specific concentration required to provide a given effect is dependent on the type of bacteria and the exposure time. Concentrations of 2–4% are used for surgical scrub preparations while wound treatment preparations are typically less than 0.05%. Chlorhexidine has a rapid immediate action. It may not be inhibited by organic debris to the same degree as povidone-iodine. It has a sustained effect of at least 6 hours. A traditionally stated advantage of chlorhexidine over povidone-iodine is its residual effect but it is unclear what, if any, clinical impact this has. The incidence of contact dermatitis is lower than that of povidone-iodine. At concentrations higher than 0.05%, chlorhexidine has been reported to be ototoxic when applied to the middle ear, and can cause ocular damage. Care should be taken when applying chlorhexidine to open wounds.

1.2.3 Patient preparation

The primary goal of patient preparation is the removal of transient microorganisms and a reduction in the number of resident flora. The degree of reduction required remains a matter of debate. Different preparations and protocols result in different levels of microbial reduction, but not on the incidence of surgical site infections.

Bathing of veterinary patients prior to clipping is controversial. It has been suggested that drying with towels may inflame the skin and liberate bacteria from pores, and wet patients can be expected to lose heat more quickly while under anaesthesia. Bathing is therefore best reserved for patients who are heavily soiled.

Clipping of the hair around the surgical site is widely accepted practice in veterinary patients. Clippers should be clean and sharp to prevent skin trauma. Blades should be changed between patients. Razors are associated with increased skin trauma and a higher rate of surgical site infections, and should not be used. Surgical clips should be wide and take account of the patient's positioning in theatre and whether any surrounding skin is going to be pulled into the surgical field during skin reconstruction procedures. It has been suggested that the rate of surgical site infection is lower if patients are clipped immediately prior to surgery, but this is not a consistent finding.

Many scrubbing protocols are reported. There appears to be little difference in efficacy between povidone-iodine and chlorhexidine. After clipping and vacuuming to remove loose hair and debris, a rough prep should be given in the prep room. A final 'sterile' prep should be given in theatre. Often sterile gloves and swabs are used, though this has not been shown to have an impact on the incidence of surgical site infection. Contact times vary between 30 seconds and 2 minutes. Preparation should start at the intended site of the surgical wound and work outwards to the clipped margins. Swabs should then be discarded and the prep repeated. The aim of scrubbing is to remove transient microorganisms and to suppress resident flora. Alternating scrub–alcohol protocols are followed. The final application of a 2% chlorhexidine and 60% isopropyl alcohol preparation has been shown to have greater efficacy than povidone-iodine alone.

1.2.4 Draping

The aim of draping is to create a barrier that prevents the spread of microorganisms from the patient into the surgical field or onto the surgeon. The drapes should be impermeable to fluids, resistant to tearing and secured to the patient. Reuseable drapes have poor barrier properties when wet, leading to strike-through. Their barrier properties are further reduced by repeated laundering, and linting of material into the surgical site is described. Disposable drapes have better barrier properties, even when wet. Their increased cost is offset by the saving in laundry and sterilisation costs. Quadrant drapes extend to the limit of the clipped hair. A second, larger surgical drape can be placed over the top of these drapes and fenestrated closer to the intended surgical site. Drapes should cover the whole of the patient and table. They can be extended to cover the instrument trolley and to shield the anaesthetist. A hanging-leg prep is used to drape extremities.

1.2.5 Surgical site infection and the use of perioperative antibiotics

A surgical site infection (SSI) occurs anywhere in the surgical field following a surgical intervention. The most common source of infection is the patient's endogenous (resident) flora. The United States Centre for Disease Control and Prevention has defined the following criteria for defining SSI.

Superficial incisional SSI

This occurs within 30 days of surgery and involves only the skin and subcutaneous tissues. Clinical signs include a superficial purulent discharge, a positive culture, superficial wound dehiscence (or surgical opening) and one of the cardinal signs of inflammation. At least one of these must be present.

Deep incisional SSI

This occurs within 30 days of surgery, or within 1 year if an implant is present. It involves the deep soft tissues (fascial and muscle layers) of the surgical incision. Clinical signs include a purulent discharge from the deep tissues, a positive culture, dehiscence (or surgical opening) of the deep incision and a deep abscess. Again, at least one of these must be present.

Organ/space SSI

This occurs within 30 days of surgery, or within 1 year if an implant is present. It may be located in any part of the body manipulated during the surgical procedure (except skin, fascia and muscle layers). Clinical signs include a purulent discharge from the organ/space, a positive culture and an abscess. Again, at least one of these must be present.

Risk factors for SSI have been described. The National Risk Council developed a classification of surgical procedures based on the expected degree of contamination (Table 1.1).

This system has been reproduced for many years in standard surgical texts and has been taught to undergraduates. SSI undoubtedly occurs more commonly with increasing levels of wound contamination. However, there remain limitations to this human classification system, which has been extrapolated for small animal patients. There is considerable overlap between categories – for example, clean orthopaedic procedures may have a higher incidence of SSI than certain clean-contaminated procedures such as elective gastrointestinal surgery. It is apparent that many other factors affect the incidence of SSI and wound healing, not least of which is surgical technique.

The duration of surgery has been shown to affect

Table 1.1 Classification of surgical procedures based on the risk of contamination.

Wound classification	Description
Clean	Non-traumatic, non-inflamed surgical wounds. Respiratory, gastrointestinal, genitourinary and oropharyngeal tracts not entered
Clean-contaminated	Surgical wounds in which respiratory, gastrointestinal or genitourinary tracts are entered under controlled conditions without unusual contamination An otherwise clean procedure in which a drain is placed
Contaminated	Operations on traumatic wounds without purulent discharge Procedures in which spillage of gastrointestinal contents or spillage of infected urine occurs Procedures in which a major break of aseptic technique occurs
Dirty	Operations on traumatic wounds with purulent discharge, devitalised tissues or foreign bodies Procedures in which a perforated viscus or faecal contamination occurs

the incidence of SSI, with the risk of infection doubling with every hour of surgery (Eugster et al., 2004). Suppression of the immune system has been correlated with the duration of surgery. Lengthy surgical procedures expose the wound to microbes for a longer period of time. Tissues are handled to a greater degree and can become traumatised or desiccated. The presence of suture material and orthopaedic implants further reduces local wound immunity.

Independent of the duration of surgery, the risk of SSI increases by 30% for each additional hour of general anaesthesia (Beal et al., 2000). Prolonged anaesthesia can result in hypotension and hypothermia, resulting in decreased wound perfusion and, hence, local immunity. Anaesthetic drugs may have a direct effect on the cells of the immune system. If lengthy diagnostic procedures are required prior to surgery, these may be more safely performed under a separate anaesthetic event.

Other reported risk factors for SSI that have been described in veterinary and human patients include the following (Eugster et al., 2004; Heldmann et al., 1999; Nicholson et al., 2002; Turk et al., 2015):

- clipping of the surgical site any time other than immediately prior to surgery
- use of propofol
- endocrinopathies
- number of people in the operating theatre
- sex of the patient
- use of immunosuppressive drugs
- persistent active infection
- hypotension
- hypothermia
- body condition
- blood loss
- suture material type
- ASA preoperative assessment score
- duration of hospital stay
- age.

Even with the best aseptic technique, it is impossible to create a sterile surgical wound. Prophylactic antibiotics are used to protect the patient from an anticipated bacterial invasion, as opposed to therapeutic antibiotics which are used to treat an established infection. The suggested indications for the use of perioperative antibiotics are when:

- the risk of an SSI is relatively high (clean-contaminated and contaminated procedures)
- the development of an SSI would be catastrophic.

The evidence base in veterinary medicine regarding prophylactic antibiotic use is poor. There is clear benefit in contaminated and dirty procedures, but their benefit in clean and clean-contaminated procedures is less clear. They would appear to be beneficial in clean orthopaedic procedures. The concern regarding their indiscriminate use is the development of bacterial resistance. Prophylactic antibiotics are not a substitute for good aseptic and surgical technique.

The chosen antibiotic should be effective against the bacteria expected to be encountered during surgery. For clean procedures, this is most commonly staphylococci and, for clean-contaminated procedures (for example, upper gastrointestinal procedures), this is most commonly Enterobacteriaceae. Cephalosporins are the prophylactic antibiotic of choice because of their broad spectrum of activity and wide safety margin. For procedures involving the caecum, colon and rectum, anaerobic coverage should be provided. The antibiotic should be in the tissues of the surgical site at the start of surgery, and effective concentrations should be maintained throughout the procedure. Typically, this means administering the antibiotic intravenously on induction, followed by repeat doses every 2 hours (Petersen and Rosin, 1995). An additional dose may be given after surgery to suppress the late growth of any bacteria not killed during surgery, and to minimise contamination from the patient's environment until the wound has sealed. If antibiotics are being used truly prophylactically, then they should not be continued beyond the immediate perioperative period unless there was a major break in aseptic technique or an unexpected change in contamination classification. The evidence base for this statement is conflicting in the veterinary literature (Aiken et al., 2015; Pratesi et al., 2015), and some surgeons routinely use oral antibiotics for several days beyond the perioperative period. Concerns about the prolonged use of prophylactic antibiotics include the development of microbial drug resistance and increased susceptibility to nosocomial infection. It is the author's preference not to continue antibiotics beyond the perioperative period unless there is a clear indication to do so.

The use of therapeutic antibiotics to treat an established SSI is well established. There is a distinction between inflamed and infected wounds. The presence of a purulent discharge marks the wound as infected. If an SSI is suspected, swabs should be taken from the wound for bacterial culture and sensitivity and broad-spectrum antibiotics started. It may be necessary to change the prescribed antibiotic based on culture and sensitivity or the response to treatment. It is important to select the correct dose and dosage interval. Concentration-dependent antibiotics are those where bacterial killing is dependent on the concentration of the antibiotic above the minimum inhibitory concentration (MIC) of the bacteria at the site of the infection. The greater the maximum concentration (Cmax), the more effective the response. Time-dependent antibiotics kill bacteria when the concentration of the drug exceeds the MIC. The optimal response is when the MIC is equal to or greater than 50% of the dosing interval. Efficacy correlates with time more than with MIC. If there is evidence of accumulated purulent material under the skin or in the deeper tissues, drainage should be established. This can be done by surgically opening part or all of the wound, or by performing surgical debridement of the wound and placing a drain. Open wounds are usually left to heal by second intention.

The management of infections associated with surgical, particularly orthopaedic, implants, can be challenging. This is largely because of the ability of bacteria to produce a biofilm that allows them to adhere to the implant and which protects them from the host's defences and from antibiotics. A biofilm has been defined as a microbially derived sessile community in which bacteria are attached to a substrate or to each other, are embedded in a matrix and exhibit altered phenotype (with regard to growth, gene expression and protein production). A biofilm begins with the covering of an implant with a conditioning film derived from the local tissue environment. Bacteria are able to reversibly adhere to this film (rather than self-implant). Certain bacteria, such as *Staphylococcus* and *Pseudomonas*, are able to create and control the biofilm environment more effectively. This binding can be rendered irreversible by the production of bacterial exopolysaccharides know as a glycocalyx. The microbes within the biofilm are sessile and are protected from the host's immune defences. In addition, bacteria within the biofilm are resistant to antibiotics. This is due to impaired perfusion of the antibiotic agent (owing to the glycocalyx), the slow bacterial growth rate (as many antibiotics work by interfering with bacterial growth and reproduction) and the adverse environment of the biofilm itself. Implant-associated surgical site infections can have catastrophic consequences. Strategies to prevent biofilm formation are being investigated, but currently successful treatment can require protracted courses of antibiotics and ultimately explantation of the implant.

There has been an explosion in the amount of interest and awareness of multidrug-resistant infections in the veterinary field. This is largely the result of the problems encountered in human hospitals with multidrug-resistant nosocomial infections. There have also been some high-profile veterinary cases which have reached the public domain. It is likely that veterinary practices will have to handle animals colonised or infected with methicillin-resistant *Staphylococcus aureus* (MRSA) or *Staphylococcus pseudintermedius* (MRSP). The British Small Animal Veterinary Association (BSAVA) has published guidelines to prevent the establishment and dissemination of MRSA and MRSP in veterinary practice (BSAVA Practice Guidelines). The key points of these are as follows.

- Effective hand hygiene before and after examining patients and the use of protective equipment such as aprons and gloves.
- Cleaning and disinfection of premises and equipment.
- The rational use of antibiotics.
- Compliance with all of the above.

MRSA/MRSP should be suspected in the following cases:

- animals from MRSA/MRSP-positive households
- animals with non-healing wounds
- animals with staphylococcal infections that are not responding to antibiotics
- nosocomial or secondary infections in high-risk patients
- animals with sepsis.

Swabs should be taken from the affected area and submitted for bacterial culture and sensitivity. Barrier nursing procedures should be implemented. The routine screening of veterinary staff and the environment is controversial. Screening is not a substitute for effective hand hygiene. Transient carriage of MRSA/MRSP is in any case more common than persistent colonisation and is most effectively controlled by hand hygiene. The role of the environment in MRSA/MRSP spread is unclear, and the significance of a positive culture is unknown.

Owing to growing public awareness of surgical site infections, nosocomial infections and MRSA/MRSP, there is a need for clinical audit of surgical site infections. Estimating the number of surgical site infections is difficult for a number of reasons. Differentiating inflammation or suture reaction from infection is critical, and the criteria for diagnosing a surgical site infection described earlier in this section need to be consistently applied.

Follow-up of patients can be an additional problem, particularly in referral centres where patients do not necessarily return to the hospital for wound checks or skin suture removal. There needs to be a system in place for flagging surgical site infections on the patient's clinical notes, and this information needs to be readily retrieved. In order to calculate infection rates, the total number and type of procedures performed also needs to be known. This allows for calculation of overall infection rates, as well as those for a given procedure.

Following on from this, infection rates can be compared between surgeons and between surgeons performing a given procedure. The results of any such audits have to be interpreted and acted upon with extreme caution. A surgeon may have a higher rate of surgical site infections owing to poor aseptic and surgical technique. Equally it could be the result of performing more difficult or lengthy procedures, of better follow-up and of being more diligent in reporting complications. Comparing the rate of surgical site infections between different hospitals is fraught with similar difficulties, as differences in defining surgical site infections, reporting and collecting data may not be standardised.

1.3 Preparation of the surgeon

Key points

- Preparation of the surgeon for theatre, surgical attire and theatre practice are somewhat controversial areas, with rules often being based on dogma rather than evidence-based studies.
- While the impact of the surgeon's attire and theatre practice may, in truth, have limited impact on the incidence of surgical site infections, most surgeons consider adherence to their basic tenets to be good practice.
- The use of antiseptics to reduce the number of microbes on the surgeon's skin is also well established, although conventional views on hand preparation have been challenged and there has been a movement from traditional hand-scrubbing techniques towards the use of alcohol-based hand rubs.
- The use of surgical gowns and gloves is now the norm in veterinary practice, and the benefits and limitations of these are discussed.

1.3.1 Surgical attire

The surgeon's theatre attire and preparation for theatre remain a controversial topic, with clinical dogma taking precedence over evidence-based studies. While there may be a paucity of clinical data to justify certain theatre practices, these can be supported on the basis of common sense. In addition, such as wearing a suit to present a lecture, having the appropriate attire in theatre can set the tone for good surgical practice.

Surgical scrubs are worn to reduce contamination of the operating room owing to shedding of microorganisms from the surgeon's skin. It is questionable whether scrub suits achieve this, particularly after repeated laundering. One advantage of surgical scrubs is that they prevent the surgeon's outdoor clothes from being contaminated by the patient's blood or other bodily fluids. Surgical scrubs should ideally not be worn in areas of the hospital other than theatre, and should never be worn outside.

Head covers are used to prevent microorganisms in the surgeon's hair contaminating the surgical field. Hair carries a higher bacterial load than hairless skin. Surgical hoods may reduce the environmental contamination compared to caps or uncovered hair. There is, however, no evidence that the use of head covers reduces the incidence of SSI.

Surgical face masks are worn to prevent direct contamination of the wound during conversation and to prevent droplets of saliva falling on to the wound. The mask acts as a barrier to bacteria, but bacteria are expelled around the edges of the mask and ultimately the environmental bacterial load is not reduced. There is no evidence that the use of surgical masks reduces the incidence of SSI.

Bacteria on the theatre floor contribute up to 15% of airborne bacteria, and walking increases the level of bacteria in the air. Shoe covers or dedicated theatre shoes are recommended to reduce the environmental contamination from outdoor footwear. These also prevent the surgeon's outdoor shoes from becoming soiled. Again, there is no evidence that the use of dedicated theatre footwear reduces the incidence of SSI.

1.3.2 Surgical hand preparation

The use of antiseptics to reduce the number of microorganisms present and, consequently, the incidence of SSI, was first demonstrated by Joseph Lister in the 19th century. The aim of surgical hand preparation is to eliminate the transient flora and reduce the number of resident flora. In addition, the antiseptic should retain its effect until the end of the procedure. There is a plethora of literature available regarding the type of antiseptic to use and the protocol to be followed. Often the information contained in the literature is conflicting, making it difficult to draw conclusions as to the best hand preparation protocol to follow. The majority of the information available is drawn from the human medical literature, with few veterinary studies available. When comparing antiseptics, most studies look at the antiseptic's ability to reduce the number of colony-forming units (CFUs) on the surgeon's hands immediately after hand preparation and defined periods of time later. Few, if any, studies look at the impact of hand preparation protocol on the incidence of SSI (Chou et al., 2016; da Silveira et al., 2016; Tanner et al., 2016).

Antiseptics traditionally used include chlorhexidine gluconate and povidone-iodine. The properties and mechanism of action of these compounds were discussed earlier in the chapter. Numerous *in vitro* and *in vivo* studies have demonstrated that chlorhexidine gluconate is superior to povidone-iodine in terms of its immediate and sustained action, and in the incidence of contact dermatitis. However, studies have failed to show any difference in the incidence of SSI and both preparations remain widely used (Tanner et al., 2016).

The recommended time for surgical hand preparation has changed over the years, with a trend towards shorter scrub times. Multiple studies have shown that shorter scrub times are as effective as longer scrub times in reducing CFUs. The current World Health Organization (WHO) suggestions for 4% chlorhexidine gluconate are 4 minutes for the first procedure of the day and 2 minutes for subsequent procedures (World Health Organization, 2009). Almost all studies discourage the use of brushes, which traumatise the skin and lead to more rapid recolonisation. Disposable sponges or combination sponge-brushes are now used almost exclusively. Despite higher bacterial counts being found under the fingernails, the efficacy of nail picks is questionable. Hands are typically rinsed after the application of the antiseptic. It is sobering to note that *Pseudomonas* species are frequently isolated from taps in hospitals. Sterile towels are used to dry wet hands after surgical hand preparation. Several methods of drying have been tested, with no difference in microbial numbers being found (Tanner et al., 2016).

There has been a trend over recent years towards the use of alcohol-based hand rubs rather than traditional scrub preparations. Numerous studies have shown the immediate action of preparations containing 60–90% alcohol to be superior to that of chlorhexidine gluconate and povidone-iodine. Alcohol-based hand rubs must comply with the European standard EN12791 to be regarded as effective for surgical hand preparation. The WHO has published a recommended procedure for the application of alcohol-based rub to dry skin, which involves keeping the forearms and hands wet with alcohol throughout the preparation (World Health Organization, 2009). Application times are much shorter than for traditional scrub preparations. One commercially available product commonly used in the veterinary industry containing a mixture of iso- and *n*-propanol, and another containing 85% ethanol, have recommended application times of 90 seconds. Older alcohol-based rubs often had chlorhexidine gluconate added to provide a persistent or sustained effect, as alcohol does not have a sustained effect (once the alcohol evaporates, it stops killing). However, it is argued that because the initial reduction in resident skin flora by alcohols is so effective that microbial rebound remains below baseline for over 6 hours, there is no requirement for these preparations to have a sustained action and that the addition of chlorhexidine gluconate is superfluous. In addition, the commonly used alcohol-based skin preparations do not alter the pH of the skin or remove oils from the skin, meaning that the stratum corneum is not damaged.

In summary, proponents of alcohol-based skin preparations argue that these products are more efficacious, in terms of immediate and sustained effect, than chlorhexidine gluconate and povidone-iodine. Application times are shorter and skin irritation is uncommon. It is estimated that 20 litres of water per surgical hand preparation are saved, and there is no potential for recontamination during rinsing. Despite these advantages, there are no studies which demonstrate a reduction in the incidence of SSI and many veterinary surgeons still choose to use traditional surgical scrub protocols (Verwilghen et al., 2011).

1.3.3 Surgical gloves

Gloves protect the patient from contamination by microorganisms on the surgeon's hands. They also protect the surgeon from infection by the patient. Surgical gloves are, however, susceptible to perforation, with latex gloves reported to be more resistant to perforation than vinyl gloves. An observational cohort veterinary study to identify the incidence and risk factors for surgical glove perforation found that at least one glove perforation occurred in 26.2% of procedures (Hayes et al., 2014). Risk factors for glove perforation include surgical times exceeding 1 hour, orthopaedic procedures, any procedure using powered instruments or orthopaedic wire, the use of polyisoprene as a glove material and being the primary surgeon. Glove perforations were detected intra-operatively in only 30.8% of cases. A second veterinary study found bacterial contamination on the outer surface of gloves as having occurred in 21% of procedures (Walker et al., 2014). The cause of the contamination was not defined and the incidence of concurrent perforation was not reported. Despite this high incidence of contamination, the incidence of SSI was low (5.1%).

Many surgeons and surgical texts advocate the practice of double-gloving (Tanner and Parkinson, 2006). The reported incidence of perforation of single gloves is 12.7–31%; for double-gloving, the reported incidence is 11.5–44% for outer gloves and 3.8–13% for inner gloves (Renberg, 2012). A meta-analysis confirmed that double-gloving significantly reduces the incidence of perforations to the innermost gloves. However, there were no studies that had the power to demonstrate that this led to a reduction in the incidence of SSI. The use of coloured indicator under-gloves was found to increase the sensitivity of intra-operative detection of tears to the outer glove from 34 to 83% (Meakin et al., 2016). Inner gloves were found to be intact in 63% of glove pairs when an outer tear occurred, and it was suggested that prompt changing of gloves following detection of a tear might reduce the incidence of contamination of the surgical site. The same meta-analysis cited above confirmed that coloured indicator gloves improved the sensitivity of intra-operative detection of tears to the outer glove, but failed to show an effect on the incidence of SSI. Open- and closed-gloving techniques are commonly used by veterinary surgeons, with no difference in the incidence of surgical site infections.

Step by step: open-gloving technique

- Use left hand to pick up the right glove by the inside of the cuff and pull it over your right hand (Fig. 1.20a).
- Hook your right thumb behind the cuff (Fig. 1.20b).
- Pick up your left glove, so that your gloved fingers touch the outside of the left cuff and your thumb (protected by the inside of the right cuff) touches the inside of the left cuff (Fig. 1.20c).
- Pull the left glove over the hand (Fig. 1.20d) and over the cuff of the gown (Fig. 1.20e).
- The gloved fingers of your left hand are then used to pull the right glove (touching only the outer part of the glove) (Fig. 1.20f) over the cuff of the gown (Fig. 1.20g).

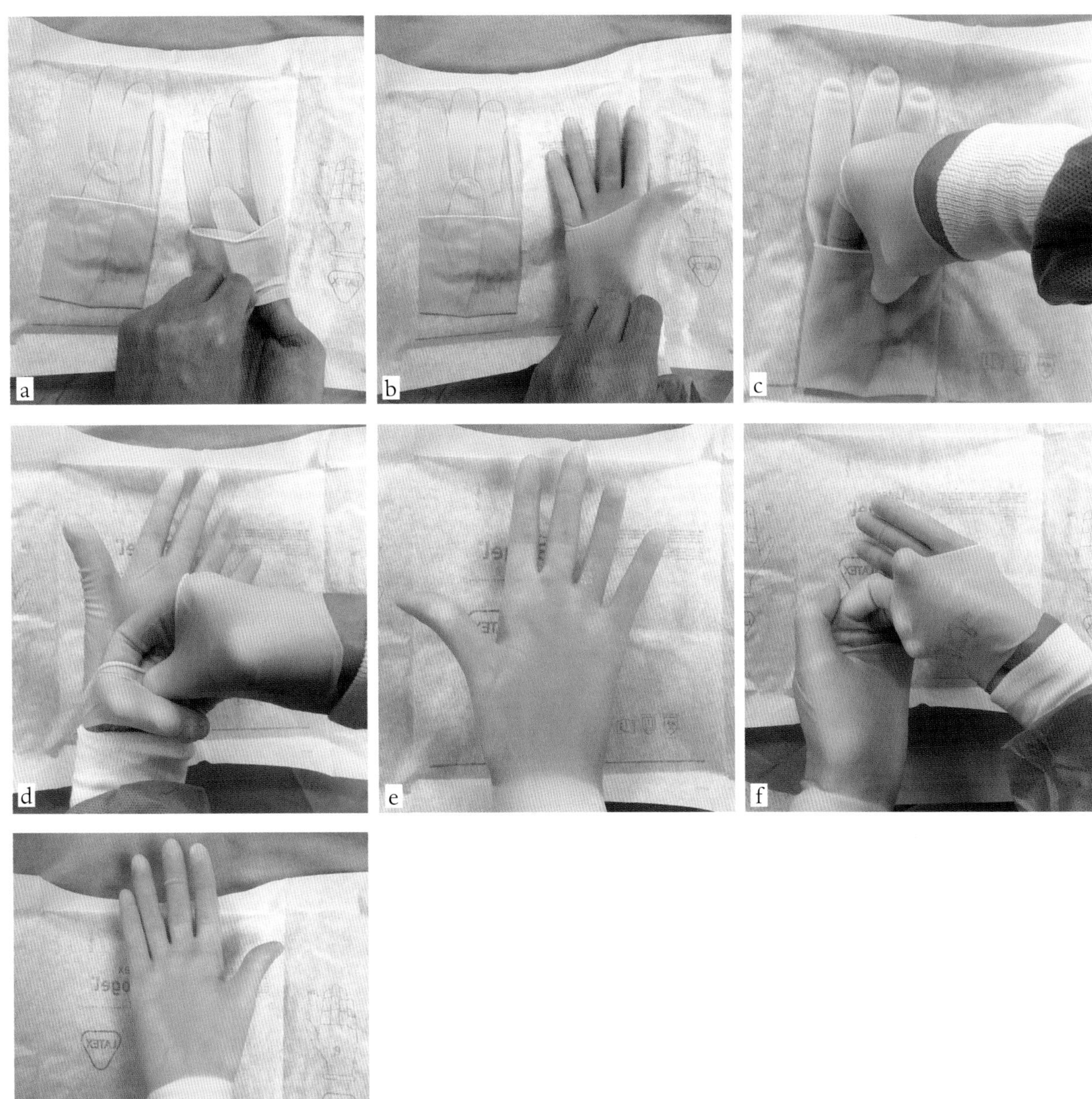

Fig. 1.20a–g
Open-gloving technique.

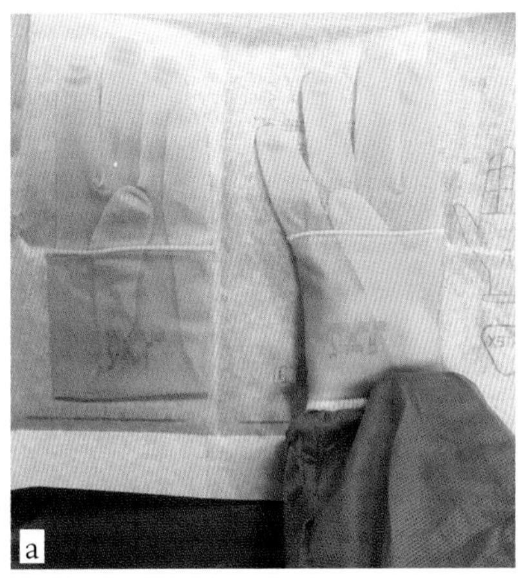
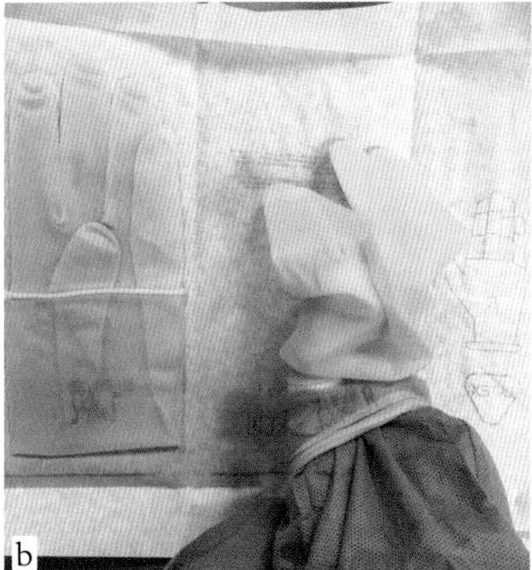
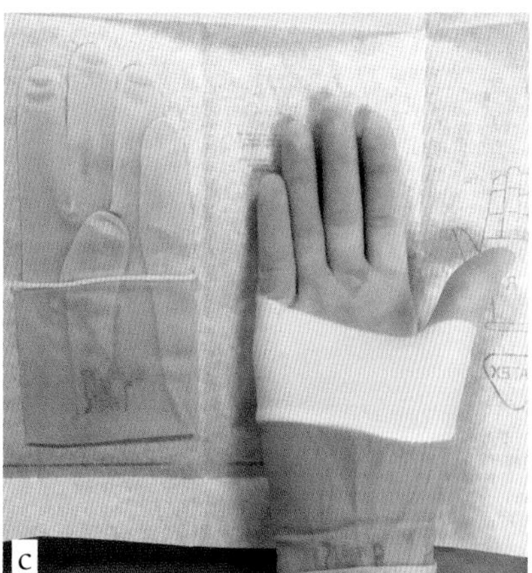
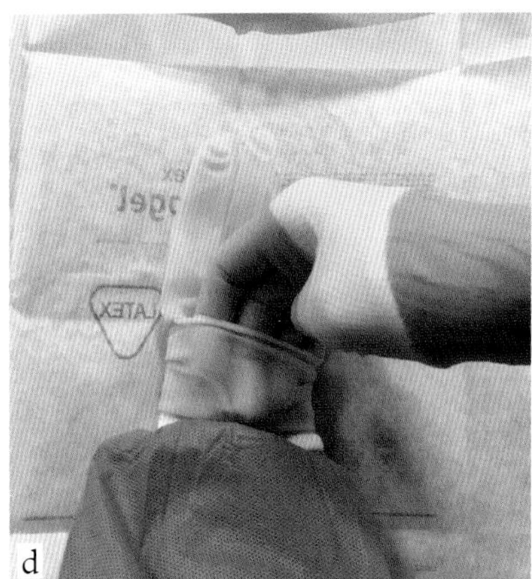
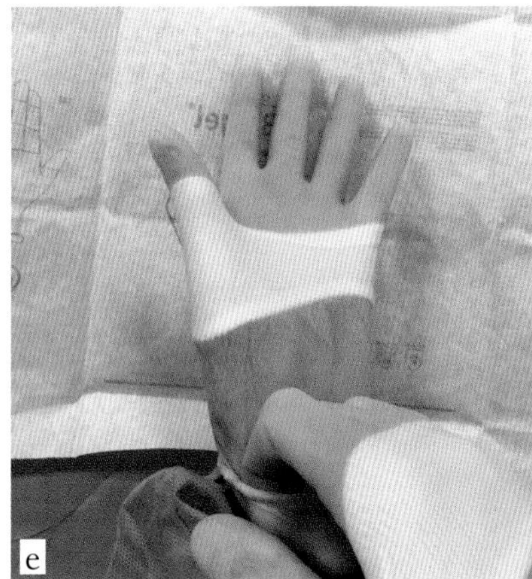

Fig. 1.21a–e Closed-gloving technique.

Step by step: closed-gloving technique

- Keep your hands within the cuffs of the gown.
- Slide your hand into the right glove, being careful to touch only the inside of the glove (Fig. 1.21a).
- Use your left hand to pull the glove over the cuff of the gown (touching only the inside of the glove) (Fig. 1.21b) while simultaneously pushing your right hand out of the gown and into the glove (Fig. 1.21c).
- Slide your left hand into the left glove, again taking care to touch only the inside of the glove.
- The gloved fingers of your right hand are hooked underneath the cuff, this time touching only the outside of the cuff (Fig. 1.21d).
- Pull the left glove over the cuff of the gown while simultaneously pushing your left hand out of the gown and into the glove (Fig. 1.21e).

References

Aiken, M.J., Hughes, T.K., Abercromby, R.H., Holems, M.A. and Anderson, A.A. (2015) Prospective, randomised comparison of the effect of two antimicrobial regimes on surgical site infection rate in dogs undergoing orthopaedic implant surgery. *Veterinary Surgery* 44, 661–667.

Beal, M.W., Brown, D.C. and Shofer, F.S. (2000) The effects of hypothermia and the duration of anaesthesia on postoperative wound infection rate in clean wounds: a retrospective study. *Veterinary Surgery* 29, 123–127.

BSAVA Practice Guidelines: Reducing the risk from MRSA and MRSP. Available at: www.BSAVA.com/resources/veterinary resources/guidelines.

Chou, P.Y., Doyle, A.J., Arai, S., Burke, P.J. and Bailey, T.R. (2016) Antibacterial efficacy of several surgical hand preparation products used by veterinary students. *Veterinary Surgery* 45, 515–522.

da Silveira, E.A., Bubeck, K.A., Batista, E.R., Piat, P., Laverty, S., Beauchamp, G., Archamboult, M. and Elce, Y. (2016) Comparison of an alcohol-based hand rub and water-based chlorhexidine gluconate scrub technique for hand antisepsis prior to elective surgery in horses. *Canadian Veterinary Journal* 57, 164–168.

Dubiel, B., Shires, P.K., Korvick, D. and Chekan, E.G. (2010) Electromagnetic energy sources in surgery. *Veterinary Surgery* 39, 909–924.

Eugster, S., Schawalder, P., Gaschen, F. and Boerlin, P. (2004) A prospective study of postoperative surgical site infections in dogs and cats. *Veterinary Surgery* 33, 542–550.

Hayes, G.M., Reynolds, D., Moens, N.M., Singh, A., Oblak, M., Gibson, T.W., Brisson, B.A., Nazarali, A. and Dewey, C. (2014) Investigation of incidence and risk factors for surgical glove perforation in small animal surgery. *Veterinary Surgery* 43, 400–404.

Heldmann, E., Brown, D.C. and Shofer, F. (1999) The association of propofol usage with postoperative wound infection rate in clean wounds: a retrospective study. *Veterinary Surgery* 28, 256–259.

Meakin, L.B., Gilman, O.P., Parsons, K.J., Burton, N.J. and Langley-Hobbs, S.J. (2016) Coloured indicator undergloves increase the detection of glove perforations by surgeons during small animal orthopaedic surgery: a randomised controlled trial. *Veterinary Surgery* 45, 709–714.

Meakin, L.B., Murrell, J.C., Doran, I.C.P, Knowles, T.G., Tivers, M.S. and Chanoit, G.P. (2017) Electrosurgery reduces blood loss and immediate postoperative inflammation compared to cold instruments for midline celiotomy in dogs: a randomised controlled trial. *Veterinary Surgery* 46, 515–519.

Nicholson, M., Beal, M., Shofer, F. and Brown, D.C. (2002) Epidemiologic evaluation of postoperative wound infection in clean-contaminated wounds: a retrospective study of 239 dogs and cats. *Veterinary Surgery* 31, 577–581.

Petersen, S.W. and Rosin, E. (1995) Cephalothin and cefazolin in vitro antibacterial activity and pharmacokinetics in dogs. *Veterinary Surgery* 24, 347–351.

Pratesi, A., Moores, A.P., Downes, C., Grierson, J. and Maddox, T.W. (2015) Efficacy of post-operative antimicrobial use for clean orthopaedic implant surgery in dogs: a prospective randomised study in 100 consecutive cases. *Veterinary Surgery* 44, 653–660.

Renberg, W.C. (2012) Preparation of the patient, operating team, and operating room for surgery. In: Tobias K.M. and Johnston S.A. (eds) *Veterinary Surgery: Small Animal.* Elsevier Saunders, St. Louis, Missouri, pp. 164–169.

Scott, J.E., Swanson, E.A., Cooley, J. and Wills, R.W. (2017) Healing of canine skin incisions made with monopolar electrosurgery versus scalpel blade. *Veterinary Surgery* 46, 520–529.

Silverman, E.B., Read, R.W., Boyle, C.R., Cooper, R., Miller, W.W. and McLaughlin, R.M. (2007) Histologic comparison of canine skin biopsies collected using monopolar electrosurgery, CO2 laser, radiowave radiosurgery, skin biopsy punch and scalpel. *Veterinary Surgery* 36, 50–56.

Tanner, J. and Parkinson, H. (2006) Double gloving to reduce surgical cross-infection. *Cochrane Database Systematic Review* 19: CD003087.

Tanner, J., Dumville, J.C., Norman, G. and Fortnam, M. (2016) Surgical hand antisepsis to reduce surgical site infection. *Cochrane Database Systematic Review* 22(1): CD004288.

Turk, R., Singh, A. and Weese, J.S. (2015) Prospective surgical site infection surveillance in dogs. *Veterinary Surgery* 44, 2–8.

Verwilghen, D., Grulke, S. and Kampf, G. (2011) Pre-surgical hand antisepsis: concepts and current habits of veterinary surgeons. *Veterinary Surgery* 40, 515–521.

Walker, M., Singh, A., Rousseau, J. and Weese, J.S. (2014) Bacterial contamination of gloves worn by small animal surgeons in a veterinary teaching hospital. *Canadian Veterinary Journal* 55, 1160–1162.

World Health Organization. (2009) *WHO Guidelines on Hand Hygiene in Health Care.* WHO Press, Geneva.

Wound management and reconstructive surgery

2

Jonathan C. Bell

Chapter summary

2.1 Principles of wound healing

Key points

- The inherent elasticity of canine and feline skin and the presence of direct cutaneous arteries (as opposed to the musculocutaneous arteries of humans) make it ideal for reconstructive procedures.
- The deep dermal plexus is the blood supply to the dermis and epidermis, and must be preserved.
- Skin is visco-elastic, and its properties of mechanical creep and stress relaxation can be utilised to facilitate wound closure.

2.1.1 Anatomy and physiology

The skin consists of a superficial epidermis and a deeper dermis. The epidermis of hair-bearing areas comprises the stratum corneum and the stratum germinativum (combined stratum cylindricum and stratum spinosum). In full-thickness skin wounds, the stratum germinativum is the source of the epithelial cells which cover the wound. Below the dermis is the hypodermis (subcutaneous tissue). The hypodermis contains adipose tissue and loose connective tissue. A thin panniculus muscle is present in the hypodermis of the head, neck and trunk. The skin is supplied by direct cutaneous vessels which run parallel to the skin within the hypodermis. The terminal branches form a rich capillary plexus known as the deep dermal (or subdermal) plexus. In areas of the skin that have a panniculus muscle, the subdermal plexus runs above and below the panniculus muscle. The deep dermal plexus must be preserved when undermining skin and creating skin flaps.

Skin contains collagen fibres (mainly type I collagen), elastin fibres and an extracellular matrix comprising mainly water and proteins. These materials confer the skin's inherent elasticity and extensibility. The skin is visco-elastic, that is, it has mechanical properties of both viscous and elastic structures. A visco-elastic material like skin exhibits hysteresis, whereby the stress–strain curve is non-linear. The skin undergoes time-dependent plastic strain while under constant stress, meaning it is stretched beyond its inherent extensibility. This property is referred to as mechanical creep, and is due to the extrusion of tissue fluid from the interstices of the collagen network. Skin also exhibits the property of stress relaxation, a term which is sometimes used interchangeably with mechanical creep, but which is actually a decrease in the level of stress under the same amount of strain. This is thought to be due to the breakage of collagen fibres and permanent plastic strain. Breakage of elastin fibres leads to a loss of the skin's elastic recoil under constant strain. Put simply, after skin has been stretched into a given position for a period of time, it no longer tends to spring back to its original position once the stress is removed. A number of the skin closure techniques discussed later in the chapter utilise these visco-elastic properties.

2.1.2 Types of wound healing

Key points

- The classical phases of wound healing, although described as separate entities, actually overlap and involve a complex series of interactions between blood cells, the extracellular matrix, parenchymal cells and cytokines.
- An understanding of the underlying mechanisms of wound healing allows the surgeon to make appropriate decisions regarding open wound management and primary wound closure.
- Although many factors affect wound healing, local factors have the greatest influence and these are directly influenced by the surgeon's surgical technique (Cornell, 2012).

A wound is a break in the continuity of the skin. It may be caused by trauma or be surgically created. First-intention healing occurs when the wound edges are sutured. This type of healing is also known as primary closure. Second-intention healing occurs when there is tissue loss and the wound edges cannot be apposed. This type of healing is also referred to as open-wound healing. Third-intention healing occurs when there is a delay in closing the wound, typically because of concerns about infection or devitalisation. Some texts refer to delayed primary closure as apposition of the wound edges within 3–5 days of injury before granulation tissue has formed, with secondary closure referring to apposition after this time in the presence of granulation tissue. Other texts use these terms interchangeably.

Wound healing involves a complex series of interactions between blood cells, the extracellular matrix, parenchymal cells and cytokines. Cytokines are chemicals released by cells within the wound. These cells have autocrine or paracrine function and direct the synthesis of compounds required for wound healing. The phases of wound healing are classically described as the inflammatory phase, the proliferative phase and the maturation and remodelling phase. Although described as separate entities, these processes overlap and occur to varying degrees depending on the nature of the open wound.

Inflammatory phase

This is sometimes referred to as the lag phase or preparatory phase, and usually lasts up to 5 days following wounding (Fig. 2.1). Bleeding occurs at the time of wounding resulting in vasoconstriction and the formation of a blood clot. The blood clot contains fibrin and fibronectin and is the basis of the provisional extracellular matrix. The provisional extracellular matrix forms a scaffold by which cells can migrate into the wound. Platelets within the clot release vasoactive compounds which result in vasodilation, and cytokines which are chemotactic for white blood cells. White blood cells leave the circulation and enter the wound bed by the processes of margination and diapedesis. The first inflammatory cell at the wound bed is the neutrophil. Neutrophils produce proteinases which debride necrotic tissue. They have a role in bacterial killing via phagocytosis and the production of free radicals. Free radical production is highly oxygen dependent. Oxygen delivery to the neutrophils occurs by diffusion across relatively short distances and requires an adequate partial pressure, emphasising the importance of preserving the wound's blood supply and maintaining perfusion. Neutrophils undergo apoptosis within a few days. Monocytes are the next cells found in the wound. These differentiate into macrophages. Macrophages have an

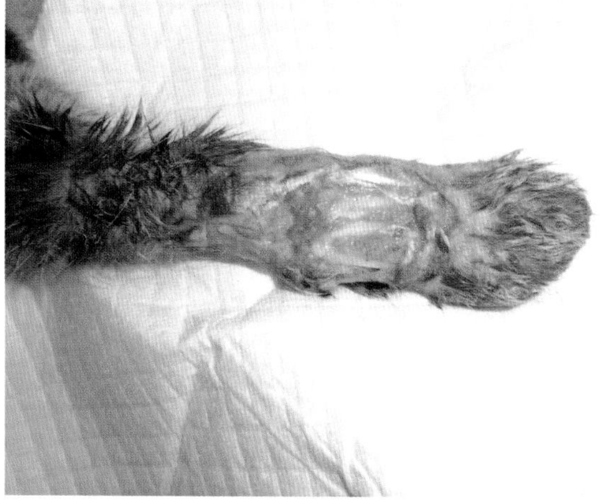

Fig. 2.1 Degloving injury in a cat. Necrotic tissue is present in the wound, along with exposed tendon and bone. This wound is in the inflammatory phase of healing.

essential role in wound healing. As well as their role in phagocytosis and wound debridement, they produce cytokines which are chemotactic for the cells necessary for the proliferative phase of wound healing. They are the primary cell in the wound within 48–96 hours.

Proliferative phase

This phase runs from approximately days 5 to 20 and its hallmark is the presence of granulation tissue (Fig. 2.2). Granulation tissue appears red and granular, and contains macrophages, fibroblasts and capillary buds. These cells bind to the provisional extracellular matrix by the virtue of specialised cell membrane receptors known as integrins and migrate across the wound.

Angiogenesis is the formation of a new capillary network and is critical for progression of wound healing. Endothelial cells migrate through the capillary membrane and form capillary buds, which migrate across the provisional extracellular matrix scaffold. This process occurs in response to a number of growth factors and wound factors such as low oxygen tension.

Fibroplasia is the proliferation of fibroblasts at the margin of the wound and their migration across the fibrin scaffold of the wound bed. They produce proteolytic enzymes such as plasminogen activator and matrix metalloproteinases (MMPs) to aid their migration. They initially produce fibronectin to form a loose extracellular matrix. The production of type III collagen follows shortly after. This occurs at around days 4–5 after wounding, and is a critical period in wound healing as it marks the start of the wound's gaining of tensile strength. The fibroblastic phase lasts 2–4 weeks. After this time, the number of fibroblasts and capillaries decreases and collagen deposition increases. The wound does not support further epithelialisation or contraction, and becomes a chronic granulating wound.

Epithelialisation is the restoration of an epithelial surface. This process begins 1–2 days after wounding. The source of epithelial cells is the wound edges in full-thickness wounds. The dermal adnexa are the source of the epithelial cells in partial thickness wounds. Epithelialisation in this case is a rapid process. Epithelial cells at the wound margin lose their attachment to the basement membrane and migrate across the wound using the extracellular matrix scaffold. In a sutured wound, the small dermal gap can be bridged within 48 hours. This process takes longer in larger open wounds, and may never be completed. The surface of open wounds that have healed by epithelialisation may be fragile and easily ulcerated (Hosgood, 2012). Hair coverage is often sparse. Sutured wounds appear healed once epithelialisation is complete. However, they may not yet have gained enough tensile strength to guarantee apposition once skin sutures are removed. This can lead to unexpected dehiscence, a phenomenon referred to as pseudo-healing.

Wound contraction is the centripetal movement of the skin edges, resulting in shrinking and sometimes closure of the wound. Fibroblasts within the wound develop smooth muscle properties and become myofibroblasts. These bind via integrins to the extracellular matrix and skin edges, pulling the skin towards the centre of the wound. Epithelial proliferation and collagen deposition occur below the stretched skin to restore normal thickness, a process referred to as intussusceptive growth. Wound contraction in the dog starts at days 5–9 and generally declines at 6 weeks. Wounds that have not closed by this time are very unlikely to do so. Excessive wound contraction can lead to distortion of body orifices and loss of normal joint movement (contracture). Animals with loose, fur-covered skin, along with puppies and kittens, have huge potential for wounds to heal by contraction, unlike the situation in humans.

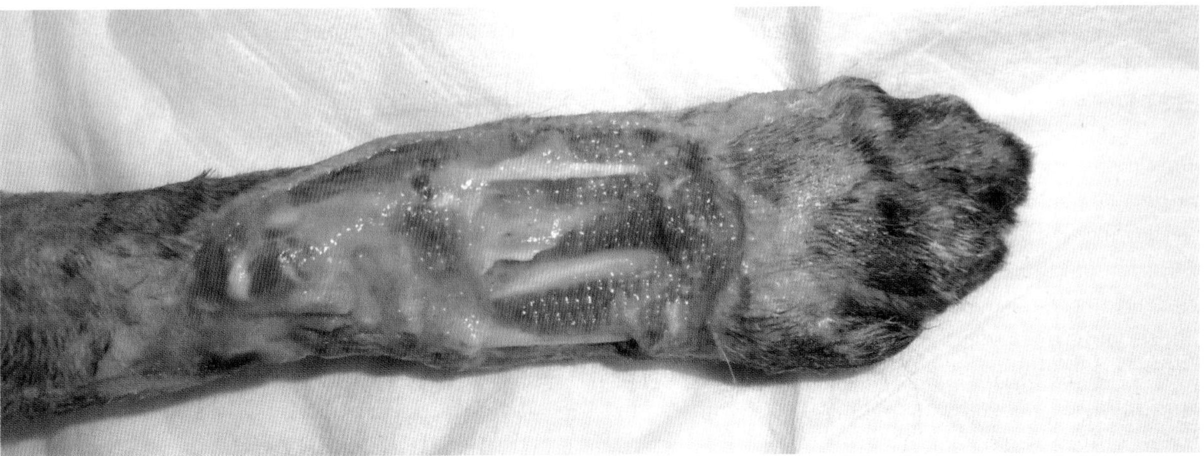

Fig. 2.2 The same wound shown in Fig. 2.1. Healthy granulation tissue is starting to fill the wound. The skin edges are healthy and attached to the wound bed. Minimal exudate is present. This wound is in the proliferative phase of healing.

Maturation and remodelling phase

This phase of wound healing is concerned with the remodelling and strengthening of collagen. Weaker type III collagen is converted to type I collagen, resulting in increased wound strength. Collagen degradation by collagenase enzymes is balanced by tissue inhibitors of metalloproteinases (TIMPs). Fibroblasts and myofibroblasts regress as tension in the wound decreases. Net collagen synthesis is complete by 4–5 weeks after the injury, but maturation continues for 12–18 months. The wound strength of canine skin is 5–10% that of normal tissue at 10–14 days, 25% at 3–4 weeks and 80% at 3 months.

There are important species differences in wound healing (Bohling et al., 2004). Feline sutured wounds have been shown to be slower to heal, being only 50% as strong as those in dogs at 7 days. Cats had lower cutaneous perfusion in the first week after surgery, followed by a more rapid gain during the second week. Cats produced less granulation tissue than dogs, with a peripheral rather than central distribution. Reduction in wound area by contraction and epithelialisation over 21 days was greater in dogs than in cats. Canine wounds closed by central pull and epithelialisation, whereas cat wounds closed by contraction of the wound edges. In both species, preservation of the subcutaneous tissues was important in second-intention healing, but less so in first-intention healing (Bohling et al., 2006). Excessive debridement of the subcutaneous tissues may, therefore, delay wound healing, particularly in cats.

Factors affecting wound healing

Both local and systemic factors can influence wound healing. Systemic factors such as poor immune function, chemotherapy, radiotherapy and age have been shown to delay wound healing. However, local wound factors are far more commonly implicated in delayed wound healing. This is important as the surgeon can directly influence many of these factors, and good surgical technique is paramount to achieving successful wound healing.

Maintaining wound perfusion is important as adequate oxygen delivery is essential for many of the stages of wound healing (Hosgood, 2006). Diffusion of oxygen in a wound is more difficult owing to large inter-capillary distances and peripheral vasoconstriction. While oxygen saturation is important, the partial pressure of oxygen is the driving force for diffusion. Every effort must be made to maintain perfusion in the face of intra-operative vasodilation (due to anaesthesia) and post-operative vasoconstriction (due to pain and hypothermia).

Necrotic tissue and foreign material both inhibit wound healing. These should be removed during surgery by sharp debridement. Haematomas and seromas disrupt the integrity of the wound, decrease diffusion and provide a medium for bacterial growth. Attention should be paid to haemostasis and minimising dead space.

Wounds containing more than 10^5 bacteria per gram of tissue are very likely to develop a surgical site infection (SSI). This threshold is lowered in the face of poor perfusion, damaged or devitalised tissue and foreign material. Clean-contaminated and contaminated wounds should have prophylactic antibiotics to decrease the risk of infection. Close attention should be paid to preserving the local blood supply, minimising tissue trauma, removing devitalised tissue and minimising the amount of foreign material, e.g. suture material, left in the wound.

Primary wound closure is preferred to second-intention healing as the sutures protect the wound from negative mechanical factors such as shear and tension which might disrupt wound healing (Fahie 2012). Second-intention healing requires the development of a bed of granulation tissue and is a slower process.

2.1.3 Open wound management

Key points

- Open wound management is a perfectly reasonable but often neglected way of managing traumatic (and occasionally surgical) wounds in veterinary practice.
- Although frequently maligned in the veterinary literature, the use of wet-to-dry dressings in conjunction with surgical debridement remains one of the quickest and most effective ways to turn a contaminated traumatic wound into a healthy granulating one.
- There is a plethora of commercial dressings available to facilitate open wound management. The evidence base for the use of these dressings is not always clear, and dressings are often selected owing to personal experience and preference. This selection should be underpinned by an understanding of the current phase of wound healing and its underlying biological mechanisms.

Open wound management is indicated when primary closure isn't possible owing to excessive tension, loss of skin, devitalised tissue or infection. Healing by second intention is a slower process than primary wound healing. The functional outcome isn't always good, with fragile epithelial coverage and excessive contraction (particularly close to joints or orifices) being problematic. Some wounds won't re-epithelialise, leaving exposed granulation tissue in the centre of the wound. Nevertheless, open wound management can be successfully employed to allow closure of large wounds in veterinary practice, and is a viable alternative to major reconstructive surgical procedures in selected cases.

Handy hints

The decision making is usually straightforward, in that if it is possible to close a wound we would generally do so. It is not uncommon for primary closure of a traumatic wound to be preceded by a period of open wound management to allow assessment of tissue viability and to control infection (third-intention healing). If a wound can't safely or physically be closed, open wound management is appropriate. Alternatively, a prolonged period of open wound management may be employed to allow a wound to contract to a size that is amenable to primary closure.

It is said there is a 'golden period' of 3–6 hours within which time traumatic wounds may be sutured. In practice, many factors influence whether or not a wound can be closed primarily. Wound edges should be fresh and vascularised with no evidence of crushing, devitalisation or the presence of debris. Clean lacerations are often suitable for primary closure. The amount of tissue damage sustained following a crushing injury may not be apparent for a few days after trauma. Puncture wounds are associated with deep tissue crushing and contamination. Anatomical degloving injuries refer to the loss of an area of skin with exposure of the underlying tissues. These occur following dragging and scraping of the skin. With a physiological degloving injury, the skin is intact but has become separated from its blood supply, with necrosis developing several days later. Crushing injuries, puncture wounds and degloving injuries do better with a period of open wound management. Wounds should not be closed primarily if there is significant skin loss, dead space or tension. Care should be taken with wounds subject to excessive motion or shearing. Dehisced surgical wounds are contaminated and treated as traumatic wounds.

Wound irrigation

Irrigation solutions are used to flush debris, loose necrotic tissue and microorganisms from the wound. The volume of solution is more important than the composition or antibiotic content. Copious volumes should be used, the old maxim being 'dilution is the solution to pollution'. Care should be taken if using antiseptic solutions, as these may be toxic to cells if they are not diluted adequately. Sterile saline may be the irrigation solution of choice, though many studies suggest that tap water is just as effective.

Handy hints

The ideal pressure for fluid administration is yet to be deduced. High pressures may be associated with tissue damage. A drip bag attached to a giving set provides low-pressure irrigation. Higher pressures can be achieved by using a 35 ml syringe and 18- or 19-gauge needle. Either is safe and effective in practice.

Topical antimicrobial agents may be applied to the wound to reduce contamination. Antibiotic ointments, silver-based dressings and hyperosmotic dressings (hypertonic saline, sugar or honey) are suitable. Systemic antibiotics should be given if the wound is heavily contaminated or infected. Ideally the antibiotic should be selected based on bacterial culture. Broad-spectrum antibiotics should be used if bacteriology is not available. Acute wound infections are usually due to one microorganism, whereas chronic wound infections are usually polymicrobial.

Wound debridement

Debridement is performed to remove contaminated and devitalised tissue from the wound. Selective debridement specifically targets necrotic tissue. Forms of selective debridement include autolytic debridement (the use of gels or dressings), enzymatic debridement and biotherapy (maggots). Non-selective debridement is a more aggressive and rapid way to remove necrotic tissue but is less precise, resulting in a degree of damage to viable tissues. Forms of non-selective debridement are surgical debridement and mechanical debridement using wet-to-dry dressings.

Surgical debridement

Surgical debridement is best done under general anaesthesia and aseptic conditions. Sharp dissection with a scalpel blade or Metzenbaum scissors should be employed to limit further tissue damage. Extension of the wound may be necessary to allow exploration of puncture wounds. For small wounds that are contaminated or devitalised, *en bloc* excision followed by primary closure of the surrounding unaffected tissues can be performed. For larger wounds that are not amenable to *en bloc* resection, layered debridement should be performed. This is the sequential removal of devitalised tissue at the wound surface, progressing to deeper tissues. Excess fat can be removed and fasciotomy may be performed to promote granulation tissue formation. Forage of exposed cortical bone allows the medullary cavity to communicate with the wound bed. Care should be taken not to remove excessive subcutaneous tissue as this can delay second-intention wound healing.

Wet-to-dry dressings

Gauze pads moistened with sterile saline are applied to the wound surface. The moisture dilutes the wound discharge and facilitates its absorption into the gauze and the outer components of the dressing. As the moisture evaporates through the dressing, the gauze dries and adheres to the wound surface and necrotic tissue. To allow adherence to the wound, the gauze should not be over-soaked. When the dressing is removed, the necrotic tissue is stripped away. This process should be repeated every 8–12 hours.

Wet-to-dry dressings have fallen out of favour for several reasons. They can be painful to remove and they are non-selective, so healthy tissues can be damaged at the same time as removal of the necrotic tissue.

Handy hints

Limiting use of wet-to-dry dressings to the inflammatory phase of wound healing, i.e. no longer than 3–5 days, is unlikely to cause significant trauma to the cells involved in the proliferative phase of wound healing.

The combination of careful surgical debridement followed by the short-term use of wet-to-dry dressings remains a cheap and highly effective way of managing necrotic wounds.

Enzymatic debridement

This is the application of proteolytic enzymes to degrade collagen bonds between the wound bed and the attached necrotic tissue. This method is usually used in patients who are not candidates for surgical debridement. It is a form of selective debridement and does not result in haemorrhage, pain or damage to viable tissues. Enzymatic debridement is a slower process than surgical debridement and can be expensive. Products available include papain-urea (Accuzyme Ointment, Healthpoint Ltd.), papain-urea, chlorophyllin copper complex (Panafil, Healthpoint Ltd.), trypsin (Granulex-V, Pfizer), collagenase (Santyl, Healthpoint Ltd.) and deoxyribonuclease with fibrinolysin (Elase, Astellas).

Autolytic debridement

Autolytic debridement refers to the body's natural processes of wound debridement by the cells within the wound. This is a form of selective debridement. These products work by retaining moisture at the wound and softening necrotic tissues, enhancing phagocytosis. Autolytic debridement is atraumatic to healthy tissues but is a slower process than surgical debridement. There is a risk of promoting infection in the presence of large amounts of necrotic tissue. In such cases, surgical debridement with or without a short period of wet-to-dry dressings is a better option.

Hydrogels contain water and are used to hydrate wounds. They also absorb and retain exudate from the wound, and are applied to the wound surface only – application to the wound edges can result in maceration of the skin. They facilitate autolytic debridement but can also be used to hydrate healthy granulation beds or partial thickness wounds. Examples of hydrogels include Intrasite (Smith & Nephew) and NuGel (Johnson & Johnson).

Hydrophilic pastes and powders – for example, Duoderm (Convatec) – are used in exudative wounds and cavities. These absorb exudate and form a gel at the wound surface, facilitating autolytic debridement.

Honey is a hygroscopic agent that can effectively reduce local oedema and retain wound fluid, promoting autolytic debridement. Its high osmolarity and acidity account for its antibacterial properties. In addition, honey produces 0.003% hydrogen peroxide which subsequently generates free radicals, accounting for its antibacterial activity. Honey is measured by its inhibin number, which is the amount of dilution up to which it will retain its antimicrobial effect. Unpasteurised honeys vary in their antibacterial properties, with manuka honey being considered the most useful of the honey products. Honey may reduce inflammation because of its antioxidant content and may stimulate lymphocyte activation, phagocytosis and cytokine release from monocytes.

Handy hints

Honey is applied liberally to the wound and covered with an absorptive dressing. The dressing may need to be changed every 8–12 hours. Care should be taken when applying honey to large open wounds because of the potential for fluid, protein and electrolyte loss.

Wound dressings

A wound dressing refers to the part of the bandage in contact with the wound (primary layer or contact layer). Dressings are classified on whether or not they adhere to the wound, their absorptive capacity and their ability to retain moisture at the wound (Campbell 2006). There are a large number of dressings from which to choose, and no dressing is perfect for every type of wound. There is in fact no clinical evidence in veterinary medicine to support the use of one dressing or wound product over another (Fahie 2007). When the veterinary surgeon is selecting a dressing or wound product, this should be done with an understanding of the stage of healing that the wound is at and the biological processes that are underpinning this, and an understanding of what is needed to be achieved in order to progress wound healing. The choice of dressing will also come down to personal preference, experience, cost and availability.

Adherent dressings

These are used for the non-selective mechanical debridement of necrotic tissue and the absorption of wound exudate. Wet-to-dry dressings are the most common example of these. The dressing material used is typically moistened gauze. These dressings are limited to the inflammatory phase of wound healing.

Non-adherent or low adherent dressings

This type of dressing is applied to healthy wounds or skin grafts, so that these tissues are not disturbed or damaged by removal of the dressing. Typically, these comprise a fabric mesh impregnated with paraffin or petrolatum (e.g. Jelonet, Smith & Nephew); Adaptic (Johnson & Johnson) is a knitted acetate fabric impregnated with petrolatum. The porous nature of these dressings allows wound exudate to pass into the absorptive (secondary) layer of the bandage. Using a topical wound gel or ointment with this type of dressing makes it semi-occlusive, providing a degree of moisture retention.

Absorptive dressings

These dressings are used to absorb fluid in exudative wounds. They are low adherent dressings, so are suitable when no further mechanical debridement is required. By retaining some of the absorbed fluid at the surface of the wound, they aid autolytic debridement.

Polyurethane foam (Allevyn, Smith & Nephew) is a highly absorptive dressing. It has a fine porous surface which is practically non-adherent. Polyurethane foams are less effective at promoting autolytic debridement than alginate and hydrocolloid dressings. They do retain some moisture at the wound surface, and can be considered to be semi-occlusive and moisture retentive.

Alginate dressings are made of alginic acid, derived from algae found in seaweed. Alginates are highly absorptive dressings and are available as sheets or ropes. They also have a topical haemostatic effect by activating prothrombin. Alginates are usually covered with an absorptive dressing to help soak up the wound exudate. Curasorb (Tyco), Nu-Derm (Johnson & Johnson) and Tegaderm Alginate (3M) are commonly used alginate dressings. Alginate dressings with antibacterial agents such as silver or manuka honey are available.

Moisture-retentive and occlusive dressings

A moist wound environment promotes autolytic debridement and many of the other processes of the proliferative phase of wound healing. The hydrocolloid and hydrogel dressings are considered moisture retentive, as are some of the absorptive dressings. Occlusive dressings are impermeable. The low oxygen tension below the dressing stimulates macrophages, fibroplasia, neovascularisation and epithelialisation. Semi-occlusive dressings allow gas and water vapour to pass through the dressing. The lower the moisture vapour transmission rate (MVTR), the more moisture retentive the dressing. The MVTR of normal skin (transdermal water loss) is 4–9 $g/m^2/h$ (this increases to 80–90 $g/m^2/h$ in open wounds). Dressings with an MVTR of less than 35 $g/m^2/h$ are considered to be moisture retentive.

Hydrogel dressings are made of water retained in a hydrophilic polymer. They are often semi-transparent to allow visualisation of the wound. They are secured to the wound with an outer bandage, forming a protective gel over the wound with limited absorptive capacity. They promote autolytic debridement and second-intention healing. These are best used on open wounds free from necrotic tissue and infection. They are usually changed every 3–4 days.

Hydrocolloid dressings have a matrix fixed to a polyurethane film or foam backing. Similar to hydrogels, they are an interactive dressing. They promote autolytic debridement and second-intention healing, and have some absorptive capacity. Like hydrogels, they should be used in wounds free from necrotic tissue and infection.

Vapour-permeable films are semi-occlusive dressings applied to minimally exudative wounds. They are not indicated for necrotic, infected or exudative wounds. Polyurethane films such as Tegaderm (3M) and OpSite (Smith & Nephew) are most commonly used. These are often used to protect sutured wounds.

Negative-pressure wound therapy

This is the application of sub-atmospheric pressure across a wound and is achieved by placing open-pore foam and drainage tubing onto the wound and covering it with an occlusive dressing. The tubing is connected to a portable suction machine. Benefits are said to include increased wound perfusion, decreased oedema, increased granulation tissue formation, decreased bacterial colonisation and the removal of wound exudate (Pitt and Stanley, 2014). While this modality has become very popular in veterinary practice, systematic reviews of its use in humans have not found evidence-based benefits.

2.2 Principles of reconstructive surgery

2.2.1 Primary wound closure

Key points

- This is the most common method of wound closure in veterinary practice.
- Successful creation and closure of surgical wounds requires correct surgical technique and an appreciation of the biological and mechanical properties of skin.
- Commonly used suture materials and patterns are described.

Successful surgical wound closure begins with correct wound creation. The least traumatic way to make a skin incision is with a scalpel blade using a fingertip grip; a pencil grip can be used for smaller incisions. Undermining, if necessary, is better performed with Metzenbaum scissors. Electrocautery and laser create bloodless incisions but cause thermal damage to the skin. An increasing number of studies are demonstrating delayed wound healing associated with the use of monopolar cautery. Meticulous haemostasis is essential for preventing problems with wound healing. This can be achieved with electrocautery, ligatures and tissue apposition. Adherence to Halsted's principles is recommended:

- gentle tissue handling
- meticulous haemostasis
- preservation of blood supply
- strict asepsis
- accurate dissection and apposition of tissues
- minimal tension
- obliteration of dead space.

Suture selection

There is quite a wide range of suture materials available in veterinary practice (Schmiedt, 2012). The choice of suture material is influenced in part by the type and location of the wound, the type of tissue being repaired and the individual characteristics of the suture material. The surgeon's choice might not always be based on science, but on personal preference and availability. The ideal suture material is suggested to have the following properties:

- easy to handle
- tensile strength to match that of the tissue into which it is being placed
- loss of tensile strength which parallels the gain in tissue strength
- good knot security
- minimal tissue reactivity
- low cost.

There is no ideal suture material, and some degree of compromise is usually necessary. The physical characteristics of a suture material determine its utility.

The configuration of a suture is the number of strands used to make it. Monofilament sutures are made from single strands, while multifilament sutures are made from multiple strands and are twisted or braided.

Suture sizes are given as either United States Pharmacopeia (USP) or metric. USP refers to a diameter range needed to produce a certain tensile strength. This range varies depending on the suture material category. Sizes are expressed with a zero after the number – more zeros indicate a smaller size. Metric sizes are determined by expressing the suture diameter in tenths of a millimetre.

The tensile strength is the maximal stress the suture will withstand before breaking. Braided suture materials generally have greater tensile strength than monofilament suture materials. Absorbable sutures lose tensile strength over time. The rate of tensile strength loss is not the same as the rate of absorption. Implanting sutures in the wound causes tensile strength loss owing to soaking. Knotted sutures have two-thirds the strength of unknotted sutures. The tensile strength of a suture does not need to exceed that of the tissue into which it is being placed. The rate at which tensile strength is lost should parallel the rate at which the sutured tissue gains tensile strength.

The knot is the weakest point of the suture. Knots function to bind two suture ends together. Knot security is all about friction, the more secure knots having the greatest friction. The basic component of a knot is the simple knot or throw. This is one revolution of one end of the suture around the other. Sutures are tied with four throws, starting with a simple throw or a surgeon's throw. The suture end is passed through a double loop with a surgeon's throw. Square knots (Fig. 2.3a) and surgeon's knots (Fig. 2.3c) generate the most friction and are the most secure. A square knot comprises two simple throws with the direction reversed on each throw. Even tension is maintained on each throw parallel to the plane of the knot. Granny knots (Fig. 2.3b) are less secure and are formed when the direction is not reversed on the second throw. Half-hitch knots (Fig. 2.3d), or sliding knots, are produced by placing tension on the long strand of a square knot in a direction perpendicular to the plane of the knot. These knots are less secure but are useful when placing a ligature in deep body cavities.

Knot security has recently been shown to be related to suture type, the number of throws, the type of

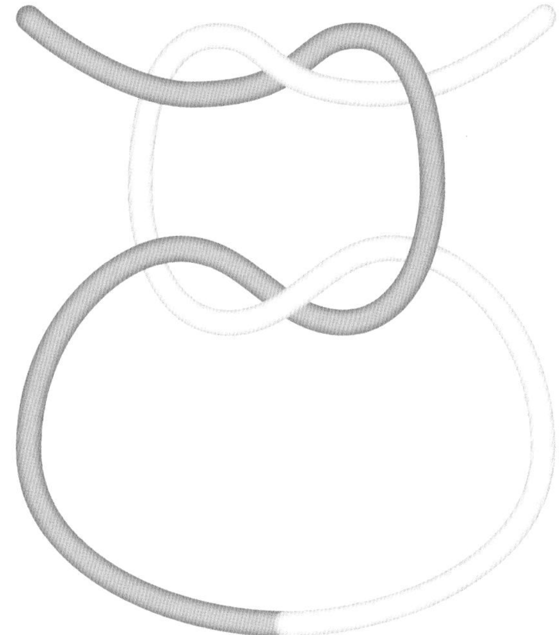

Fig. 2.3a Square knot.
Illustrator: Elaine Leggett

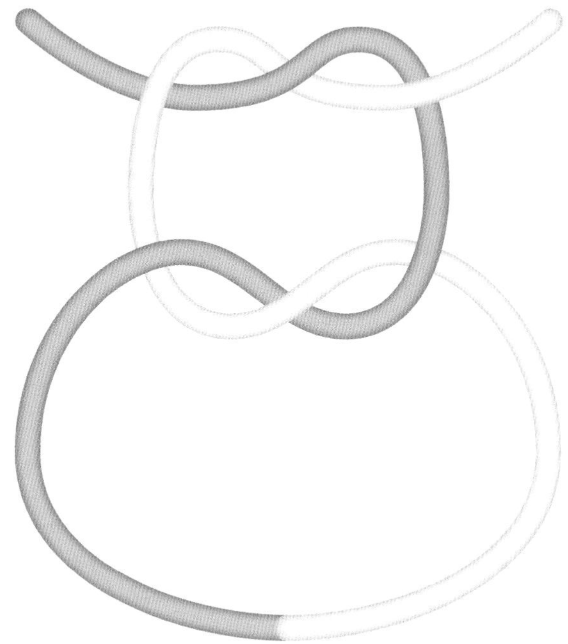

Fig. 2.3b Granny knot.
Illustrator: Elaine Leggett

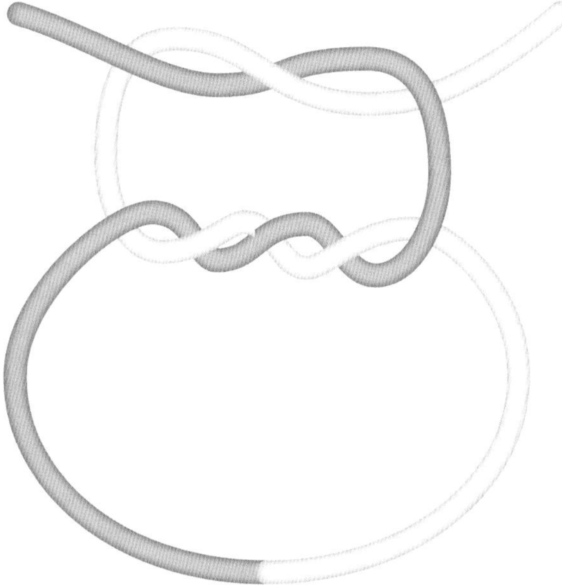

Fig. 2.3c Surgeon's knot.
Illustrator: Elaine Leggett

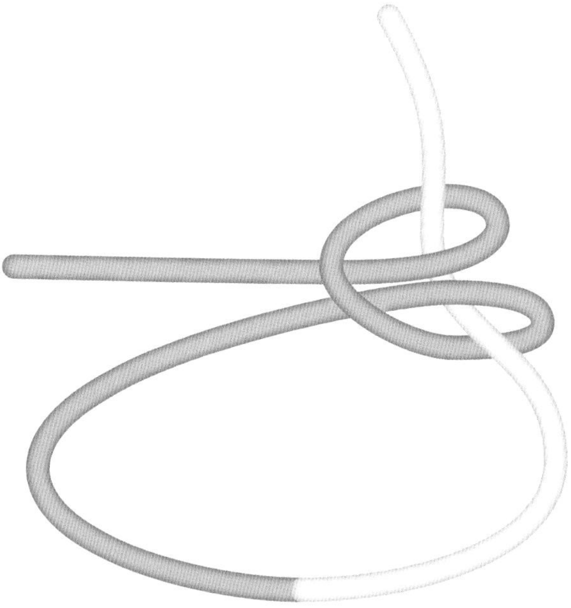

Fig. 2.3d Half-hitch knot.
Illustrator: Elaine Leggett

suture pattern and surgeon experience (Marturello et al., 2014). For most suture types, four throws provides adequate knot security and there was no advantage found to using a greater number of throws. In fact, for certain suture types, three throws were adequate. The synthetic non-absorbable suture materials had the poorest knot security. Knots ending a simple continuous suture pattern were less secure than those starting it or simple interrupted sutures. There was no difference in knot security between simple interrupted knots and knots starting simple continuous patterns. It has previously been suggested that additional throws are added to square knots at the beginning and end of simple continuous patterns (Rosin and Robinson, 1989).

Sutures have been developed with barbs to eliminate the problems associated with knots. Several studies have shown that barbed sutures provide equivalent tensile strength to normal sutures (Ehrhart et al., 2013; Kieves and Krebs, 2017; Templeton, 2015). One study showed that barbed sutures enabled faster skin closure (Law, 2017).

Plasticity allows the suture material to stretch and retain its new shape and length to accommodate tissue swelling. Elasticity allows the suture to return to its normal shape and length once the swelling has resolved, thus maintaining tissue apposition. Most sutures are elastic, with few being plastic. Memory is the ability of a suture to return to its original shape after deformation by tying. Sutures with high memory, such as monofilament sutures, can be stiff, difficult to handle and have poor knot security.

Suture handling is related to its pliability, i.e. how easily it can be bent. The coefficient of friction is a measure of slipperiness. Braided sutures have a high coefficient of friction and exert tissue drag. They are, however, easier to handle and have better knot security.

All sutures cause a degree of tissue inflammation. Natural suture materials are absorbed by proteolysis, which causes a significant tissue response. Synthetic suture materials are absorbed by hydrolysis, which causes minimal reaction. Braided sutures have high capillarity, which means they absorb and retain fluid and bacteria. This can result in greater tissue reactions and may promote infection. The volume of suture material in the wound has an effect on the tissue reaction. The surgeon should avoid using sutures of too large a diameter and tying bulky knots.

Recently, sutures have been coated with triclosan to provide antibacterial properties. Studies suggest this lowers the incidence of SSI.

Suture materials

Suture materials may be absorbable or non-absorbable, natural or synthetic, and braided or monofilament. Absorbable sutures lose their tensile strength within 60 days. These sutures are usually applied below the skin. Non-absorbable sutures are not degraded in living tissues and retain their tensile strength. They are used for skin closure and under the skin when a permanent suture is desired. Table 2.1 summarises the properties of the commonly used veterinary sutures.

Suture needles

Suture needles may be straight or curved. Straight needles are not used commonly, but occasionally may be used for placement of certain skin sutures. Curved needles are used more commonly as these are more suited to small or deep surgical fields. Swaged needles are supplied with suture in single-use sterile packs; these have the advantages of being sharp and causing less tissue drag. Non-swaged needles are almost obsolete. Taper needles have a fine point that penetrates and spreads tissue during needle passage. These maintain the small size of the needle hole and are best suited for use in visceral organs. Taper-cut needles have an oval body and

Table 2.1. Properties of commonly used sutures in veterinary practice.

Suture	Brand name	Configuration	Tensile strength	Absorption
Surgical gut	Catgut	Natural, absorbable	50% at 7–10 days, 0% at 10–21 days	Proteolysis, 70–90 days
Polyglactin 910	Vicryl	Synthetic, absorbable, braided but coated	60% at day 14, 8% at day 28	Hydrolysis by 60–90 days; 35 days for Vicryl Rapid
Lactomer	Polysorb	Synthetic, absorbable, braided but coated	80% at day 14, 30% at day 21	Hydrolysis by 56–70 days
Polydioxanone	PDS	Synthetic, absorbable, monofilament	74% at day 14, 58% at day 28, 41% at day 42	Hydrolysis by 180–210 days
Glycomer 631	Biosyn	Synthetic, absorbable, monofilament	75% at day 14, 40% at day 21	Hydrolysis by 90–110 days
Poliglecaprone 25	Monocryl	Synthetic, absorbable, monofilament	20–30% at day 14	Hydrolysis by 90–120 days
Polygytone 6211	Caprosyn	Synthetic, absorbable, monofilament	0% by 21 days	Hydrolysis by 56 days
Silk	Mersilk	Natural, non-absorbable, braided	Low	Degraded over 2 years
Monofilament nylon	Ethilon, Monosof	Synthetic, non-absorbable, monofilament	High	67% after 11 years
Polypropylene	Prolene, Surgipro	Synthetic, non-absorbable, monofilament	Moderate	None

reverse cutting point to allow greater ease of tissue penetration. Cutting needles have a triangular tip and are used for placing sutures in tougher tissue, such as skin. Conventional cutting needles have the cutting surface on the concave surface of the needle, whereas reverse-cutting needles have the cutting surface on the convex surface of the needle. Conventional cutting needles may result in a larger suture hole, which in turn may increase the risk of suture pull-through.

Suture patterns

Simple interrupted sutures provide secure closure and allow precise adjustments of tension along the wound. They are easy to apply but take longer to do than continuous suture patterns; they also use more suture material. Simple continuous suture patterns are quick and easy to perform and promote suture economy, but they don't allow precise adjustments of tension as do simple interrupted sutures. Excessive tension can lead to puckering and strangulation of the skin.

Subcutaneous tissues are best closed with an absorbable monofilament suture; an interrupted or continuous pattern can be used. Because polyglactin 910 is coated, it is perfectly suited for this purpose. Excess adipose tissue can be closed in two layers: the superficial layer can be used to close the dermis and pull the skin edges together. For continuous suture patterns, the recommended number of throws at the beginning and end of the suture depends on the suture type and size. Excessive throws should be avoided as the bulky knot can cause tissue reaction. Synthetic suture ends should be cut to 3–4 mm in length. When using needle-holders, they should not be applied to any portion of the suture within the knot.

Skin closure can be performed with intradermal or subcuticular sutures. A horizontal pattern incorporates the dermis only. A vertical pattern includes the dermis and subcutaneous tissues. Absorbable monofilament (or coated braided) sutures are used. Cutaneous sutures may be interrupted or continuous. A Ford interlocking pattern is easy to apply and provides extra security. Monofilament nylon or polypropylene is used. One study showed that subcuticular monofilament sutures had higher tissue reactivity initially than simple interrupted skin sutures, but ultimately achieved a better cosmetic result (Sylvestre et al., 2002).

Dog-ears are a minor cosmetic problem that resolves with time. If necessary, any of the following techniques can be used to remove these: apex cutaneous suture; removal of one or two triangles; extension of fusiform incision; removal of arrowhead-shaped piece of skin; and half-Z correction.

2.2.2 Tension-relieving techniques

Key points

- These techniques facilitate primary wound closure when there is mild to moderate skin tension.
- They are not suitable for the closure of large defects, where skin flaps or free skin grafts are more appropriate.
- The surgeon must have an understanding of tension lines and shear forces.
- Some of these techniques utilise the previously described visco-elastic properties of skin.

Surgical principles

Skin wounds should be closed primarily wherever possible. All wounds should be closed with minimal tension and should allow a return to function of the affected area with no morbidity (Stanley, 2012).

Atraumatic surgical technique should be employed when handling skin. Fine instruments should be used and skin edges and flaps should be handled with stay sutures or spay hooks. When harvesting flaps or grafts, donor and recipient beds should be protected with moistened swabs. Adequate amounts of skin should be clipped and prepped to prevent hair entering the surgical site. Excess skin can be temporarily brought into the surgical field with towel clamps. The patient should be positioned in such a way as to reduce tension at the wound site. This may involve the use of sandbags.

Wounds should never be closed by direct apposition if the tension is so great as to result in ischaemic necrosis and suture cut-out. Tension is determined by the pull of collagen and elastin in dermal and hypodermal tissues. Tension lines are well described in dogs, but there is large variation in elasticity of the skin between different parts of the body and between the same parts of the body in different breeds. Wounds should ideally be closed along tension lines and not perpendicular to them. Wounds in highly mobile areas are subject to shear forces; this necessitates a more robust closure than for a corresponding wound not subject to shear, and possibly immobilisation of the wound.

Techniques for relieving tension

Undermining

Separating the skin from its underlying tissue attachments frees up its full elastic potential. Undermining is performed by a combination of blunt and sharp dissection using Metzenbaum scissors. Care must be taken to preserve the deep dermal plexus; this is done by undermining deep to the panniculus muscle (or deep to the hypodermis if this is not present). The skin adjacent to the wound must be healthy to allow successful undermining.

Tension-relieving sutures

These sutures alleviate tension on the suture line by distributing it over a wider area. Strong subcutaneous sutures effectively do this, as well as closing dead space and providing tissue apposition. Stent sutures, far-near-near-far / far-far-near-near sutures and mattress sutures are commonly used in the skin. Horizontal mattress sutures may compromise blood supply to the wound edges; vertical mattress sutures tend to cause eversion of the skin edges and are best used as stent sutures.

Skin-stretching techniques

These methods utilise the skin's inherent properties of mechanical creep and stress relaxation. Pre-tensioning sutures are placed to influence an existing wound, whereas pre-suturing is placed prior to a planned excision. Commonly used techniques include loose placement of a simple continuous skin suture or continuous intradermal suture, which is then tightened on a daily basis, or plication of the skin with Lembert sutures. Commercially available kits with Velcro straps can be used.

Walking sutures

These are placed by undermining the wound edges and placing simple interrupted sutures between the dermis and underlying fascia. Sutures are placed at the furthest point from the wound edges and used to advance (walk) the skin edges to the centre of the wound. They distribute tension throughout the skin. If placed correctly, they result in temporary skin dimpling. Too many sutures can lead to vascular compromise and excess foreign material in the wound.

Relaxing incisions

Mesh expansion (multiple punctate relaxing incisions). The skin is undermined and 1 cm full-thickness incisions are made in a row parallel to the wound, 1 cm apart and 1 cm from the wound edge. Further staggered rows can be added as necessary. These small wounds further utilise the skin's elastic potential and heal by epithelialisation. Making the incisions too long or placing them too close together can lead to vascular compromise. Mesh expansion should not be used in skin flaps.

Simple relaxing incision. This is essentially a bipedicle advancement flap. An incision is made parallel to the long axis of the wound. The width is equal to the width of the wound, and the length:width ratio should not exceed 4:1. The skin is undermined and moved into the deficit. The relaxing incision can be closed or left to heal by second intention. This technique is useful for closing defects near an orifice or joint.

V–Y-plasty. This is used to close defects near structures that would be distorted by primary closure. A V-shaped incision is made with the point away from the wound. The skin is undermined and advanced to close the defect in the shape of a Y.

Z-plasty (Fig. 2.4). This makes additional skin available by changing the direction of tension. It is used for closing a cicatrix or any nearby wound. A Z-shaped incision is made with the central limb perpendicular to the wound. Two triangular flaps are created from the common central limb. These triangular flaps are then undermined and transposed. Tension is relieved along the central limb (perpendicular) and increased in the skin parallel to the wound. There must be sufficient lax skin parallel to the wound for this technique to be successful. The central limb must be at least 3 cm from the wound, all limbs should be of equal length and the angle between the central limb and arms should be 60°. For correcting a cicatrix, the central limb is along the length of the scar.

M-plasty. This is used at the end of fusiform incisions where the skin availability may be limited. It is most commonly used for bilateral mastectomy and areas where closure is compromised by an orifice. The final suture line is Y-shaped.

Geometric wound closure

Closing *crescent-shaped defects* in a straight line can result in dog-ears if there is a discrepancy between the length of each edge of the wound. If the difference is less than 20%, the wound edges can be fudged together by suturing midpoints. Alternatively, the wound can be closed from both ends or from the centre. The resulting dog-ears can be excised. A half bow-tie technique can be used for wound edge discrepancies greater than 20%.

Triangular defects. These are closed as a Y, starting from each corner of the triangle and working towards the centre. The central portion of the Y is closed with a half-buried mattress suture.

Rectangular and square defects. These are closed from each corner, resulting in an X-shaped wound. Half-buried mattress sutures are used at the junction of suture lines. Alternatively, these defects can be closed with paired rotational flaps.

Circular defects. These can be closed in a variety of ways:

- linear closure with excision of dog-ears
- conversion to a fusiform shape
- division into three arcs with a 3-point closure
- combined V-plasty.
- O- to S-plasty.

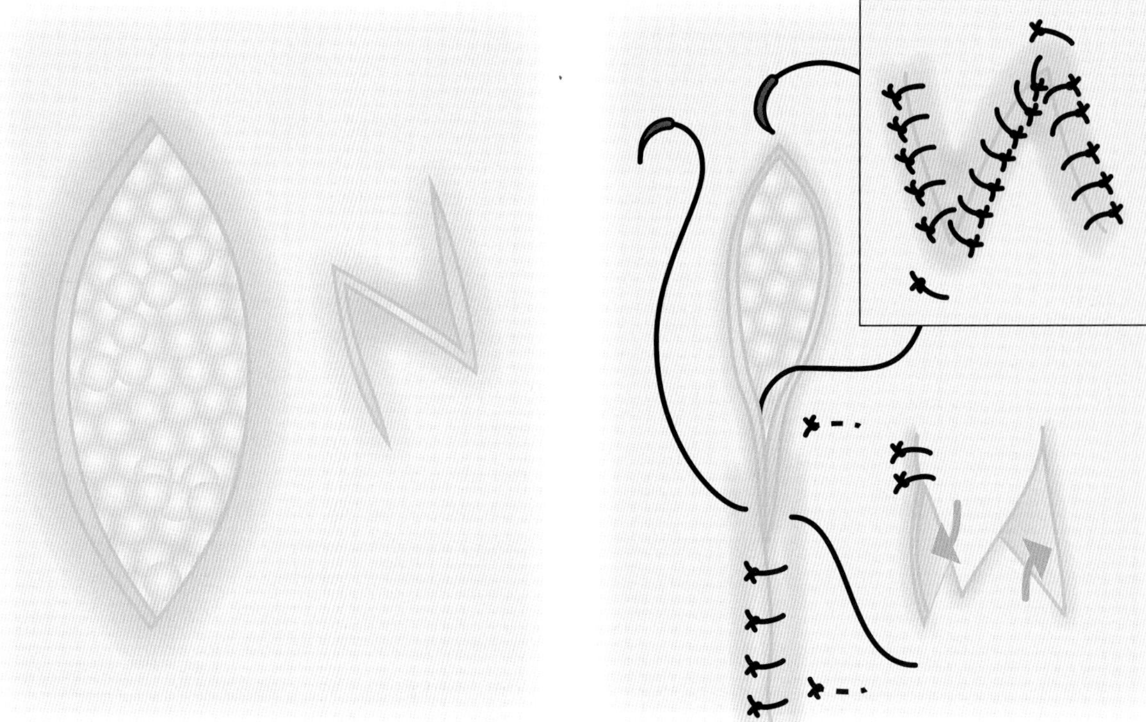

Fig. 2.4 Z-plasty. To reduce tension in direction x (direction x = 90 degrees to skin incision), a skin incision is made perpendicular to the wound. Two skin incisions are made at 60° to the first incision to create two equilateral triangles. These triangles of skin are undermined and transposed to give an increase in length in the direction of x, thus relieving tension. *Illustrator: Elaine Leggett*

2.2.3 Random or subdermal plexus flaps

Key points

- The inherent elasticity of canine and feline skin lends itself well to the creation of skin flaps that can be mobilised to close larger skin defects.
- Random flaps are commonly used in veterinary patients.
- The deep dermal plexus must be preserved to ensure viability of the flap.
- Local flaps (such as advancement, rotation and transposition flaps) are most commonly used, with distant flaps being less commonly employed.
- Complications are not uncommon but are often amenable to relatively conservative management.
- The incidence of complications can be reduced by understanding the blood supply to the skin and by meticulous surgical technique.

Subdermal plexus flaps are full-thickness tongues of skin that are detached from the skin adjacent to the wound along three of four quadrants and then advanced or rotated into the wound (Hunt, 2012). In this way, an area of skin with abundant elasticity (donor site) is moved into an area where there is insufficient skin for closure (wound bed or recipient site). Successful use of skin flaps requires meticulous surgical technique, preservation of the flap's blood supply and a tension-free closure (Pavletic, 2010). Fine instruments should be used. Dissection should be sharp whenever possible. Skin flaps should be manipulated with stay sutures to prevent crushing injury to their edges. Moist swabs should be used to prevent desiccation of the donor and recipient sites during flap creation and closure.

The blood supply to random flaps is via the deep dermal (subdermal) plexus. In order to preserve this blood supply, flaps must be undermined deep to the panniculus muscle (Fig. 2.5). In areas of the body where this isn't present, flaps must be undermined as close as possible to the underlying fascia. If the skin is intimately associated with the deeper tissue, this too may need to be incorporated into the flap. Flap survival has been shown to be enhanced by staged development. This is referred to as the delay phenomenon. The use of axial-pattern flaps has rendered the delay phenomenon less useful clinically.

There are no strict guidelines in regard to safe flap dimensions, only general recommendations. Flaps should be large enough to cover the recipient site while allowing the donor site to be closed. Flaps should have a base slightly wider than the width of the flap: if the base is too narrow the flap's blood supply might be

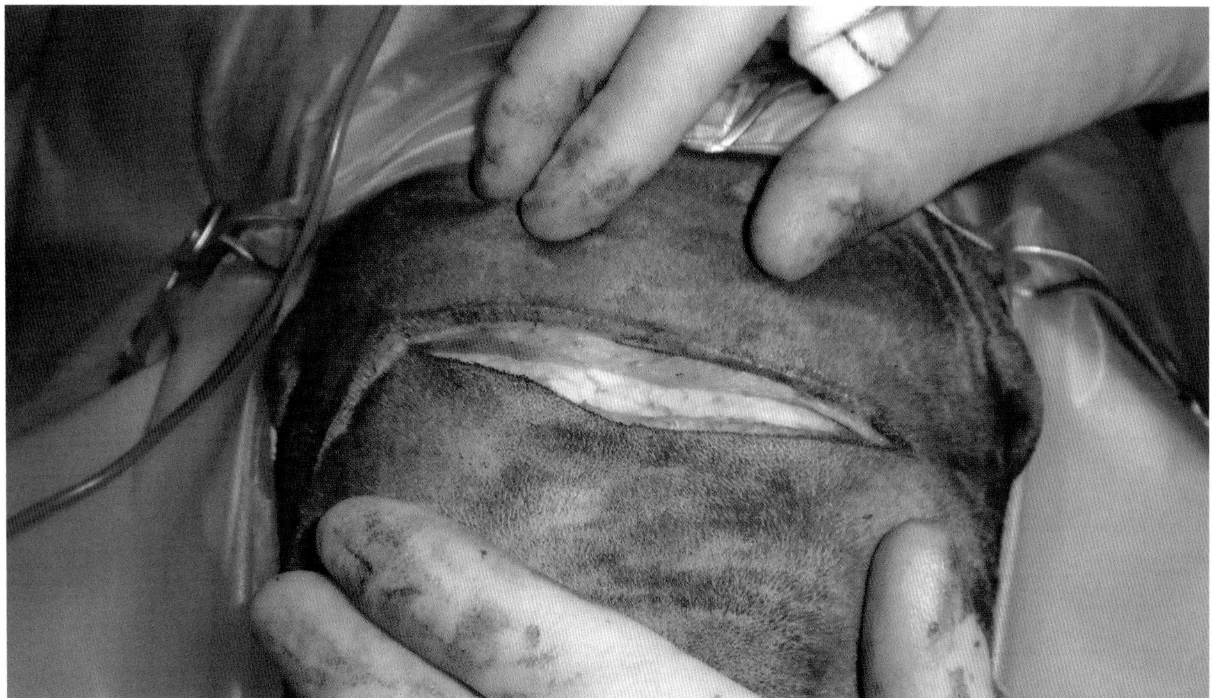

Fig. 2.5 The panniculus muscle can be seen in the hypodermis. Skin flaps must be undermined deep to this muscle in order to preserve the deep dermal plexus.

compromised. There are no guidelines available for the specific length:width ratio possible. The longer the flap, the greater the risk of vascular compromise to the flap's extremities.

Flaps should be closed in two or three layers. It is essential that there is no tension on the flap. Care must be taken when using flaps around the limbs, first to ensure that the flap will not be exposed to excessive shearing forces, and second to ensure that movement of the limb doesn't distort the base of the flap with resulting vascular compromise. Drains and light compression bandages can be placed to counteract dead space and prevent fluid accumulation.

Local flaps are developed adjacent to the recipient bed. These include advancement flaps, rotational flaps, transposition and interpolation flaps, and skin-fold flaps. These are the most commonly used skin flaps in practice. Distant flaps are created using skin that is distant to the recipient bed. The skin is then transferred either directly to the recipient site (hinge flaps or pouch flaps; Fig. 2.6a,b) or indirectly (tubed flaps). These are used for closure of extremity wounds.

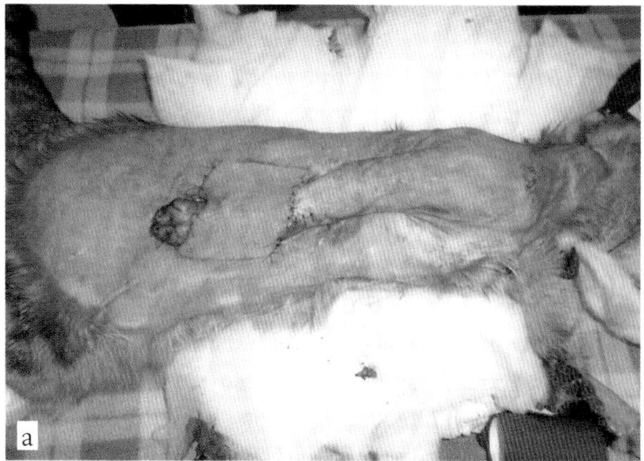

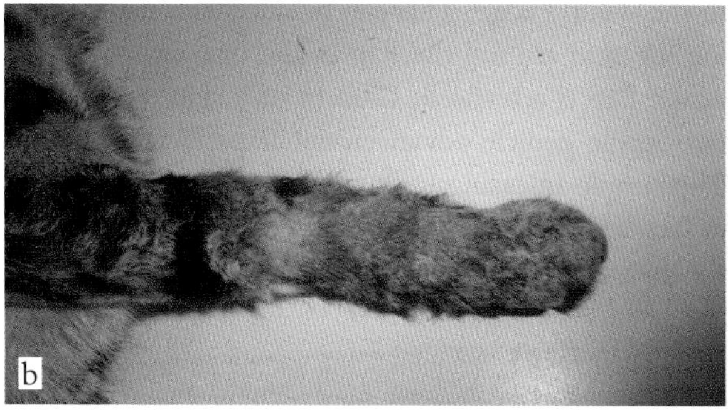

Fig. 2.6a,b Distant direct flap in a cat with a degloving injury to its paw and subsequent pancarpal arthrodesis. Paired full-thickness incisions are made in the cat's flank to create a pouch of skin (effectively a bipedicle flap). The paw is transferred to the pouch, which is sutured to the edges of the wound. A body dressing was used to immobilise the limb and the patient was hospitalised. After 10 days, the flap was divided in quarters every 2–3 days and sutured to the wound edges. The functional and cosmetic outcome was excellent. This is an excellent alternative to a free skin graft in compliant, smaller patients.

Advancement flaps

Two skin incisions are made perpendicular to the wound leaving a single base (single pedicle advancement flap; Figs. 2.7, 2.8a,b). The incisions should diverge to leave a slightly wider base. The length of the flap is generally equal to that of the wound, but should be made longer if necessary to ensure a tension-free

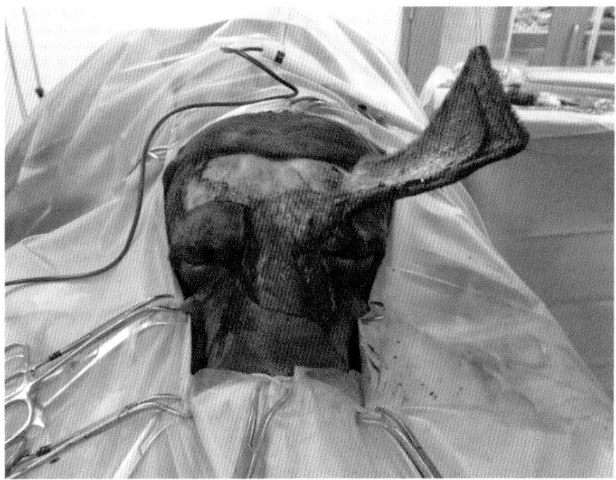

Fig. 2.11a Transposition flap used to close a facial deficit following excision of a mast cell tumour. This flap utilised the abundant elastic skin perpendicular to the wound.

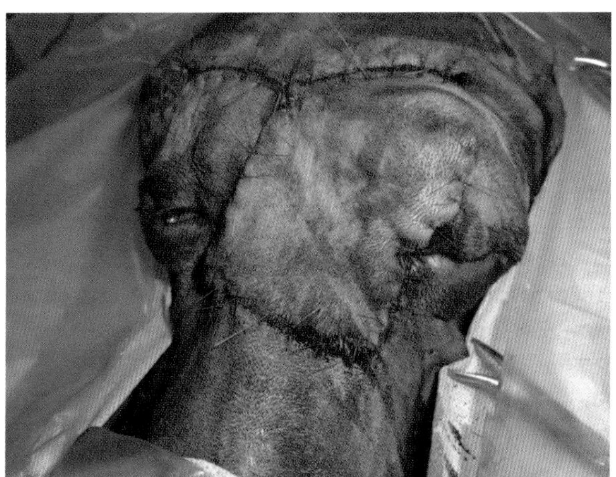

Fig. 2.11b The donor site was closed primarily. Transposition flaps are extremely useful for closing skin defects on the head and face.

durable flaps, and are used to close brachial, elbow, axillary, sternal, inguinal, thigh and stifle defects.

Complications of subdermal plexus flaps

Seroma formation is more likely to occur when flaps are created on the lateral flank or thorax. The incidence can be reduced by careful surgical technique, the use of drains and bandages and exercise restriction after surgery. Seromas should be surgically drained to allow adherence of the flap to the recipient site.

Flap dehiscence may be due to poor surgical technique, excessive tension or flap necrosis (Figs. 2.13, 2.14). Flaps should be kept moist and handled with stay sutures or skin hooks. Tension is usually due to failure to create an adequately sized flap. Seroma formation or excessive shear forces can prevent flap adherence to the recipient site.

Flap necrosis occurs due to inadequate perfusion. This may be due to creation of too narrow a pedicle, damage to the subdermal plexus during flap creation, thrombosis of the subdermal plexus, pressure due to bandages, self-trauma or excessive flap rotation. Necrotic tissue should be debrided to allow more rapid second-intention healing.

Skin defects due to flap dehiscence or necrosis are often best managed as open wounds for a short period of time. Small defects can be left to heal by second intention, while larger defects may be amenable to primary closure owing to the elasticity of the donor skin that has been brought into the wound and the visco-elastic

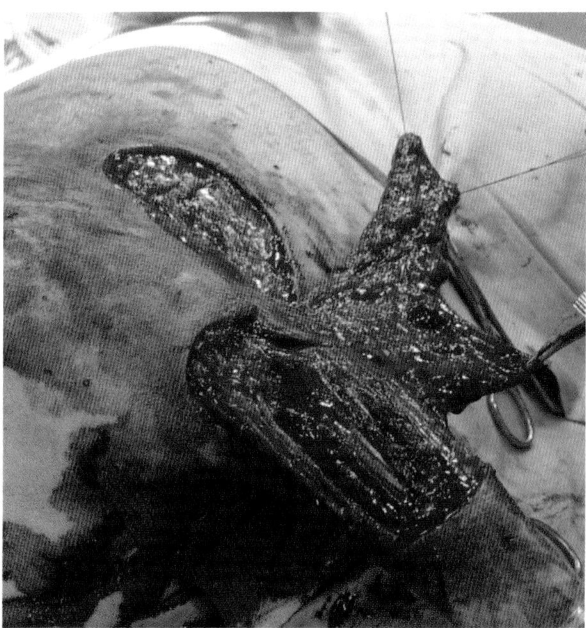

Fig. 2.12a Elbow skin fold flap used to close an antebrachial wound following resection of a soft tissue sarcoma. The flap retains its attachment to the medial brachium.

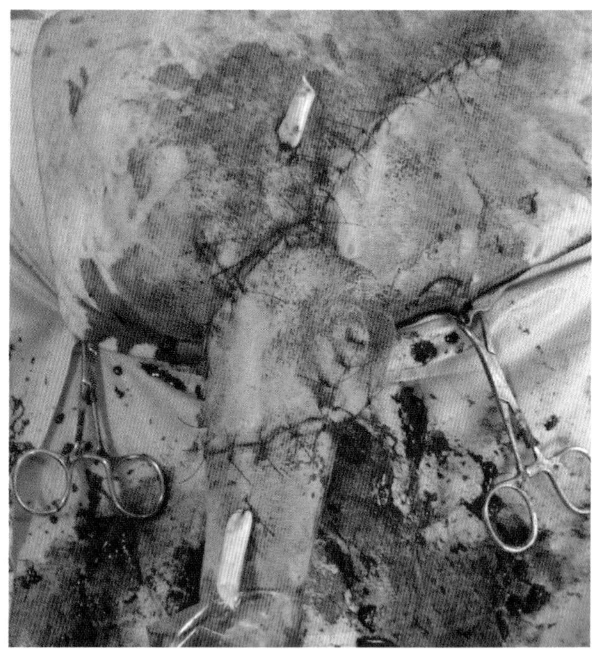

Fig. 2.12b Note the U-shaped appearance of this flap.

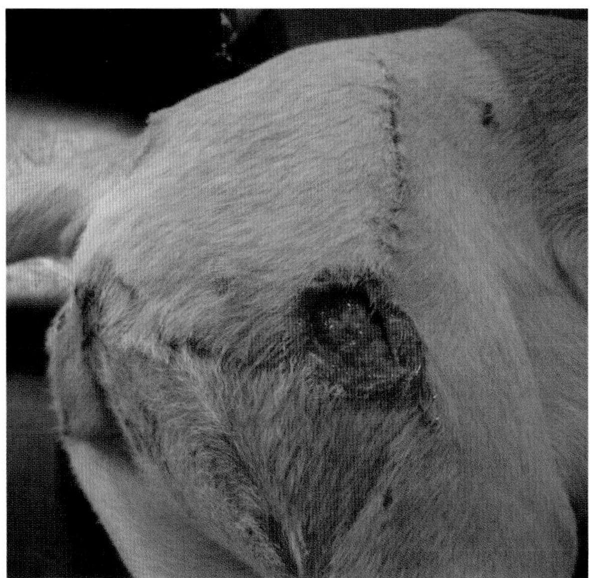

Fig. 2.13 Wound dehiscence following closure with a transposition flap. Dehiscence occurred owing to tip necrosis. This smaller wound eventually healed by second intention.

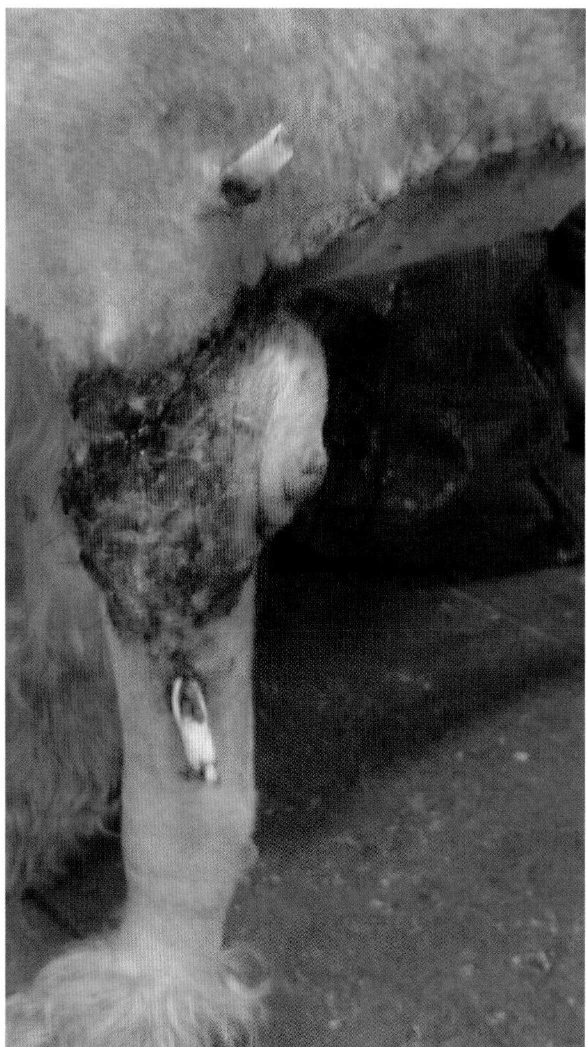

Fig. 2.14 Epidermal necrosis of an elbow skin fold flap. After debridement, it was evident that the dermis was viable. This flap eventually healed and re-epithelialised.

properties of the adjacent skin (creep-and-stress relaxation). Larger defects may require closure with a second skin flap.

2.2.4 Axial-pattern flaps

Key points

- The blood supply to these flaps is based on a direct cutaneous artery and vein, rather than just the subdermal plexus (Wardlaw and Lanz, 2012).
- Axial-pattern flaps have greater survivability than random flaps, and larger areas of skin can be elevated and mobilised.
- The location and anatomical landmarks of the commonly used axial-pattern flaps are described in this and other veterinary texts, and these can be referred to when a large skin defect is encountered.

These flaps incorporate a direct cutaneous artery and vein in their pedicle. This allows for creation of a larger flap with more consistent survival. These flaps can be rotated up to 180°. Peninsular flaps have intact skin at their base, while island flaps do not. These flaps can be placed directly over bone, tendons and ligaments (unlike free skin grafts). Long flaps do not require a two-stage procedure to improve circulation (by the delay phenomenon) and the overall survival rate of axial-pattern flaps is high. Mean survival of these flaps is estimated to be 50% greater than that for subdermal plexus flaps. Axial-pattern flaps based on the thoracodorsal artery and caudal superficial epigastric artery are most commonly described. Tip necrosis is a common complication of these flaps, but overall survival rates are high (Aper and Smeak, 2003, 2005). Cats have a lower density of tertiary and higher vessels than dogs, which means their cutaneous perfusion is lower and skin wound healing is slower than in dogs. A recent retrospective study of axial-pattern flaps in 73 cases found a complication rate of 89% (Field et al., 2015). Complications included dehiscence, swelling, necrosis, infection, discharge and seroma. In spite of this very high complication rate, 93% of patients were found to have a successful outcome although an additional surgical procedure was required in one-third of cases.

Wide margins of skin need to be clipped and aseptically prepared. Ideally, both the donor site and recipient site should be within the surgical field. The surgical technique principles for harvesting these flaps are the same as those for subdermal plexus flaps. It is critical that the direct cutaneous artery and vein supplying the flap are identified and preserved. This requires a full appreciation of regional anatomy and careful dissection when approaching the region of the blood vessels.

Once created, the flap can be tacked into position in the recipient bed with simple interrupted subcutaneous sutures. The subcutaneous tissues and skin are then closed. Interrupted suture patterns may be preferable to continuous suture patterns. Walking sutures should not be used as these may compromise the flap's blood supply. Drains are almost always used to manage dead space and prevent seroma formation. Closed-suction drains are usually preferred to Penrose drains.

Guidelines for axial-pattern flap development

Caudal auricular artery

- Vessel originates in a depression between the base of the vertical ear canal and the wing of the atlas.
- Flap is centred over the wing of the atlas and the width is one-third of the lateral cervical area.
- Flap may extend to the spine of the scapula.
- Useful for facial and pinnal defects.

Cervical cutaneous branch of omocervical artery

- Vessel originates in the region of the superficial cervical lymph node in the cranial shoulder depression.
- Caudal incision along the spine of the scapula.
- Cranial incision is the same distance from the cranial edge of the scapula (cranial shoulder depression) as that of the scapular spine.
- Flap may extend to the contralateral shoulder joint.
- Useful for head, neck, shoulder and axillary defects.

Thoracodorsal artery (Figs. 2.15a,b and 2.16a,b)

- Vessel originates at the caudal shoulder depression parallel to the dorsal point of the acromion
- Cranial incision along the spine of the scapula; the caudal incision is the same distance from the caudal edge of the scapula (caudal shoulder depression) as that of the scapular spine.
- Flap may extend to the contralateral shoulder joint.
- Useful for thoracic, shoulder, forelimb and axillary defects.

Superficial brachial artery

- Vessel originates at the flexor surface of the elbow.
- Cranial and caudal incisions run parallel to the humerus centred on the anterior third of the flexor surface of the elbow.
- Flap may extend to the greater tubercle.
- Useful for antebrachial and elbow defects.

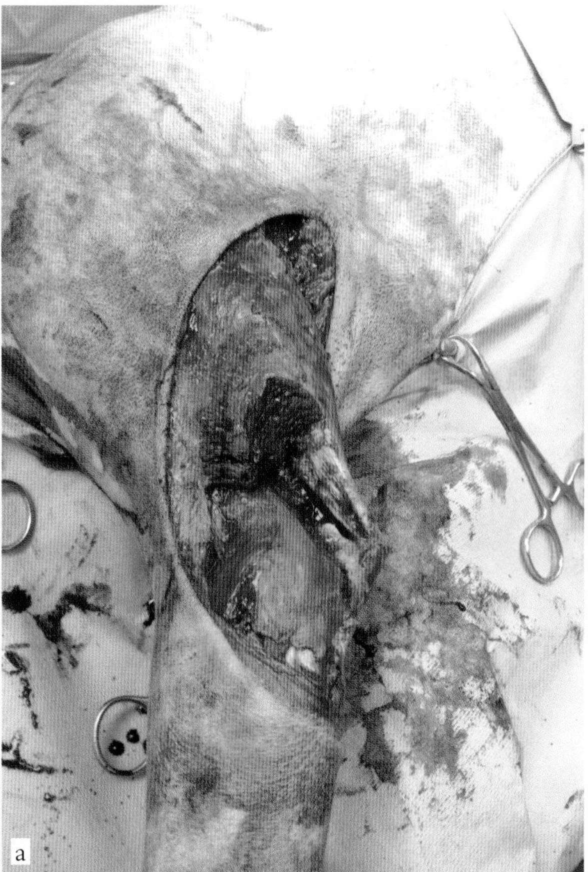

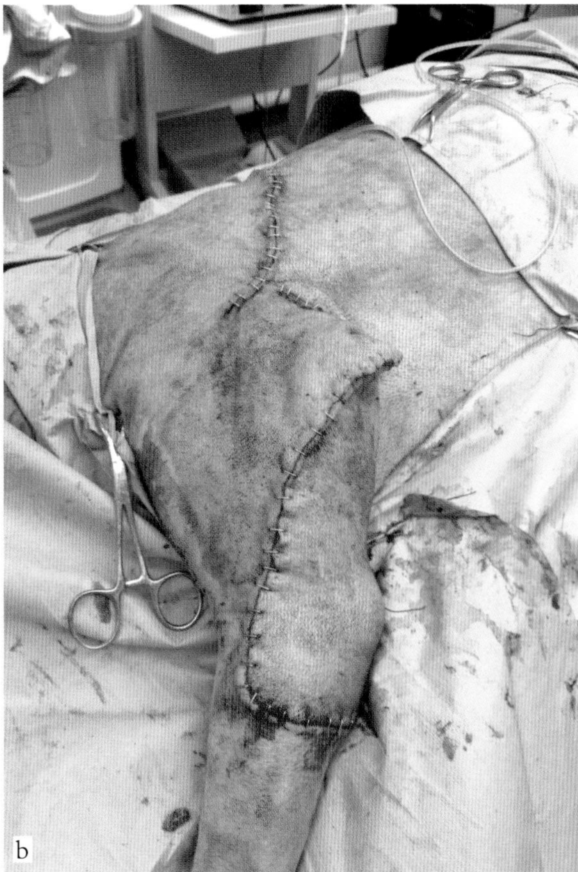

Fig. 2.15a,b Thoracodorsal axial-pattern flap used to close an extensive defect over the elbow following resection of a soft tissue sarcoma.

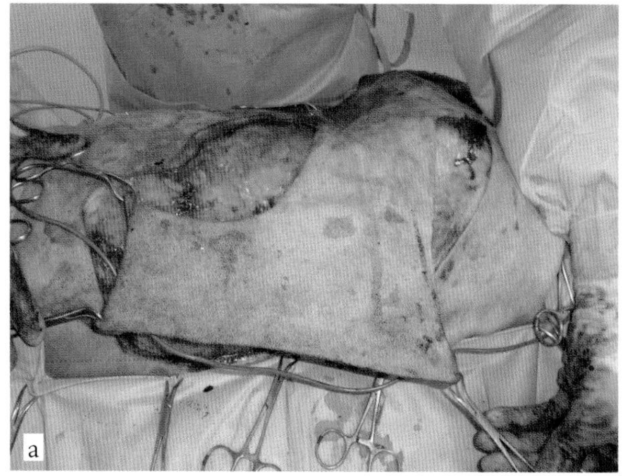

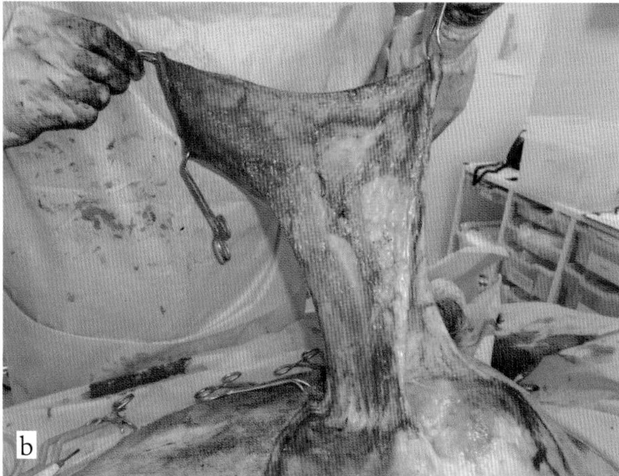

Fig. 2.16a,b The thoracodorsal axial-pattern flap can be elevated in a hockey-stick configuration to increase the quantity of skin available.

Cranial epigastric artery

- Vessel originates from the hypogastric region.
- Medial incision is along the abdominal midline.
- Lateral incision is the same distance from the mammary teats as the medial incision.
- Flap may extend to the fourth mammary teat.
- Useful for sternal defects.

Caudal superficial epigastric artery (Fig. 2.17)

- Vessel originates from external inguinal ring.
- Medial incision is along the abdominal midline (the base of the prepuce must be included in the male dog).
- Lateral incision is the same distance from the mammary teats as the medial incision.
- Flap may extend to the second mammary teat.
- Useful for flank, thigh, stifle, perineal and preputial defects.

Deep circumflex iliac artery (dorsal branch)

- Vessel originates cranioventral to the wing of the ilium.
- Caudal incision is halfway between the cranial edge of the wing of the ilium and the greater trochanter.
- Cranial incision is parallel to the caudal incision, the same distance from the cranial edge of the wing of the ilium.
- Flap may extend dorsal to the contralateral flank fold.

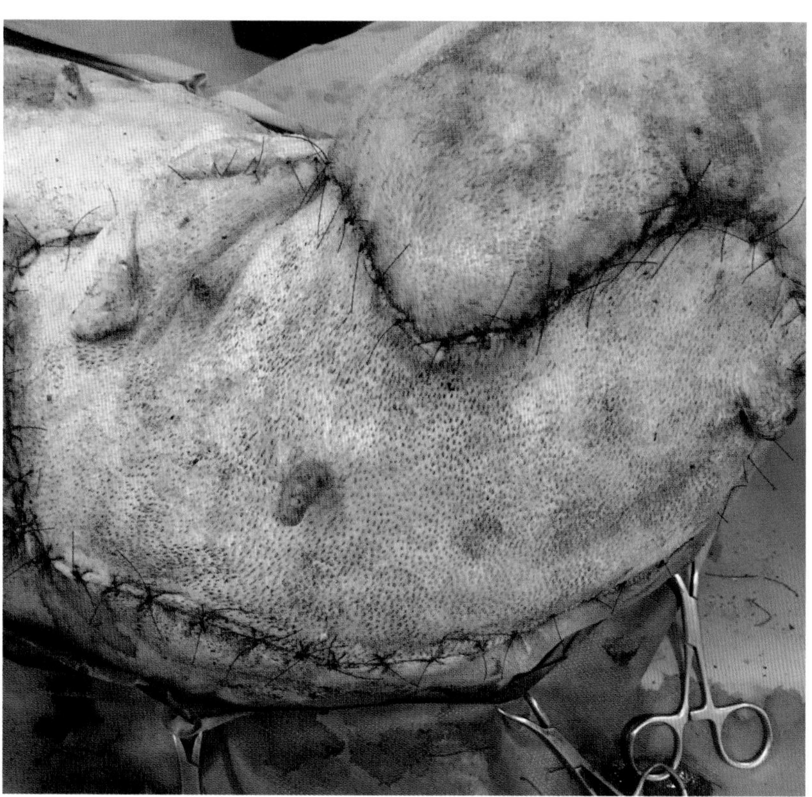

Fig. 2.17 Caudal superficial epigastric flap used to close a large thigh defect. Note the use of mesh expansion in the adjacent skin to reduce tension.

- Useful for thoracic, lateral abdominal wall, flank, thigh and greater trochanter defects.

Deep circumflex iliac artery (ventral branch)

- Vessel originates cranioventral to the wing of the ilium.
- Caudal incision starts halfway between the cranial edge of the wing of the ilium and the greater trochanter, and extends distally anterior to the cranial border of the femur.
- Cranial incision is parallel to the caudal incision, the same distance from the cranial edge of the wing of the ilium.
- Flap may extend proximal to the patella.
- Useful for lateral abdominal wall, pelvic and sacral (as an island flap) defects.

Genicular artery

- Vessel originates over the medial stifle joint, the base of the flap extending 1 cm above the patella to 1.5 cm below the tibial tuberosity.
- Cranial and caudal incisions extend caudodorsally parallel to the femur.
- Flap may extend to the base of the greater trochanter.
- Useful for lower limb defects between the stifle and tarsus.

Reverse saphenous conduit flap (Fig. 2.18a,b)

- Flap incorporates branches of the saphenous artery and medial saphenous vein, which supply the overlying skin by direct cutaneous branches.
- Division of the vascular connections to the femoral artery and vein proximally allows reverse flow from cranial branches of the saphenous artery and perforating metatarsal artery, and cranial branches of the medial and lateral saphenous veins distally.
- Proximal incision is located at the central third of the medial thigh at the level of the patella.
- Incisions extend distally 0.5–1 cm cranial and caudal to the saphenous vessels.
- The peroneal artery and vein may need to be divided.
- Base of the flap is at the level of the tarsus.
- Useful for metatarsal defects.

Lateral caudal arteries

- Vessels located lateral and ventral to transverse processes.
- Dorsal or ventral skin incision with dissection along deep caudal fascia.

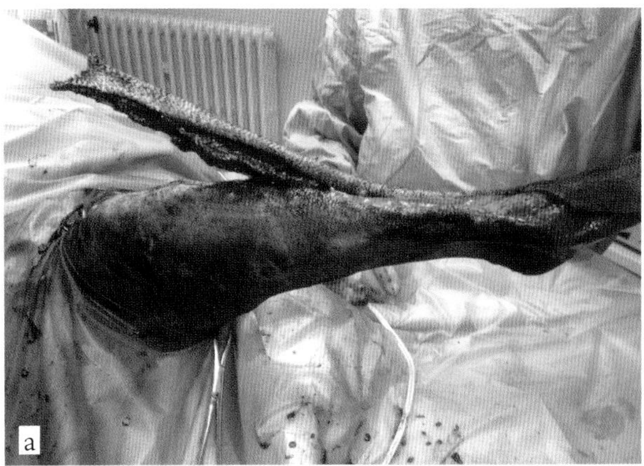

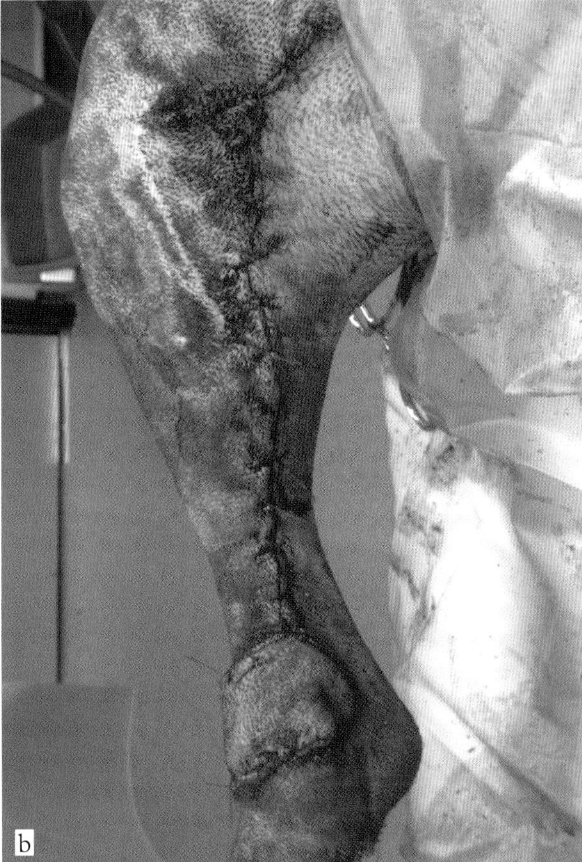

Fig. 2.18a,b Reverse saphenous conduit flap used to close a wound over the plantar tarsus/metatarsus. The flap is connected to the wound by a short bridging incision. This flap is an alternative to free skin grafts for the closure of wounds distal to the tarsus.

- Amputation of tail at 3rd to 4th intervertebral space, preserving skin.
- Useful for perineal and caudodorsal trunk defects.

2.2.5 *Muscle and omental flaps*

Key points

- The availability of axial-pattern flaps renders myocutaneous flaps less useful in veterinary patients.

- Muscle flaps are useful for reconstruction of body wall defects.
- The commonly used muscle flaps and their vascular supply are described.
- The benefits of omentum in wound healing are reviewed.

Myocutaneous flaps are those in which skeletal muscle and the overlying skin are elevated simultaneously (Wardlaw and Lanz, 2012). These are used in humans, who lack direct cutaneous arteries. The musculocutaneous arteries exiting the muscle surface supply the overlying skin. Myocutaneous flaps are less useful in dogs and cats, which have an abundance of loose skin for random flaps and direct cutaneous arteries that can be incorporated into axial-pattern flaps.

Muscle flaps are more clinically useful. These are typically used for reconstruction of body wall defects following trauma or oncological resections, and for hernia repairs. Muscle flaps are classified according to their vascular supply:

- Type I:
  - There is one dominant vascular pedicle.
  - Type I muscles can be elevated and pivoted on this pedicle.
- Type II:
  - There is one dominant vascular pedicle near the origin or insertion, with a minor pedicle supplying the muscle belly.
  - Type II muscles are likely to survive following ligation of the minor pedicle, providing the major pedicle is intact.
- Type III:
  - There are two dominant pedicles supplying approximately half the muscle belly.
  - Ligation of one vascular pedicle may or may not compromise the part of the muscle belly it supplies.
- Type IV:
  - Smaller segmental vascular pedicles supply the muscle between its origin and insertion.
  - Survival is inconsistent following muscle elevation.
- Type V:
  - There is one dominant vascular pedicle at the muscle insertion, with segmental pedicles entering near its origin.
  - The muscle will survive providing its dominant pedicle is intact.
  - Survival based on the segmental pedicles would be less consistent.

A number of muscle flaps are used clinically, including the latissimus dorsi, external abdominal oblique, cranial and caudal sartorius, temporalis, flexor carpi ulnaris, semitendinosus and transverse abdominis.

Latissimus dorsi

- This is a type V muscle. The thoracodorsal and lateral thoracic arteries supply the dorsal and ventral portions of the muscle. There are segmental branches to the dorsal part of the muscle from the intercostal arteries.
- The origin of the muscle is the superficial leaf of the lumbodorsal fascia, and the insertion is an aponeurosis medially on the triceps muscle.
- The ventral border of the muscle is identified and elevated from the thoracic wall. Segmental branches of the intercostal arteries are ligated. The muscle is separated from its terminal attachments on the terminal ribs and its origin on the superficial leaf of the lumbodorsal fascia is incised.
- This muscle is most commonly used to close thoracic wall defects.

External abdominal oblique

- The cranial branch of the cranial abdominal artery supplies this muscle, and is accompanied by the cranial hypogastric nerve and a satellite vein.
- The costal component of the muscle originates segmentally from ribs 4–5 to rib 13.
- The lumbar component of the muscle originates in the thoracolumbar fascia along the iliocostalis muscle.
- The aponeurosis is ventral and caudal, contributing to the external rectus fascia, the external inguinal ring and the prepubic tendon.
- This muscle is approached via a paracostal incision 5 cm caudal to rib 13.
- The caudal and ventral fascial edges are incised, leaving a 1 cm margin attached to the muscle. The lumbar component is undermined and the neurovascular pedicle, which runs caudal to rib 13, is identified and preserved. The dorsal lumbar attachments are severed to the level of rib 13.
- This muscle is most commonly used for ventral abdominal wall and caudal thoracic wall defects.

The use of the omentum to augment wound healing is well established. Its extensive vascular and lymphatic supply gives it angiogenic, immunogenic and adhesive properties that can restore blood supply, improve drainage and control infection. The omentum is subdivided into the greater and lesser omentum. The greater omentum arises from the greater curvature of the stomach and extends to the level of the urinary bladder. It is a double peritoneal sheet that folds back on itself. Between these ventral and dorsal leaves is a pocket called the omental bursa or lesser peritoneal cavity. There is a single opening to the omental bursa, the epiploic foramen, which is bordered ventrally by the portal vein and dorsally by the caudal vena cava. The splenic portion of the greater omentum is often referred to as the gastrosplenic ligament. The veil portion of the greater omentum contains the left lobe of the pancreas.

The omentum can be accessed through either a midline coeliotomy or a left paracostal abdominal approach. Most intra-abdominal and abdominal wall defects can be closed without lengthening the omentum. Stage 1: lengthening of the omentum can be performed by incising the dorsal leaf at its attachment to the pancreas. This doubles the length of the omentum and enables its use for thoracic wall defects. Stage 2: lengthening requires an inverted-L incision to be created in the left side of the omentum caudal to the gastrosplenic ligament. This incision extends two-thirds of the width and two-thirds of the length of the omental sheet. Omental vessels are ligated and there is a risk of vascular compromise. When tunnelling the omentum, care must be taken not to twist, tear or compress it.

2.2.6 Free skin grafts

Key points

- Free skin grafts comprise only dermis and epidermis and ultimately derive their vascular supply from the recipient site wound bed.
- Successful engraftment or 'take' requires the graft to be immobilised for around 2 weeks with bandages.
- Dressing management is intensive, and technical errors can contribute to graft failure.
- The ready availability of skin flaps in veterinary patients tends to limit the use of free skin grafts to distal extremity wounds.
- Full-thickness skin grafts are easily harvested, are most durable and have the best survival rates.

Introduction

A skin graft is a segment of epidermis and dermis removed from the body and transferred to a recipient site (Bohling, 2012). Survival depends on re-establishment of a vascular supply through engraftment or 'take'. In cats and dogs, skin grafts are mainly used for extremity wounds.

Graft failure is most commonly due to separation of the graft from its bed owing to fluid accumulation, infection or movement. Incorrect surgical technique in harvesting the graft and incorrect post-surgical management, particularly in respect to bandaging, contribute to graft failure.

Grafts require vascular ingrowth, so must be placed on either a fresh surgical wound or healthy granulation tissue. Stratified squamous epithelial surfaces, irradiated tissues, avascular fat, chronic granulation tissue, and bone, cartilage, tendon or nerve denuded of overlying granulation tissue are all unsuitable surfaces. Several studies have shown that grafts will take when placed directly onto surgical wounds containing bones and tendons, without having to wait for a bed of granulation tissue to form (Tong and Simpson, 2012). This makes skin grafts ideal for use on extremity wounds following procedures such as tumour resection.

Engraftment

Successful graft take requires two separate but interrelated processes to occur: adherence and nutrition. Adherence is established by a network of fibrin strands. During phase I, fibrin forms links between collagen and elastin on the graft and recipient bed. These fibres polymerise, resulting in gain in strength. This is greatest within the first 8 hours. Phase II begins after 72 hours. The fibrinous network is invaded by fibroblasts, leukocytes and phagocytes and is converted to a fibrous adhesion. A fibrous union is present by day 10. Collagen maturation is responsible for graft contraction.

Nutrition of the graft occurs initially by a process known as *plasmatic imbibition*. Serum, erythrocytes and neutrophils leak from recipient vessels and accumulate under the graft. Graft vessels dilate and pull fibrinogen-free, serum-like fluid and cells into the graft by capillary action. This process keeps the graft vessels dilated and nourishes the graft. Haemoglobin and its breakdown products give the graft a purple or cyanotic appearance. Diffusion of fluid into the interstitial space causes oedema.

The next stage of nutrition is the anastomosis of cut graft vessels and recipient vessels, a process known as *inosculation*. This is commonly seen between 48 and 72 hours. The fibrin network provides a scaffold for vascular ingrowth. Anastomoses and capillary blood flow have an inhibitory effect on further vascular proliferation. Blood flow continues to increase and is normal by day 5 or 6.

Vascular ingrowth of capillaries from the recipient bed into the dermis or pre-existing graft vessels occurs at a daily rate of 0.5 mm. Graft vessels not involved in inosculation or ingrowth degenerate. Maturation of vessels begins within 48 hours.

Grafts are initially pale. During the first 48 hours they are purple and oedematous. As inosculation begins and inflow exceeds outflow, the graft may appear congested; this gives way to a lighter hue by 72–96 hours. The graft is red to pink by days 7–8 if survival is complete. A more normal skin colour is seen by day 14.

Types of graft

Grafts are classified according to either the depth of skin harvested or the extent of wound coverage. Full-thickness grafts comprise the epidermis and the whole of the dermis. Partial-thickness grafts comprise the epidermis and part of the dermis; full-thickness grafts are the most commonly used grafts – these are easy to harvest and don't require special instrumentation. Many texts describe a 90–100% take, and these grafts provide the best durability and hair regrowth (and consequently the best cosmetic appearance). A recent study found that these grafts had a higher success rate in cats than in dogs, and that skin grafts applied to the antebrachium carried a poorer prognosis (Riggs et al., 2014). Partial-thickness grafts are used when donor skin is at a premium. They require a special instrument called a dermatome to harvest them. They are more fragile, less durable and have sparse hair regrowth. The donor site heals by epithelialisation. Sheet grafts are most commonly used and provide coverage of the entire wound. Pinch, punch, stamp and strip grafts provide partial coverage. These are less commonly used in veterinary practice.

Full-thickness skin grafts

The ideal donor site should have durable skin of appropriate thickness and have a hair colour and density similar to that of the recipient site. The donor site should have easily mobilised skin to allow for an easy and cosmetic closure. The flank is an ideal donor site. A swab can be used as a template of the wound. An increase of 0.5–1 cm should be added to the dimensions to allow for

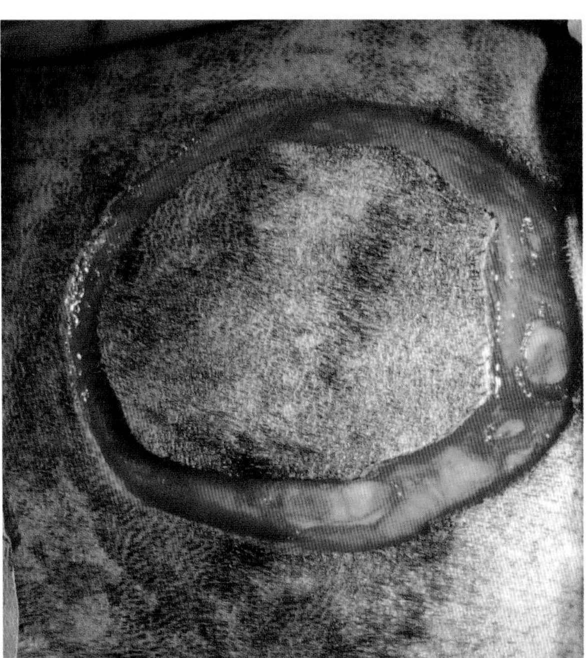

Fig. 2.19a A full-thickness skin incision is made in the donor site to harvest the graft.

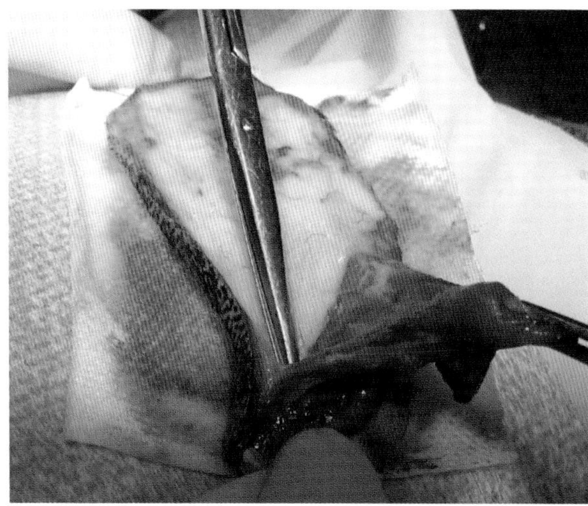

Fig. 2.19b Hypodermic tissues are removed by sharp dissection.

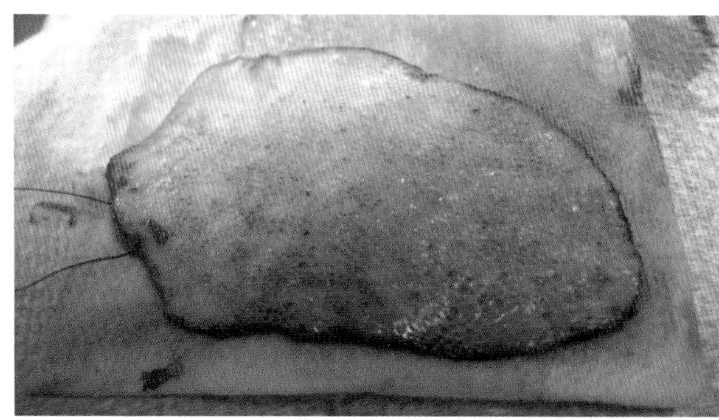

Fig. 2.19c Graft following removal of the hypodermis. Hair follicles are visible within the dermis. The suture marks the top of the graft.

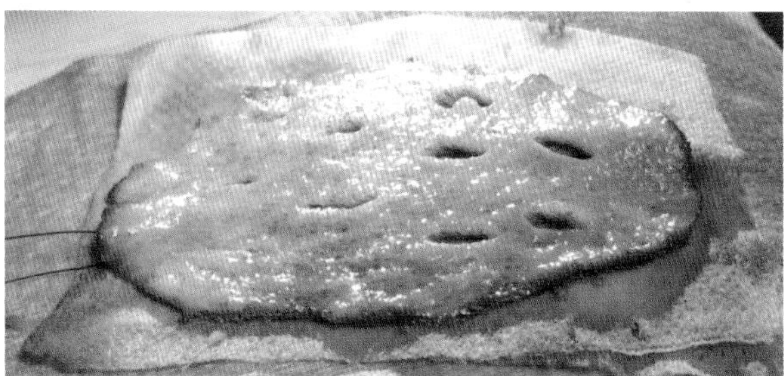

Fig. 2.19d Staggered 1 cm incisions are made to mesh the graft.

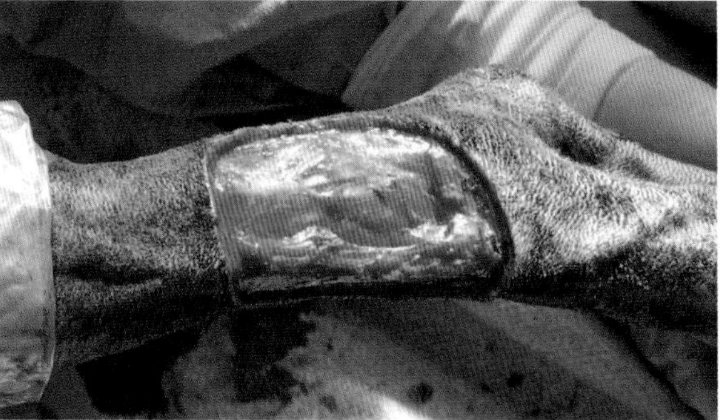

Fig. 2.19e A fresh surgical wound is a suitable site for graft placement.

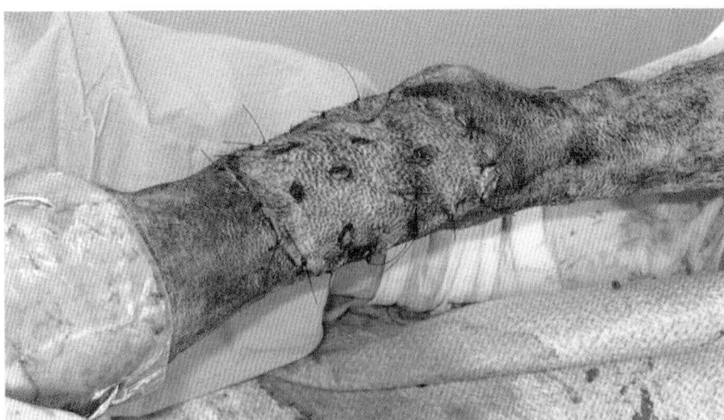

Fig. 2.19f Graft sutured into position with simple interrupted sutures of monofilament nylon.

graft contraction. A full-thickness skin incision is made around the template at the donor site (Fig. 2.19a), and the graft is excised. A suture can be placed at the top of the graft so that the surgeon will remember which way is up; this is important to ensure that hair regrows in the right direction. The hypodermic fat and panniculus muscle (if present) are then removed by sharp dissection (Fig. 2.19b,c). This is best done with the graft stretched over a roll of sterile bandage or the surgeon's finger. Following removal of the hypodermis, staggered rows of 1 cm incisions are made in the graft to mesh it (Fig. 2.19d). Meshing improves drainage and conformity of the graft to the wound. The graft is then sutured or stapled to the wound bed (Fig. 2.19e,f). The graft must be stretched so that it conforms precisely to the wound bed. The edges of the graft slightly overlap the wound edges to allow for graft contraction. The stab incisions are allowed to open slightly to provide drainage.

Graft bandages

The correct application of an appropriate dressing is critical in ensuring survival of the graft. A non-adherent contact layer should be used, which should cover the whole of the graft and be applied evenly. Staples or sutures can be used to tack the dressing in place. Some authors recommend applying an antibiotic ointment to the contact layer. Suitable contact layers include knitted cellulose acetate mesh impregnated with petrolatum emulsion (Adaptic, Johnson & Johnson) or a polyurethane foam (Allevyn, Smith & Nephew). This contact layer can be covered with sterile surgical swabs to increase the absorptive capacity. Two or more layers of cast padding secured with gauze roll make up the secondary layer of the bandage. At this stage, the bandage should be firm. The outer layer of the bandage is a self-adherent elastic wrap. Additional immobilisation in the form of a splint may be necessary, particularly if the graft is overlying a joint. A spica bandage should be used in cats with extremity grafts. Vacuum-assisted closure has been described as a method of securing skin grafts (Ben-Amotz et al., 2007; Or et al., 2017; Stanley et al., 2013).

The earliest a bandage should be changed is 48 hours after graft placement. Ideally, it is safer to wait for 72 hours to ensure that the critical period of revascularisation is not disturbed. Sedation or general anaesthesia may be necessary to prevent inadvertent damage to the graft during removal of the dressing. The contact layer can be adhered as a result of dried blood binding the granulation tissue to the interstices of the dressing; such areas should be softened with warm saline prior to gentle removal. Bandages should be changed every 3–4 days until the graft has taken (usually 14 days). Bandages can be left on for longer if there are any concerns that the patient might traumatise the graft. Kennel rest with only limited lead exercise for toileting is mandatory while the dressing is in place, to prevent motion at the graft site.

2.3 Surgical drains

Key points

- Surgical drains are used to evacuate fluid from the subcutaneous space and body cavities and to obliterate dead space.
- Latex Penrose drains are passive – that is, they rely on gravity for drainage and are placed commonly in subcutaneous tissues.
- Active drains rely on a vacuum or other suction device to achieve drainage, and are more efficient than passive drains.
- Adherence to the principles of drain placement helps to reduce the incidence of complications.
- The use of drains should be avoided where possible, and they should not be left in place any longer than necessary.

Drains may be used either prophylactically or therapeutically (Campbell 2012). They can remove accumulations of fluid that might provide a media for bacteria; they can relieve pressure that might compromise tissue perfusion and ventilation; and they can evacuate inflammatory mediators, bacteria, necrotic tissue and foreign material. Latex rubber, polyethylene, polyvinylchloride and silicone rubber are commonly used materials. All drains incite an inflammatory response and decrease tissue resistance to bacterial colonisation. PVC and silicone rubber are the more inert materials.

2.3.1 Open passive drains

Penrose drains (Fig. 2.20) are made from latex rubber and are the most commonly used drain in veterinary practice. They rely on capillary action, gravity, overflow and fluctuations in pressure within the space occupied by the drain. Drainage occurs along the outside of the tube. Its shape provides a high surface area:volume ratio; fenestration is therefore contraindicated. Penrose drains should not be used with suction or in body cavities.

The proximal end of the drain is placed in the deep tissues and can be secured to the exit point by a simple interrupted monofilament nylon skin suture. Using a buried suture is not advisable because the drain can tear around the suture during removal, leaving a fragment *in situ*. The distal end of the drain exits the skin and is secured by a simple interrupted monofilament nylon skin suture. Exiting the drain at both ends is not advisable because it precludes having the drain in the deep tissues and creates an entry point for bacteria. The exception to this is the inguinal and axillary regions, where a single exit point may act as a one-way valve. Some texts advise protecting the drain with an absorbent dressing, which acts as a barrier to bacteria and protects the skin.

2.3.2 Closed active drains

Suction drains consist of a tube connected to a vacuum or other suction device. Fenestrations in the tip of the tube allow fluid to enter the lumen. The fenestrated end of the tube must be in an airtight cavity. Advantages of active suction drains include decreased risk of contamination and excoriation. The volume of fluid produced by the wound can be quantified. The negative pressure created by the drain helps to close dead space and promote tissue apposition. These drains are very easy to manage and patients can be discharged from the hospital with these drains in place. Suction may be continuous or intermittent. The reservoir should be emptied every 6 hours with intermittent suction. Commercial suction drains are available, e.g. compressible grenade bulbs on fenestrated silicone Jackson–Pratt drains (Fig. 2.20). One study showed that grenade-type drains are safe and consistent, operating with lower suction while providing ongoing drainage with minimal fluid production (Halfacree et al., 2009). Laminar flow through a drain is described by Poiseuille's law:

$$F = dP\pi r^4 / 8nL$$

where F is the laminar flow, dP is the pressure gradient, r is the radius of the drain, n is the viscosity of the fluid and L is the length of the drain.

This means that doubling the diameter of the drain increases flow 16 times, and halving the length doubles the flow. Compressible grenades start to lose suction as they fill to 20–30% of their capacity.

2.3.3 Principles of drain placement

- The proximal end of the drain should be placed in the deepest part of the cavity to be drained.
- Passive drains must be dependent; active drains do not need to be.
- Drains should not exit through the incision as this increases the risk of infection and dehiscence.
- Drains should be placed from the inside to the outside to minimise the potential for contamination of the wound by external flora. To facilitate this, the drain is grasped with forceps which are then tunnelled subcutaneously to the exit point. A stab incision is made on to the forceps.

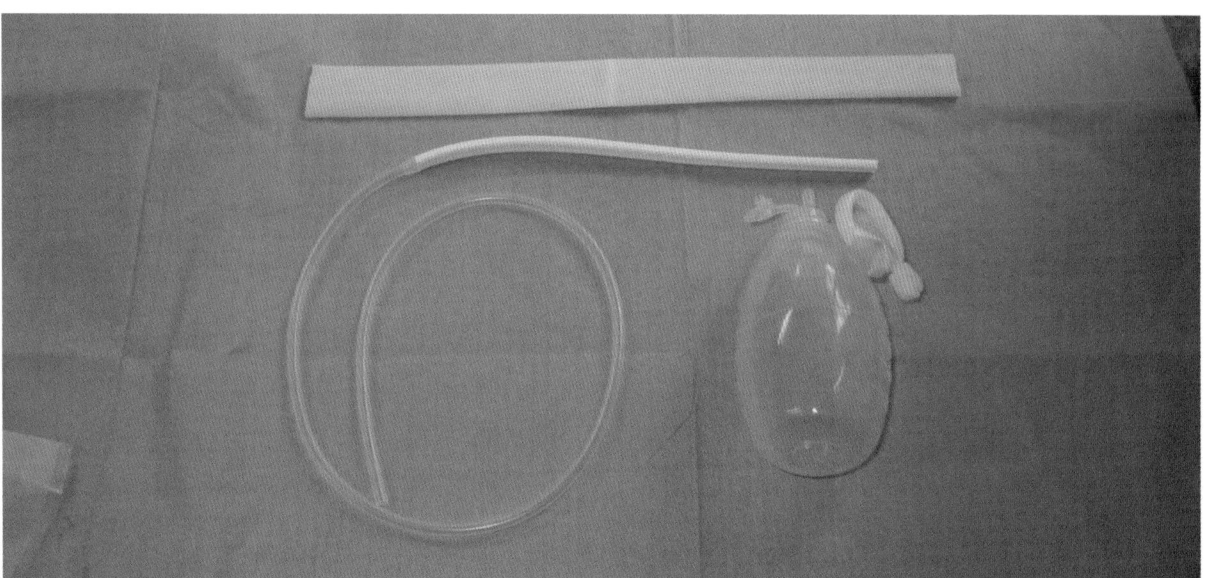

Fig. 2.20 Commercially available Penrose drain and fenestrated Jackson–Pratt drain with compressible grenade bulb.

- The exit hole in the skin should be the same width as an active suction drain and slightly wider than a passive drain.
- The exit site should be covered with a dressing to reduce the risk of ascending infection and to absorb exudate from the drain.
- Drain removal is dependent on the quantity and quality of fluid produced.
- The risk of bacterial colonisation increases with time, so drains should be removed as soon as possible. All drains induce fluid production, so zero fluid is unlikely.
- Drains should be removed in a single, smooth motion after removal of any anchoring sutures. The exit hole is left to heal by second intention.

2.3.4 Complications of surgical drains

Drains may fail for the following reasons:

- inadequate diameter
- poor positioning, particularly passive drains
- blockage
- retrograde contamination
- loss of negative pressure
- dislodgement.

Drains are foreign material and consequently decrease the tissue resistance to infection. They also provide a route of entry to the wound, and this is of particular concern in the hospital environment. Adding a drain to a clean site turns it into a clean-contaminated site. A recent study found a 15.6% infection rate in clean surgeries where a closed suction drain had been used (Bristow et al., 2015). Pressure bandages should be used rather than drains to prevent dead space expansion wherever possible. The risk of infection can be reduced by:

- using the smallest size and number of drains possible
- choosing a flexible drain
- using a closed drain
- removing the drain as soon as possible
- following proper surgical technique
- avoiding flushing blocked drains.

Drains shouldn't be placed in sites of tumour resection owing to the risk of seeding of tumour cells, although the veterinary evidence base for this is scant. However, if drains are to be placed, the exit hole should be placed close to the incision so that it can be included in the radiation field or resected during revision surgery.

Erosion into anastomotic sites, large vessels and hollow organs has been reported, so care must be taken when placing drains close to these structures. One veterinary study reported two cases of post-surgical haemorrhage related to active suction drain placement (Lynch et al., 2011). It was suggested that the use of low-pressure drains such as the Jackson–Pratt and silicone grenade may reduce the risk of this occurring.

References

Aper, R.L. and Smeak, D. (2003) Complications and outcome after thoracodorsal axial-pattern flap reconstruction of forelimb skin defects in 10 dogs (1989–2001). *Veterinary Surgery* 32, 378–384.

Aper, R.L. and Smeak, D.D. (2005) Clinical evaluation of caudal superficial epigastric artery axial-pattern flap reconstruction of skin defects in 10 dogs (1989–2001). *Journal of the American Animal Hospital Association* 41, 185–192.

Ben-Amotz, R., Lanz, O.I., Miller, J.M., Filipowitz, D.E. and King, M.D. (2007) The use of vacuum-assisted closure therapy for the treatment of distal extremity wounds in 15 dogs. *Veterinary Surgery* 36, 684–690.

Bohling, M.W., Henderson, R.A., Swaim, S.F., Kincaid, S.A. and Wright, J.C. (2004) Cutaneous wound healing in the cat: a macroscopic description and comparison with cutaneous wound healing in the dog. *Veterinary Surgery* 33, 579–587.

Bohling, M.W., Henderson, R.A., Swaim, S.F. Kincaid, S.A. and Wright, J.C. (2006) Comparison of the subcutaneous tissues in cutaneous wound healing in the dog and cat. *Veterinary Surgery* 35, 3–14.

Bohling, M.W. (2012) Skin grafts. In: Tobias, K.M. and Johnston, S.A. (eds) *Veterinary Surgery: Small Animal*. Elsevier Saunders, St. Louis, MO, pp. 1270–1290.

Bristow, P.C., Halfacree, Z.J. and Baines, S.J., (2015) A retrospective study of the use of active suction wound drains in dogs and cats. *Journal of Small Animal Practice* 56, 325–330.

Campbell, B.G. (2006) Dressings, bandages and splints for wound management in dogs and cats. *Veterinary Clinics of North America Small Animal Practice* 36, 759–791.

Campbell, B.G. (2012) Bandages and drains. In: Tobias, K.M. and Johnston, S.A. (eds) *Veterinary Surgery: Small Animal*. Elsevier Saunders, St. Louis, MO, pp. 221–230.

Cornell, K. (2012) Wound healing. In: Tobias, K.M. and Johnston, S.A. (eds) *Veterinary Surgery: Small Animal*. Elsevier Saunders, St. Louis, MO, pp. 125–134.

Ehrhart, N.P., Kaminskaya, K., Miller, J.A. and Zaruby, J.F. (2013) In vivo assessment of absorbable knotless barbed suture for single layer gastrotomy and enterotomy closure. *Veterinary Surgery* 42, 210–216.

Fahie, M.A. and Shettko, D. (2007) Evidence-based wound management: a systematic review of therapeutic agents to enhance granulation and epithelialisation. *Veterinary Clinics of North America Small Animal Practice* 37, 559–577.

Fahie, M.A. (2012) Primary wound closure. In: Tobias, K.M. and Johnston, S.A. (eds) *Veterinary Surgery: Small Animal*. Elsevier Saunders, St. Louis, MO, pp. 1197–1209.

Field, E.J., Kelly, G., Pleuvry, D., Demetriou, J. and Baines, S.J. (2015) Indications, outcome and complications with axial pattern skin flaps in dogs and cats: 73 cases. *Journal of Small Animal Practice* 56, 698–706.

Halfacree, Z.J., Wilson, A.M. and Baines, S.J. (2009) Evaluation of in vitro performance of suction drains. *American Journal of Veterinary Research* 70, 283–289.

Hosgood, G. (2006) Stages of wound healing and their clinical relevance. *Veterinary Clinics of North America Small Animal Practice* 36, 667–685.

Hosgood, H. (2012) Open wounds. In: Tobias, K.M. and Johnston, S.A. (eds) *Veterinary Surgery: Small Animal.* Elsevier Saunders, St. Louis, MO, pp. 1210–1220.

Hunt, G.B. (1995) Skin-fold advancement flaps for closing large sternal and inguinal wounds in cats and dogs. *Veterinary Surgery* 24, 172–175.

Hunt, G.B., Tisdall, P.L., Liptak, J.M., Beck, J.A., Swinney, G.R. and Malik, R. (2001) Skin-fold advancement flaps for closing large proximal limb and trunk defects in dogs and cats. *Veterinary Surgery* 30, 440–448.

Hunt, G.B (2012) Local or subdermal plexus flaps. In: Tobias, K.M. and Johnston, S.A. (eds) *Veterinary Surgery: Small Animal.* Elsevier Saunders, St. Louis, MO, pp. 1243–1255.

Kieves, N.R. and Krebs, A.L. (2017) Comparison of leak pressures for single-layer simple continuous suture pattern for cystotomy closure using barbed and monofilament suture material in an ex vivo canine model. *Veterinary Surgery* 46, 412–416.

Law, A.Y. (2017) Biomechanical testing and histologic examination of intradermal skin closure in dogs using barbed suture device and non-barbed monofilament suture. *Veterinary Surgery* 46, 59–66.

Lynch, A.M., Bound, N.J., Halfacree, Z.J. and Baines, S. (2011) Postoperative haemorrhage associated with active suction drains in two dogs. *Journal of Small Animal Practice* 52, 172–174.

Marturello, D.M., McFadden, M.S., Bennett, R.A., Regetly, G.R. and Horn, G. (2014) Knot security and tensile strength of suture materials. *Veterinary Surgery* 43, 73–79.

Or, M., Van Goethem, B., Kitshoff, A., Koenraadt, A., Schwarzkopf, I. and Bosmans, T. (2017) Negative pressure wound therapy using polyvinyl alcohol foam to bolster full-thickness mesh skin grafts in dogs. *Veterinary Surgery* 46, 389–395.

Pavletic, M.M. (2010) *Atlas of Small Animal Wound Management and Reconstructive Surgery*, 3rd edn. Wiley-Blackwell, Ames, IA.

Pitt, K.A. and Stanley, B.J. (2014) Negative pressure wound therapy: experience in 45 dogs. *Veterinary Surgery* 43, 380–387.

Riggs, J., Jennings, J.L., Friend, E.J., Halfacree, Z., Nelissen, P., Holmes, M.A. and Demetriou, J.L. (2014) Outcome of full-thickness skin grafts used to close skin defects involving the distal aspects of the limbs in cats and dogs: 52 cases (2005–2012). *Journal of the American Veterinary Medicine Association* 247, 1042–1047.

Rosin, E. and Robinson, G.M. (1989) Knot security of suture materials. *Veterinary Surgery* 18, 269–273.

Schmiedt, C.W. (2012) Suture material, tissue staplers, ligation devices and closure methods. In: Tobias K.M. and Johnston, S.A. (eds) *Veterinary Surgery: Small Animal.* Elsevier Saunders, St. Louis, MO, pp. 187–200.

Stanley, B.J. (2012) Tension-relieving techniques. In: Tobias, K.M. and Johnston, S.A. (eds) *Veterinary Surgery: Small Animal.* Elsevier Saunders, St. Louis, MO, pp. 1221–1242.

Stanley, B.J., Pitt, K.A., Weder, C.D., Fritz, M.C., Hauptman, J.G. and Steficek, B.A. (2013) Effects of negative pressure wound therapy on healing of free full-thickness skin grafts in dogs. *Veterinary Surgery* 42, 511–522.

Sylvestre, A., Wilson, J. and Hare, J. (2002) A comparison of 2 different suture patterns for skin closure of canine ovariohysterectomy. *Canadian Veterinary Journal* 43, 699–702.

Templeton, M.M. (2015) Ex vivo biomechanical comparison of v-loc® absorbable wound closure device and standard polyglyconate suture for diaphragmatic herniorraphy in a canine model. *Veterinary Surgery* 44, 65–59.

Tong, T. and Simpson D. J. (2012) Free skin grafts for immediate wound coverage following tumour resection from the canine distal limb. *Journal of Small Animal Practice* 53, 520–525.

Wardlaw, J.L. and Lanz, O.I. (2012) Axial pattern and myocutaneous flaps. In: Tobias K.M. and Johnston S.A. (eds) *Veterinary Surgery: Small Animal.* Elsevier Saunders, St. Louis, MO, pp. 1256–1269.

Case 2.1

Fig. 2.21 shows injuries sustained to the skin of the ventral abdomen following a dog attack.

- How would you describe the wound and what are your immediate concerns? What would your initial treatment be?

There is extensive trauma to the skin of the ventral abdomen, inguinal regions, medial thighs and prepuce. There are multiple puncture wounds with a moderately sized open wound in the right inguinal region. Bite wounds cause crushing and shearing injuries to the tissues below the skin. Damage to the skin's blood supply can lead to necrosis of the skin, a physiological degloving injury. Bite wounds also result in inoculation of bacteria into the deeper tissues. This can lead to local infection and, in some cases, to systemic infection and sepsis. These patients are likely to be in pain. Initially the patient should be supported with intravenous fluids and given broad-spectrum antibiotics and analgesics. Urination may be painful and a urinary catheter should be placed to prevent urinary retention.

Fig. 2.22 shows the same patient 48 hours later.

- Describe the changes in the wound and how you would manage it.

There has been loss of skin in the left and right inguinal regions owing to avascular necrosis. The underlying fat and muscle are discoloured, suggesting that they are also devitalised. The prepuce and ventral abdominal skin are black and

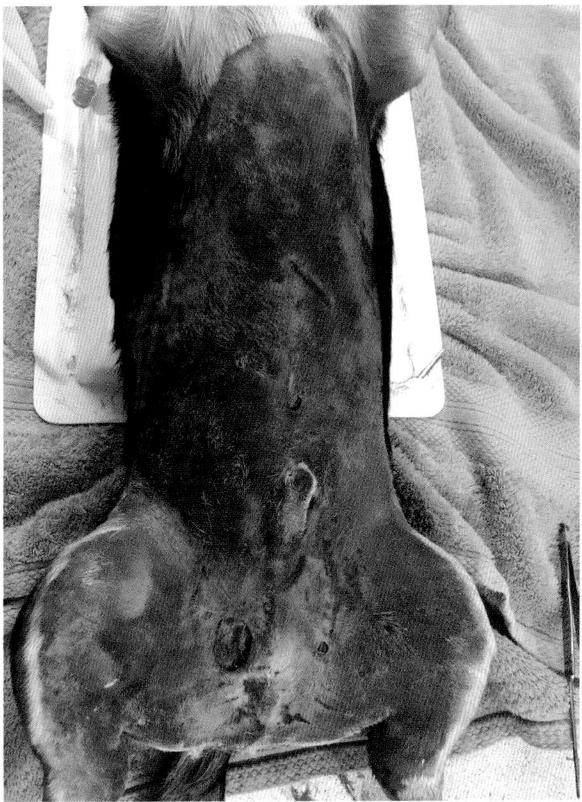
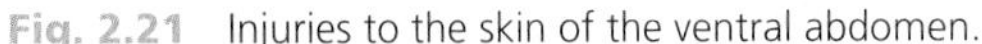

Fig. 2.21 Injuries to the skin of the ventral abdomen.

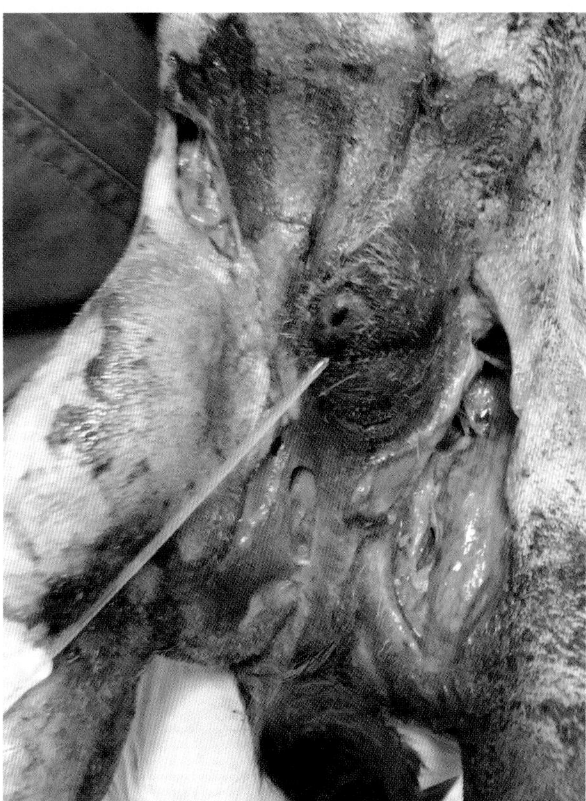

Fig. 2.22 Patient from Fig 2.21, 48 hours later.

non-viable. There is a moderate exudate from the wound. Pitting oedema is present in the pelvic limbs which might be due to infection, impaired venous/lymphatic drainage or both. This wound is still in the inflammatory phase of healing. The presence of extensive necrotic and contaminated tissue means that wound healing won't progress further without debridement. Given the size and location of the wound, as well as the amount of necrotic tissue present, layered surgical debridement is the most appropriate treatment option.

Fig. 2.23 shows the same wound after surgical removal of all necrotic tissue.

- What do you want to achieve in terms of wound healing and what would you do to promote this?
- What additional problems do you foresee in this patient and how might you overcome them?

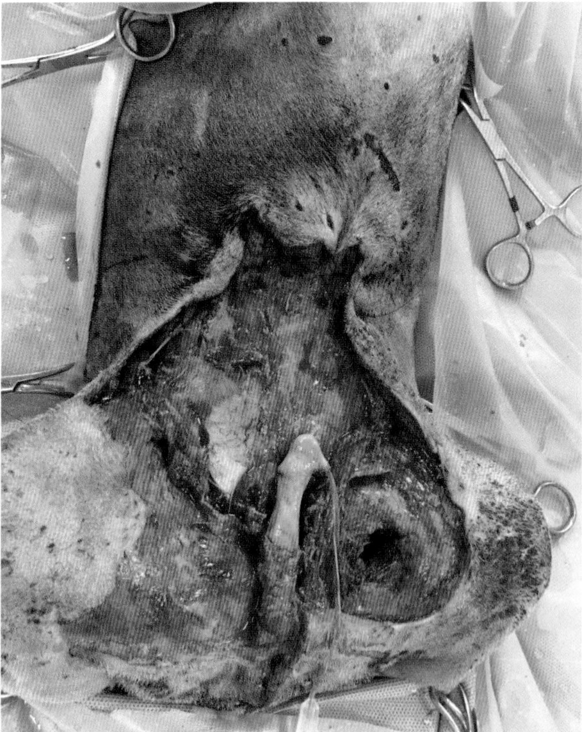

Fig. 2.23 Same wound from Fig 2.21 after surgical removal of all necrotic tissue.

Although the wound is now healthier in appearance, it is still in the very early stages of wound healing. The wound is likely to be exudative and fluid may not be retained at the wound surface, resulting in desiccation. The wound is also subject to further contamination and trauma. A dressing needs to be applied to protect the wound and to promote the proliferative phases of wound healing. A moisture-retentive dressing will prevent desiccation and promote autolytic debridement and granulation. The dressing should be absorbent to prevent maceration of the wound. In this patient, a non-adherent silicone contact layer with a highly absorbent backing was used. Wounds in this area are difficult

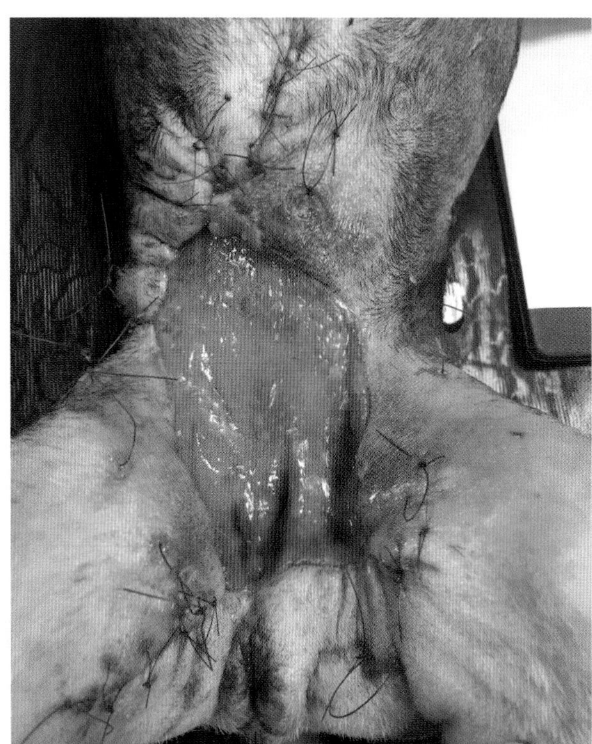

Fig. 2.24 Same wound from Fig 2.21 after 10 days of open wound management.

to apply dressings to, and in this patient a tie-over dressing was used to secure the dressing to the wound surface. Loops of monofilament nylon were placed in the skin around the wound and the dressing was sutured onto the loops. This technique enabled regular dressing changes without having to anaesthetise the patient. An additional concern in this patient is the combination of ventral abdominal and medial thigh skin defects. These wounds are subject to considerable shearing forces owing to limb movement. In this patient, the inguinal skin folds were still present. By dividing the attachments of the inguinal folds on the dorsal trunk, the resulting flap, with its single attachment to the lateral thigh, could be rotated to close the medial thigh defects. The penile mucosa is exposed and this patient will require penile amputation and scrotal urethrostomy. These procedures were performed a few days after the initial surgical debridement.

Fig. 2.24 shows the same wound after 10 days of open wound management.

- Describe the appearance of the wound.
- What are the options available to facilitate wound healing and what would you do at this stage?

The wound is now starting to granulate and the skin edges appear viable. The inguinal skin fold flaps have healed well, resulting in good coverage of the medial thighs. The options for wound closure at this stage are continued open wound management or reconstruction of the wound with skin flaps. The defect is still large, and a considerable amount of local skin would need to be mobilised to fully close the defect. An important consideration is that the blood supply to the regional skin might still be suboptimal, increasing the risk of flap necrosis and failure. A second consideration is that the amount of local skin available is limited, meaning that any closure technique might be done under tension. The patient and client were both coping well with open wound management, and it was a far safer option to allow an extended period of second-intention healing than to attempt further reconstruction.

Fig. 2.25 shows the wound several weeks after surgery. The wound has been managed on an outpatient basis with tie-over dressings. There has been a significant reduction in the size of the defect owing to wound contraction. The exposed granulation tissue was healthy in appearance and the patient was coping extremely well. Closure of the wound with a local skin flap could be considered at this point. Equally reasonable is continued open wound management. This wound went on to heal by second intention. This case emphasises the benefit of early and aggressive surgical debridement followed by a longer period of open wound management. Open wound management should never be underestimated, and even extensive wounds such as this can heal in this manner. Attempting to close wounds such as this with large and complicated skin flaps is not always the best option, and the temptation to do so should be avoided.

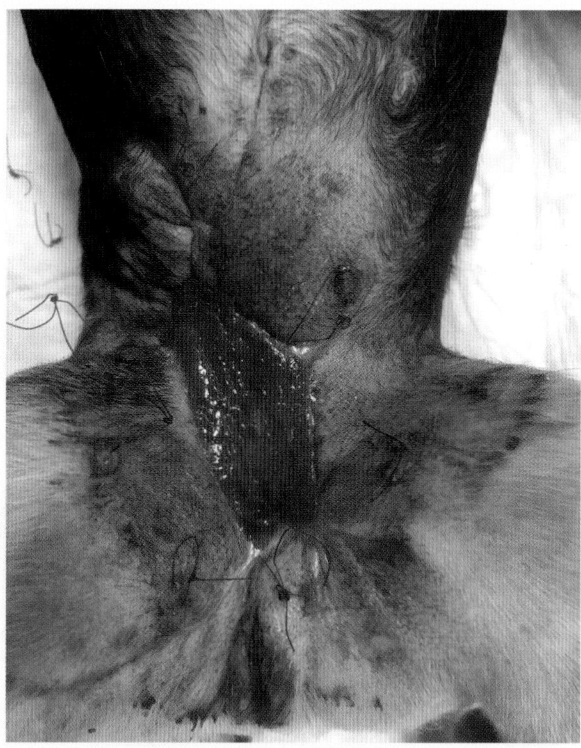

Fig. 2.25 Wound from Fig 2.21 several weeks after surgery.

Case 2.2

Fig. 2.26 shows a dog with a soft tissue sarcoma in the skin overlying the sternum. The mass is to be excised with wide margins as shown.

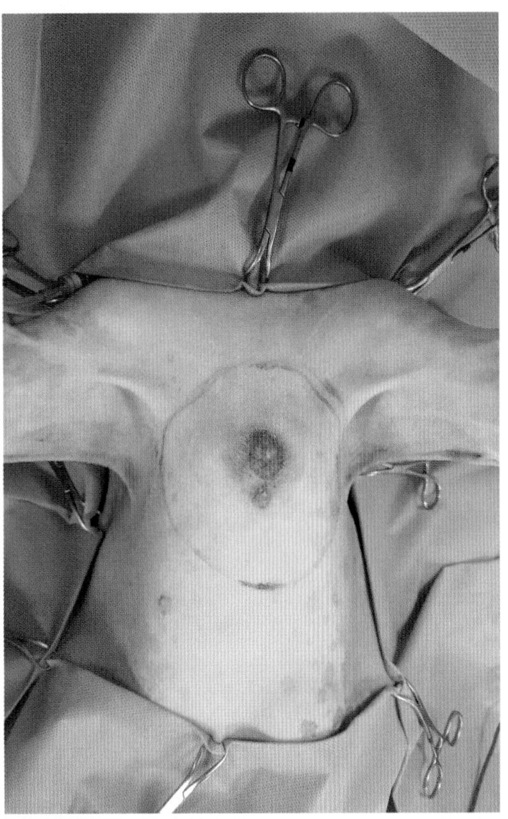

Fig. 2.26 A dog with a soft tissue sarcoma in the skin overlying the sternum.

- Aside from ensuring that you achieve adequate lateral and deep surgical margins, what would your considerations be in terms of closing the resulting surgical wound?

The direction of tension lines should be ascertained by moving the skin edges in different directions. The wound is adjacent to the thoracic limbs and axillae, so the influence of shear forces should be considered. The predicted wound edges should be brought into apposition to assess whether primary closure is feasible. The skin defect in this case is likely to be too wide to allow primary closure without the skin edges being under tension. Utilising tension-relieving techniques such as undermining or mesh expansion should be considered, but are unlikely be sufficient to overcome tension unless it is borderline. Tissue expanders could be used to utilise the skin's properties of mechanical creep and stress relaxation. However, these will prolong the time to surgery and may still not utilise sufficient skin to allow closure. Ideally this wound would be closed with a local skin flap. This will enable the wound to be closed immediately following tumour excision.

Fig. 2.27 shows the skin defect following wide excision of the tumour.

- What types of skin flap are available to close the skin defect in this area?
- What are the limitations of these flaps and how might these be overcome?

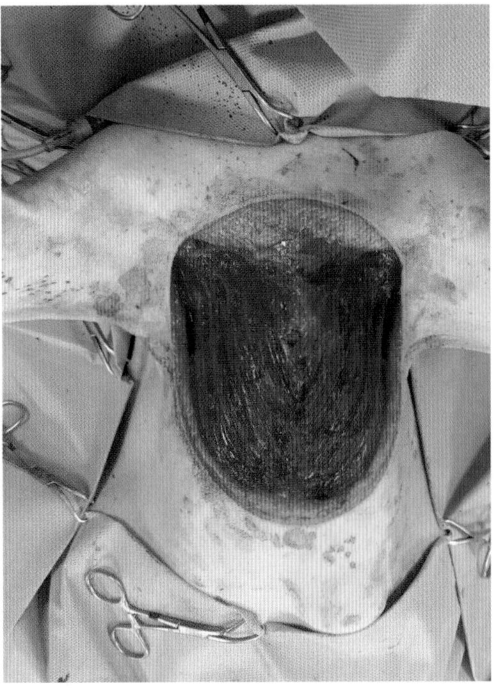

Fig. 2.27 Skin defect from Fig 2.26 following wide excision of the tumour.

Skin flaps may be random (subdermal) or axial pattern. For a skin defect of this size an axial-pattern flap is a better choice. These flaps are based on a direct cutaneous artery and, as such, have a better blood supply, allowing a larger area of skin to be mobilised. Unfortunately in the case of this defect there are no locally available axial-pattern flaps and therefore a random flap will have to be used. These flaps have lower survivability than axial-pattern flaps as their blood supply is derived from the subdermal plexus rather than a direct cutaneous artery. A random flap in this area would need to be rotated into the defect as there is too much tension to allow advancement of the skin edges in either direction.

These problems were overcome in this case by utilising bilateral elbow skin fold flaps. The elbow skin fold comprises two layers of skin and has four attachments: medial and lateral brachium and dorsal and ventral trunk. In this case the attachments to the medial and lateral brachium were excised and the resulting subdermal plexus flap, with its base being the dorsal trunk attachment, was advanced and rotated into the sternal defect. This was performed bilaterally. Skin fold flaps have a robust blood supply and, by severing the attachments between the body and thoracic limb, tension and shearing forces caused by limb movement are eliminated. In addition, 'unfolding' the flap provides a large surface area of skin with which to cover the defect.

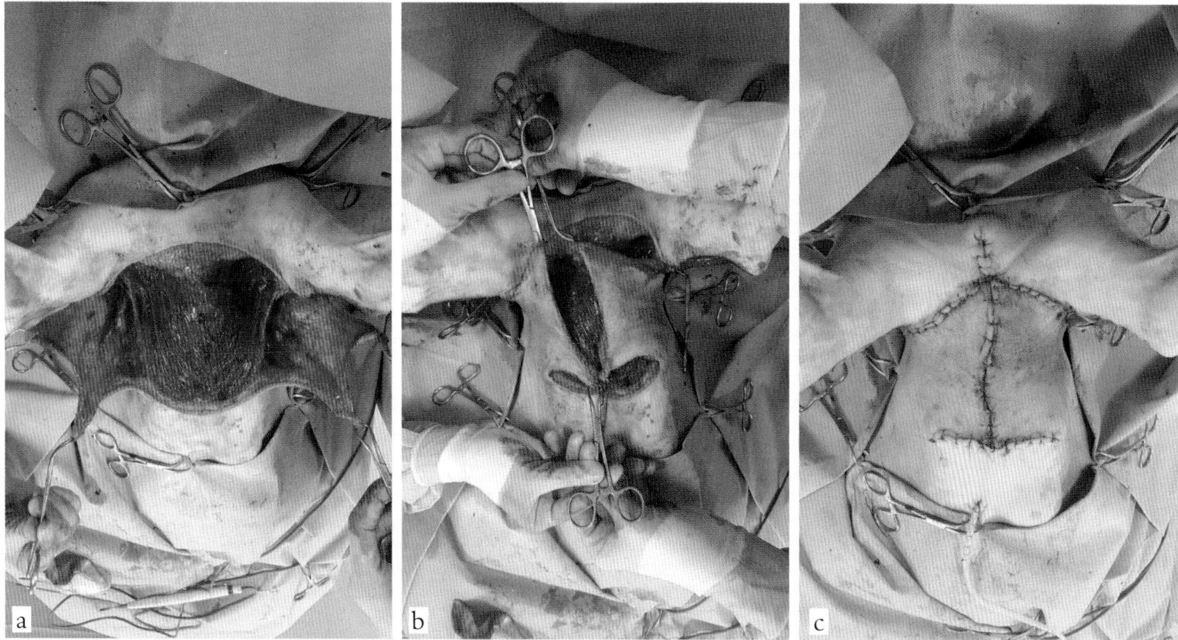

Fig. 2.28a–c Immediate post-surgical appearance following reconstruction.

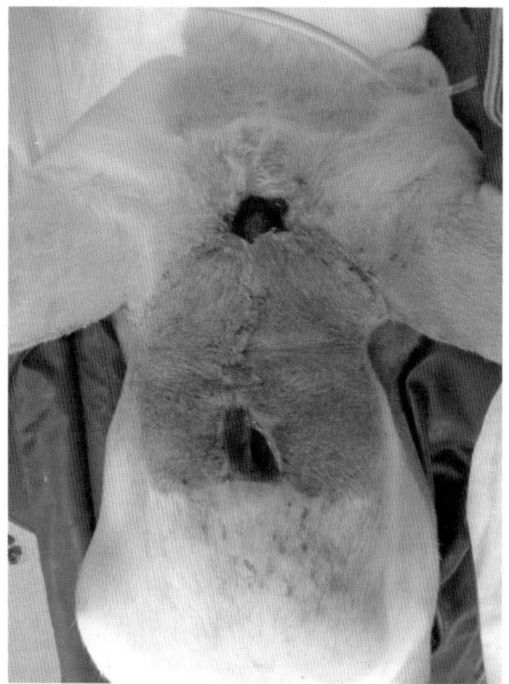

Fig. 2.29 Appearance of the wound 2 weeks after surgery.

Fig. 2.28a–c shows the immediate post-surgical appearance following reconstruction.

- What are the potential complications of this surgery, and what would you do to minimise them?

The main complications associated with subdermal plexus flaps are oedema, seroma formation, inflammation, infection, necrosis (particularly of the tip of the flap) and dehiscence owing to tension. It was necessary in this case to close the cranial portion of the wound in a linear fashion, and the confluence of four suture lines increases the risk of dehiscence. Tension-relieving sutures could be utilised in this portion of the wound. Many of the above complications can be prevented by careful handling of the flap. It is especially important that the subdermal plexus is preserved during dissection of the flaps. A vacuum drain has been placed in this case to reduce the risk of seroma formation. Strict rest is important while the flap heals, and a protective collar or body suit should be used to prevent self-trauma.

Fig. 2.29 shows the appearance of the wound 2 weeks after surgery.

- Describe the appearance of the wound. What factors have caused or contributed to these complications, and how would you manage them?

There are two small open wounds, one at each end of the wound. These have arisen owing to a combination of tension and tip necrosis of the skin flaps. The previously described confluence of suture lines is another risk factor for dehiscence. These wounds are best left to heal by second intention. Both wounds have a mild exudate but otherwise are healthy in appearance. A non-adherent, absorbent dressing is appropriate. Both wounds healed uneventfully by second intention.

Surgery of the gastrointestinal tract

3

Ana Marques

Chapter summary

Surgery of the gastrointestinal tract presents numerous challenges. Clinical signs are often vague and clinical examination will not necessarily help the surgeon in identifying the affected organ. Diagnostic imaging is therefore essential to achieve a final diagnosis in most cases.

Surgery of the gastrointestinal tract is considered a clean-contaminated procedure and perioperative antibiosis is therefore indicated. Antibiotics are administered intravenously at the time of induction of the anaesthesia and repeated every 2 hours for up to 12 hours postoperatively. The author uses cefuroxime (22 mg/kg).

Complications of gastrointestinal surgery can be devastating and life-threatening. The use of good surgical principles to minimise tissue trauma and surgical contamination and maximise primary intention healing is key to success and an uneventful postoperative recovery.

3.1 Salivary gland

Key points

- Salivary gland diseases are uncommon in small animals.
- Pathologies reported in the literature include trauma, rupture, inflammation, necrosis, foreign body, sialoliths and neoplasia.
- Diagnosis can be challenging and often requires a combination of cytology, imaging and surgery.

3.1.1 Anatomy and physiology

In dogs and cats there are four pairs of major salivary glands: the parotid gland, the mandibular gland, the sublingual gland and the zygomatic gland (Fig. 3.1). These all drain into the oral cavity and have as their main function the production of saliva. Saliva is used in small animals for lubrication of ingesta, cleansing of the oral cavity, buffering of weak acids, reduction of bacterial growth and protection of the surface epithelium.

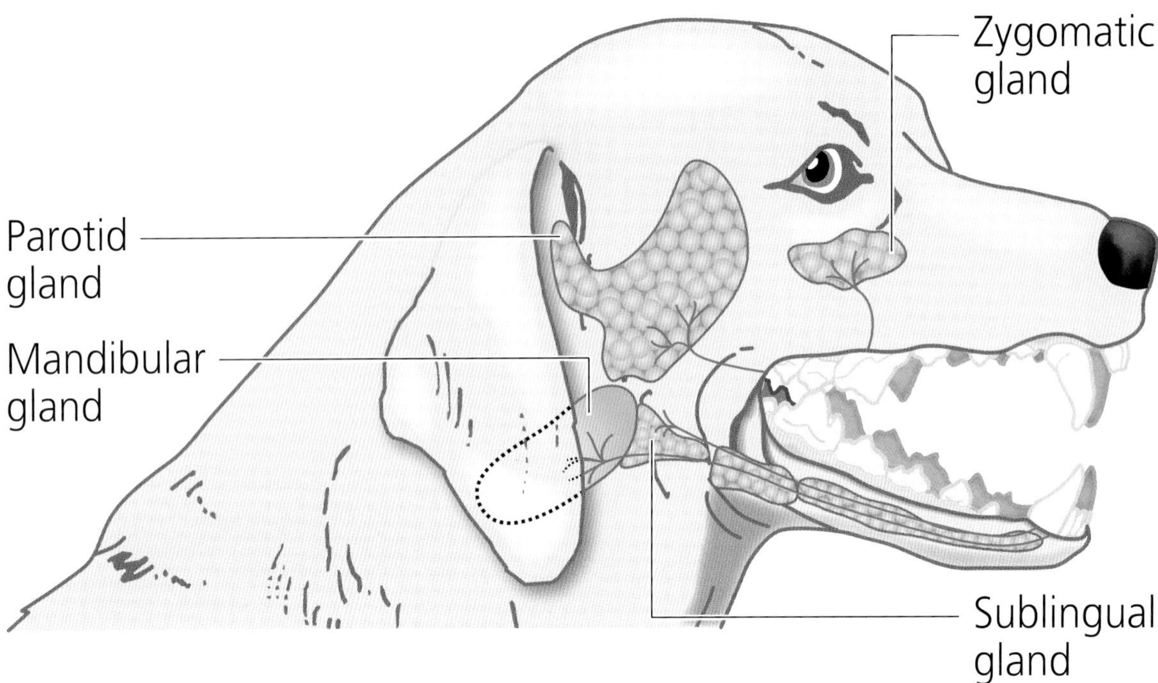

Fig. 3.1 Major salivary glands in the dog. *Illustrator: Elaine Leggett*

In dogs, it is also particularly important in aiding thermoregulation through panting.

The flow of saliva is decreased following sympathetic stimulation and increased following parasympathetic stimulation (Ritter et al., 2012).

3.1.2 Sialoadenosis

Sialoadenosis is a bilateral, non-painful enlargement of the salivary glands. It most commonly affects the mandibular salivary gland and its cause is unknown (Boydell et al., 2000; Sozmen et al., 2000). The clinical signs have an acute presentation and include vomiting, gulping, gagging, lip smacking, hyporexia and anorexia (Alcoverro et al., 2014). The condition, although idiopathic, has been associated with an unusual form of limbic epilepsy and it is responsive to treatment with phenobarbital. A case of sialoadenosis associated with an oesophageal foreign body has been reported (Gilor et al., 2010). A case of an acute transient swelling of the submandibular glands after general anaesthesia has been recently reported, but resolved without requiring treatment with phenobarbital (Cattai et al., 2017). The diagnosis is made by exclusion and by response to phenobarbital. Histopathologic analysis of affected salivary glands showed no consistent abnormalities (Sozmen et al., 2000). Treatment with phenobarbital typically results in clinical improvement in the first 72 hours, complete resolution of the clinical signs within one week and decrease in the size of the salivary glands within two to four weeks. The dose varies from 2 to 6 mg/kg, twice daily, and it can be tapered (Alcoverro, 2014). Lifelong therapy may be required.

3.1.3 Sialoadenitis and necrotising metaplasia

Sialoadenitis and necrotising sialometaplasia are inflammatory conditions of the salivary glands that can progress to necrosis. Affected animals have painful, enlarged salivary glands and clinical signs similar to those observed in sialoadenosis. An association with oesophageal disease has been reported in the literature; it is hypothesised that an afferent vagal reflex may be involved, and that the mechanism of disease is similar to the neural pathogenesis suggested for hypertrophic osteopathy (Schroeder and Berry, 1998). Diagnosis is made by histopathology, but computed tomography (CT) and magnetic resonance imaging (MRI) are sensitive for glandular changes (Cannon et al., 2011). On histopathology, affected glands present lobular necrosis, inflammation, squamous metaplasia, infarction and hypertrophy of the ductal epithelium (Mukaratirwa et al., 2015). Treatment is targeted at the primary oesophageal disorder. Response to phenobarbital administration has also been reported.

3.1.4 Sialocele

Sialocele, or salivary mucocele, is a subcutaneous collection of saliva in a sublingual (ranula), cervical, periorbital or pharyngeal location (Glen, 1972; Waldron and Smith, 1991). Most cases are considered idiopathic although several causes have been reported such as trauma (Adams et al., 2011; Guthrie and Hardie, 2014; Yoon et al., 2017), foreign bodies (Goldsworthy et al., 2013; Marques et al., 2008; Philp et al., 2012), sialoliths (Han et al., 2016; Lee et al., 2014; Ryan et al., 2008), neoplasia (Spangler and Culbertson, 1991) and others (Clarke and L'Eplattenier, 2010; Termote, 2003; Vallefuoco et al., 2011).

The diagnosis is made by fine needle aspiration biopsy of a non-painful swelling and retrieval of a viscous, clear or blood-tinged fluid. In chronic cases, the fluid may have lost its viscosity. On cytology, moderate numbers of non-degenerate neutrophils and irregular clumps of homogeneous pink–violet-staining mucin are observed. A mucin-specific stain (Periodic Acid Schiff) can be used to confirm the presence of saliva (Ritter et al., 2012).

In most parotid and zygomatic sialoceles, the swelling is located in close proximity to the affected salivary gland. In cervical sialoceles, the swelling often is in a ventral midline location, making it challenging to identify the affected salivary gland. To aid diagnosis the animal can be placed in dorsal recumbency, and the swelling tends to shift to the side of the affected salivary gland. Alternatively, diagnostic imaging can be performed.

Sialography entails injection of an iodine-based contrast agent through a salivary duct followed by radiography. The technique allows visualisation of the salivary duct and gland on a radiograph and potentially detects contrast leakage, duct obstruction or abnormal gland appearance greatly aiding diagnosis (Fig. 3.2). For duct cannulation (Table 3.1), the author uses a blunt lacrimal cannula. CT sialography has also been successfully developed (Kneissl et al., 2011). The author has applied this technique in several clinical cases, with good results. The advantage of CT over radiography is avoiding superimposition of local structures. Ultrasonographic evaluation of sialoceles has shown that the findings vary depending on the chronological stage of the disease (Torad and Hassan, 2013). MRI has been used to report variation in the anatomic location of the salivary glands and to successfully diagnose salivary gland disease and aid surgical planning (Boland et al., 2013; Durand et al., 2016).

Table 3.1 Anatomic location of the major salivary gland papillae.

Salivary gland	Anatomic location of papillae
Zygomatic	Caudal aspect of last upper molar tooth
Parotid	1 cm rostral to zygomatic papilla
Mandibular	Sublingual caruncle
Sublingual	Sublingual caruncle

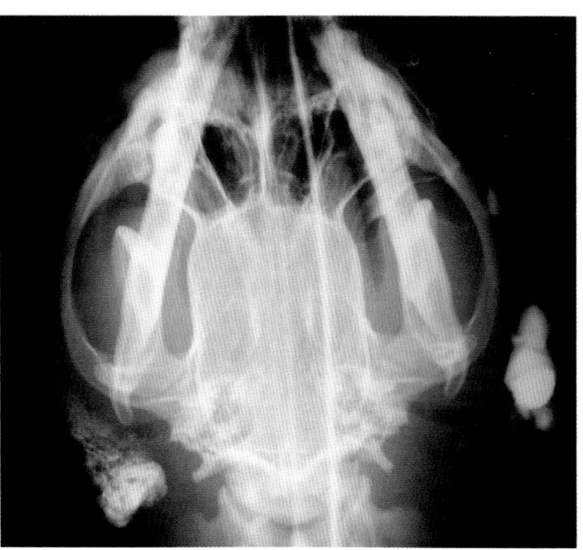

Fig. 3.2 Ventrodorsal radiograph showing bilateral parotid sialography (right and left markers absent). The parotid gland at the bottom of the image has a normal uptake of contrast showing a glandular appearance. Dense accumulation of contrast can be appreciated in the area of the contralateral gland, highly suggestive of pathology.

Treatment entails removal of the affected salivary gland (sialoadenectomy) and drainage and exploration of the sialocele. In most cases this can be done as an elective procedure. The exception can be animals that present with pharyngeal sialoceles. These swellings are formed in the caudodorsal or lateral pharynx just rostral to the level of the epiglottis and can cause laboured breathing or upper airway obstruction (Benjamino et al., 2012). Emergency relief can be provided by either draining the sialocele (stab incision) or performing a temporary tracheostomy in severe cases. The origin of the sialocele is usually the mandibular or sublingual salivary gland, and these will require resection to avoid recurrence.

Handy hints

Both mandibular and sublingual salivary glands share a common capsule and therefore are required to be removed together as a single structure. Both glands are commonly named as the mandibular–sublingual salivary gland complex.

Sialoadenectomy of the mandibular–sublingual salivary gland complex can be performed through either a lateral or ventral approach. The sublingual salivary gland is composed of monostomatic and polystomatic portions. The polystomatic component is more cranial and better approached through a ventral approach (Papazoglou, 2015; Ritter et al., 2006). This approach is preferred by the author. The lateral approach is simpler and also offers good results, providing both ducts of the salivary glands are identified and ligated.

Step by step: ventral approach for sialoadenectomy of the mandibular–sublingual salivary gland complex

- The animal is positioned in dorsal recumbency.
- An incision is made starting 4–5 cm caudal to the mandibular ramus, on the affected side, and extending rostrally towards the mandibular symphysis (Fig. 3.3a).
- After incision of the platysma muscle, the mandibular salivary gland can be identified just rostral to the bifurcation of the jugular vein.
- The salivary gland complex is then bluntly dissected surrounding the capsule (Fig. 3.3b).

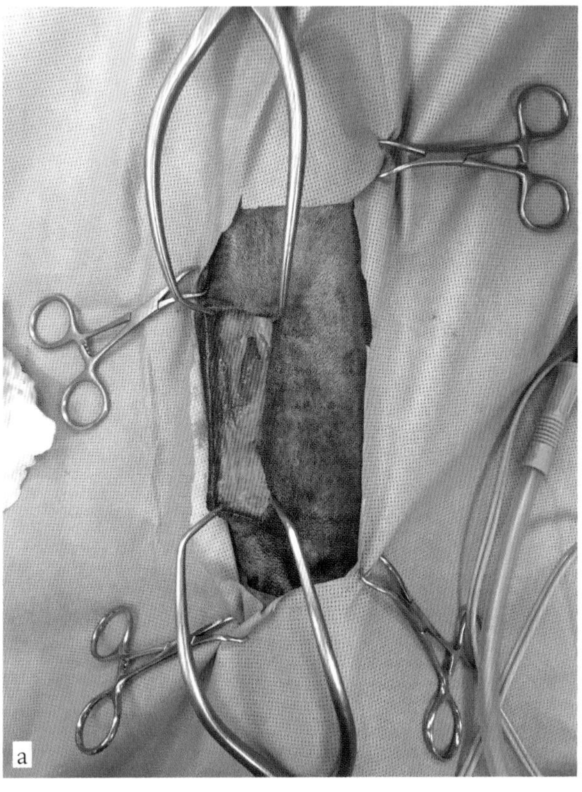

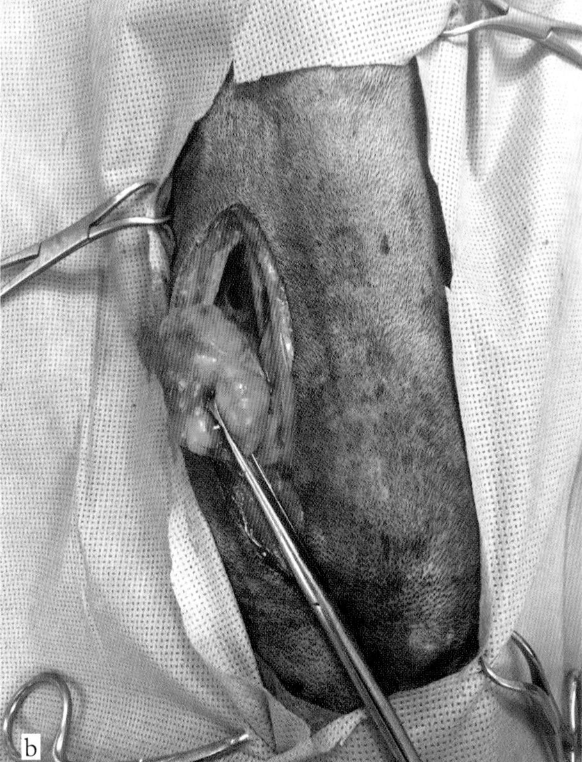

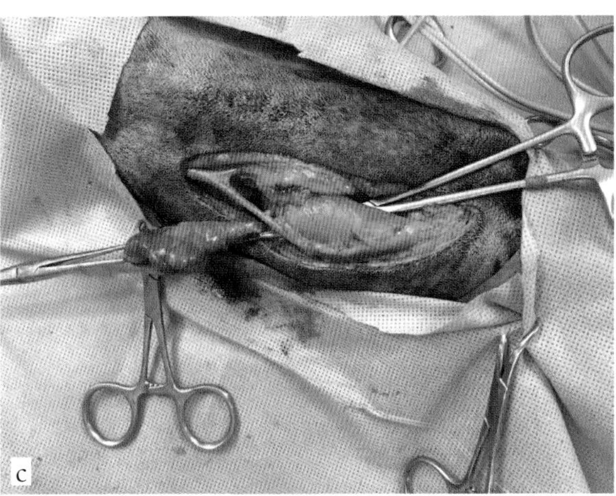

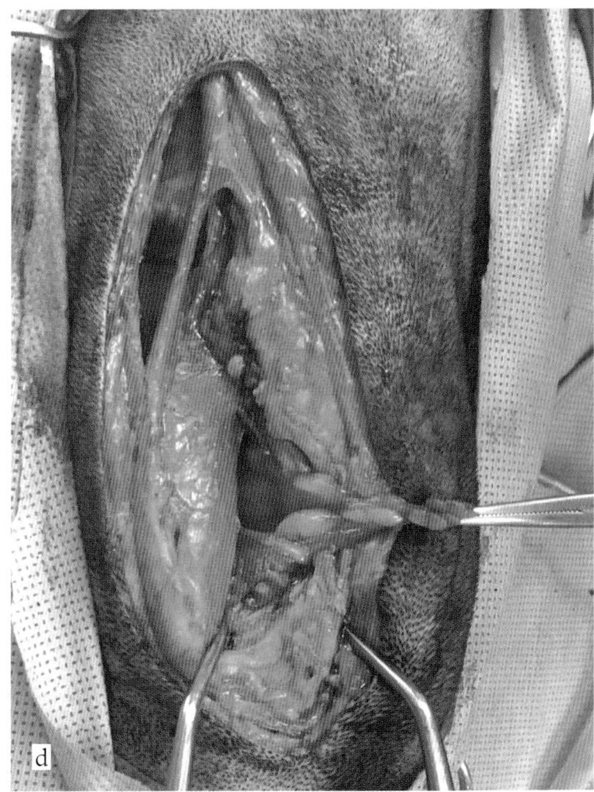

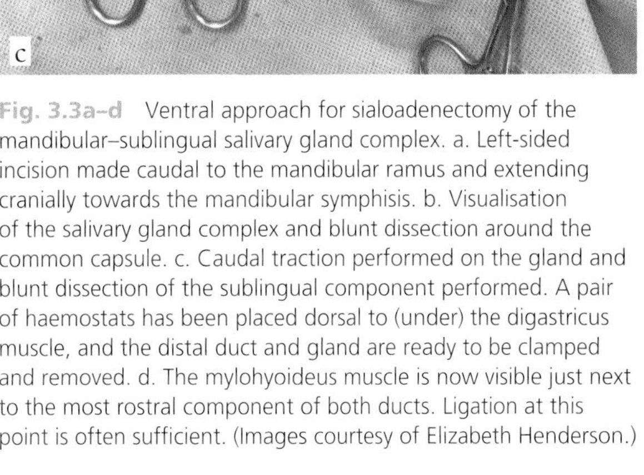

Fig. 3.3a–d Ventral approach for sialoadenectomy of the mandibular–sublingual salivary gland complex. a. Left-sided incision made caudal to the mandibular ramus and extending cranially towards the mandibular symphisis. b. Visualisation of the salivary gland complex and blunt dissection around the common capsule. c. Caudal traction performed on the gland and blunt dissection of the sublingual component performed. A pair of haemostats has been placed dorsal to (under) the digastricus muscle, and the distal duct and gland are ready to be clamped and removed. d. The mylohyoideus muscle is now visible just next to the most rostral component of both ducts. Ligation at this point is often sufficient. (Images courtesy of Elizabeth Henderson.)

- Caudal retraction is then performed to allow dissection of the sublingual component located under (dorsal to) the digastric muscle.
- Forceps are used to clamp the ducts, and the caudal component of the gland is removed (Fig. 3.3c).
- The forceps and ducts are then pulled under the digastric muscle.
- Blunt dissection is then continually rostrally to the level of the lingual nerve. In most cases, ligation of the ducts at this level and resection of the caudal remainder of the gland is sufficient (Fig. 3.3d).
- When a ranula is present, dissection may be continued rostrally to the lingual nerve and under the mylohyoid muscle so that all glandular tissue can be removed up to the level of the sublingual caruncle.
- The ducts are then ligated as rostrally as possible and transected.
- The sialocele can then be drained.

Step by step: lateral approach for sialoadenectomy of the mandibular–sublingual salivary gland complex

- The animal is positioned in lateral recumbency with the affected side upmost.
- An incision is made just cranial to the bifurcation of the jugular vein.
- The salivary gland complex is identified and bluntly dissected surrounding the capsule.
- Caudal retraction is performed and both salivary ducts are identified and bluntly dissected to the level of the digastricus muscle (Fig. 3.4).
- At this level, the ducts are ligated and all glandular tissue caudal to the ligation point are resected.
- A recent study describes tunnelling under the digastricus to increase duct exposure and completeness of resection (Marsh and Adin, 2013).

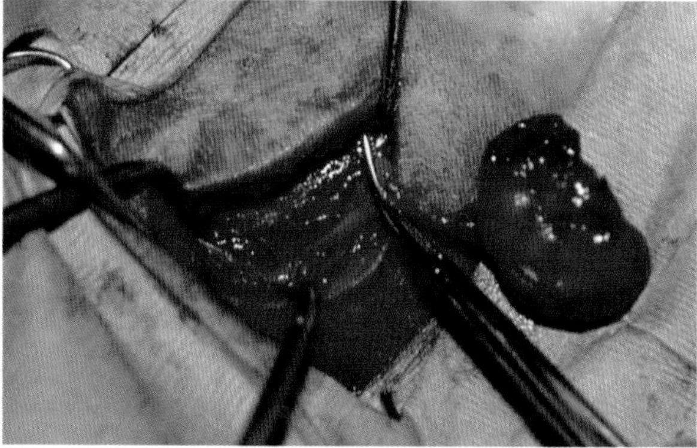

Fig. 3.4 Lateral approach for sialoadenectomy of the mandibular–sublingual salivary gland complex. Caudal retraction of the complex; both ducts are identified, dissected and clamped ready for ligation.

Zygomatic sialoadenectomy is made via a horizontal incision through the skin and subcutaneous tissues just over the dorsal aspect of the zygomatic arch. Variations of the technique have been reported, such as a modified lateral orbitotomy (Bartoe et al., 2007).

Parotid sialoadenectomy is a challenging procedure (Proot et al., 2016). Dissection extends to the region of the horizontal ear canal and therefore facial nerve paralysis can be a common complication. A meticulous dissection close to the horizontal ear canal is advised to minimise this complication.

Step by step: zygomatic sialoadenectomy

- The animal is positioned in lateral recumbency with the affected side upmost, or in sternal recumbency with a beanbag under the head and neck area.
- An incision through the skin and subcutaneous tissues is made just over the dorsal aspect of the zygomatic arch.
- The aponeurosis of the masseter muscle is reflected ventrally and the orbital fascia is reflected dorsally.
- A portion of the zygomatic arch may require resection to gain access to the gland.
- Orbital fat is then dissected and retracted to gain access to the gland.
- The gland is then gently bluntly dissected and retracted dorsally so that its blood supply (a branch of the infraorbital, the malar artery) can be ligated.

Step by step: parotid sialoadenectomy

- The animal is positioned in lateral recumbency.
- A skin incision is made over the vertical ear canal starting below the external acoustic meatus and extending ventrally to the level of the caudal angle of the mandible.
- The platysma and parotidoauricularis muscles are then incised to expose the glandular tissue (Fig. 3.5a).
- The gland is gently dissected from caudal to rostral.
- The dissection should be particularly meticulous close to the horizontal ear canal, to spare the facial nerve if possible.
- Several small vessels are encountered and will require ligation.
- Dissection is continued ventrally until the duct is identified and ligated (Fig. 3.5b).

Complications following sialoadenectomy are infrequent, and include seroma formation, haemorrhage and recurrence of the sialocele (Kaiser et al., 2016). In the author's experience, seroma is a relatively common complication but it is self-limiting and is reabsorbed

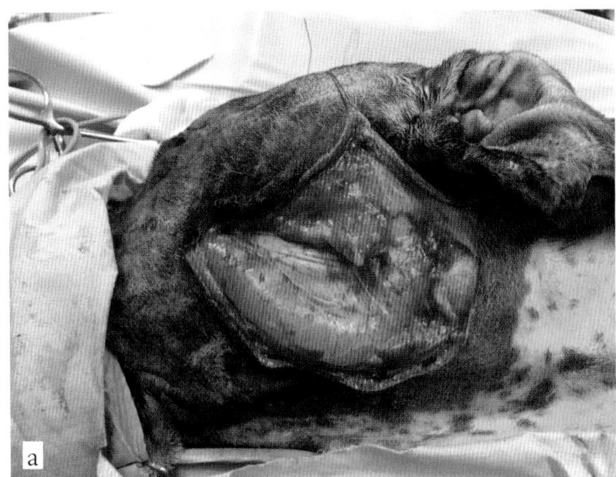

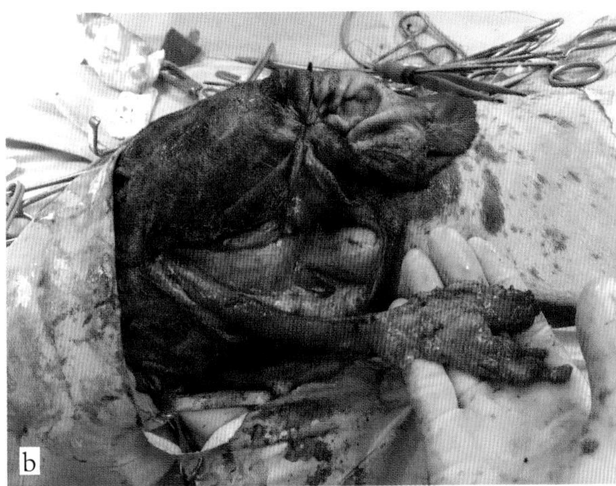

Fig. 3.5a,b Parotid sialoadenectomy. a. Parotid glandular tissue and dilated duct identified after incising the platysma and parotidoauricularis muscles. b. Parotid gland and duct completely dissected just before duct ligation.

after two to three weeks with restricted exercise and a combination of cold and hot packing. Recurrent sialocele is best managed by revision surgery with increased exposure and identification and resection of the remnant salivary tissue (Tsioli et al., 2013). Other techniques have been published, including the use of a sclerosing agent (Stuckey et al., 2012) and radiation therapy (Poirier et al., 2017).

3.1.5 Sialoliths

Sialoliths are most often associated with the parotid duct, but have also been reported in other salivary glands. Stone components include calcium, oxalate, phosphate, magnesium, carbonate, ammonium and non-mineral proteinaceous material. Diagnosis can be made by palpation, radiography or CT. Treatment involves sialoadenectomy and exploration and lavage of the sialocele (Han et al., 2016; Lee et al., 2014; Ryan et al., 2008; Suh et al., 2015).

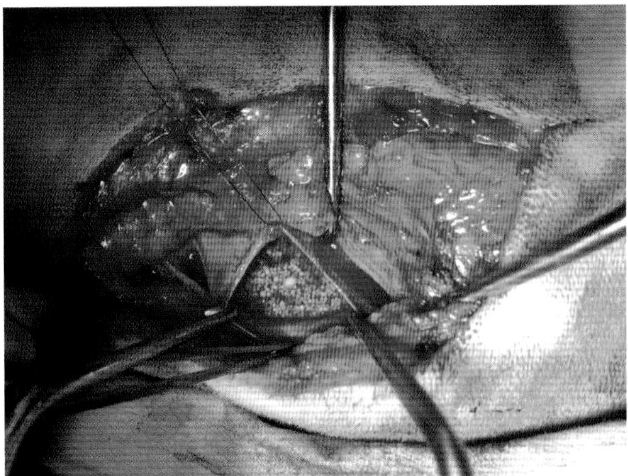

Fig 3.6 Exploration of a sialocele after sialoadenectomy showing several sialoliths.

Handy hints

The author has found sialoliths in some cases when exploring the sialocele (Fig. 3.6). For this reason, exploration and lavage of the sialocele (rather than just drainage) is always advised.

3.1.6 Neoplasia

Neoplasia of the salivary glands is uncommon, with a reported incidence of 0.17%. Most tumours are of epithelial origin, with the majority being adenocarcinoma or acinic carcinoma. The mandibular and parotid salivary glands are most commonly affected, but others have also been reported (Kishimoto et al., 2015; Lenoci and Ricciardi, 2015; Mason et al., 2001). Regional lymph node involvement is possible, but distant metastasis is less common. Clinical signs vary and may include the presence of a firm swelling, halitosis, dysphagia and exophthalmos. Diagnosis includes fine needle aspiration biopsy or incisional biopsy of the mass and associated lymph node. Full staging with blood work and ultrasound scan may be indicated. Advanced imaging is very useful in aiding surgical planning. The owner should be made aware of the goals of surgery, which usually include cytoreduction, diagnosis, palliation, metastectomy and, rarely, curative intent. Adjuvant therapy may be indicated postoperatively (Hammer et al., 2001; Militerno et al., 2005; Ritter et al., 2012; Sozmen et al., 2003).

3.2 Oesophagus

Key points

- Oesophageal surgery is associated with a high complication rate compared to other surgeries of the gastrointestinal tract. Absence of a serosal layer, lack

of local omentum available to augment the surgical site, presence of segmental blood supply, constant movement caused by deglutition and respiration and the presence of local tension are thought to be responsible for the higher risk of complications.
- To maximise healing, the surgeon should follow strict surgical principles including gentle tissue manipulation, minimisation of contamination, appropriate selection of suture material, judicious use of electrocautery, good tissue apposition, minimal disruption of the submucosal intramural plexus, patching of the surgical area with viable tissues (muscle and pericardium) and minimisation of postoperative movement through placement of a gastrostomy tube.
- Animals with oesophageal disorders may present with respiratory signs such as pneumothorax or pneumonia, and require stabilisation prior to surgical intervention.
- Patients with oesophageal perforation, severe trauma or pneumonia should receive antibiotic treatment.

3.2.1 Surgical anatomy

The oesophagus begins dorsal to the cricoid cartilage of the larynx and follows the trachea caudally. Proximally, the oesophagus is located on the left side of the trachea and dorsal to the trachea further caudally. It enters the thoracic cavity via the thoracic aperture and leaves via the oesophageal hiatus of the diaphragm. The cervical section is accompanied by the common carotid artery, the vagosympathetic trunk and the recurrent laryngeal nerves. The thoracic section is accompanied by the right and left vagus nerves. The oesophageal wall is composed of four layers – mucosa, submucosa, muscularis and adventitia. The blood supply to the cervical oesophagus is predominately from the thyroid artery, and two-thirds of the thoracic oesophagus is supplied by the bronchoesophageal artery, aortic branches and dorsal intercostal arteries; the caudal thoracic oesophagus is supplied by the left gastric artery. An intramural plexus is present in the submucosal layer. The oesophagus is innervated by sympathetic and parasympathetic trunks of the vagus nerve and recurrent laryngeal nerves (Evans and de Lahunta, 2013; Kyles, 2012).

3.2.2 Foreign body

Oesophageal foreign bodies are commonly reported in small animals. In dogs, bones are most commonly diagnosed. In cats, fishhooks, needles and strings are most frequently found. Small breeds and, in particular, terriers are most affected (Rodríguez-Alarcón et al., 2010). The foreign body will often lodge at the thoracic inlet, heart base or caudal oesophagus, as these structures restrict oesophageal dilation. Clinical signs include regurgitation, swallowing disorders, retching, gagging, excess salivation, restlessness, lethargy and inappetence (Jankowski et al., 2013) and can be acute or chronic. More severe clinical signs can be present in the case of oesophageal perforation, abscessation, pleuritis, mediastinitis, pneumomediastinum, pneumothorax, peritonitis, pneumoperitoneum and fistula formation (broncho-oesophageal or trachea-oesophageal) (Keir et al., 2010; King, 2001; Seiler et al., 2001).

Most foreign bodies are diagnosed on plain radiographs (Fig. 3.7). Radiographs should also be closely observed for signs of mediastinal or thoracic disease. Contrast radiography using an iodine-based contrast agent can aid diagnosis. Oesophagoscopy is the golden tool that can be used to confirm the diagnosis, retrieve or help retrieve the foreign body, check for perforations and evaluate the oesophageal mucosa (Fig. 3.8a–c) (Kyles, 2012).

Treatment should always start with attempted

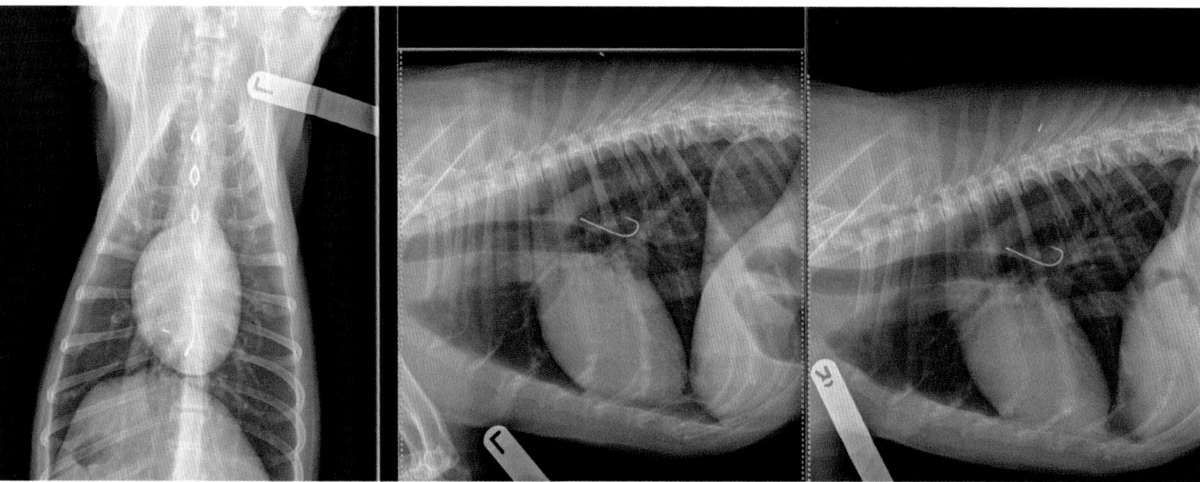

Fig. 3.7 Right and left lateral and ventrodorsal radiographs showing an oesophageal foreign body (fishhook) at the heart base.

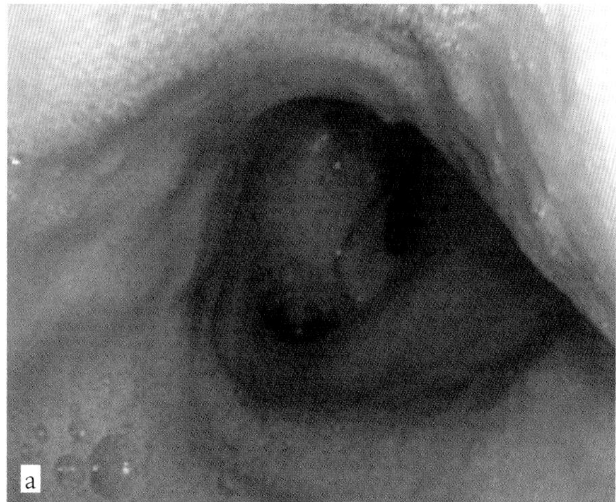

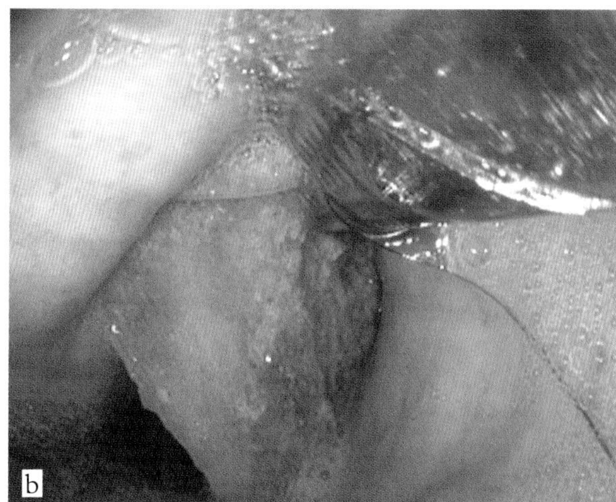

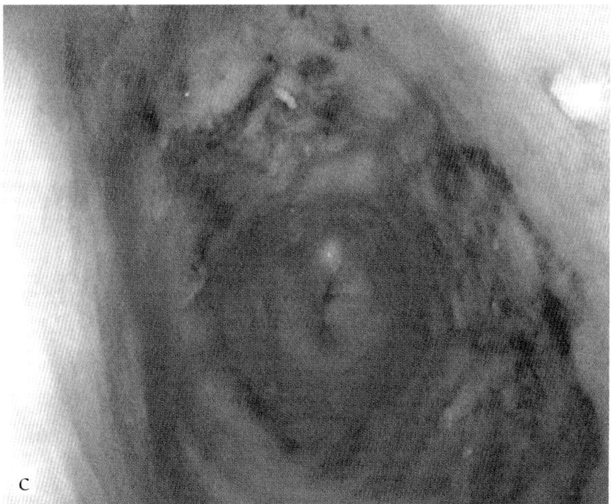

Fig. 3.8a–c Oesophagoscopy for diagnosis and removal of an oesophageal foreign body. (Images courtesy of Jennifer Cartwright.)

retrieval using an oesophagoscope or with fluoroscopy using grasping forceps (Moore, 2001). A recent study showed that endoscopic removal of fishhooks lodged in the proximal oesophagus is successful, but that oesophageal perforation occurred in approximately half of all cases; these all survived to discharge (Binvel et al., 2017). If the foreign body is firmly lodged, retrieval should not be forced as it may result in perforation. If the foreign body is smooth, a balloon catheter can be used for retrieval by passing it beyond the foreign body, inflating the balloon and gently applying cranial traction. If retrieval is not possible, the foreign body should be pushed, if possible, into the stomach because gastrotomy carries much fewer risks than oesophagotomy. Anaesthetic parameters such as oxygen saturation, blood pressure and ventilation should be closely monitored. One study showed that the success of endoscopic removal is adversely affected by the duration of clinical signs prior to presentation (Juvet et al., 2010).

If oesophagoscopy or fluoroscopy fails, surgical retrieval via a cervical, thoracic or abdominal approach is required. If the foreign body is caudal to the base of the heart, removal via gastrotomy through a ventral midline coeliotomy is possible (Aertsens et al., 2016). A recent study comparing oesophagoscopy and oesophagotomy for removal of oesophageal foreign body showed no difference in outcome (Deroy et al., 2015). Another study looking at risk factors in dogs treated for oesophageal foreign body obstruction showed that the risk of death was significantly higher with surgery and that 100% of dogs died if surgery was recommended but declined (Burton et al., 2017). The approach to the different regions of the oesophagus is summarised in Table 3.2.

Handy hints

All oesophagotomies should be augmented to maximise healing of the surgical site. The sternohyoid muscle can be used in the cervical oesophagus, the pericardium in the thoracic oesophagus and the omentum in the caudal oesophagus.

Step by step: approach to the cervical oesophagus

- The animal is positioned in dorsal recumbency.
- Place a towel underneath the neck area.

Table 3.2 Approaches to the different regions of the oesophagus.

	Cervical	Cranial thoracic	Caudal
Approach	Ventral midline cervical	Intercostal thoracotomy R 3rd, 4th, 5th L 3rd, 4th	Ventral midline coeliotomy Gastrotomy

- A ventral cervical midline incision is performed, beginning at the larynx and extending caudally to the manubrium.
- The platysma muscle and subcutaneous tissues are incised and retracted.
- The paired sternohyoid muscles are separated and retracted to expose the trachea (Fig. 3.9a).
- The trachea is retracted to the right to allow visualisation of the oesophagus.
- Other local structures can also now be visualised, such as the thyroid gland, the cranial and caudal thyroid artery, the recurrent laryngeal nerve and the carotid sheath.
- A stomach tube is passed orally to the level of the oesophageal obstruction.
- An incision is performed, if possible, immediately caudal to the foreign body and it is removed (Fig. 3.9b).
- The oesophagotomy is closed with an interrupted suture pattern in one or two layers using 1.5 or 2.0 metric polydioxanone.
- If a two-layer pattern is chosen, the first layer encompasses the mucosa and submucosa with the knots turned into the oesophageal lumen. The second layer can then encompass the muscularis and adventitia, with the knots turned to the outside (Fig. 3.9c).
- The surgical site is augmented and the surgical wound is lavaged and closed in three layers: muscle layer, subcutaneous layer and skin.

Step by step: approach to the cranial oesophagus

- The animal is positioned in lateral recumbency with the affected side upmost.
- Place a towel underneath the intercostal space to be incised.
- A stomach tube is passed orally to the level of the oesophageal obstruction.
- In left intercostal thoracotomy, the oesophagus is identified dorsal to the brachiocephalic trunk.
- In right intercostal thoracotomy, the oesophagus is identified just dorsal to the trachea in the mediastinum. The azygos vein can be dissected and retracted or ligated to maximise exposure.
- An incision is performed, if possible immediately caudal to the foreign body and it is removed.

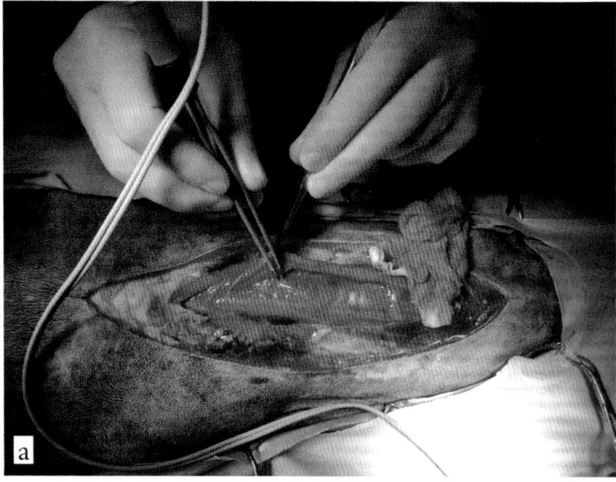

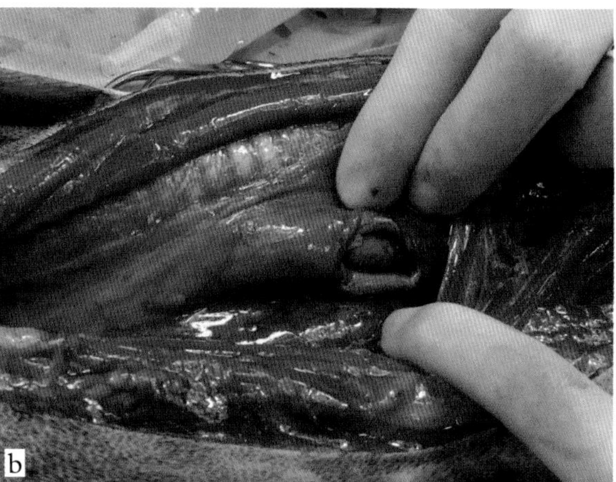

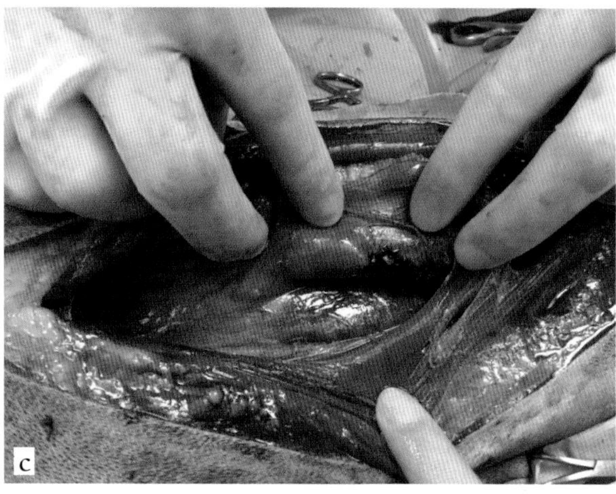

Fig. 3.9a–c Ventral approach to the oesophagus. (Images courtesy of Jon Hall.) a. The paired sternohyoideus muscles are separated and retracted to expose the trachea. b. An oesophagotomy has been done and the foreign body removed. The oesophagostomy tube has been advanced to facilitate closure. c. The oesophagotomy has been closed in a single layer using simple interrupted sutures.

- The oesophagotomy is closed with an interrupted suture pattern in one or two layers using 1.5 or 2.0 metric polydioxanone.
- If a two-layer pattern is chosen, the first layer encompasses the mucosa and submucosa and the knots are turned into the oesophageal lumen.
- The second layer can then encompass the muscularis and adventitia with the knots turned to the outside.
- A thoracostomy drain is placed before closure of the thoracic cavity.
- The thoracic cavity is lavaged and closed in four layers. Several circumcostal sutures are placed, approximately 0.5–1.0 cm apart, using 3.0 or 4.0 metric polydioxanone depending on the animal size; closure of the muscle layers using 2.0 or 3.0 metric polydioxanone; closure of the subcutaneous layer and skin.
- Fluid and air are drained from the thoracic cavity using the thoracostomy drain.

Handy hints

The thoracostomy drain can be maintained for up to 72 hours postoperatively to monitor air and fluid production, which are likely to increase in the case of surgical dehiscence.

Step by step: approach to the caudal oesophagus

- The animal is positioned in dorsal recumbency.
- A ventral midline exploratory coeliotomy is performed.
- In most cases the foreign body can be removed via a gastrotomy.
- A caudal median sternotomy or diaphragmatic myotomy may be useful to increase exposure of the cranial abdomen.
- The foreign body is removed and the gastrotomy closed and omentalised (see gastrotomy section).
- If a caudal median sternotomy or diaphragmatic myotomy has been performed, a thoracostomy drain should be placed before closure of the median sternotomy or apposition of the diaphragm.
- The abdomen is lavaged and routinely closed in three layers.

In cases where oesophageal perforation is present, the area should be debrided, sutured and augmented by a local muscle flap or omentum. Some cervical perforations may only require local drainage and be allowed time to heal by second intention. Dogs treated for more extensive oesophageal lesions, as well as those undergoing oesophagectomy or resection and anastomosis, are more likely to develop postoperative complications (Sutton et al., 2016). Oesophageal resection and anastomosis is rarely indicated and carries much higher risks. However, it has been reported with success in a few cases in the literature (Cariou and Lipscomb, 2011).

Handy hints

Cases involving severe oesophageal trauma or perforation should have samples collected for bacteriological analysis at the time of surgical intervention, so that appropriate antibiotic therapy can be instituted. Prophylactic antibiotic therapy is initiated at the time of presentation, and changed according to the bacteriology and sensitivity results.

After foreign body removal, antacids (H2 antagonist; proton pump inhibitor) should be administered to minimise oesophagitis. Antibiotics may be indicated depending on the level of contamination. If no perforation is present, a soft diet is given for 7 days. In cases where perforation or severe trauma is present, no oral intake is given and nutritional support is given via a gastrostomy tube for 10 days.

Complications following endoscopic foreign body removal include perforation, oesophageal stricture, oesophageal diverticulum, peri-oesophageal abscess, pneumothorax, pleural effusion and respiratory arrest. The presence of bony foreign bodies, a bodyweight of less than 10 kg and oesophageal or gastric foreign bodies in place for more than 3 days are significant risk factors for complications (Gianella et al., 2009).

3.2.3 Stricture

Oesophageal stricture is most commonly acquired and results from severe circumferential oesophageal injury extending into the muscular layer of the oesophagus (Glazer and Walters, 2008). The damaged tissue heals by fibrosis and wound contracture, resulting in a narrow lumen and potential obstruction (Fig. 3.10) (Kyles, 2012). The most common cause in dogs and cats is oesophageal reflux during anaesthesia (Adami et

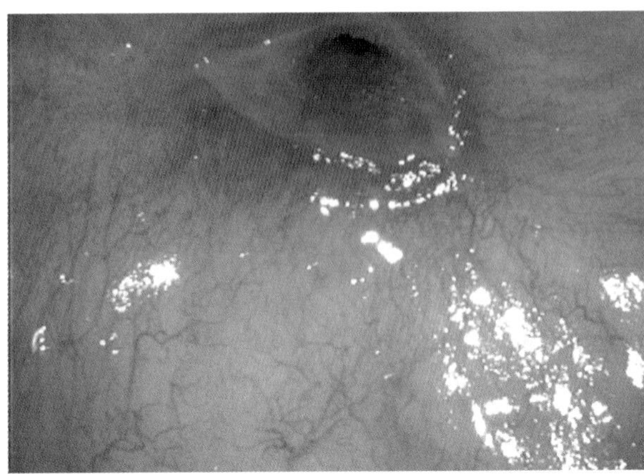

Fig. 3.10 Oesophagoscopy showing an oesophageal stricture. (Image courtesy of Nicki Read.)

al., 2011). A recent study showed that the prevalence of reflux events in cats during anaesthesia is similar to that of dogs (Garcia et al., 2017). Another study showed that large, deep-chested dogs have a higher frequency of gastro-oesophageal reflux in comparison to other breeds (Anagnostou et al., 2017).

The main clinical sign is regurgitation (usually 3 weeks after an anaesthetic). The diagnosis is made with positive contrast oesophagography or oesophagoscopy, but fluoroscopy can also be useful. Post-anaesthetic oesophageal strictures can occur at any site in the oesophagus and may be single or multiple.

One study showed that pre-anaesthetic administration of cisapride and esomeprazole decreased the number of reflux events in anaesthetised dogs, but administration of esomeprazole alone was associated with no acid and weakly acidic reflux in most dogs (Zacuto et al., 2012). Another study showed that the preoperative administration of omeprazole was effective in reducing the incidence of gastro-oesophageal reflux during anaesthesia in dogs (Panti et al., 2009).

The preferred method of treatment includes ballooning or bougienage (Sellon and Willard, 2003). Surgery should be advised only in cases where more conservative methods have failed.

Bougienage consists of conical dilation (increasing diameter) to push open a stricture (Bisset et al., 2009); balloon dilation involves inflating a balloon catheter within the stricture. Both techniques can be performed with endoscopic or fluoroscopic guidance. Balloon dilation uses a radial stretch force while bougienage uses a longitudinal shearing force. For this reason, bougienage is thought to be more aggressive and indicated for oesophageal perforation. Most animals require repeat dilation with a range of one to eight procedures (Harai et al., 1995; Leib et al., 2001), and for bougienage a median of three for dogs and five for cats (Bissett et al., 2009). The main complications of balloon dilation include perforation and recurrence. A good outcome is reported in 71–88% of cases (Leib et al., 2001). Following the procedure, animals should receive H2 receptor antagonists, proton pump inhibitors, sucralfate and prokinetic drugs to increase reduced oesophageal sphincter tone and gastric emptying. Corticosteroids are often prescribed to avoid scar tissue formation, but evidence supporting their efficacy is lacking. Intra-lesional injection of triamcinolone acetonide has also been reported in the literature (Fraune et al., 2009).

Stenting has been used to treat oesophageal strictures. Even though the technique is minimally invasive, safe and technically effective, the implant is unpredictably tolerated in dogs and significant complications have been reported (Lam et al., 2013).

Surgical options include simple oesophagoplasty (transverse closure of a longitudinal incision), resection anastomosis, patch oesophagoplasty (pericardium, diaphragm muscle, sternothyroideus) and oesophageal substitution (use of inverse skin graft or jejunal segment graft). Surgical correction is unfortunately associated with a high incidence of recurrence and dehiscence, and is therefore never advised as a first line of treatment.

3.2.4 Diverticulum

Oesophageal diverticulum is rare. In small animals, diverticula are classified as epiphrenic (arising between the heart base and diaphragm) and can often be associated with a broncho-oesophageal fistula (Della Ripa et al., 2010). The diverticulum can be impacted with food and cause oesophagitis, ulceration and subsequent stricture. Peridiverticulitis (inflammation surrounding the diverticulum) can cause a broncho-oesophageal fistula and adhesions to adjacent lung lobes.

Clinical signs include regurgitation, retching, gagging, gulping, generalised pain, hypersalivation, weight loss and anorexia. Respiratory distress may be associated with the presence of a broncho-oesophageal fistula or aspiration pneumonia. Lameness associated with secondary hypertrophic osteopathy has been reported. Some diverticula can be incidental (Kyles, 2012). Plain radiographs may show ingesta or an air-filled dilation in the caudal oesophagus. Positive contrast radiography is useful in delineating the diverticulum. Secondary broncho-oesophageal fistula can result in consolidation of a lung lobe and may be seen on positive contrast oesophagography. Oesophagoscopy can be useful, but care must be taken as perforation of the diverticulum may occur. CT may also be useful (Park et al., 2012).

A small diverticulum can be treated conservatively with a soft diet fed from a height. A large diverticulum usually requires surgical management through a lateral intercostal thoracotomy and excision of the diverticulum using a thoraco-abdominal stapler (TA™) (Pavletic, 1994). If a broncho-oesophageal fistula is present, lung lobectomy may be required. Large and multiple diverticula may require more extensive procedures, such as partial oesophageal resection or inlay patch, or oesophageal resection and anastomosis, and carry a grave prognosis. Single, small diverticula carry a good prognosis (Kyles, 2012).

3.2.5 Neoplasia

Oesophageal neoplasia is rare in small animals. In dogs the most reported primary tumours include squamous cell carcinoma, leiomyosarcoma, osteosarcoma, fibrosarcoma and undifferentiated sarcoma (Ranen et al., 2008). Benign tumours include leiomyoma and plasmocytoma. The most commonly affected site is the caudal oesophagus. In cats, squamous cell carcinoma is the most common tumour. Para-oesophageal tumours can also invade the oesophagus. In dogs, most cases of oesophageal osteosarcoma, fibrosarcoma and undifferentiated sarcoma are associated with *Spirocerca lupi*, a nematode found in tropical and subtropical areas. *Spirocerca* nodules can degenerate into malignant sarcomas (Nivy et al., 2014).

Clinical signs include regurgitation, vomiting and megaoesophagus (Arnell et al., 2013). Hypertrophic osteopathy has been reported, particularly with *Spirocerca*-induced oesophageal sarcoma (Kyles, 2012).

Diagnosis can be made by radiography, contrast studies and advanced imaging. Haematology may show microcytic anaemia due to chronic blood loss and neutrophilia. *S. lupi* ova can be detected in the faeces of dogs with oesophageal sarcoma. Oesophagoscopy allows direct visualisation of the lesions and cytological evaluation.

Most oesophageal tumours are advanced at the time of diagnosis, and metastases are seen in more than 50% of cases. For this reason, surgery is rarely indicated but palliation can be provided by placement of a gastrostomy tube. Partial oesophagectomy followed by chemotherapy has been reported in the management of sarcoma, with survival ranging from 2 to 16 months (Ranen et al., 2004). Trans-endoscopic oesophageal mass ablation in dogs with spirocercosis-associated oesophageal neoplasia has been reported as an alternative to open surgery (Shipov et al., 2015; Yas et al., 2013). In most cases the prognosis for oesophageal tumours is very poor.

3.3 The stomach

Key points

- The stomach is a very well-vascularised organ with good healing properties.
- Its location in the cranial abdomen and underneath the rib cage can make surgical management challenging, especially in deep-chested breeds.
- Abnormalities of the stomach, in particular some gastric foreign bodies, may be incidental findings. For this reason, a full exploratory coeliotomy should always be performed before addressing the gastric pathology.

3.3.1 Anatomy

The stomach is divided into the cardia, fundus, body, pyloric antrum and pylorus (Fig. 3.11) and is composed of four layers: mucosa, submucosa, muscularis and serosa. The gastric (lesser curvature) and gastro-epiploic (greater curvature) arteries supply the stomach and are derived from the coeliac artery. The short gastric arteries arise from the splenic artery and supply the greater curvature. A hepatogastric ligament attaches the stomach to the liver (Fossum, 2013).

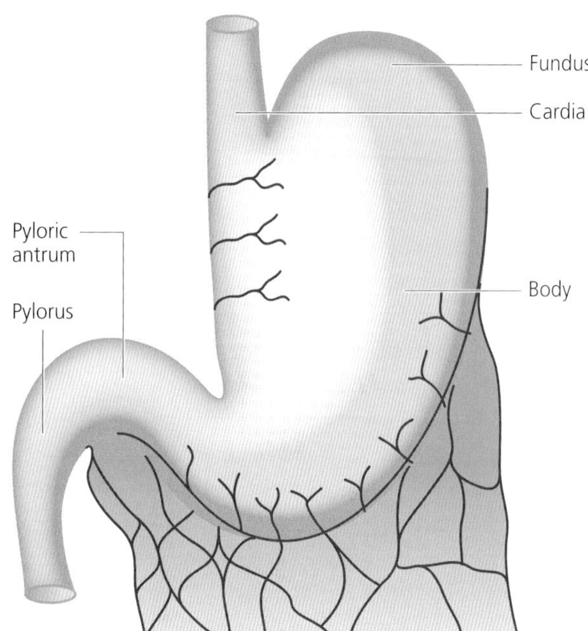

Fig. 3.11 Anatomical areas of the stomach.

3.3.2 Surgical principles

A full exploratory coeliotomy should be performed when operating on the stomach. Increased exposure can be accomplished by performing a long incision (xiphisternum to the pubic brim), removal of the falciform fat, usage of abdominal retractors and good theatre lighting. Further exposure can be achieved by performing a caudal median sternotomy or a diaphragmatic myotomy. Tissue contamination can be minimised by packing sterile laparotomy swabs soaked in warm sterile saline, and by tenting the stomach up with stay sutures before starting an incision. The submucosa layer is the holding layer for the whole of the gastrointestinal tract, and it should be closed using an appositional pattern (simple continuous or simple interrupted). When a two-layer pattern is used for closure, an inverting pattern can be used in the outer layers (muscularis and serosa). When performing abdominal surgery, both local and general lavage should be performed and all fluid suctioned. All swabs and small instruments should be counted at the beginning of the procedure and just before closure of the abdominal cavity, to minimise the chances of a gossypiboma (retained foreign object).

3.3.3 Hiatal hernia

The oesophageal hiatus is formed by the medial portion of the lumbar crus of the diaphragm. The opening allows passage of the oesophagus, associated blood vessels and vagosympathetic trunk (Evans and de Lahunta, 2013). Hiatal hernia refers to herniation of abdominal contents through the oesophageal hiatus.

Four types of hiatal hernia have been described in the human literature, and the classification system is summarised in Table 3.3. In small animals, the majority of reported hernias are type I and congenital in origin, and are therefore seen more commonly in young animals. An unusual type III hiatal hernia has been reported in a great Dane (Gordon et al., 2010). Affected breeds include Chinese Shar-Pei, English bulldog, French bulldog and great Dane and also cats (Gordon et al., 2010; Guiot et al., 2008; Reeve et al., 2017). One recent study showed that prevalence is higher than expected in the French bulldog (Reeve et al., 2017).

Table 3.3 Types of hiatal hernia described in the human literature.

Hiatal hernia classification	
Type I/sliding	Intermittent movement of the gastro-oesophageal junction into the thoracic cavity
Type II/para-oesophageal	Gastro-oesophageal junction remains in normal position and a portion of the fundus herniates
Type III	Elements of types I and II
Type IV	Herniation of abdominal organs other than the stomach

Acquired type I hiatal hernia has been reported as a result of trauma or in breeds with severe upper

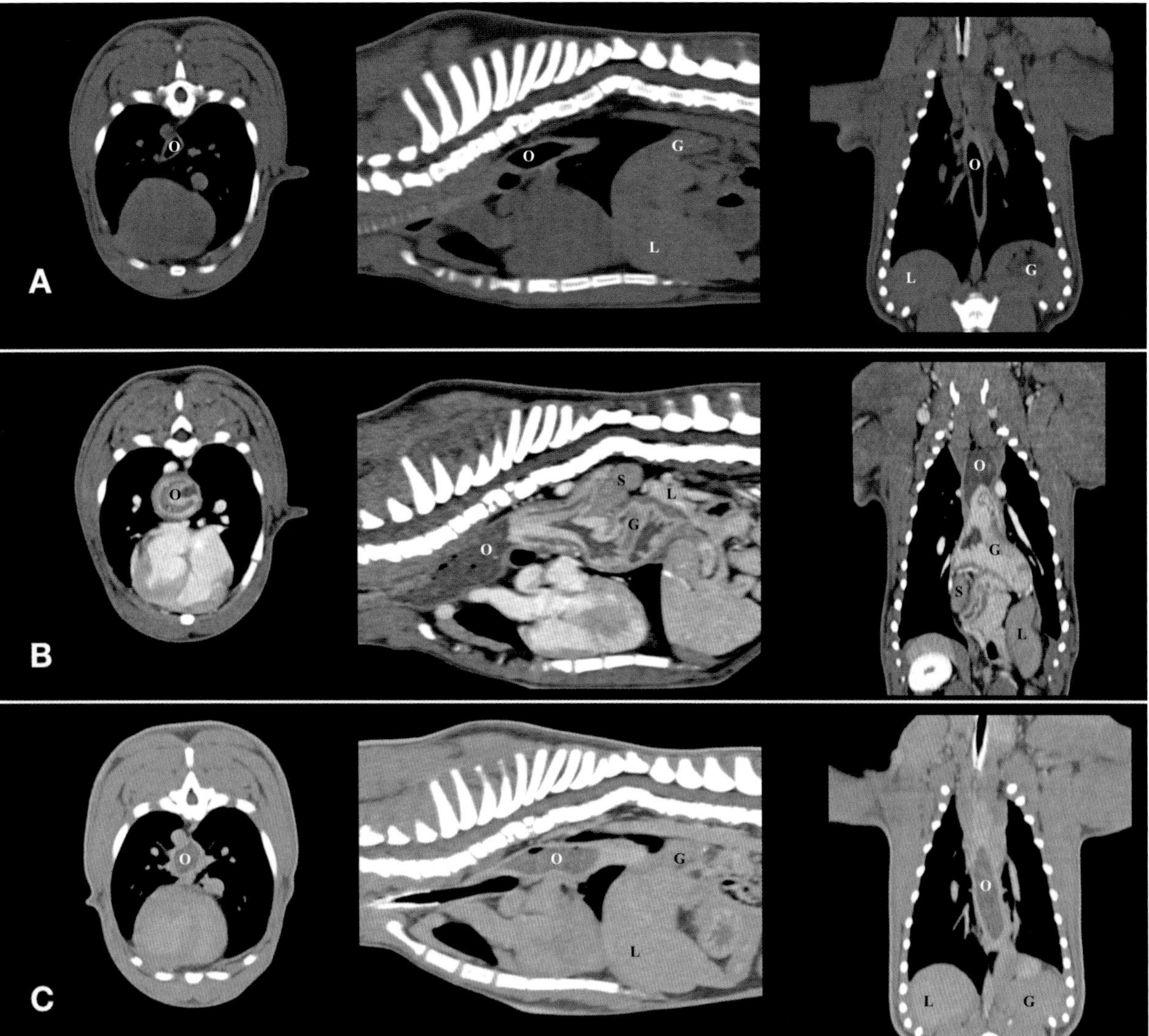

Fig. 3.12a–c Transverse, sagittal and dorsal plane CT views of the thorax and cranial abdomen. a. Soft tissue window before contrast injection, representing normal anatomy. b. Post-contrast administration study showing a hiatal hernia with herniated stomach, liver and spleen. c. All abdominal organs returned to their anatomical position and the oesophagus is fluid filled.

O, oesophagus; G, stomach; S, spleen; L, liver. (Images courtesy of the imaging department at the University of Edinburgh.)

respiratory effort, such as brachycephalic breeds or animals with laryngeal paralysis. These animals have decreased intrathoracic pressure during inspiration that may contribute to oesophageal reflux and hiatal herniation (Cornell, 2012a).

Clinical signs vary and can include regurgitation, anorexia, hypersalivation, vomiting, dysphagia, haematemesis and respiratory distress (Prymak et al., 1989).

The diagnosis can be made with plain radiographs and positive contrast oesophagograms. Fluoroscopy is useful in the diagnosis of dynamic cases (Fig. 3.12) and minimises the level of restraint required in animals with respiratory distress (Levine et al., 2014). Reflux oesophagitis occurs concurrently and may be diagnosed on oesophagoscopy (Reeve et al., 2017).

In stable cases, medical therapy should be attempted first and trialled for up to one month. Para-oesophageal hiatal hernia and large, sliding hiatal hernia should be considered for prompt surgical treatment (Sivacolundhu et al., 2002).

The goals of medical management are to (1) reduce the secretion of gastric acid, which provides protection to the oesophageal mucosa and (2) increase the rate of gastric emptying whilst augmenting the tone of the lower oesophageal sphincter. Drugs commonly used include famotidine, ranitidine, cimetidine, omeprazole and sucralfate. Sucralfate can decrease the absorption of the other drugs, and therefore administration should be separated by 2 hours. Metoclopramide increases gastric emptying and the tone of the lower oesophageal sphincter, and is advisable.

Several surgical procedures have been described for the management of hiatal hernia. The author advises using the following procedures in conjunction: reduction of the oesophageal hiatus (phrenoplasty), oesophagopexy and left-sided gastropexy. All procedures are performed through a ventral midline abdominal approach. There are no set standards regarding optimal hiatal size, and therefore clinical judgement will have to be used.

Step by step: surgical management of hiatal hernia

- A ventral midline coeliotomy is performed.
- The left lobes of the liver are medially retracted to expose the oesophageal hiatus (Fig. 3.13a).
- The hernia is reduced (Fig. 3.13b).
- The left triangular ligament (ligament between the left lobe of the liver and the diaphragm) is transected.
- A stomach tube is passed to help identify and manipulate the cardia.
- Phrenoplasty: the oesophageal hiatus is identified and reduced by placing interrupted sutures between the diaphragmatic muscle using 1.5 or 2.0 metric polypropylene. Leave a 1 cm gap so that the vagus nerve does not become entrapped (Fig. 3.13c).
- Oesophagopexy: using a dry swab, the oesophageal wall is gently wiped until it appears red. Interrupted sutures are placed between the outer layers of the oesophagus (adventitia and muscularis) and the diaphragm. These sutures should be placed approximately 0.5 cm apart and 360° around the oesophagus using 1.5 or 2.0 metric polypropylene. Try to visualise the vagus nerve so that it does not become entrapped (Fig. 3.13d).
- Incisional left-sided gastropexy: a 2 cm incision is made in the seromuscular layer of the fundic region of the stomach, and a 2 cm incision is made in the left body wall. The edges of the incisions are sutured together with simple continuous patterns using 2.0 or 3.0 metric polydioxanone (Fig. 3.13e).

Handy hints

In an incisional gastropexy, first start the most dorsal suture line at its cranial extent then start the ventral suture line at its cranial extent. Complete the dorsal suture line and then complete the ventral suture line. This will maximise your visualisation during the procedure. Lavage the abdominal cavity, omentalise the pexy site and close the abdomen in three layers.

Postoperatively, animals need to be monitored for complications including recurrence, gastric dilatation and volvulus (Aslanian et al., 2014) and pneumothorax. Regurgitation may persist due to inflammation, but sudden deterioration may indicate failure and requirement for revision surgery. The best postoperative prognosis appears to be associated with the oesophagopexy technique (Lorinson and Bright, 1998). Recent evidence suggests that the clinical signs of sliding hiatal hernia improve following surgery but do not consistently resolve (Mayhew et al., 2017).

3.3.4 Gastric outflow disease

Gastric outflow disease, or pyloric outflow obstruction, may be congenital or acquired. Congenital obstructions are usually muscular in origin and occur most commonly in brachycephalic breeds younger than 1 year of age, and are commonly referred to as pyloric stenosis. Acquired obstructions may be mucosal or a combination of mucosal and muscular in origin. Acquired obstructions occur most commonly in small breeds (<10 kg). Studies have shown that brachycephalic breeds that present with respiratory signs may have concurrent pyloric outflow obstructions. It has been hypothesised that chronic air dilation of the stomach occurring secondary

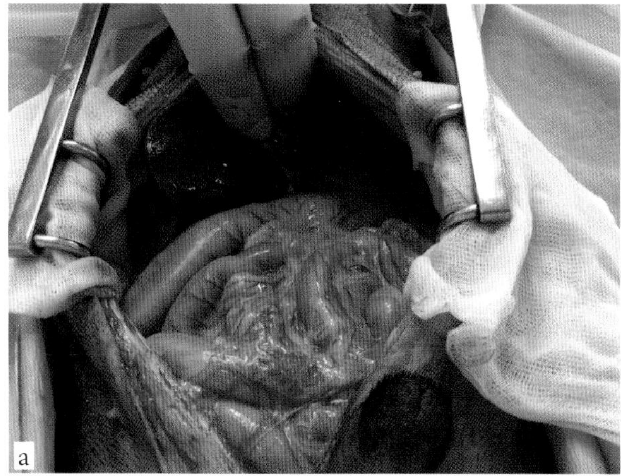

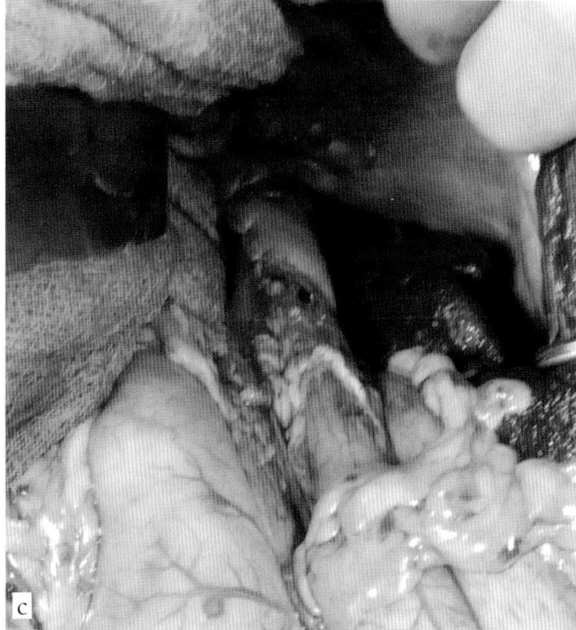

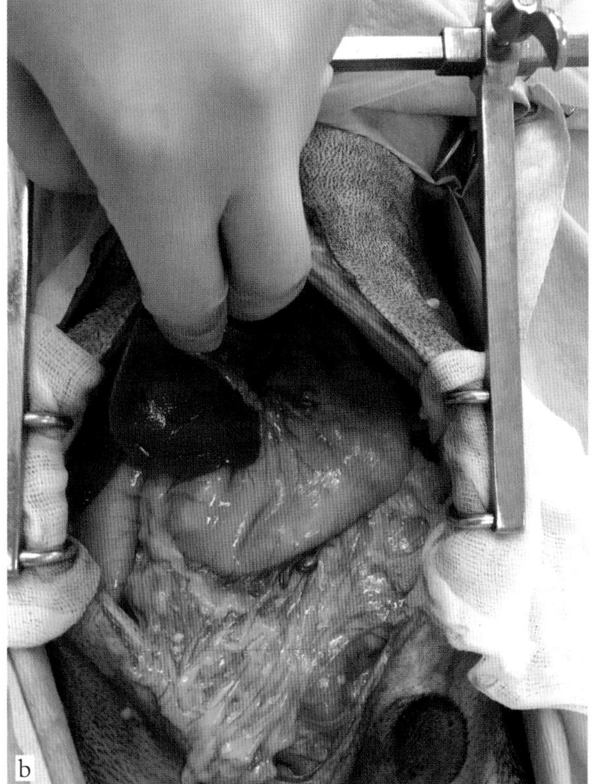

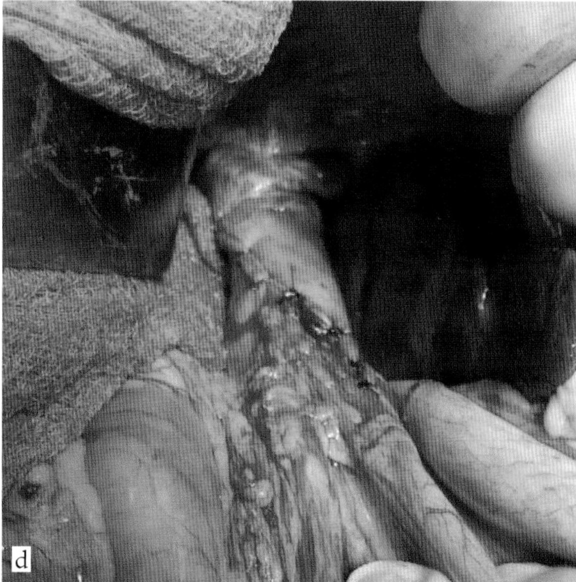

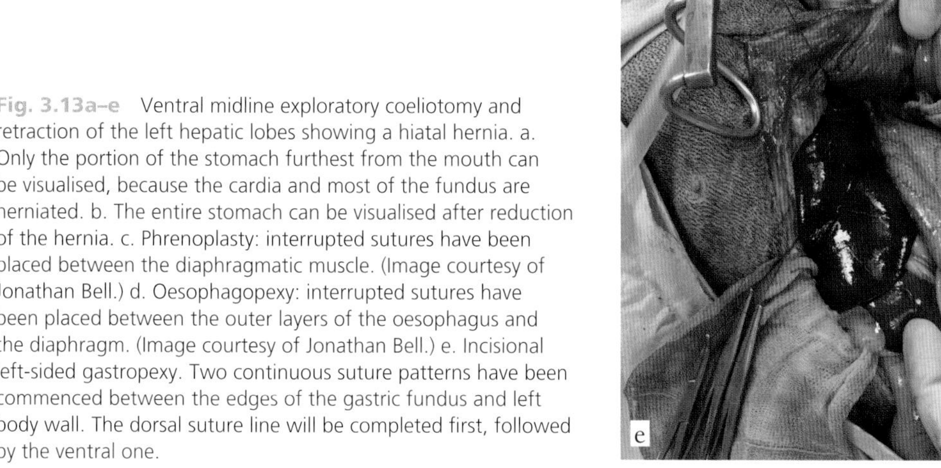

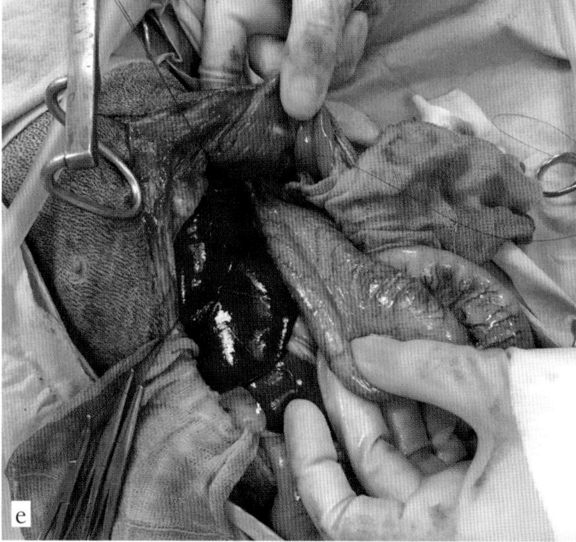

Fig. 3.13a–e Ventral midline exploratory coeliotomy and retraction of the left hepatic lobes showing a hiatal hernia. a. Only the portion of the stomach furthest from the mouth can be visualised, because the cardia and most of the fundus are herniated. b. The entire stomach can be visualised after reduction of the hernia. c. Phrenoplasty: interrupted sutures have been placed between the diaphragmatic muscle. (Image courtesy of Jonathan Bell.) d. Oesophagopexy: interrupted sutures have been placed between the outer layers of the oesophagus and the diaphragm. (Image courtesy of Jonathan Bell.) e. Incisional left-sided gastropexy. Two continuous suture patterns have been commenced between the edges of the gastric fundus and left body wall. The dorsal suture line will be completed first, followed by the ventral one.

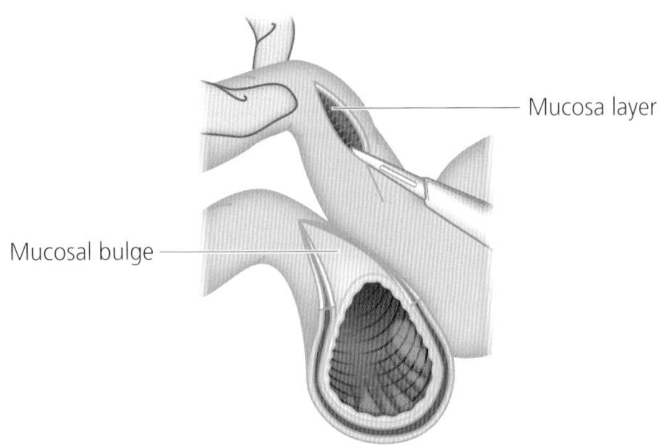

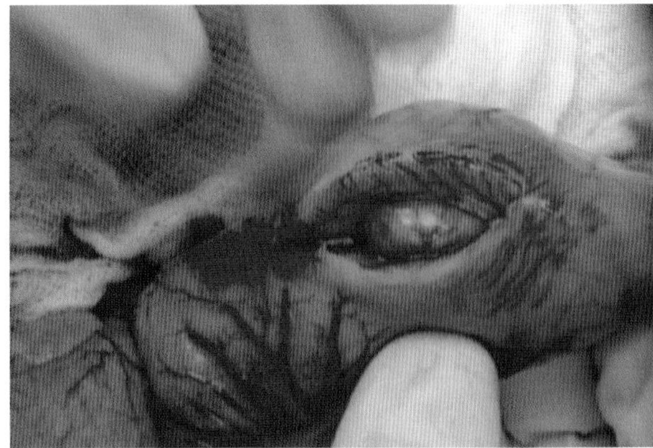

Fig. 3.14 Fredet–Ramstedt pyloromyotomy. *Illustrator: Elaine Leggett*

to upper respiratory difficulties leads to increased intragastric pressure, secondary secretion of gastrin and gastric acid and the resultant production of cholecystokinin and secretin, which have a trophic effect on the antral and pyloric mucosa (Cornell, 2012a).

Clinical signs can include chronic intermittent vomiting containing partially digested food, regurgitation and hypersalivation.

The diagnosis is suggested when survey radiographs show delayed gastric emptying of over 8 hours. Contrast radiographs may show a distended stomach or narrowing of the pyloric region (apple core appearance). Ultrasound may be useful in assessing the thickness of the pyloric layers. In cases of mucosal hypertrophy, endoscopy may readily identify the problem area and allow biopsy collection.

Most cases require surgical management. However, correction of dehydration, electrolyte imbalance, oesophagitis and potential aspiration pneumonia takes priority. Several procedures have been described depending on the severity of the disease and the specific pyloric layer affected. In cases of muscular hypertrophy alone, a Fredet–Ramstedt pyloromyotomy (longitudinal incision in the seromuscular layer) may be used to increase the pyloric outflow tract diameter. In cases of mucosal or combined mucosal and muscular hypertrophy, a transverse (Heineke–Mikulicz) or Y–U advancement pyloroplasty is indicated (Randolph, 1975). In children, the Heineke–Mikulicz procedure has not always been satisfactory because of inadequate size and distortion of the muscular gastroduodenal funnel, and thus Y–U advancement pyloroplasty has been developed (Randolph, 1975). Both these techniques require entering of the lumen and facilitate a full-thickness biopsy collection.

The outcome after surgical correction of benign conditions of the pylorus is very good with a good to excellent response to surgery in greater than 80% of affected animals (Cornell, 2012a).

Step by step: Fredet–Ramstedt pyloromyotomy (Fig. 3.14)

- A ventral midline coeliotomy is performed.
- The pylorus is identified and a longitudinal incision is made through the seromuscular layer in a hypovascular area.

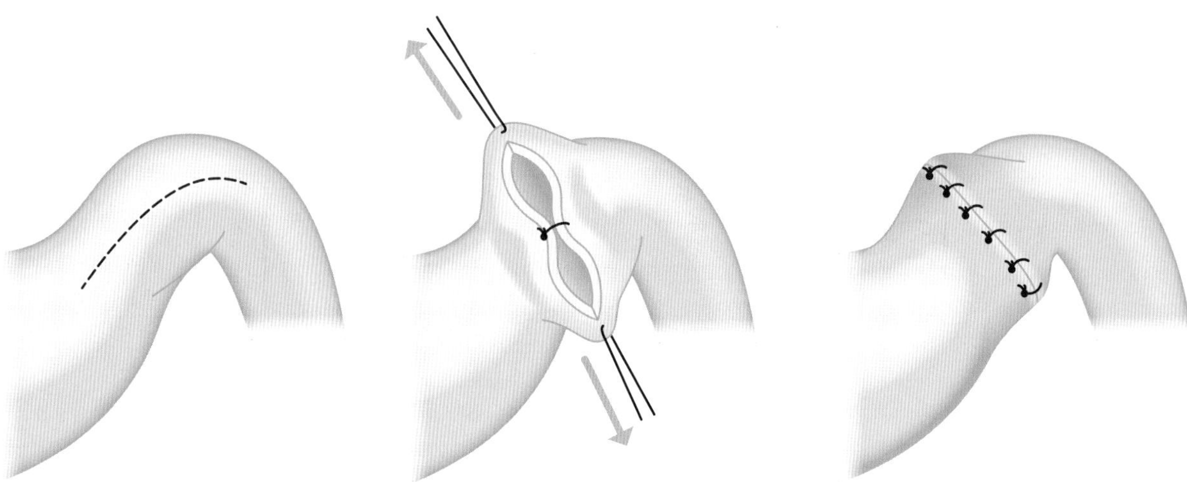

Fig. 3.15 Heineke–Mikulicz pyloroplasty. *Illustrator: Elaine Leggett*

- The muscularis should be completely incised in order that the muscosa can bulge through the incision site.
- The abdominal cavity is lavaged and the abdominal cavity is closed in three layers.

Step by step: Heineke–Mikulicz pyloroplasty (Fig. 3.15)

- A ventral midline coeliotomy is performed.
- A longitudinal full-thickness incision is made in the ventral surface of the pylorus.
- Stay sutures are placed at the centre of the incision and traction is applied so that it is oriented transversally.
- The incision is closed transversally using 2.0 or 3.0 metric polydioxanone sutures in a simple interrupted pattern.
- A watertight seal closure should be achieved.
- The abdominal cavity is lavaged, the suture line is omentalised and the abdominal cavity is closed in three layers.

Step by step: Y–U pyloroplasty

- A ventral midline coeliotomy is performed.
- A 'Y'-shaped, full-thickness incision is made in the pylorus with the arms of the 'Y' parallel to the lesser and greater curvature of the stomach and the 'leg' into the pylorus/duodenum (Fig. 3.16a).
- The base of the central flap is sutured to the distal end of the duodenal incision with a simple interrupted suture using 2.0 or 3.0 metric polydioxanone (Fig. 3.16b).
- The remainder of the flap can then be sutured using the same pattern. The end result should be a 'U'-shaped flap (Fig. 3.16c).
- A watertight seal closure should be achieved.
- The abdominal cavity is lavaged, the suture line is omentalised and the abdominal cavity is closed in three layers.

3.3.5 Foreign body

Gastric foreign body is one of the most common indications for gastrotomy in small animals. Dogs are more commonly affected, as they tend to be less selective in what they ingest. Foreign bodies can be singular or multiple, blunt or sharp and linear or non-linear. Examples include fishhooks, sewing needles, bones, sticks, wooden skewers, pebbles and magnetic material (Garneau and McCarthy, 2015). Linear foreign bodies can present a particular challenge because these are often anchored to the stomach and continue into the small intestine (Hobday et al., 2014; Hunt et al., 2004; Pratt et al., 2014).

Clinical signs can vary from absent to vomiting, regurgitation, abdominal distension, abdominal pain and electrolyte and acid–base abnormalities. One study showed that dogs with a linear foreign body were more likely to have a history of vomiting, anorexia, lethargy and pain on abdominal palpation. They were also more likely to require intestinal resection and anastomosis and require a longer hospitalisation time (Hobday et al., 2014). Another study looking at dogs with gastrointestinal foreign bodies found that the most common electrolyte and acid–base abnormalities were hypochloraemia (51.2%), metabolic alkalosis (45.2%), hypokalaemia (25%) and hyponatremia (20.5%). No significant association was found between electrolyte or acid–base abnormalities and the site of the foreign body (Boag et al., 2005).

Diagnosis can be made by radiography (plain or contrast), abdominal ultrasound, endoscopy or by more advanced imaging modalities such as CT scan. The

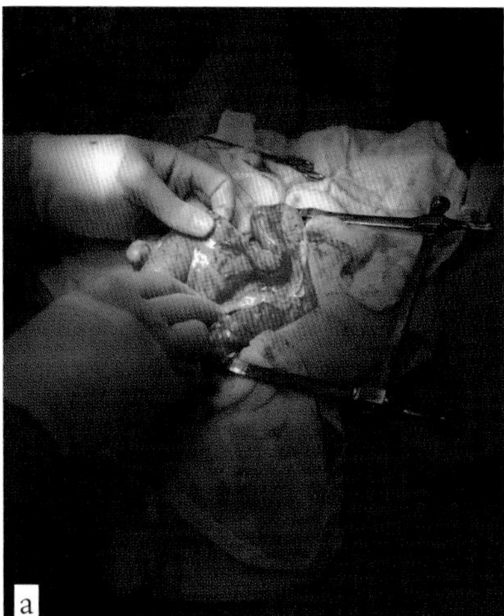

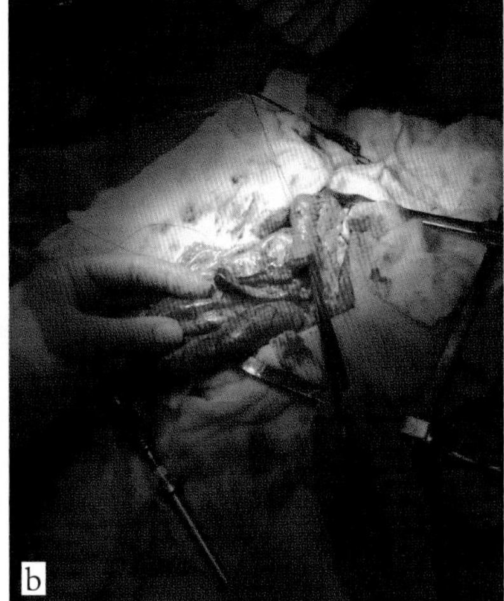

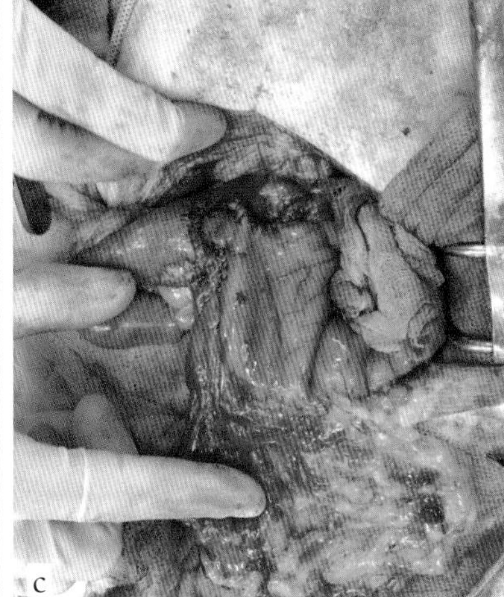

Fig. 3.16a–c Y–U pyloroplasty. (Images courtesy of Jon Hall.) a. A Y-shaped incision is made in the pylorus, with the arms of the 'Y' parallel to the lesser and greater curvature of the stomach and the 'leg' into the pylorus/duodenum. b. The full-thickness incision is completed. c. The flap is sutured in place with the base of the central flap sutured to the distal end of the duodenal incision.

presence of free gas in a survey abdominal radiograph indicates perforation and the likelihood of peritonitis. One study showed that ultrasonography alone could be used to make the diagnosis and may be a more appropriate choice than survey radiography (Tyrrell and Beck, 2006).

Endoscopic removal of foreign bodies has become more popular, and the success rate is high even if the foreign body is sharp (Binvel et al., 2017; Pratt et al., 2014). Equipment and technical experience greatly influence the success rate. Surgical management is indicated when endoscopic retrieval fails or is not available, or when there are radiographic or ultrasonographic signs of perforation or peritonitis. The procedure of choice is gastrotomy through a ventral midline exploratory coeliotomy.

Handy hints

The length of the incision depends on the size of the foreign body, and instruments used to manipulate and retrieve the foreign body should be separated from the remaining pack and considered contaminated. The author usually changes gloves after foreign body retrieval.

Step by step: gastrotomy for foreign body removal

- A ventral midline coeliotomy is performed.
- The stomach is isolated by packing sterile laparotomy swabs soaked in sterile saline.
- An avascular area of the stomach is chosen to be incised (usually in the fundic region) and is exteriorised by placing two stay sutures and tenting them up with haemostats (Fig. 3.17a).
- An incision is made with a no. 11 scalpel blade, making sure that it goes through all the gastric layers.
- The incision is enlarged as required using Metzenbaum scissors (Fig. 3.17b).
- The foreign body is removed.
- The gastric wall is closed in one or two layers using either polydioxanone or polyglecaprone-25 in a taper-cut needle.
- For single-layer closure an appositional pattern is used, such as a simple interrupted or a simple continuous pattern.
- For a double-layer closure an appositional pattern is used in the mucosa and submucosa, such as a

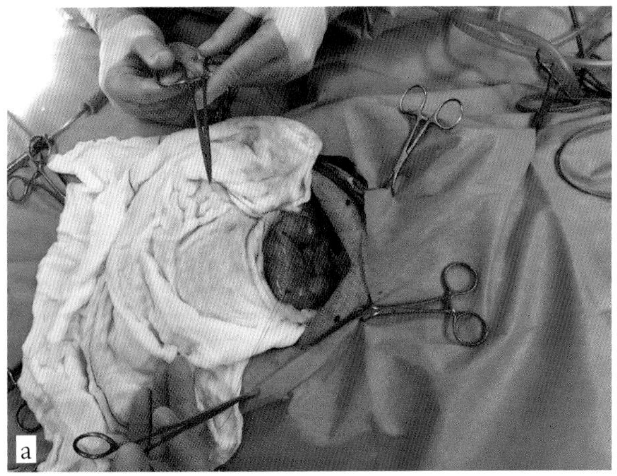

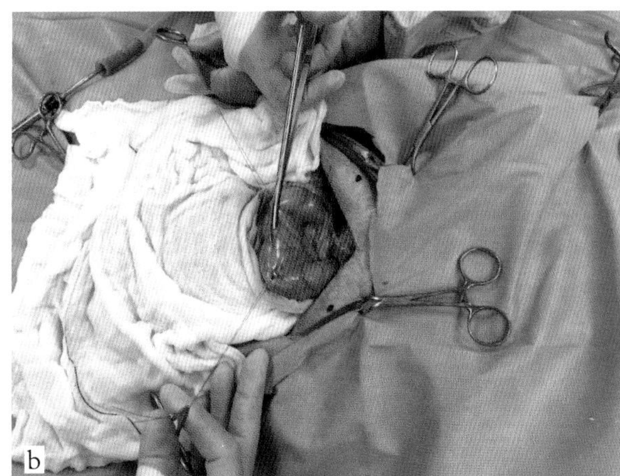

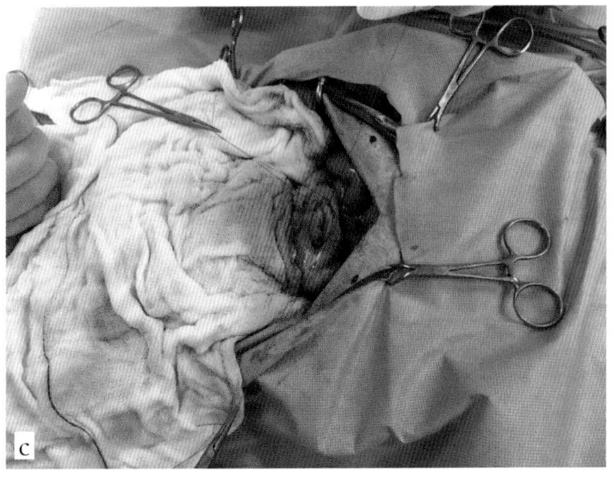

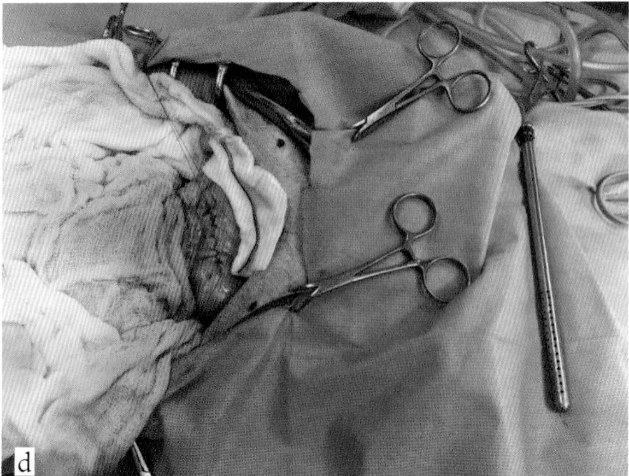

Fig. 3.17a–d Gastrotomy for foreign body removal. (Images courtesy of Samantha Woods.) a. An avascular area of the stomach is chosen to be incised, and is exteriorised by placing two stay sutures and tenting them up with a haemostat. b. A full-thickness incision has been performed with a no. 11 scalpel blade and is being enlarged with Metzenbaum scissors. c. The mucosa and submucosa layers are being apposed with a simple continuous pattern. d. The seromuscular layer has been closed with an inverting pattern.

simple interrupted or simple continuous pattern; an inverting pattern is used in the seromuscular layer, such as a Cushing or Lembert pattern (Fig. 3.17c,d).
- A watertight seal closure should be achieved.
- The abdominal cavity is lavaged, the suture line is omentalised and the abdominal cavity is closed in three layers.

Postoperative care includes analgesia, anti-acids and prokinetic agents such as metoclopramide if regurgitation occurs. Feeding can be initiated with a bland diet as soon as the animal is fully recovered from its anaesthetic.

The prognosis is usually good for a simple gastrotomy. Complications include regurgitation, postoperative ileus and dehiscence of the surgical site with secondary peritonitis. One study showed that large or giant-breed dogs with a gastric foreign body were approximately five times more likely to develop gastric dilatation and volvulus in comparison to a similar dog with no gastric foreign body (de Battisti et al., 2012).

3.3.6 Dilatation and volvulus

Gastric dilatation and volvulus (GDV) is a life-threatening condition that most commonly affects large breeds and, in particular, deep-chested dogs. In GDV the stomach rotates on its axis, usually clockwise, trapping air in the lumen and increasing intra-gastric pressure. The results of one study suggest that the gaseous gastric distension is not the result of aerophagia (Van Kruiningen et al., 2013). Severe gastric distension causes compression of the caudal vena cava, decreasing venous return to the heart and cardiac output. The end result is a mixture of portal hypertension, systemic hypotension, hypovolaemic shock and cardiogenic shock.

With continuing collapse of the gastric capillaries, gastric wall necrosis, bacterial translocation (stomach and other hypo-perfused areas) and perforation can occur. Pressure on the diaphragm from the distended stomach makes inspiration more difficult and further decreases oxygen delivery (Cornell, 2012a).

The impact of GDV on cardiac function is multifactorial. Inadequate coronary vessel flow, coupled with the production of myocardial depressant factor, results in myocardial ischaemia and subsequent cardiac arrhythmias, further decreasing systemic perfusion (Sharp and Rozanski, 2014).

The cause of GDV is not completely understood. Specific risks factors identified in dogs include pure breed and large or giant breed; increased thoracic depth-to-width ratio; history of gastric dilatation and volvulus in a relative; feeding fewer meals per day; eating rapidly; decreased food particle size; aggressive or fearful temperament; increased hepatogastric ligament length; and exercise or stress after a meal (Bell, 2014; Gazzola and Nelson, 2014; Glickman et al., 2000a,b; Harkey et al., 2017; Raghavan et al., 2004). Previous splenectomy has been suggested as a risk factor, but different studies show contradictory results (Goldhammer et al., 2010; Grange et al., 2012; Maki et al., 2017; Sartor et al., 2013). For this reason, the current recommendation remains to perform gastropexy at the time of splenic removal only in cases considered high risk or with a family history of GDV.

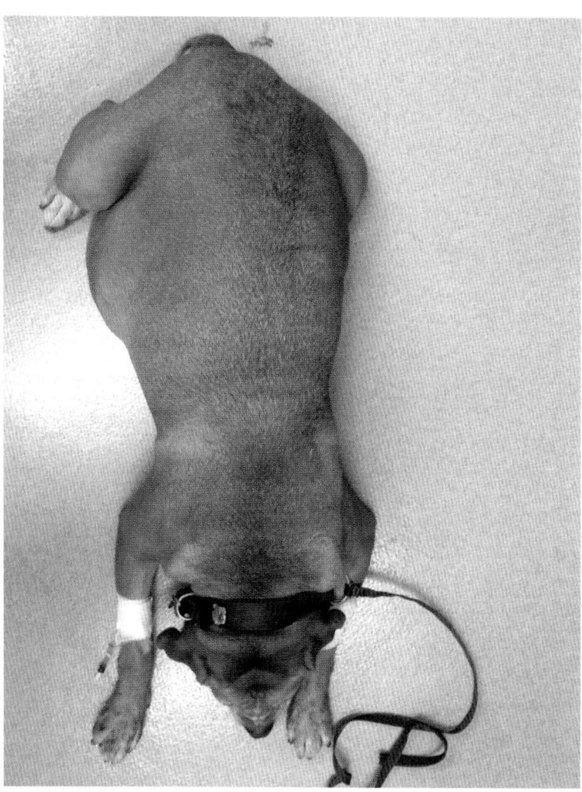

Fig. 3.18 Abdominal distension and collapse in a dog with GDV. (Image courtesy of Jon Hall.)

Clinical signs include abdominal distension, unproductive retching, restlessness and hypersalivation. Shock may also be present with pale mucous membranes, increased capillary refill time, weak or absent peripheral pulses, bradycardia and cold temperature (Fig. 3.18). The diagnosis is made based on the history, signalment and clinical examination findings. A recent paper looked at differentiation between gastric dilatation and volvulus. A method of measuring gastric distension is described which has highlighted that gastric dilation secondary to food engorgement can be marked and that there is a large degree of overlap between dogs with gastric dilation and volvulus. In patients with food engorgement, the degree of gastric dilation was not associated with increased blood lactate concentration, suggesting no compromise of oxygen delivery (Humm and Bartfield, 2017). More importantly, animals with gastric dilation only were effectively treated with

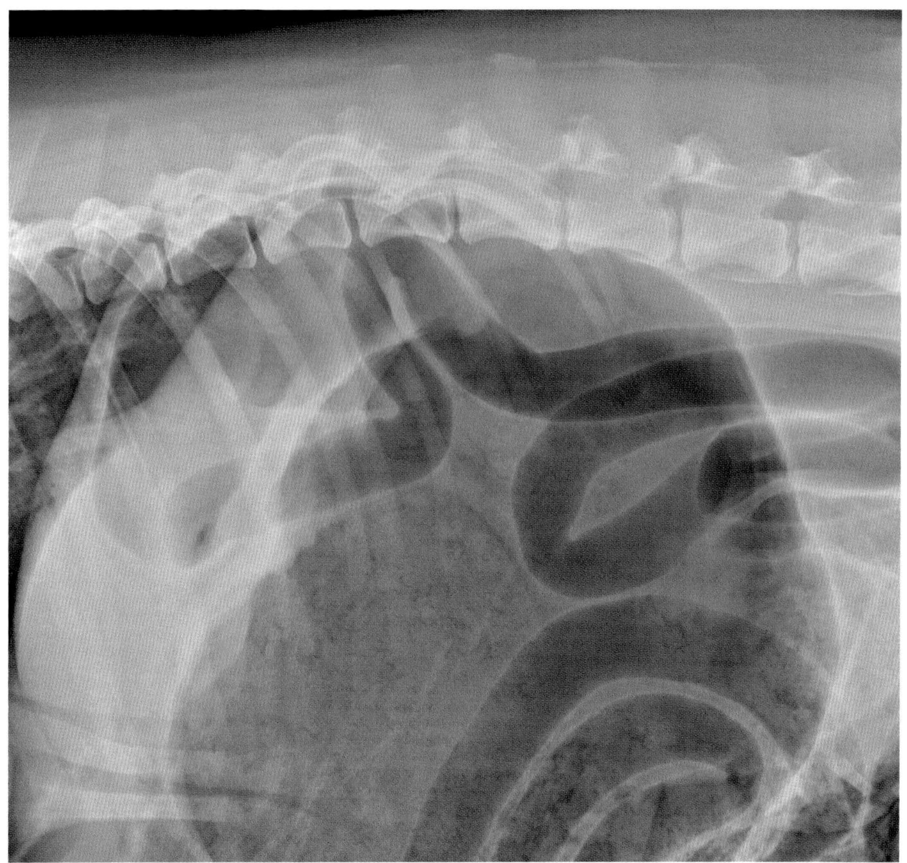

Fig. 3.19 Right lateral radiograph showing gastric dilation and a reverse 'C' sign indicating the presence of gastric volvulus.

intravenous fluids and analgesia and none developed GDV. Even though that study is retrospective and incorporates a relatively small population sample, it raises an important point in distinguishing between dilation and GDV. This can be done by performing a right lateral radiograph and looking for signs of torsion including a double bubble, a reverse 'C' or a Popeye sign (Fig. 3.19). These changes are the result of seeing air in the pylorus that is separated from air in the body of the stomach by a soft tissue density. Another important radiographic abnormality is the presence of a pneumoperitoneum, which indicates gastric perforation and likely necrosis and a poorer prognosis. However, we must be careful in interpreting this finding if trocharisation of the stomach has occurred previously. Other reported radiographic findings include a small vena cava, oesophageal dilation, microcardia and aspiration pneumonia (Green et al., 2012).

Rarely, dogs may develop chronic intermittent gastric dilation with partial volvulus. Clinical signs include weight loss, chronic vomiting, lethargy and abdominal pain. This is not an emergency situation and can be challenging to diagnose. A combination of radiography, ultrasonography and endoscopy may be required to detect altered positioning of gastric landmarks. Affected animals responded well to a right-sided gastropexy (Paris et al., 2011).

Medical management of the condition aims at stabilisation of the animal. Fluid therapy is the most critical component before surgery. Two large-bore catheters should be placed in the cephalic or jugular vessels and shock doses (90 ml/kg/h) of crystalloids should be administered. Colloids can be concurrently administered to help support oncotic pressure. If hypotension persists after appropriate volume expansion, vasopressor therapy may be administered (Cornell, 2012a). Gastric decompression is attempted next, with orogastric intubation (do not forget to pre-measure the tube to the last rib). If resistance is met and the tube cannot be advanced, trocharisation can be considered. Both techniques have been associated with low complication and high success rates (Goodrich et al., 2013).

The animal should be monitored regularly (every 10–15 minutes) for signs of systemic improvement meeting at least 2 of 3 criteria: (1) capillary refill time 1–2 seconds, pink mucous membrane colour, strong femoral pulse quality; (2) heart rate (HR) ≤150/min; and (3) indirect arterial systolic blood pressure (SBP) >90 mmHg. Oxygen therapy can be delivered flow-by to increase oxygen saturation of haemoglobin. An electrocardiogram should be continuously monitored and cardiac arrhythmias should be treated if these result in pulse deficits or poor peripheral perfusion or are likely to progress to fibrillation.

Once stabilisation has been achieved, treatment should progress with surgical intervention. Timing is critical, as delaying surgery may result in gastric necrosis and perforation. The goals of surgery are to reposition the stomach, remove devitalised or necrotic tissue, check the spleen and create a permanent adhesion between the pyloric antrum and the right body wall.

A full exploratory coeliotomy incision is performed and the stomach is de-rotated (Fig. 3.20a). The stomach is fully emptied by repeated orogastric intubation guided by the surgeon. Gastric lavage may be required to remove food or thick gastric content. A full exploration of the abdominal cavity is followed and the stomach and spleen are assessed for viability. To assess gastric viability the surgeon inspects the serosal layer looking at the colour, peristalsis, texture (thinning of the wall) and whether it bleeds when nicked (Fig. 3.20b). For splenic viability, the surgeon looks at the colour after de-rotation and whether the supply vessels appear patent or thrombotic/avulsed. If a non-viable area of the stomach is present (black or green in colour, or thinned wall), a partial gastrectomy should be performed. If a small area of questionable viability is present, gastric invagination can be considered by performing an inverting suture pattern (Fig. 3.20c). If the spleen is non-viable, a splenectomy should be performed. After dealing with devitalised tissue, a permanent adhesion must be created. For this, a right-sided gastropexy should be performed. Several techniques have been described, but the authors prefer the incisional gastropexy. This technique is simple and fast and an effective way of creating a strong and permanent adhesion (Allen and Paul, 2014; Benitez et al., 2013; Przywara et al., 2014). Tube gastropexy techniques have also been used with success (Belch et al., 2017).

Step by step: gastrectomy for resection of necrotic tissue or a mass lesion

- The stomach is isolated by packing sterile laparotomy swabs soaked in sterile saline.
- The area of the stomach to be resected is identified.
- The vessels supplying this portion of the stomach are ligated: branches of the right and left gastric artery and vein (lesser curvature) and left gastro-epiploic artery and vein (greater curvature).
- Any omental attachments are removed.
- If possible, stay sutures are placed around the area to be resected and the stomach is tented up (Fig. 3.21). This will minimise spillage, but is not always possible depending on the area requiring resection and the extent of tissue to be resected.
- The affected area is resected, leaving a normal and actively bleeding area to suture.
- The gastric wall is closed in one or two layers as described for the gastrotomy technique.

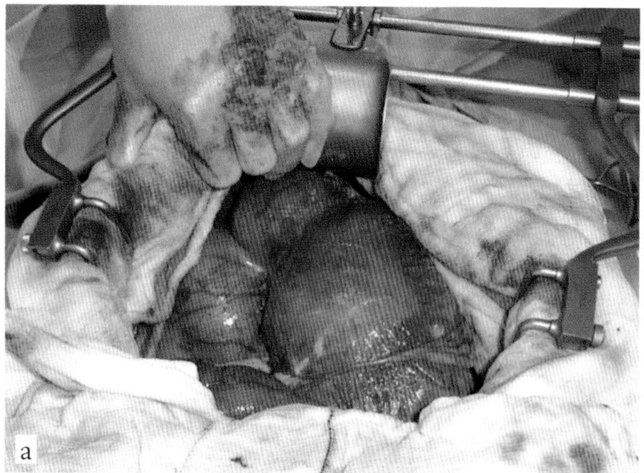

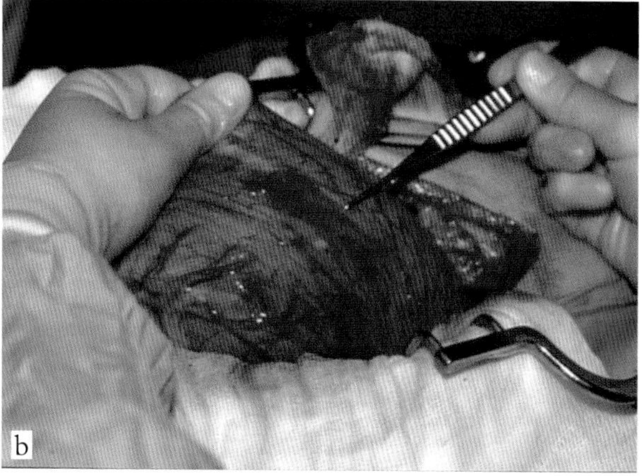

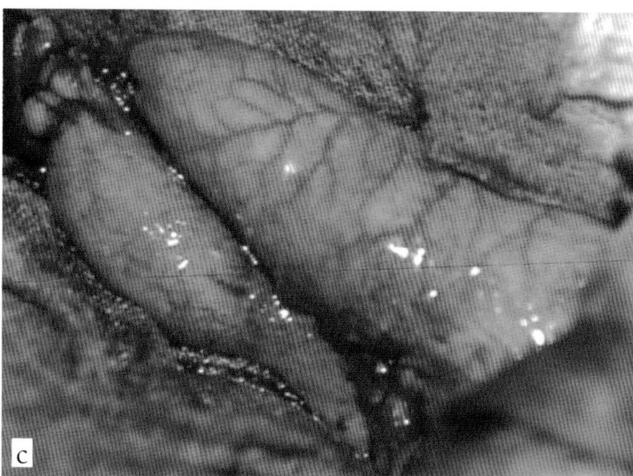

Fig. 3.20a–c Surgical management of GDV. a. 90° rotation of the stomach in a clockwise direction with the pylorus located in cranial midline. b. Bleeding observed after nicking the serosal layer of the stomach with a no. 10 scalpel blade, suggesting the presence of gastric viability. c. Gastric invagination performed by placing an inverting suture pattern, with the entire necrotic wall now in contact with gastric secretions. (Image courtesy of the University of Edinburgh.)

Step by step: invagination of necrotic gastric tissue

- This technique does not require opening of the gastric lumen.
- However, it can be used only when a small area of necrosis is present.

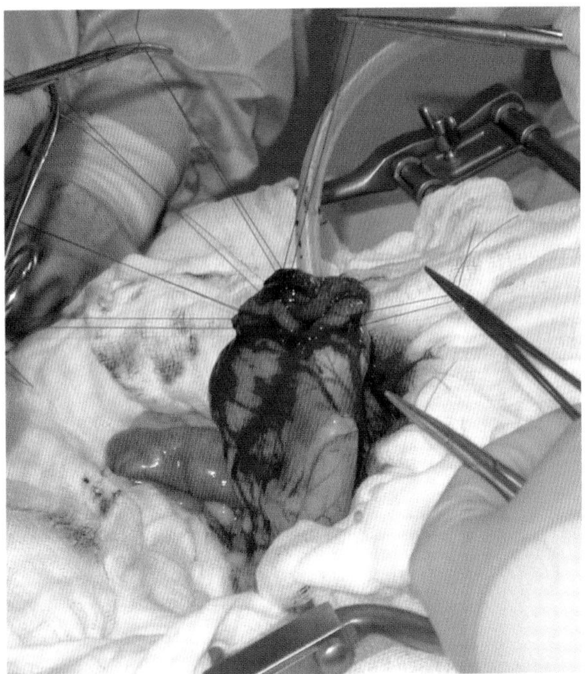

Fig. 3.21 Gastrectomy performed for removal of an adenocarcinoma. Stay sutures are placed around the resected area to minimise spillage. The mass has been removed and gastric wall is ready for closure.

- A full-thickness continuous suture pattern is placed followed by an inverting pattern (Fig. 3.20c).
- Sutures should be placed in healthy tissue, invaginating the whole necrotic area.

Step by step: incisional gastropexy

- An incision is made in the seromuscular layer of the gastric antrum (Fig. 3.22a).
- An incision is made in the ventrolateral abdominal wall (Fig. 3.22b).
- The incision length depends on the size of the dog, but generally 2–3 cm will suffice.
- The edges of the incisions are sutured together in simple continuous patterns using 2.0 or 3.0 metric polydioxanone (Fig. 3.22c).

Handy hints

During an incisional gastropexy, first start the most dorsal suture line at its cranial extent then start the ventral suture line at its cranial extent. Complete the dorsal suture line and then complete the ventral suture line. This will maximise your visualisation during the procedure.

Step by step: tube gastropexy

- A purse-string suture is placed in a hypovascular area of the gastric antrum; the suture is left untied (Fig. 3.23a).

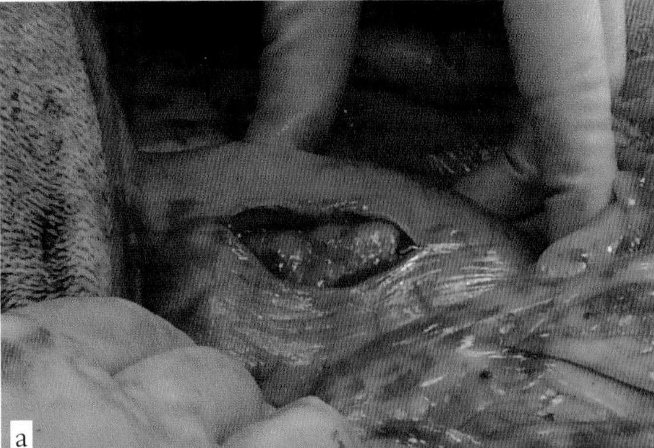

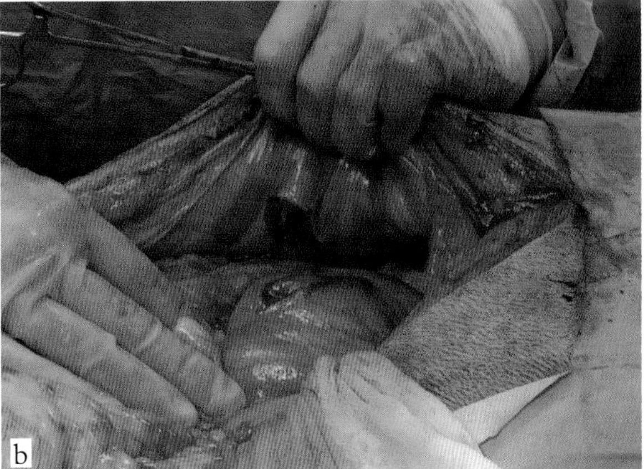

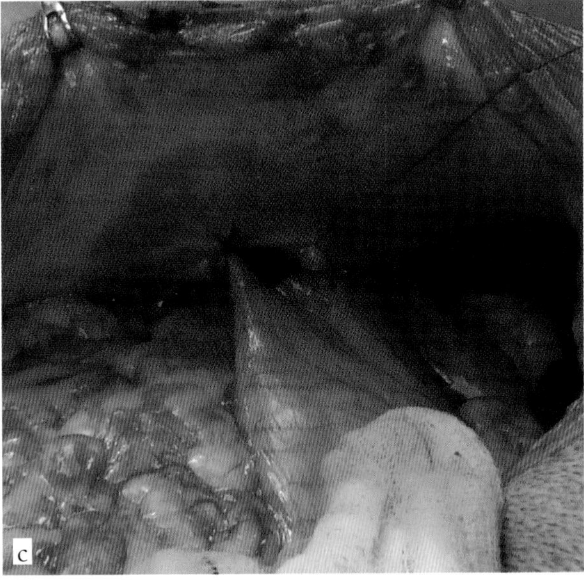

Fig. 3.22a–c Right-sided incisional gastropexy. a. An incision has been made in the seromuscular layer of the gastric antrum. b. An incision has been made in the ventrolateral abdominal wall. c. The edges of the incisions are sutured together in two continuous patterns. (Image courtesy of Samantha Woods.)

- A full-thickness stab incision is made in the centre of the purse-string suture.
- A full-thickness stab incision is made in the right body wall, caudal to the last rib and lateral to the ventral midline.
- A mushroom-tip feeding tube is passed through the

right body wall and the purse-string suture into the gastric lumen (Fig. 3.23b).

- The purse-string suture is tied.
- Four sutures are pre-placed through the seromuscular layer of the stomach antrum and the right body wall using 2.0 or 3.0 metric polydioxanone (Fig. 3.23c).
- Traction is applied in the feeding tube so that the stomach is then close to the body wall, and the sutures are tied.
- The tube is secured to the skin using a Roman sandal pattern (Fig. 3.23d).
- A bandage is placed around the dog's abdomen, and an Elizabethan collar is advised to prevent premature tube removal.

Handy hints

If a tube gastropexy is performed for feeding purposes in an animal not suffering from GDV, it should be placed in the fundic stomach region (left-sided) and attached to the left body wall. This will not prevent pyloric rotation. A gastric tube has to be left in place for 7–10 days. Premature removal could cause leakage of gastric contents into the abdominal cavity, resulting in septic peritonitis.

Therapy in the postoperative period is focused on maintaining tissue perfusion, along with intensive monitoring for prevention and early identification of ischaemia-reperfusion injury (IRI) and consequent potential complications such as hypotension, cardiac arrhythmias, acute kidney injury (AKI), gastric ulceration, electrolyte imbalances and pain. In addition, early identification of patients in need of re-exploration owing to gastric necrosis, abdominal sepsis or splenic thrombosis is crucial (Cornell, 2012a). Early treatment with intravenous (IV) lidocaine bolus (2 mg/kg), followed by constant-rate infusion (CRI: 0.05 mg/kg/min) for 24 hours following presentation decreased the occurrence of cardiac arrhythmias and AKI, and hospitalisation time (Bruchim et al., 2012). Antacids should be administered and, if ileus is present, prokinetic agents such as metoclopramide (CRI: 0.5 mg/kg/h) can be considered. Feeding can be initiated hours after surgery with small amounts of a bland diet.

Despite appropriate medical and surgical treatment, the reported mortality rate in dogs with GDV is high (10–28%). Dogs with GDV involving gastric necrosis or that develop AKI have higher mortality rates (Bruchim and Kelmer, 2014). Other factors that have been associated with mortality include the presence of

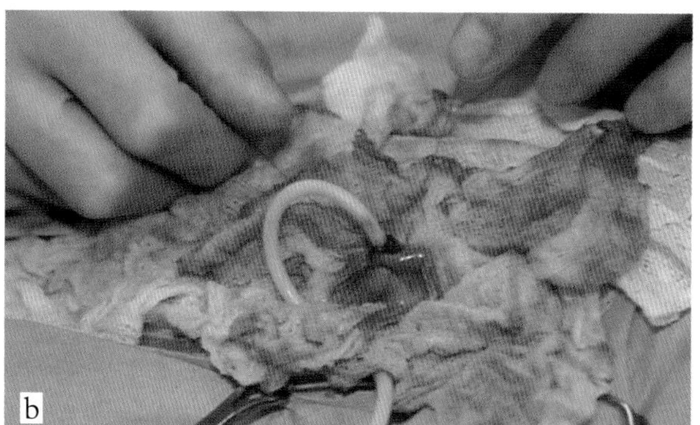

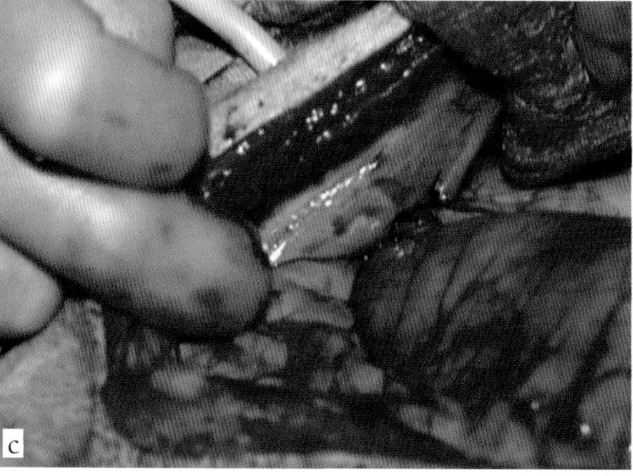

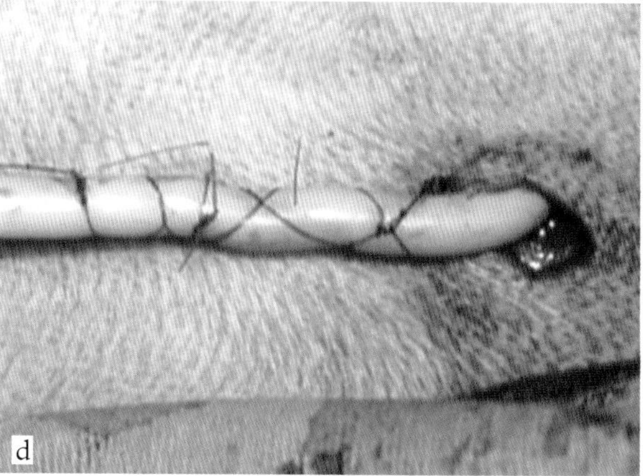

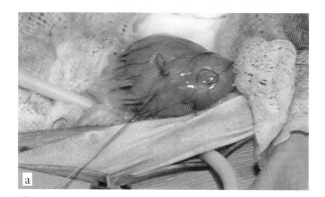

Fig. 3.23a–d Tube gastropexy. (Images courtesy of the University of Edinburgh.) a. A purse-string suture is placed in a hypovascular area of the gastric antrum; the suture is left untied. b. A mushroom-tip feeding tube is passed through the right body wall and the purse-string suture into the gastric lumen. c. Four sutures are pre-placed through the seromusular layer of the stomach antrum and the right body wall using 2.0 or 3.0 metric polydioxanone; the sutures have been tied. d. The tube is secured to the skin using a Roman sandal pattern.

clinical signs for more than 6 hours and the occurrence of hypotension, peritonitis, sepsis and disseminated intravascular coagulation (Beck et al., 2006; Mackenzie et al., 2010). Biochemical parameters evaluated as prognostic indicators include lactate. A preoperative plasma concentration <6.0 mmol/l has been associated with 99% survival rate, while a cut-off value of 9.0 mmol/l has been associated with a good prognosis. An absolute change in lactate pre- and post-resuscitation >4.0 mmol/l has been associated with 86% survival. Also, a percentage of change in lactate concentration >42.5% has been associated with 100% survival and a final lactate measurement <6.4 mmol/l has been associated with 91% survival (Beer et al., 2013; Green et al., 2010; Mooney et al., 2014; de Papp et al., 2002; Verschoof et al., 2015; Zacher et al., 2010). Myoglobin concentration at the time of diagnosis has also been evaluated as a prognostic factor. In one study, an initial cut-off value of 168 ng/ml was 60% sensitive and 84% specific for prediction of survival (Adamik et al., 2009).

Prophylactic gastropexy in high-risk breeds has been discussed; open, laparoscopic and endoscopic techniques have been described (Dujowich et al., 2010: Haraguchi et al., 2017; Loy et al., 2016; Mayhew and Brown, 2009; Rawlings et al., 2002; Steelman-Szymeczek et al., 2003). One study looking at the effects of laparoscopically assisted gastropexy on gastrointestinal transit in dogs showed no effect (Balsa et al., 2017). Complications can occur with any surgical procedure. The benefits and risks should be fully discussed with clients and considered on a case-to-case basis.

3.3.7 Neoplasia

The most common gastric neoplasms in dogs and cats are carcinoma/adenocarcinoma and lymphosarcoma, respectively (Cornell, 2012a). Other tumours have been reported, including gastrointestinal stromal tumour (GIST) and gastric extramedullary plasmocytoma (Von Bavo et al., 2012).

The incidence of gastric carcinoma in the general population is reportedly low. However, certain breeds including Tervuren, Bouvier des Flandres, Groenendael, collie, standard poodle and Norwegian elkhound have been identified as having an increased risk of developing the disease (Seim-Wikse et al., 2013). Median age at presentation ranges from 8 to approximately 10 years (Hugen et al., 2017). The most common clinical sign is vomiting, but others including anorexia, melaena and weight loss have also been reported. The disease is mostly located in the lesser curvature or pyloric antrum. Morphologically it has been described as taking one of three forms: (1) diffuse infiltration of the stomach wall with thickening, termed linitis plastic (leather bottle), resulting in a scirrhous stomach wall that may be difficult to biopsy, especially via endoscopy; (2) groups of ulcerated mucosal plaques; or (3) discrete polypoid masses. Histologically, classification ranges from a diffuse disease with randomly arranged epithelial cells to a distinct glandular form. Metastasis is common, with the regional lymph nodes, liver and lung being the most common sites (Swann and Holt, 2002). The long-term prognosis for most cases of gastric carcinomas is poor. However, surgical resection may palliate cases suffering from gastric outflow obstruction.

Lymphoma in cats is the most common gastric tumour, and can be solitary or represent one site of systemic involvement. The median age of affected cats is 9–13 years. Clinical signs are similar to those reported with other gastric tumours, including vomiting, weight loss, anorexia and occasionally diarrhoea (Gustafson et al., 2014). Imaging is indicated in animals with suspected gastric neoplasia to include radiography, ultrasound, endoscopy and, potentially, CT scan. Endoscopic biopsies are partial thickness and may be insufficient to provide a diagnosis. The treatment of choice for gastric lymphoma is chemotherapy. Surgery may be indicated for diagnostic purposes, or to offer palliation in cases with an obstructive pattern (Gualtieri et al., 1999) (Fig. 3.24).

The prognosis depends on the tumour classification. Intermediate and high-grade lymphomas are usually rapidly progressive and fatal despite treatment, and cats with low-grade (well-differentiated small cell) lymphoma have a median survival time of 704 days with chemotherapy (Cornell, 2012a).

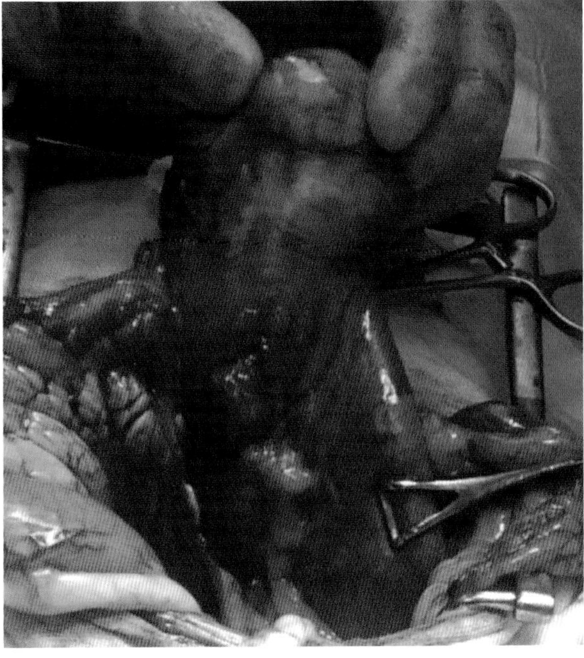

Fig. 3.24 Gastric neoplasia confirmed during exploratory coeliotomy. (Image courtesy of Jonathan Bell.)

3.4 Small intestine

Key points

- Surgery of the small intestine is commonly performed in practice. Indications for intestinal surgery include foreign body removal, biopsy and management of ulcerative or mass lesions.
- A wide variety of electrolyte and acid–base derangements is found in dogs with gastrointestinal obstructions. Hypochloraemia and metabolic alkalosis are common in these cases, and can be seen with both proximal and distal obstructions (Boag et al., 2005).
- High intestinal obstructions are historically accompanied by more severe acid–base derangements.
- In complete obstruction, the production of fluid into the intestinal lumen is increased and its absorption, together with electrolytes, is decreased, leading to possible hypovolaemic shock.
- Stabilisation of patients with small intestinal obstruction prior to surgery is often required and may include administration of crystalloids, colloids and potassium supplementation (infusion should not exceed 0.5 mEq/kg/h) (Cornell, 2012a).
- The surgical principles described for gastric surgery should be applied when operating on the small intestine. Following good surgical principles, and watertight and effective tissue apposition, minimises the likelihood of surgical dehiscence and septic peritonitis.

3.4.1 Anatomy

The small intestine comprises the duodenum, jejunum and ileum, and extends from the pylorus to the ileocolic junction. It is the longest portion of the alimentary canal, having an average length, in the living animal, of 3.5 times the length of the body (Evans and de Lahunta, 2013). The duodenum is relatively immobile, which can present challenges during surgical dissection (Fig. 3.25). Its most proximal portion contains the intramural component of the common bile duct and the pancreatic duct, which open into the duodenum at the major duodenal papilla (Fig. 3.26). Another pancreatic duct also opens into the minor duodenal papilla (distally to the major duodenal papilla) (Evans and de Lahunta, 2013).

Nearly all the intestinal blood supply originates from the cranial mesenteric artery which, in conjunction with intestinal lymphatics and the mesenteric plexus, is located at the root of the mesentery. The cranial mesenteric artery divides into 12–15 jejunal arteries that anastomose with each other in arcades and form the vasa recta within the intestinal wall (vascular network beneath the serosa and submucosa). The duodenal branches from both the cranial and caudal pancreatico-duodenal arteries supply the duodenum. The ileum is supplied on its mesenteric side by ileal branches from

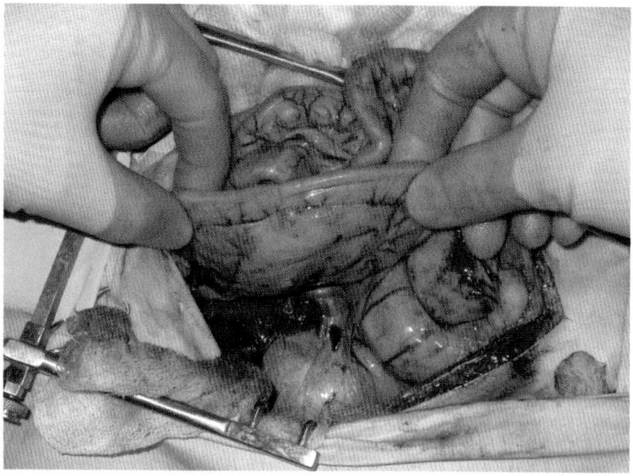

Fig. 3.25 Meso-duodenal sling by manipulation of the duodenum. Cranially, mobilisation of the duodenum is impaired by the insertion point of the common bile duct, pyloric region and close proximity to the pancreatic body. Caudally, mobilisation of the duodenum is impaired by the duodeno-colic ligament. (Image courtesy of the University of Edinburgh.)

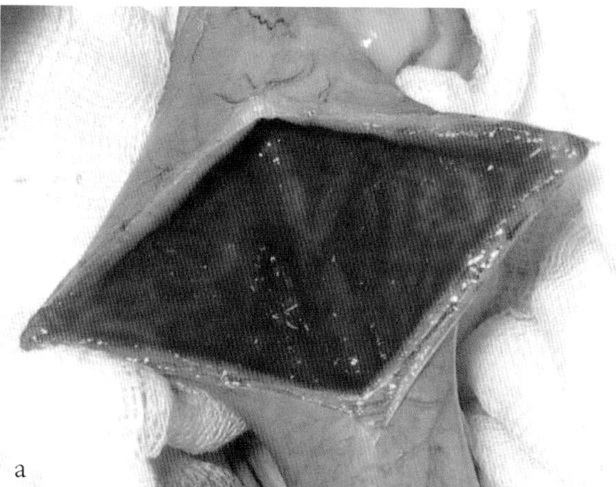

a

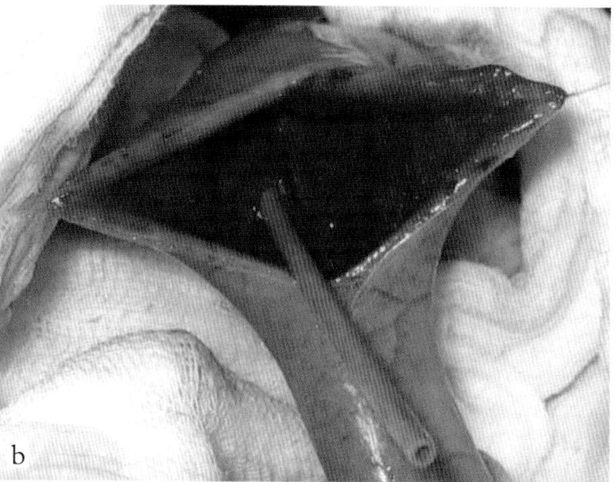

b

Fig. 3.26a,b Major duodenal papilla at the proximal part of the duodenum. (Images courtesy of Jonathan Bell.)

the ileocolic artery and, on its anti-mesenteric side, it is supplied by the anti-mesenteric ileal branches of the caecal artery (Evans and de Lahunta, 2013). Venous drainage is provided by the portal vein.

Six lymph nodes are present in the root of the mesentery, draining the local lymphatics. Some smaller lymph nodes may also be in contact with local gut. The hepatic and colic lymph nodes also drain some intestinal lymph. Nerve fibres to the mesenteric portion of the small intestine originate from the vagus and splanchnic nerves. In dogs, lymphoid tissue is grouped to form aggregated follicles, also known as Peyer's patches, throughout the small intestine.

The wall of the small intestine has four layers: mucosa, submucosa, muscularis and serosa. The mucosa is ruged into villi, which increase the surface area about 8-fold in the dog and 15-fold in the cat. It contains two cell types: columnar cells, which have as their main function absorption, and goblet cells, which have as their main function mucus production.

Intestinal motility is represented by segmental contractions that mix, and peristaltic contractions that move the ingesta aborally (away from the mouth). Rhythmic segmentation is random contractions of small areas of the intestinal smooth muscle (stimulated by local stretch reflexes and the vagus nerve) that can occur when the intestine is full, to slow down forward motion of food and allow more effective digestion and absorption. Between meals, the intestinal smooth muscle has a different electromechanical activity that drives residual undigested material throughout the intestinal tract. Reduced peristaltic contractions lead to ileus, and reduced segmental contractions may result in diarrhoea.

3.4.2 Surgical principles

The surgical principles described for gastric surgery also apply for the remaining gastrointestinal tract. In the same way, a full exploratory coeliotomy should be considered to maximise visualisation and identification of possible concurrent pathologies. The whole gastrointestinal tract should be evaluated.

Intestinal viability is assessed using the parameters previously described, including colour, thickness, presence of peristalsis and haemorrhage (when nicked). Objective measurements of viability have been described, including fluorescein infusion and surface oximetry (Alkukhun et al., 2017; MacDonald et al., 1993; Tollefson et al., 1995). The results of these methods are operator dependent and can be variable. The author would always opt for resection of a questionable area of intestine rather than relying on the result of these two techniques. Their use may be considered when the area to be resected is too extensive to be compatible with life or will probably result in short bowel syndrome.

The intestine heals in three phases – lag, proliferative and maturation. The lag phase lasts 3–4 days and is the most critical phase of healing, since dehiscence and breakdown are most likely to occur in the first 72–96 hours. All strength in the surgical wound at this stage comes from the surgical incision, which makes the technique crucial to avoiding leakage and dehiscence.

The suture material used for intestinal closure should be monofilament, synthetic and absorbable and should survive the expected intestinal healing time. The author prefers to use polydioxanone for the whole of the gastrointestinal tract, although polyglecaprone-25 has also been used successfully.

Closure of the intestinal wall should be done in a single layer using an appositional suture pattern, such as simple interrupted or simple continuous. These patterns maximise primary healing of the submucosa (holding layer) and minimise the likelihood of dehiscence.

Sutures should be placed close to each other and with adequate tension, without crushing the tissue, to provide a watertight seal. A taper-cut needle is advised. Everted mucosa can be trimmed or a modified Gambee pattern may be used.

A functional end-to-end anastomosis using a gastrointestinal stapler (GIA™) or a thoraco-abdominal stapler (TA™ 55) can be performed with a high success rate (Fig. 3.27). Although very reliable, these devices are expensive and therefore should be chosen carefully. Their use may be particularly justifiable in animals with septic peritonitis where the risk of dehiscence is considered higher (Davis et al., 2018; Duell et al., 2016). Risk factors for dehiscence of stapled functional end-to-end anastomosis include inflammatory bowel disease, location of the anastomosis (higher risk in the large bowel) and intra-operative hypotension (Snowdon et al., 2016).

Regular skin staples have also been successfully used to close an enteral anastomosis, although the author would personally not recommend their use (Coolman et al., 2000).

3.4.3 Omental wrapping

The omentum is a mesothelial membrane with extensive vascular and lymphatic supply that exhibits angiogenic, immunogenic and adhesive properties. It helps in restoring blood supply, controlling infection and establishing lymphatic drainage. For this reason, omentum is routinely wrapped around a new enterotomy/enterectomy closure. The author prefers to wrap omentum around the suture line rather than suturing it to it (Fig. 3.28). If you decide to place sutures, make sure they do

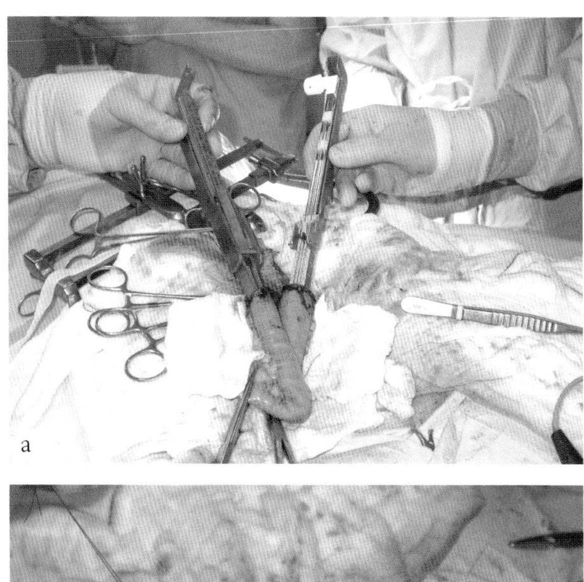

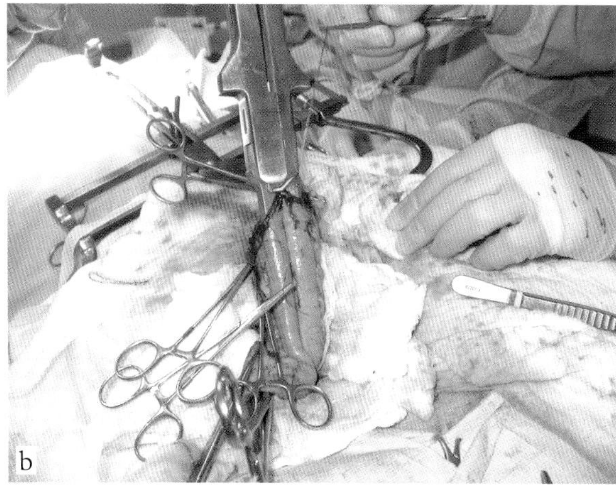

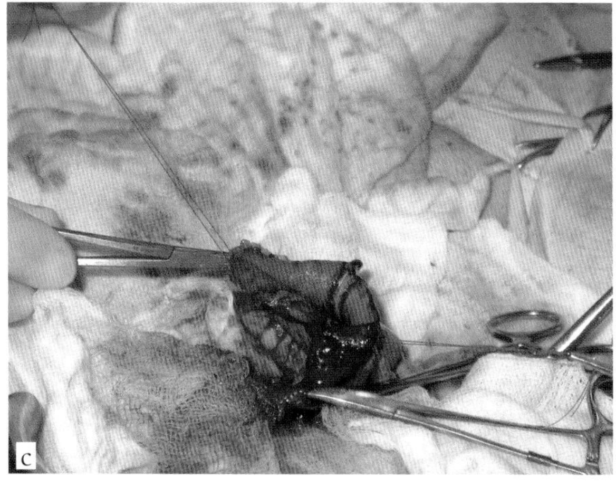

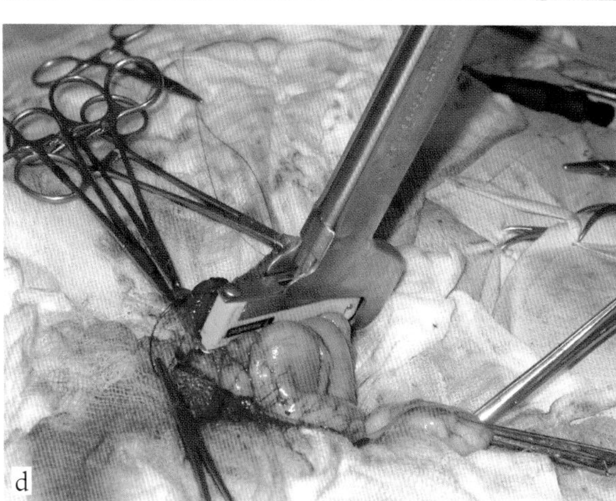

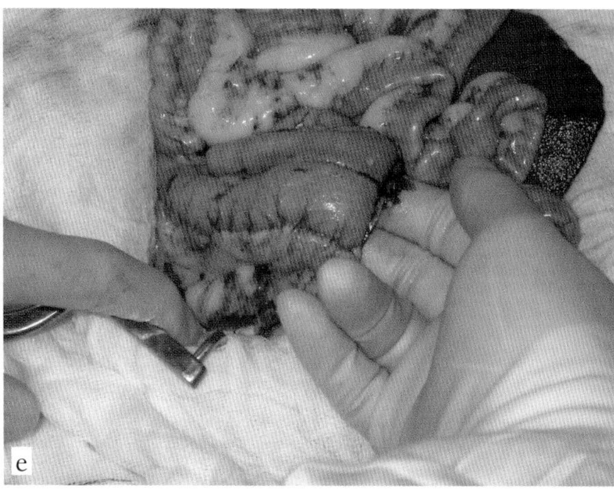

Fig. 3.27a–e Functional end-to-end stapled anastomosis. a. Each arm of the GIA™ stapler is placed in healthy intestinal loops (after resection of compromised tissue), with the staples and blade pointing towards the anti-mesenteric side of each intestinal loop. Both arms are approximated and locked, and the staple gun is fired leaving two staple lines on each side of the anastomosis and creating the anastomosis with an inbuild blade. b. The stapler gun has been fired and the new anastomosis can be seen. c. The GIA™ stapler has been removed, and an opened cul-de-sac of the new anastomosis can be visualised. d. A TA™ 55 stapler is used to close the cul-de-sac, firing two rows of staples. e. Completed anastomosis.

not occlude the omental vascular supply. Omentum has been shown to plug large duodenal defects and produce healing through a process of inflammation, granulation, vascularisation and fibrosis (Katsikas et al., 1977; Raj et al., 1997). However, omentalisation will not prevent leakage in all cases and it should not be used as a replacement for good surgical principles.

3.4.4 Serosal patching

Serosal patching is used to reinforce an intestinal repair, and involves suturing the anti-mesenteric surface of a healthy loop of intestine to the enterotomy closure site by placing sutures encompassing the submucosa layer of both loops. The jejunum is classically used for this technique due to its ease of mobilisation (Fig. 3.29). A recent study showed that serosal patching did not protect dogs from either postoperative septic peritonitis or failure to survive (Grimes et al., 2013). The author chooses serosal patching over omentalisation only in cases where the omentum is severely compromised or contaminated.

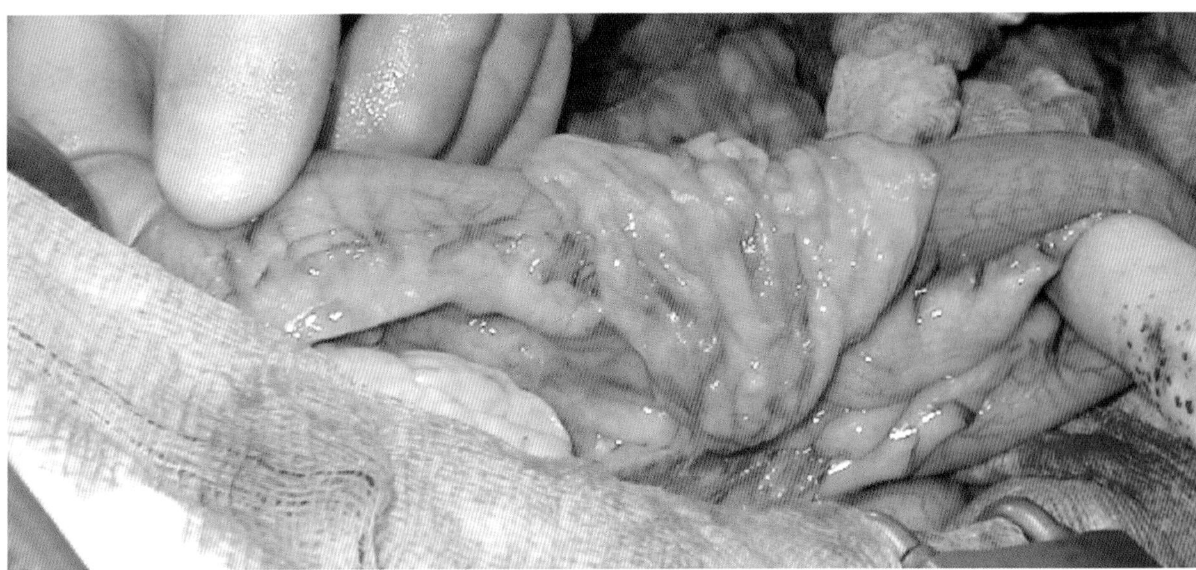

Fig. 3.28 Omentum ready to be wrapped around an enterotomy site.

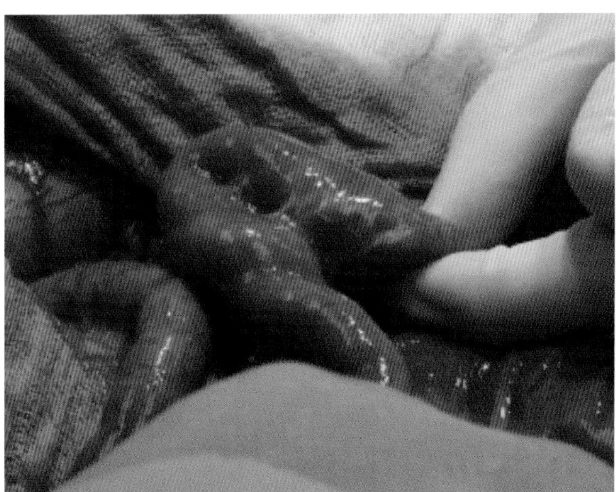

Fig. 3.29 Exploratory coeliotomy showing an area where jejunal serosal patching had previously been performed.

3.4.5 Foreign body

Foreign bodies (FBs) are a common cause of partial or complete intestinal obstruction. Clinical signs vary with their location, duration and severity and may include vomiting, jaundice and abdominal pain (Hayes, 2009; Sharma et al., 2011). Obstructive non-linear FBs compromise the local blood supply by luminal distension, leading to intestinal wall oedema and progressive necrosis. This contributes to ileus and an increase in the number of pathogenic intra-luminal bacteria, leading to the breakdown of the mucosal barrier and systemic endotoxaemia (Ellison, 2001).

Plain radiographs classically show the presence of multiple gas-distended loops of bowel (Fig. 3.30). As a guideline, we can compare the maximum small intestinal diameter and the height of the body of the 5th lumbar vertebra (L5) at its narrowest point: a small intestinal diameter/L5 ratio of 1.6 is considered the upper limit of normal. Animals with a ratio >2.0 are very likely to have an intestinal obstruction. A recent study showed this measurement to have a sensitivity and specificity of 66% (Ciasca et al., 2013). Contrast radiography can be used in the diagnosis. Contrast material usually reaches the small bowel in 12 hours post-ingestion and up to 24 hours for more distal obstructions. Abdominal ultrasonography has shown greater accuracy, fewer equivocal results and provided greater diagnostic confidence compared with radiography. The ultrasonographic presence of moderate-to-severe jejunal diameter enlargement (due to lumen dilation >1.5 cm) should prompt a thorough search for the cause of small intestinal obstruction (Sharma et al., 2011).

Treatment includes stabilisation of any fluid or electrolyte imbalance followed by an enterotomy or, in cases of perforation or questionable intestinal viability, an enterectomy is performed. The prognosis is usually good.

Linear foreign bodies produce a unique form of intestinal obstruction. The foreign body typically anchors itself at the base of the tongue or pylorus, and peristaltic waves carry the remainder of the foreign body aborally. The intestine progressively gathers into accordion-like pleats along the object. As peristalsis continues, the object becomes taut and embedded in the mesenteric aspect of the intestinal lumen. If left untreated, the intestine eventually becomes devitalised and develops multiple perforations (Brown, 2012). Clinical signs in the dog can be more severe, with frequent reports of anorexia, vomiting, lethargy and abdominal pain (Hobday et al., 2014). Diagnosis is made by abdominal

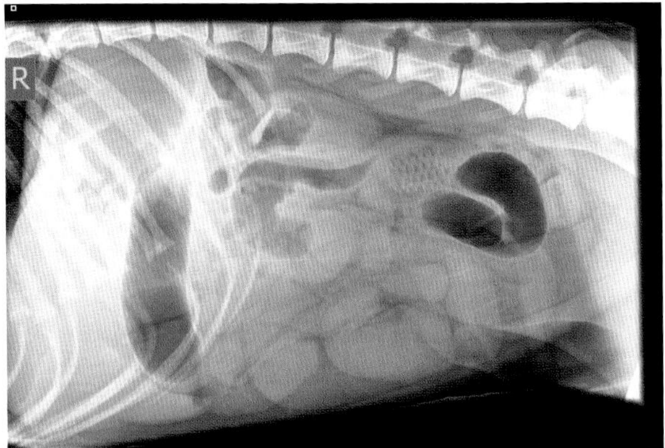

Fig. 3.30 Lateral abdominal radiograph showing distention of intestinal loops due to an intestinal foreign body. (Image courtesy of Jon Hall.)

palpation and plain abdominal radiographs, where the small bowel appears plicated and gathered in the cranial to mid-ventral abdomen (Fig. 3.31). Contrast radiographs may make the diagnosis more obvious.

Treatment is surgical in the vast majority of cases, and entails multiple enterotomies or enterectomies. Pulling a linear foreign body out through a single proximal enterotomy can cause friction of the object against the intestinal mesenteric border, and occult perforations may develop. It is preferable to remove the object in short segments via multiple enterotomies on the anti-mesenteric border. A technique has been described for removal of linear foreign bodies via a single enterotomy incision, tying the linear foreign body to a rubber catheter and milking it aborally until retrieval via the anus (Anderson et al., 1992). However, this technique may not be effective for linear objects that have caused more severe plication or are knotted or matted and cannot be advanced aborally (Muir and Rosin, 1995).

During surgery, the plicated bowel is isolated from the remainder of the abdominal contents and multiple enterotomies are performed to locate and remove

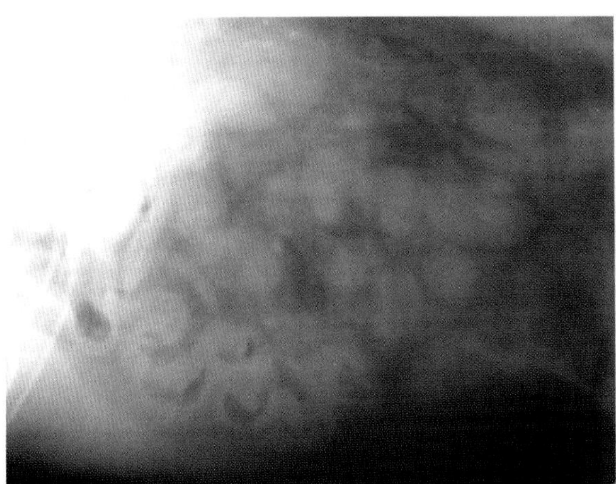

Fig. 3.31 Lateral abdominal radiograph showing plication of the small bowel. (Image courtesy of University of Edinburgh.)

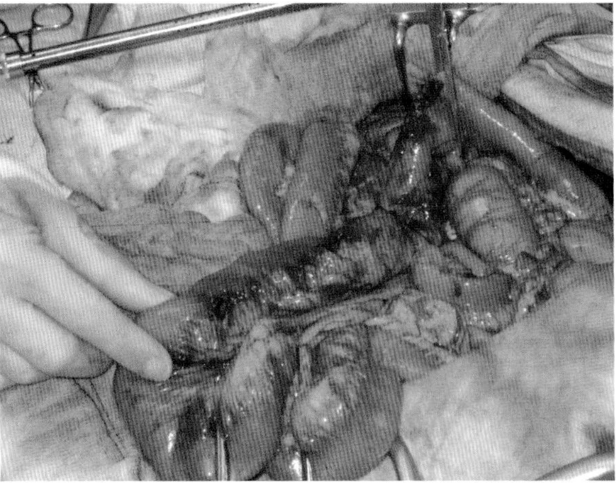

Fig. 3.32 Linear foreign body. An enterotomy has been performed to remove part of the foreign body. Several mesenteric ulcers have been identified and the intestine has been prepared for resection anastomosis. (Image courtesy of Samantha Woods.)

the foreign body (Fig. 3.32). If perforations or necrosis are present, resection anastomosis of the affected area should be performed. When large or multiple areas of intestinal necrosis are present, clinical signs associated with short bowel syndrome may occur; these include secretory diarrhoea and malabsorption.

The precise percentage of small intestinal length that can be removed without causing short bowel syndrome is not known. In the human case, 40–50% can be removed safely but when >75% is removed, nutritional status cannot be maintained on enteral nutrition alone (Yanoff and Willard, 1989). In five experimental dogs, resection of 85% of the small intestine did not affect their ability to live for 11–24 months with no special therapy (Cuthberston et al., 1970). If massive resection of the small intestine is required, nutritional support until adaptive changes in the intestine can occur should be anticipated. These adaptive changes include increased bowel diameter, crypt and villus mucosal cell hyperplasia, an increase in villus height and crypt depth, and an increase in the number of epithelial cells per unit length of the villus. In the interim, antidiarrhoeals may be necessary, as well as antibacterial therapy, to limit bacterial overgrowth (Bebchuk, 2002; Yanoff and Willard, 1989). Fibre (10–15%) stimulates adaptive changes in the intestine, modulates motility, increases water reabsorption and binds excess bile salts that may cause secretory diarrhoea.

Intestinal dehiscence is the most significant and potentially devastating complication, and has been associated with an 80% mortality rate in dogs and cats versus a 7.2% mortality rate in cases with no dehiscence (Wylie and Hosgood, 1994). It has also been shown that the survival rate is negatively correlated with multiple intestinal procedures. For this reason, it is imperative to obey good surgical principles and to perform a single enterotomy or enterectomy whenever feasible.

Step by step: enterotomy and biopsy

- A ventral midline coeliotomy is performed.
- The segment of bowel to be removed is isolated from the other abdominal contents and packed with moistened laparotomy swabs (Fig. 3.33a).
- The intestinal contents are milked away from the area to be resected, and non-crushing forceps (Doyens) or the assistant's fingers are applied to occlude the intestinal lumen proximal and distal to the planned incision area (Fig. 3.33b).
- The anti-mesenteric area of the intestine just proximal to the FB is incised (Fig. 3.33c).
- The incison is enlarged, if required, with Metzenbaum scissors to ensure that no intestinal wall is torn whilst removing the FB.
- The foreign body is removed using the instruments selected.
- The enterotomy is closed in a single layer using an appositional suture pattern, such as simple interrupted

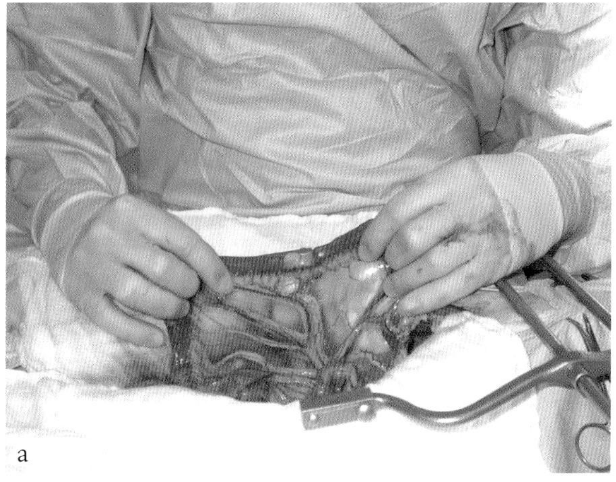
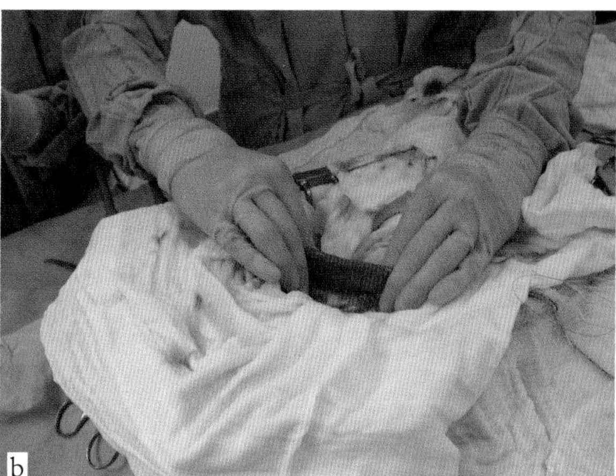
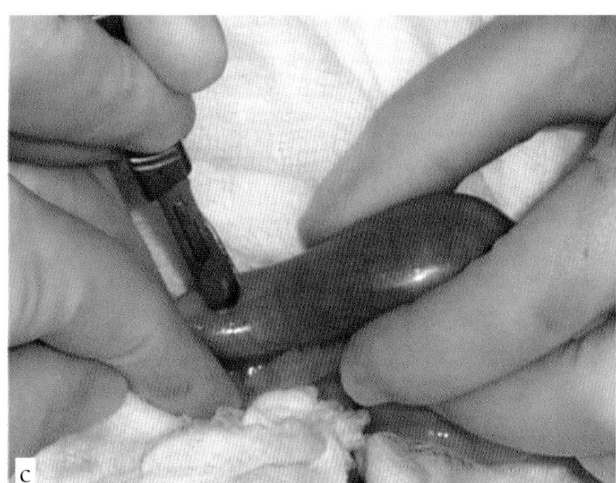
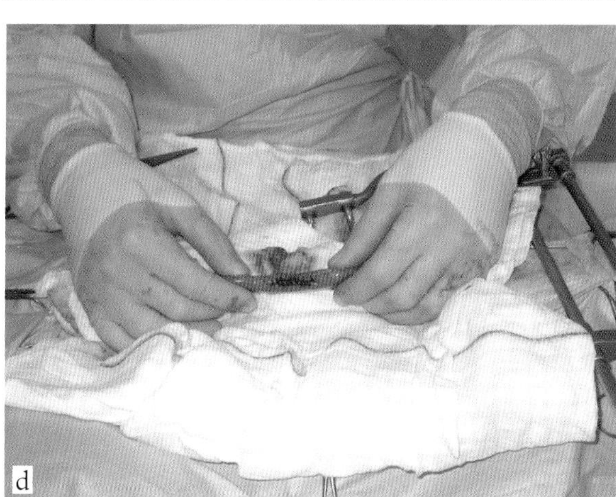
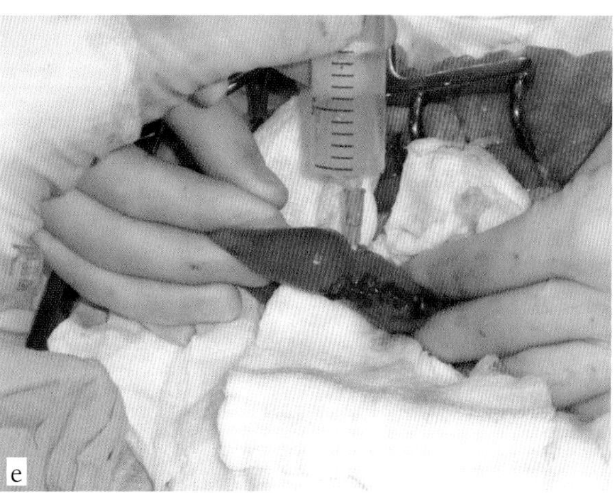

Fig. 3.33a–e Small intestinal enterotomy, biopsy. a. The intestinal loop to be biopsied is isolated from the abdominal cavity and packed with moistened laparotomy swabs. b. The intestinal contents are milked away from the area to be resected, and the assistant's fingers are applied to occlude the intestinal lumen proximal and distal to the planned incision area. c. An anti-mesenteric area of the intestine is incised. d. The enterotomy has been closed with a single continuous suture pattern. e. A leakage test is performed by injecting sterile saline into the intestinal lumen using a 25-g needle (orange), away from the suture line and checking for leakage of saline through the suture line. (Images courtesy of the University of Edinburgh.)

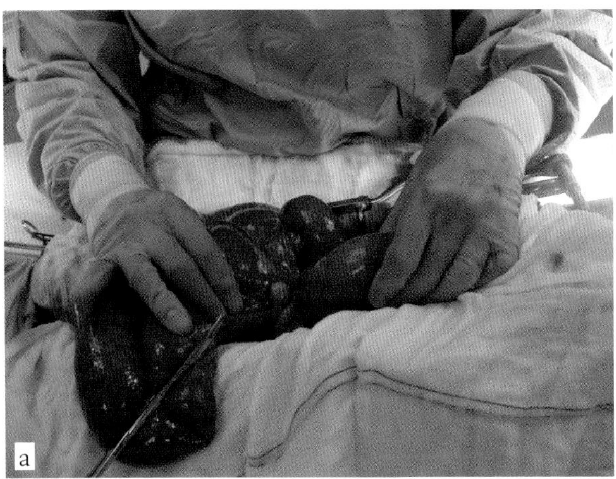

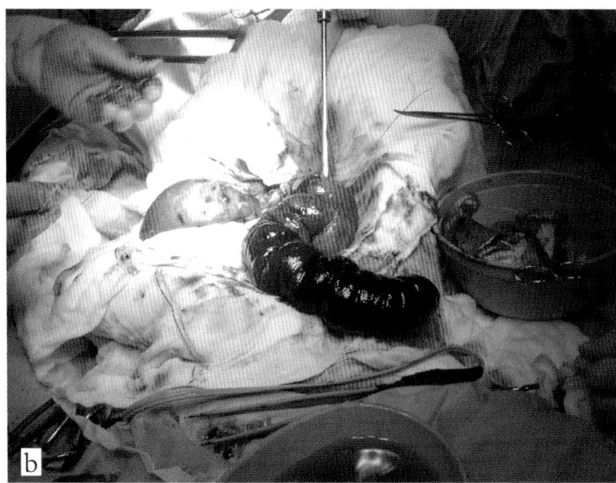

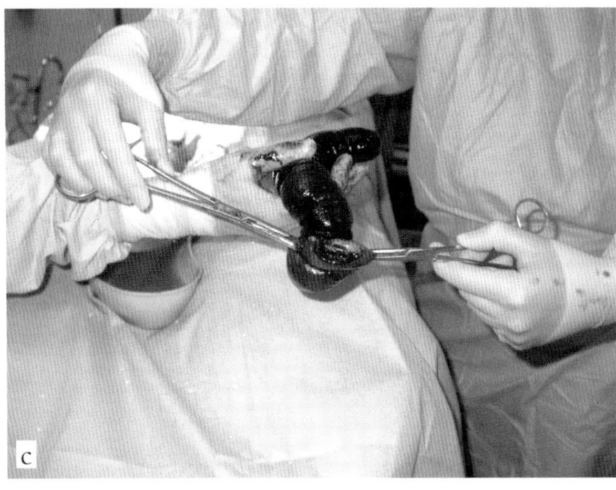

Fig. 3.38a–c Intussusception. a. Intussusception at the ileocolic junction before reduction. b. Intussusception following reduction, showing necrosis of the intussusceptum (caecum). c. The compromised area of the bowel has been resected.

long-term medical management may be required (Fernandez et al., 2017).

Enteroplication can be considered according to the surgeon's preference regarding decreasing the likelihood of recurrence. For this technique, adjacent bowel loops are placed side by side and in a series of gentle turns, to avoid kinking. Complete plication of the jejunum and ileum is recommended, as recurrence can appear away from the original site. The loops of intestine are sutured to each other through the antimesenteric border with interrupted sutures, ensuring that the submucosa layer is incorporated, using 1.5 metric polydioxanone. Complications associated with the technique may be life-threatening and include obstruction, strangulation, perforation and generalised septic peritonitis (Applewhite et al., 2001). The author performs enteroplication only when recurrence is identified intra-operatively.

3.4.8 Neoplasia

Tumours of the small intestinal tract are often focal, annular lesions that can cause partial or complete obstruction (Fernandez et al., 2017). The tumours most commonly diagnosed in the dog include adenocarcinoma, leiomyoma, lymphoma and leiomyosarcoma. Lymphoma is the most common tumour in the cat (Fig. 3.39) (Gieger, 2011). Feline gastrointestinal lymphoma is classified as high grade (large cell), intermediate grade or low grade (small cell) according to the cell morphology and mitotic rate (Pohlman et al., 2009; Valli et al., 2000). In cats with intermediate or large-cell gastrointestinal lymphoma, perforation post-chemotherapy can occur. It is unknown in this subset

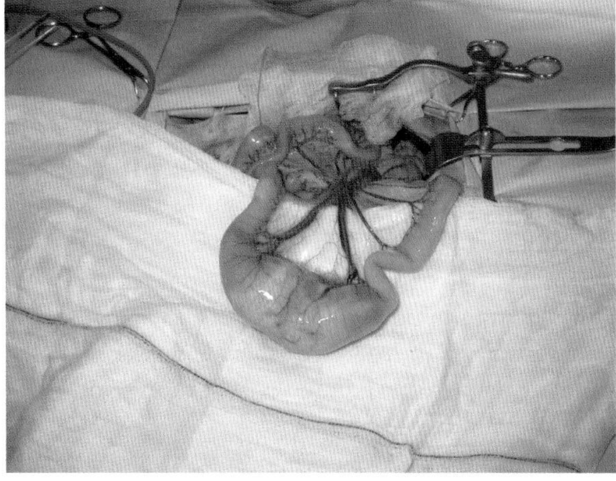

Fig. 3.39 Obstructive lymphoma in the small intestine of a cat. Enlarged mesenteric lymph nodes are also present.

of animals whether surgical resection would decrease this risk (Crouse et al., 2017).

Surgical resection of benign tumours is indicated, and it carries a good prognosis. For malignant tumours, the prognosis depends on the presence or absence of metastasis at the time of surgical intervention (Crawshaw et al., 1998).

3.5 Large intestine

Key points

- Surgery of the large bowel is relatively common. Indications include resection of obstructive tumours, management of idiopathic megacolon, colopexy and caecal impaction or inversion.
- The bacterial flora exponentially increases from the small to the large bowel, and a large anaerobic population is present.
- The blood supply of the large intestine is linear, and surgical procedures entering the intestinal lumen are considered contaminated.
- Some factors have been shown to negatively affect colonic wound healing, including tissue hypoperfusion, wound tension, poor apposition, infection, distal obstruction, hypovolaemia, zinc deficiency, iron deficiency, blood transfusion, medications such as cisplatin, immunodeficiency, poorly controlled diabetes and icterus (Williams, 2012).
- A full evaluation of the animal, stabilisation when required and adherence to strict surgical principles are key to minimising potentially devastating surgical complications.

3.5.1 Anatomy

The large intestine comprises the caecum, colon (ascending, transverse and descending) and rectum.

The majority of the colon receives its irrigation from the cranial mesenteric artery. The cranial mesenteric artery branches as the common colic artery, which subdivides into: ileocolic artery – irrigates caecum; ileocolic artery and right colic artery – irrigate ascending colon; right colic and middle colic artery – irrigate transverse colon; middle colic artery – irrigates proximal half of descending colon; left colic branch of caudal mesenteric – irrigates distal half of descending colon; and cranial rectal artery – irrigates most distal portion of descending colon and rectum. All these arteries connect to the colon via the vasa recta. Venous drainage is via the portal vein.

Autonomic innervation to the colon is from the cranial and caudal mesenteric plexuses, which course with the mesenteric vasculature to the intestine.

Like the small intestine, the large intestinal wall is composed of four layers: mucosa, submucosa, muscularis and serosa. The mucosa is composed of columnar and cuboid epithelial cells arranged in crypts and interspaced with goblet cells. Solitary lymphoglandular complexes are found instead of villi or aggregated lymphatics (present in the small intestine), through which the colonic glands discharge. In the cat, these complexes are found only in the caecum.

3.5.2 Surgical principles

Large bowel surgery is considered contaminated due to the high number of intra-luminal bacterial flora. Bowel cleansing prior to surgery is contraindicated, as this turns faecal material into liquid slurry which is more likely to leak and contaminate the surgical field. Perioperative antibiosis is recommended with an extended anaerobic spectrum. The author often uses a combination of cefuroxime and metronidazole, with administration commenced 48 hours preoperatively and continuing postoperatively for up to 10 days.

Omentalisation is advised to maximise wound healing, as in the small intestinal tract.

Colonic closure can be performed with a single- or double-layer closure, similar to the stomach. Monofilament long-lasting suture material should be used in a taper-cut needle. A single-layer continuous pattern is similar in terms of safety to a two-layer technique, but because it's easier to perform it may be preferable (Garcia-Osogobio et al., 2006). The author prefers a single-layer closure.

Stapling devices can also be used in the large bowel. An end-to-end circular stapler has been used successfully in open and laparoscopic surgery (Fig. 3.40a–f) (Julian et al., 1989). These devices are expensive, and their use should be considered on a case-by-case basis.

3.5.3 Caecal resection/typhlectomy

Typhlectomy may be indicated in the presence of impaction, subclinical impaction, perforation, inversion, severe inflammation or neoplasia (Clark and Wise, 1994; Eastwood et al., 2005; Guffy et al., 1970; Kapatkin et al., 1992; Maas et al., 2007; Westgarth et al., 2013). The ileocolic junction should be preserved if possible unless the disease extends into this area.

If the caecum is inverted, it should be everted prior to resection. For resection, the ileocaecal fold is dissected freeing the caecum from the ileum (be careful not to damage the anti-mesenteric ileal vessels). Atraumatic clamps are placed across the base of the caecum and,

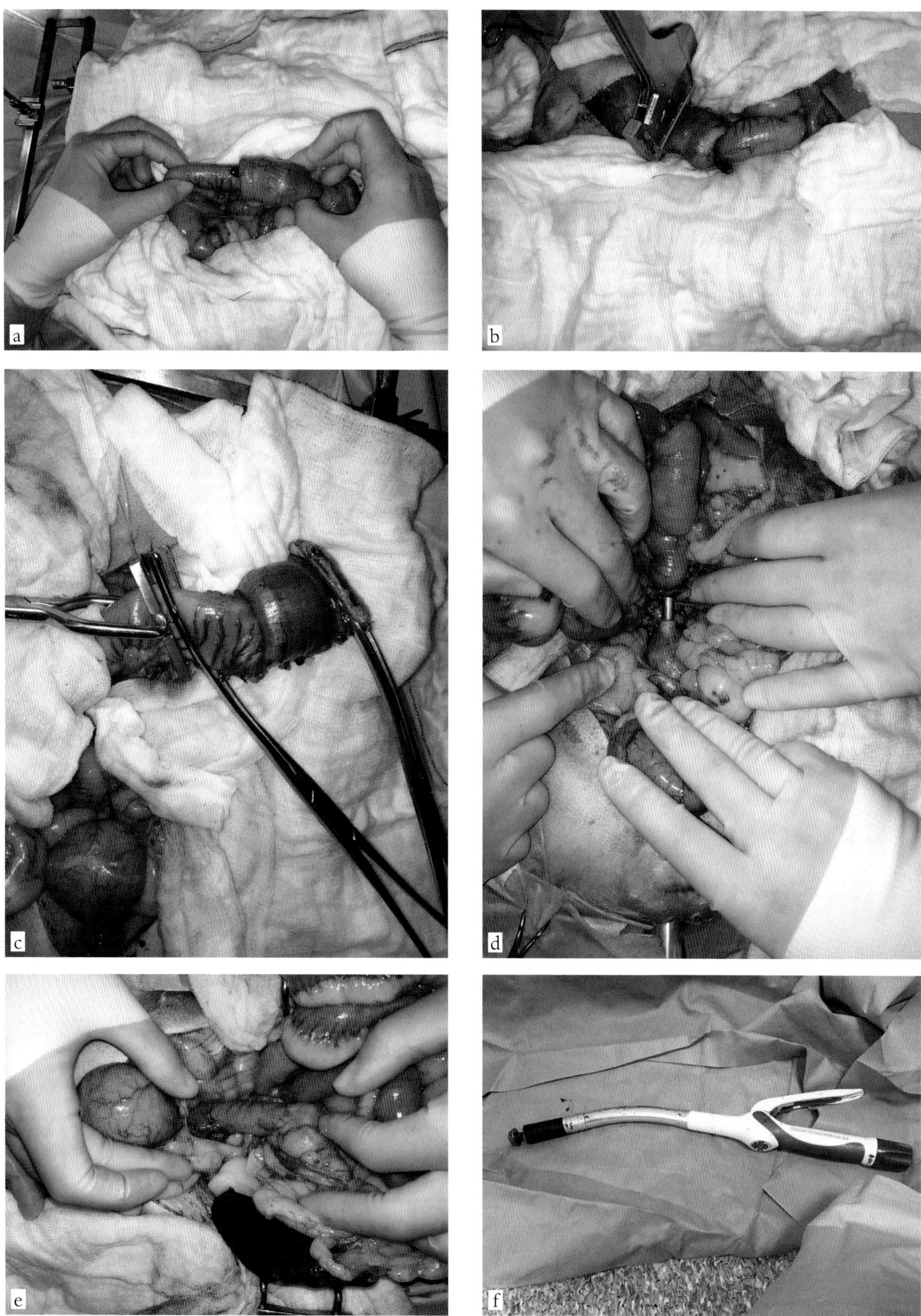

Fig. 3.40a–f Colonic mass resection and end-to-end anastomosis. a. Colonic mass causing a non-reducible intussusception at the ileocolic junction. b The caudal intestine is sealed using a 3.5 mm TA™ stapler and transected proximal to the staple line (after ligation of the vasa recta). c. A purse-string suture is placed proximal to the proximal transection line. d. The circular stapler is inserted per rectum and the anvil is pushed through the staple line and secured to the proximal purse-string suture, which is tied. The stapler is fired, creating a new end-to-end anastomosis. e. Circular staple line after completion of the procedure. f. An end-to-end circular stapler.

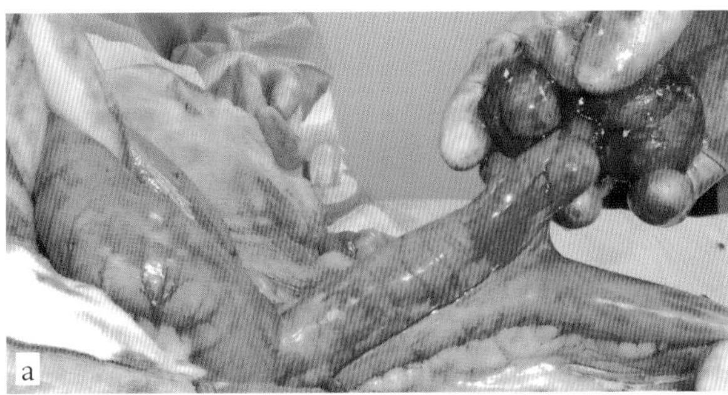

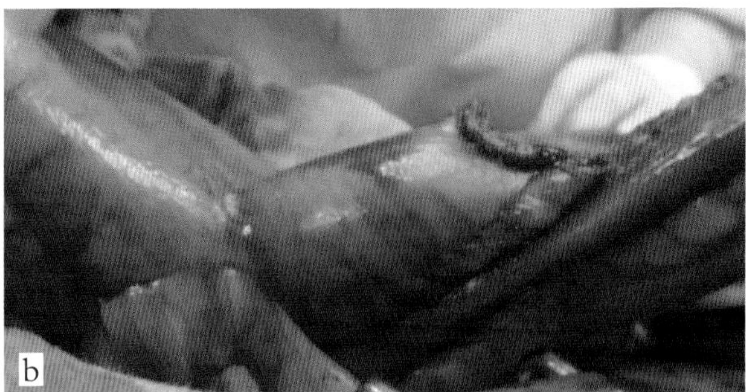

Fig. 3.41a,b Typhlectomy. (Images courtesy of Jonathan Bell.) a. Caecal mass identified during exploratory coeliotomy; the ileocaecal fold has been dissected, freeing the caecum from the ileum. b. A thoraco-abdominal surgical stapler has been used to complete the procedure; the stapler line is visible.

after resection, a Parker–Kerr suture pattern is used to close the wound (Williams, 2012). Alternatively, a single- or double-layer closure as described for closure of the stomach can be used. A thoraco-abdominal stapler can also be used (Ullman, 1994) (Fig. 3.41a,b).

3.5.4 Colonic biopsy and colostomy

Colonic biopsy can be performed to aid in the diagnosis of diffuse or focal disease. The biopsy technique is similar to that described for the small bowel, but the colonic lumen has a wider diameter and transverse closure of a longitudinal incision is seldom required. Colotomy is rarely indicated. Colonic foreign bodies have travelled throughout the whole of the small intestine and will probably pass with defaecation. A full exploration of the abdominal cavity should always be performed to check for lesions or perforations located in a proximal direction.

Step by step: colotomy and biopsy

- A ventral midline coeliotomy is performed.
- The segment of bowel to be removed is isolated from the other abdominal contents, and packed with moistened laparotomy swabs.
- The colonic contents are milked away from the area to be resected, and non-crushing forceps (Doyen) or the assistant's fingers are applied to occlude the intestinal lumen proximal and distal to the planned incision area.
- The desired anti-mesenteric area of the colon is incised.
- The colotomy is closed in a single layer using an appositional suture pattern such as simple interrupted or simple continuous, using 1.5 metric polydioxanone.
- Sutures should be placed close to each other and with adequate tension without crushing the tissue, to provide a watertight seal.
- A leakage test is performed by injecting sterile saline into the intestinal lumen using a 25-g hypodermic needle (orange), away from the suture line and checking for leakage of saline through the suture line.
- If leakage is present, the colonic closure is patched with simple interrupted sutures.
- The abdominal cavity is lavaged, the suture line is omentalised and the abdominal cavity is closed in three layers.
- For biopsy, a full-thickness elliptical incision is performed after the colotomy using Metzenbaum scissors.
- Alternatively, a full-thickness suture is placed through the intended biopsy site (no colotomy performed) and an elliptical incison is made around the suture to remove the sample.

3.5.5 Colectomy

Colectomy refers to resection of part or the entire colon. Indications for this procedure include megacolon, neoplasia, perforation, trauma and chronic intussusception. When the ileocaecal valve is preserved, the procedure is called subtotal colectomy; when the ileocaecal valve is resected the procedure is called total colectomy.

Step by step: total and subtotal colectomy

- A ventral midline coeliotomy is performed.
- The segment of bowel to be removed is isolated from the other abdominal contents, and packed with moistened laparotomy swabs (Fig. 3.42a).
- The vasa recta supplying the segment to be removed are double ligated and divided as close to the intestinal wall as possible (Fig. 3.42b).
- After milking the intestinal contents away from the area to be resected (when possible), crushing forceps are applied to the area being removed and non-crushing forceps (Doyen) or the assistant's fingers applied to the intestinal area that will remain (Fig. 3.42c).

- A sufficiently lengthy cuff of healthy tissue must be left to facilitate closure.
- For subtotal colectomy (preservation of the ileocaecal valve), the proximal site to be resected is 1–2 cm distal to the ileocolic junction.
- For total colectomy (resection of the ileocaecal valve), the proximal site to be resected is 1–2 cm proximal to the ileocaecal fold.
- The distal transection site is at the junction of the rectum and colon: 2 cm cranial to the pelvic brim; 1 cm caudal to where the caudal mesenteric artery penetrates the serosa.
- The intestine to be removed is incised using a new no. 11 scalpel blade in a slight diagonal shape, so that the mesenteric borders are longer than the anti-mesenteric (Fig. 3.42d).
- The affected segment is discarded with its associated crushing forceps, and the bowel is assessed for any possible luminal disparity.
- If luminal disparity is present, this can be addressed using different techniques:
  - Sutures are spaced further apart on the segment with greater diameter.
  - The intestine is transected with the smaller luminal diameter at an angle.
  - An incision is performed in the anti-mesenteric side, also known as 'spatulation'.
  - The diameter of the larger loop is reduced by suturing it as if it were a 'cul-de-sac'.
- The colectomy is closed in a single layer using an appositional suture pattern such as simple interrupted or simple continuous, using 1.5 metric polydioxanone.
  - For a simple interrupted pattern:
    - The first two sutures are placed, one in the mesenteric side and the other in the anti-mesenteric.
    - The gaps are filled so that the sutures are placed close to each other and with adequate tension without crushing the tissue, to provide a watertight seal.
  - For a simple continuous pattern:
    - A suture line is started in the mesenteric side and another one is started on the anti-mesenteric (Fig. 3.42e).
    - One suture line is completed until it meets the other, and the same technique is repeated on the other side (Fig. 3.42f).
- Sutures should be placed close to each other and with adequate tension without crushing the tissue, to provide a watertight seal.
- A leakage test is performed by injecting sterile saline into the intestinal lumen using a 25-g needle (orange), away from the suture line and checking for leakage of saline through the suture line.
- If leakage is present, the intestinal closure is patched with simple interrupted sutures.
- The abdominal cavity is lavaged, the suture line is omentalised and the abdominal cavity is closed in three layers (Fig. 3.42g).

3.5.6 Colopexy

Colopexy entails fixation of the colon to the abdominal wall (left side), and is indicated for management of severe or recurrent rectal prolapse. The procedure also reduces rectal sacculation seen in animals with perineal hernia. Colopexy can be performed using an abrasion technique (rubbing the colon and abdominal wall with a dry swab) or by performing a partial-thickness incision through the seromuscular layer of the colon and abdominal wall. The author prefers the former technique.

Step by step: colopexy

- A ventral midline coeliotomy is performed.
- The segment of colon to be fixated is isolated from the other abdominal contents, and packed with moistened laparotomy swabs.
- With a dry swab, the anti-mesenteric area of the colon to be fixated and a similar area in the left lateral body wall are rubbed until red (usually 2–3 cm will suffice).
- The abraded area of the colon and the left body wall are sutured together with a simple continuous suture pattern, using 1.5 metric polypropylene (non-absorbable suture material) (Fig. 3.43).
- The suture bites should ideally reach the submucosa layer but not the intestinal lumen.
- The abdominal cavity is lavaged, the suture line is omentalised and the abdominal cavity is closed in three layers.

3.5.7 Megacolon

Megacolon is an end-stage obstipation characterised by colonic hypomotility and a permanent increase in the diameter of the colon (Fig. 3.44).

Megacolon has been categorised as congenital or acquired, primary or secondary, intrinsic or extrinsic, functional or mechanical, and dilated or hypertrophic.

In dogs, megacolon is described as acquired (secondary) or idiopathic (primary). The acquired form can be the result of a mechanical or functional obstruction. Examples of mechanical obstruction include pelvic canal stenosis (due to pelvic fractures with narrowing of >45% of the pelvic canal), neoplasia, foreign body and perineal hernia. This form of the disease has

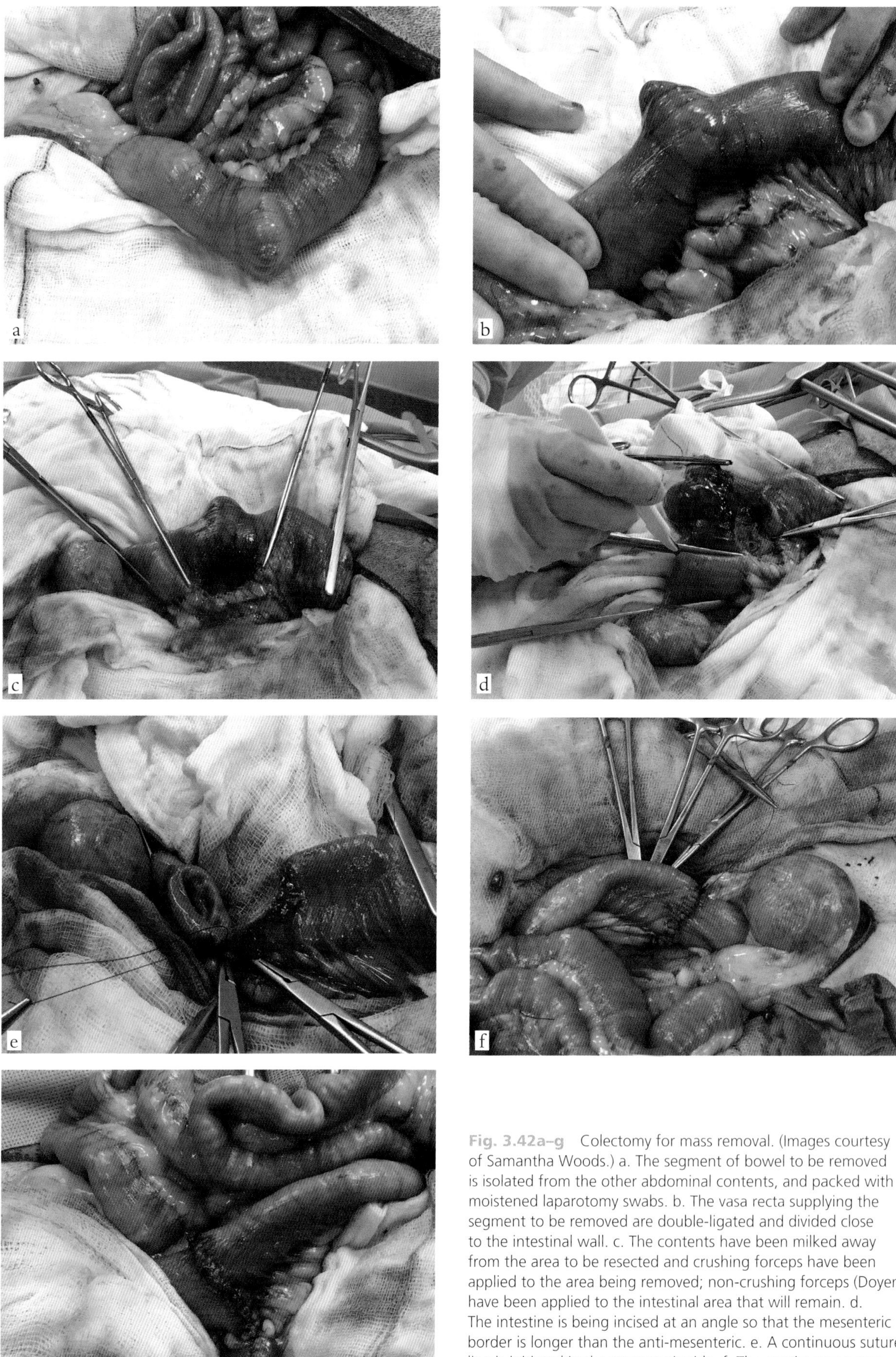

Fig. 3.42a–g Colectomy for mass removal. (Images courtesy of Samantha Woods.) a. The segment of bowel to be removed is isolated from the other abdominal contents, and packed with moistened laparotomy swabs. b. The vasa recta supplying the segment to be removed are double-ligated and divided close to the intestinal wall. c. The contents have been milked away from the area to be resected and crushing forceps have been applied to the area being removed; non-crushing forceps (Doyen) have been applied to the intestinal area that will remain. d. The intestine is being incised at an angle so that the mesenteric border is longer than the anti-mesenteric. e. A continuous suture line is initiated in the mesenteric side. f. The continuous suture line is completed and meets the other one started at the anti-mesenteric side. g. Closure of the mesenteric defect.

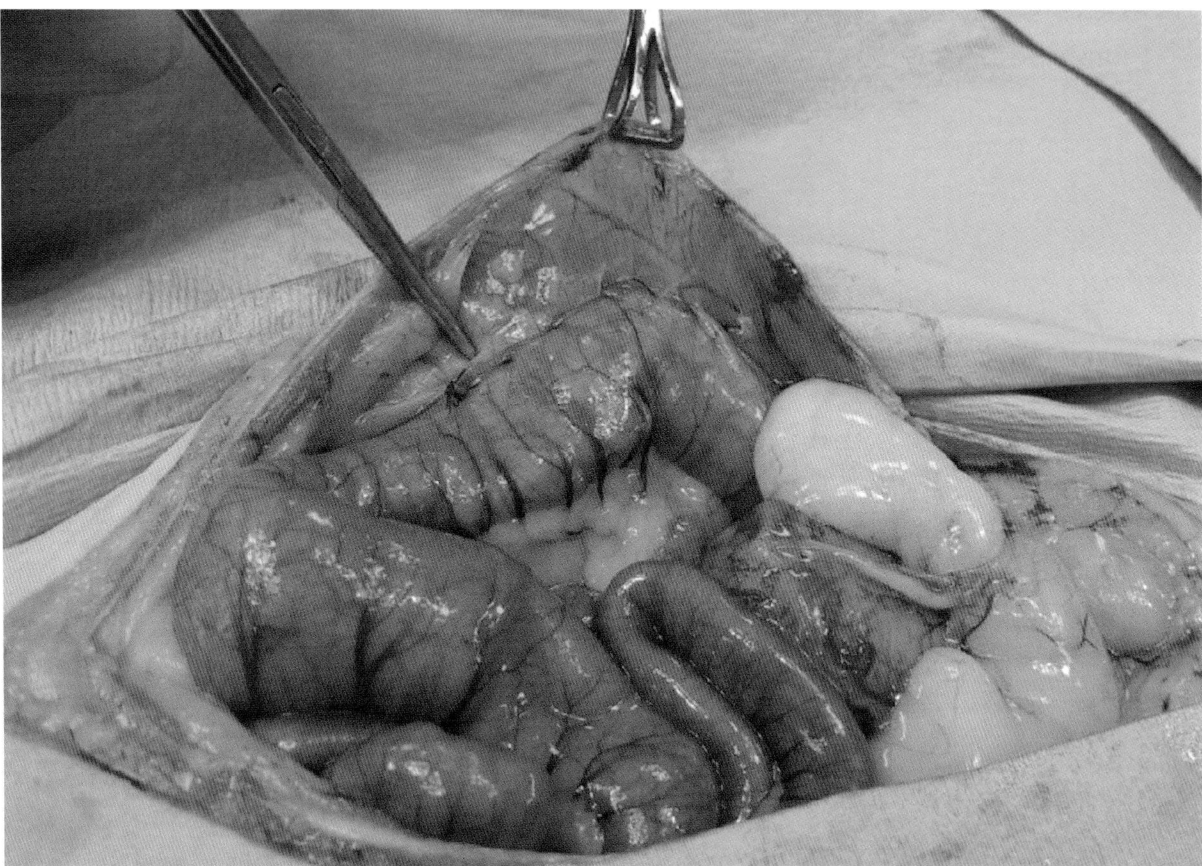

Fig. 3.43 Abrasion colopexy performed with a simple continuous pattern using polypropylene. (Image courtesy of University of Edinburgh.)

also been termed hypertrophic megacolon (Williams, 2012).

Functional causes include neuromuscular dysfunction such as spinal cord disease, pelvic nerve injury, dysautonomia, metabolic disease and autonomic ganglioneuritis.

In the cat, idiopathic megacolon is the most common diagnosis, occurring in approximately 60–70% of the cases reported in the literature (Bertoy, 2001; Washabau and Holt, 1999). Breeds affected include Siamese, domestic short hair and domestic long hair. Older animals are over-represented. Idiopathic megacolon is thought to be due to a generalised dysfunction of the longitudinal and circular smooth muscle, but its full pathophysiology is unknown (Washabau and Stalis, 1996).

Diagnosis is usually made when clinical signs are severe and the condition is chronic and irreversible, since it is difficult for owners to know their cat's normal defaecation pattern. Clinical signs include tenesmus, pain on defaecating, constipation, obstipation and an enlarged abdomen. More severe cases may present with anorexia, vomiting, weight loss and dehydration. Systemic signs may manifest from disruption of the mucosal barrier and absorption of toxic luminal products such as those produced by *Clostridia* spp. (Williams, 2012). Ruling out all other causes of intractable constipation results in a diagnosis of idiopathic megacolon. A complete physical examination, including a rectal examination, should be performed to assess any evidence of distal colonic or rectal stricture, tumour or presence of a perineal hernia. A neurologic examination should be performed with specific emphasis on the function of the sacrocaudal spinal cord. Although laboratory data are usually normal in cases of megacolon, these tests (complete blood cell count, serum chemistry and urinalysis) should be performed to rule out other causes of constipation and to help identify any complicating conditions before pursuing other more invasive diagnostic procedures (Bertoy, 2001).

Radiography is used primarily to rule out obstructive diseases, such as pelvic fracture malunion, sacrocaudal spinal trauma or deformities and intramural or mural colonic or recto-anal obstructive lesions (Fig. 3.45). However, it is also useful to assess the degree of colonic dilation. A ratio of maximal diameter of the colon to L5 length >1.48 is a good indicator of megacolon (sensitivity 77%, specificity 85%) (Trevail et al., 2011).

Most cases of feline megacolon are chronic (>6 months is considered irreversible) and require surgical

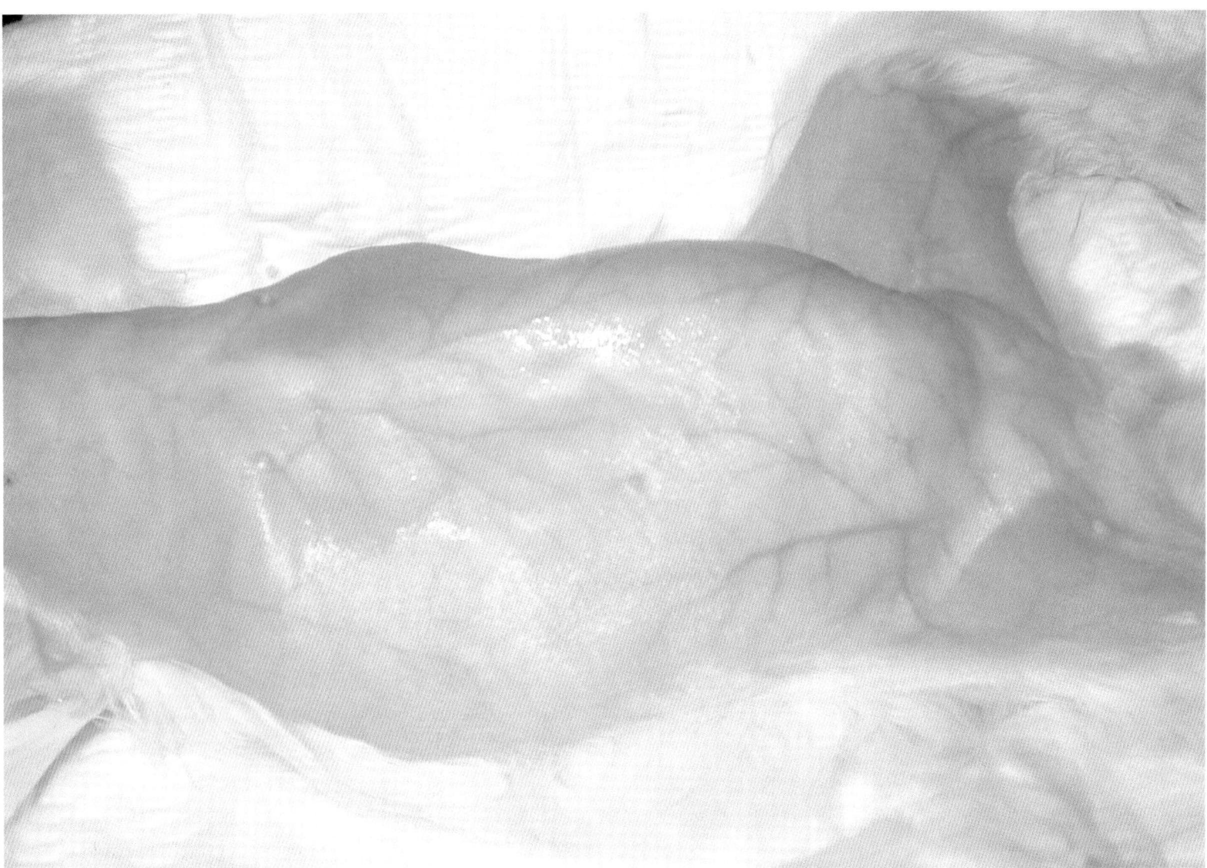

Fig. 3.44 Cat in dorsal recumbency showing abdominal distension due to presence of megacolon.

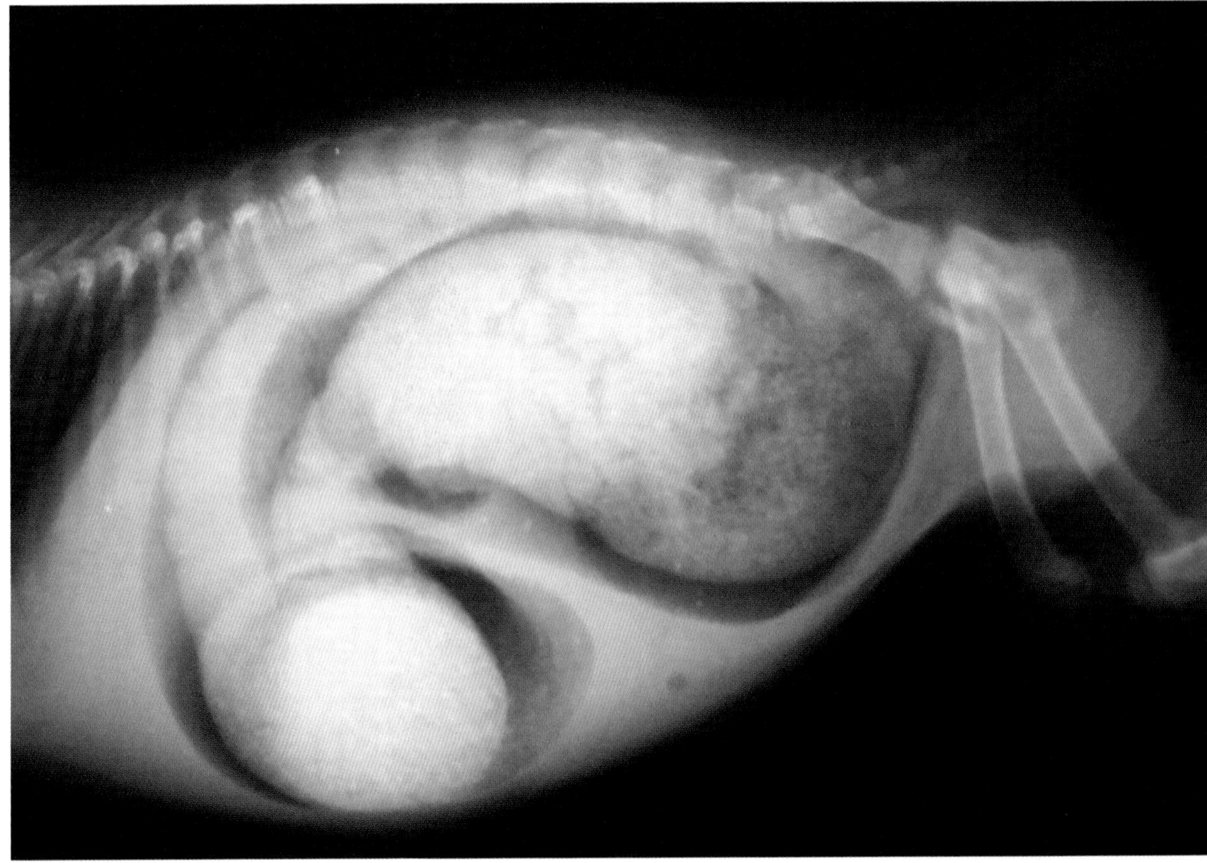

Fig. 3.45 Lateral abdominal radiograph of a puppy with atresia ani and secondary megacolon.

intervention that entails total or subtotal colectomy. Medical therapy is supportive and palliative, addressing fluid, electrolyte and acid–base imbalance. Faecoliths can be manually removed or by using stool softeners and enemas. Intravenous antibiotics should be given prior to manual evacuation, as disruption of the mucosa is inevitable. Long-term medical management includes stool softeners (lactulose), high-fibre diets, periodic enemas and prokinetics such as cisapride (stimulates contraction of smooth muscle in the descending colon) (Bertoy, 2001; Williams, 2012). Phosphate enemas should never be used in cats as these cause rapid dehydration, hypocalcaemia, hypophosphataemia and death.

Surgery of idiopathic megacolon entails total or subtotal colectomy (Fig. 3.46a–d). Loose stools are expected in the initial postoperative period. When the ileocolic junction is removed, poorly formed stools and faecal incontinence can be observed up to 3 months postoperatively (Bertoy et al., 1989; McCready and Beart, 1979). With adequate diet, improvement is gradually observed.

The prognosis for cats undergoing subtotal colectomy is fair to good, and recurrence of constipation is uncommon.

3.5.8 Neoplasia

Large intestinal tumours account for approximately 30–60% of all intestinal tumours (Morello et al., 2008). Adenomas are the most common benign tumour, while adenocarcinoma, lymphosarcoma and leiomyosarcomas are the most common malignant tumour of the intestine (Guilford and Strombeck, 1996; Morello et al., 2008). The lesions may be pedunculated, infiltrative (diffuse) with an uneven surface or annular (Sapierzyński, 2006; Selting, 2013; Spuzak et al., 2017; Willard, 2005). The clinical signs of neoplastic lesions in the large intestine include the presence of blood in the stool, obstructed defaecation, painful defaecation and tenesmus (Danova et al., 2006; Morello et al., 2008; Terragni et al., 2006).

Surgical resection is indicated when metastases are absent, and for non-lymphomatous lesions (Desmas et al., 2017). In the dog, the median survival time after resection of colorectal adenocarcinomas is 6–22 months. The median survival time for cats undergoing subtotal colectomy for colonic adenocarcinoma is 138 days compared with 68 days for those receiving mass resection alone. Chemotherapy significantly increases survival time, but the presence of metastasis at the

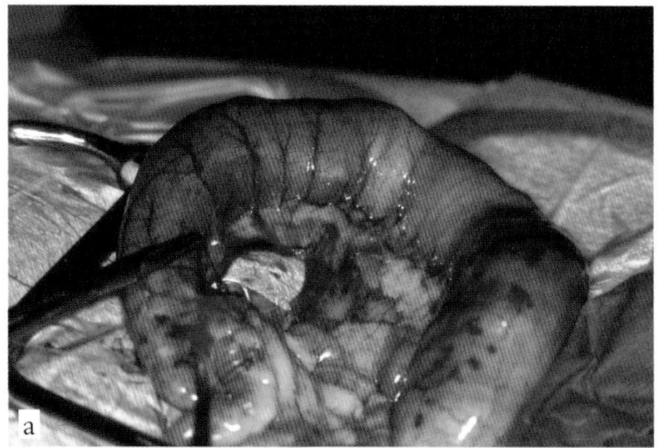

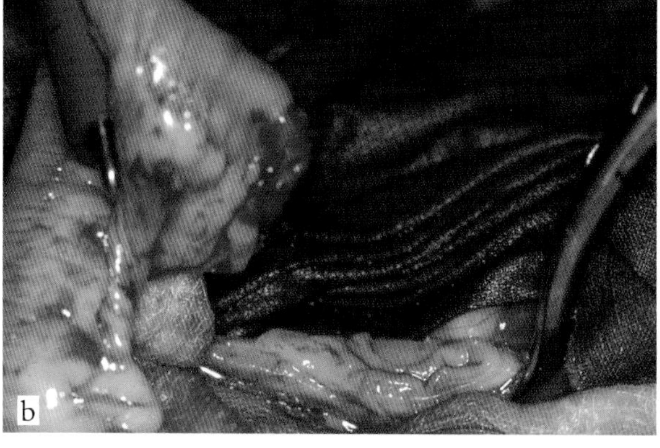

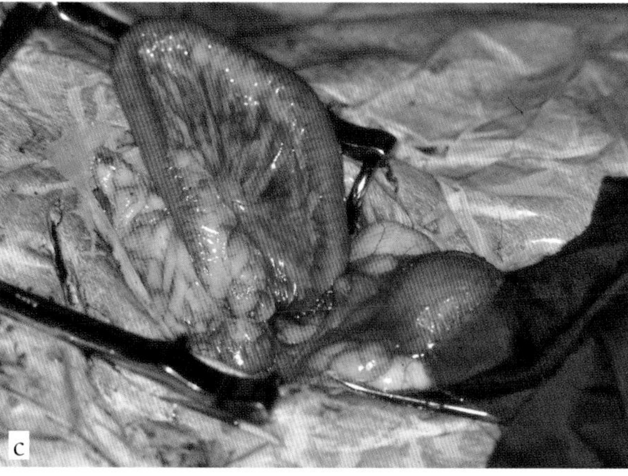

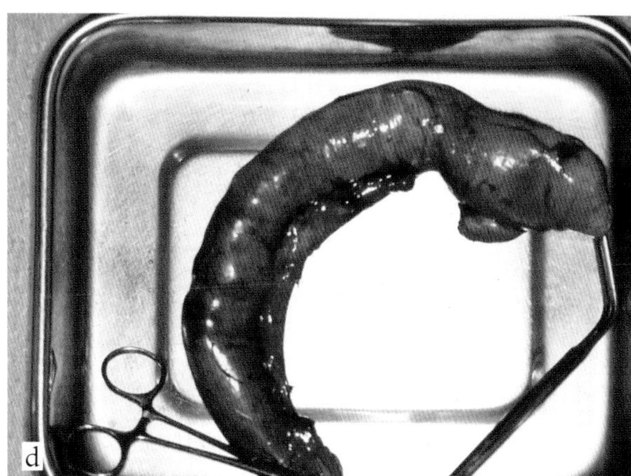

Fig. 3.46a–d Total colectomy for management of megacolon. a. Ligation of vasa recta in the affected segment of the colon. b. Luminal disparity between the ileum and colon. c. Ileocolostomy anastomosis completed. d. Segment of colon resected, including the ileocaecal valve. (Images courtesy of the University of Edinburgh.)

time of surgery decreased the mean survival time as expected (Williams, 2012).

3.6 Rectum and anal canal

Key points

- Surgery of the rectum is complicated due to its location and high bacterial load (Nucci et al., 2014).
- Indications for surgery include neoplasia, rectal stricture, diverticulum, perforation, fistula and trauma.
- Surgical preparation aims at minimising faecal flow during and after the procedure, and reducing the bacterial load.
- Food is withheld or a low-residue, high calorie diet is offered for 24–48 hours. Enemas up to 12 hours prior to surgery can be used (if no obstruction present).
- Perioperative antibiosis is recommended, with an extended anaerobic spectrum. The author often uses a combination of cefuroxime and metronidazole, starting administration 48 hours preoperatively and continuing postoperatively for up to 10 days.

3.6.1 Anatomy

The rectum comprises an intra-peritoneal and a retroperitoneal portion. The retroperitoneal portion is located below the second coccygeal vertebra in the dog, being slightly more caudal in the cat. This portion of the rectum lacks a serosal layer, which has implications for surgical healing. In the dog, the cranial rectal artery provides most of the blood supply to the terminal colon and rectum. This artery needs to be preserved, unless the intra-pelvic rectum is resected. In the cat, the intra-pelvic rectum is supplied by the middle and caudal rectal artery between other vessels, rendering preservation of the cranial rectal artery less critical (Evans and de Lahunta, 2013).

The anal sphincter has an internal and external component. The internal anal sphincter is a caudal thickening of the circular smooth rectal muscular layer. The external anal sphincter is a large, circumferential band of skeletal muscle that encourages maximal distention of the rectum for faecal storage while maintaining faecal continence.

The anal sacs lie between the two anal sphincters on either side of the anus. The anal canal is supplied by branches of the internal pudendal artery. The blood supply to the external anal sphincter derives from the perineal arteries (Evans and de Lahunta, 2013).

Parasympathetic fibres of the pelvic plexus are excitatory to the rectum and inhibitory to the internal anal sphincter (defaecation phase). Sympathetic fibres from the hypogastric nerves are inhibitory to the rectum and excitatory to the internal anal sphincter (storage phase). The caudal rectal branch of the pudendal nerve supplies motor innervation to the external anal sphincter (conscious control), and the perineal branch provides sensory innervation. Damage to the pudendal nerve may result in faecal incontinence (Aronson, 2012).

3.6.2 Surgical principles

Several approaches have been described, including a ventral approach, a dorsal inverted-U approach, mucosal eversion, a lateral approach and a trans-anal rectal pull-through with or without a combined abdominal approach (Aronson, 2012; Fossum, 2013). All these approaches present limitations and technical challenges. The trans-anal rectal pull-through offers a better exposure and the potential to remove mid-rectal lesions impossible through an abdominal approach.

Step by step: trans-anal rectal pull-through

- The animal is positioned in ventral recumbency with the hind limbs elevated.
- The rectum is everted with stay sutures placed cranially to the mucocutaneous junction (at least 1.5 cm cranial to junction if possible) (Fig. 3.47a).
- Caudal traction is applied in the cranial rectum using the stay sutures.
- A full-thickness 360° resection line is started but not completed.
- Stay sutures are placed and cranial dissection is performed along the external wall, freeing the rectum from its pelvic attachments with Metzenbaum scissors (Fig. 3.47b).
- Dissection as far as the caudal rectal artery is possible.
- Dissection cranial to the second caudal vertebra results in entering the abdominal cavity.
- Longitudinal incision into the rectal wall being resected may be required to identify healthy tissue beyond the lesion.
- The diseased rectum is transected in stages, and the anastomosis closed in stages with a simple interrupted suture pattern using 1.5 metric polydioxanone (Fig. 3.47c).

Handy hints

Vessels are ligated as encountered with either electrocautery or ligatures. A degree of capillary haemorrhage is expected throughout the procedure and can decrease visualisation. The use of cold saline

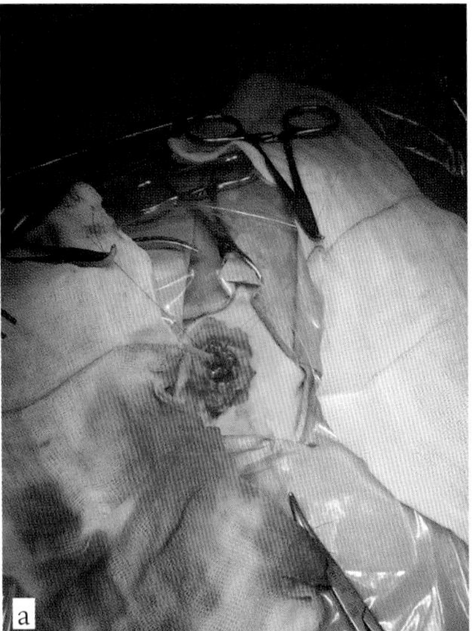

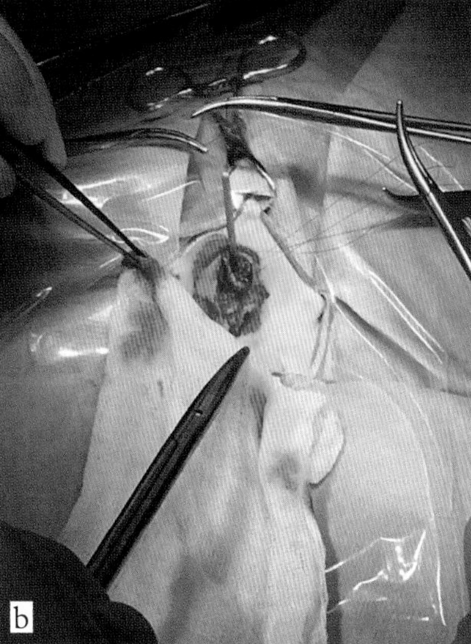

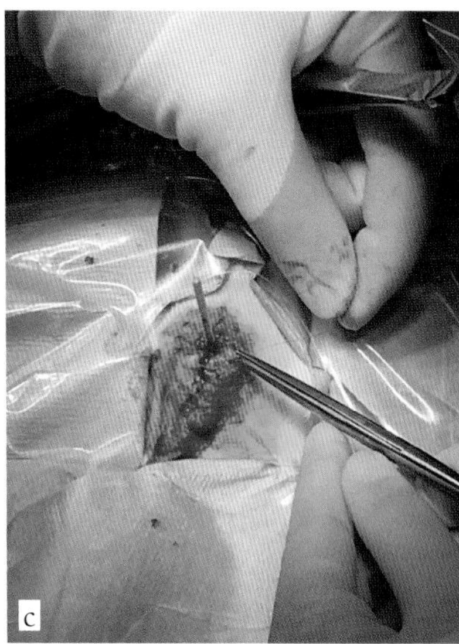

Fig. 3.47a–c Trans-anal rectal pull-through. (Images courtesy of Jon Hall.) a. The rectum has been everted with stay sutures, placed cranially to the mucocutaneous junction. b. A full-thickness 360° resection line has been started; stay sutures have been placed ready for cranial dissection to commence. c. The anastomosis has been closed with a simple interrupted pattern.

(previously chilled in the fridge) can help in decreasing haemorrhage and improving visualisation.

Faecal incontinence is encountered in some animals following rectal pull-through (Nucci et al., 2014). Other complications include dehiscence, tenesmus and stricture formation (Fossum, 2013). The severity and degree of complications depend on the area resected, extent of resection and appearance and location of the original lesion (Aronson, 2012; Morello, 2008). A full description of rectal surgery is beyond the scope of this chapter. Further reading is suggested by the author (Aronson, 2012; Fossum 2013; Morello et al., 2008; Nucci et al., 2014).

3.6.3 Anal and rectal prolapse

Anal prolapse occurs when the mucosa layer protrudes through the anal orifice. Rectal prolapse occurs when all layers of the rectum protrude through the anal orifice as an elongated cylindrical mass (Fig. 3.48a) (Aronson, 2012). Predisposing factors include diseases of the genito-urinary and gastrointestinal tracts, including parasitism, typhlitis, colitis, proctitis, tumours of the colon, rectum or anus, rectal foreign bodies, perineal hernia, cystitis, prostatitis, urolithiasis and dystocia (Aronson, 2012; Besalti and Ergin, 2012; de Battisti et al., 2013; Landon et al., 2007; Ober et al., 2016; Odendaal and Cronje, 1983). Depending on the duration of the prolapse, the tissue may be compromised or necrotic.

Diagnosis of the initial cause should be attempted. Faecal analysis, complete blood count, chemistry panel, urinalysis, urine culture, abdominal and thoracic radiographs and ultrasonography may be indicated.

Treatment depends on the cause and amount of viable tissue. Anal prolapse is easily reduced manually with saline or lubricant. In severe cases, the author uses a 50% dextrose solution to decrease tissue swelling and facilitate reduction. After reduction, a purse-string suture is inserted at the mucocutaneous junction to narrow the anal sphincter (3–5 days) (Fig. 3.48b). Sufficient width of aperture must be left to allow the animal to defaecate. A low-residue diet and a laxative such as lactulose can be used to facilitate defaecation.

In cases of rectal prolapse where tissue is healthy, manual reduction is performed, the same way as in cases of anal prolapse. When a purse-string is not sufficient to provide resolution, a colopexy can be considered (see colopexy, section 3.5.6.). In cases where the prolapsed tissue is severely traumatised or necrotic, resection of the affected segment and anastomosis is required. Prognosis depends on the cause of the prolapse and the presence or absence of necrosis.

Step by step: resection of a necrotic rectal prolapse

- The animal is placed in dorsal recumbency.
- The necrotic rectum is identified and a probe placed through the lumen (Fig. 3.49a).
- Three or four equidistant stay sutures are placed through all layers of the prolapsed rectum, just cranial to the transection site.
- The necrotic tissue is transected in stages, caudal to the stay sutures (Fig. 3.49b).
- The resected areas are then apposed with simple interrupted sutures, placed approximately 2 mm apart using 1.5 metric polydioxanone (Fig. 3.49c).

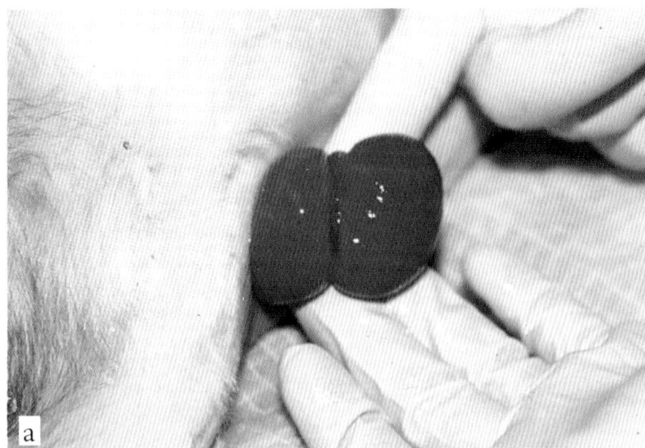
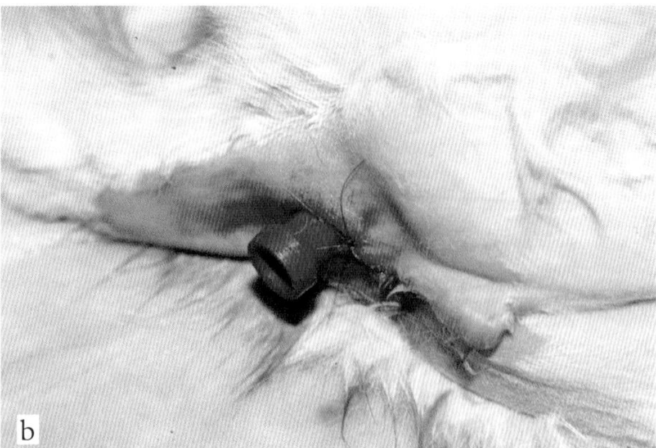

Fig. 3.48a,b Rectal prolapse. (Images courtesy of the University of Edinburgh.) a. Rectal prolapse with congested but viable rectal tissue. b. The prolapse has been reduced and a purse-string suture placed and tied around a blood sampling tube cap to prevent complete occlusion of the anal orifice and allow defaecation through the purse-string.

- Once all stages are completed, the anastomosis is checked for gaps and patched accordingly.
- The stay sutures are removed and the new anastomosis is gently placed within the anal or pelvic canal.

3.6.4 Rectal stricture

Rectal stricture can occur secondary to surgery, inflammation, trauma, foreign body, fistula, malformation or neoplasia (Lamoureux et al., 2017; Webb et al., 2007). Older animals are more commonly affected, probably due to the higher incidence of rectal disease.

Clinical signs may vary depending on the cause and the degree of narrowing; tenesmus, dyschezia, haematochezia and passage of ribbon-like faeces are commonly reported.

Diagnosis can be made through clinical examination and diagnostic imaging including rectal examination, positive contrast studies and endoscopy. Biopsy may be indicated.

Treatment depends on the underlying cause and degree of narrowing. Mild, non-neoplastic cases may be amenable to bougienage, digital bougienage or balloon dilation with or without concomitant intralesional injection of triamcinolone (Lamoureux et al., 2017; Webb et al., 2007). Repeated treatments may be required.

In more severe cases, surgical resection may be indicated. The approach depends on the exact location of the lesion. Rectal pull-through would be the author's choice for circumferential strictures. Surgical complications include tenesmus, wound dehiscence, infection, incontinence and recurrence of the stricture. Prognosis depends on the underlying cause and degree of resection (Aronson, 2012).

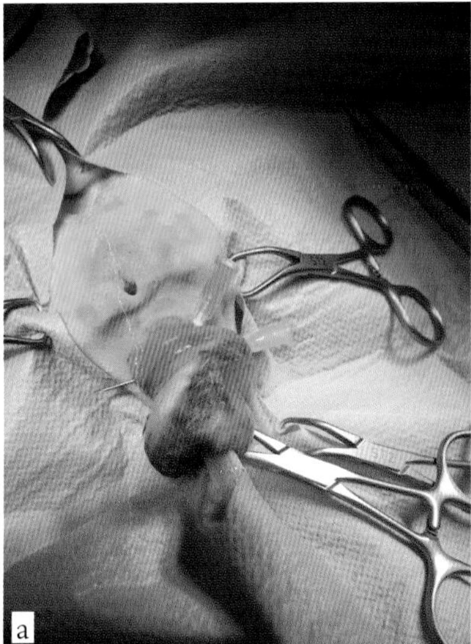
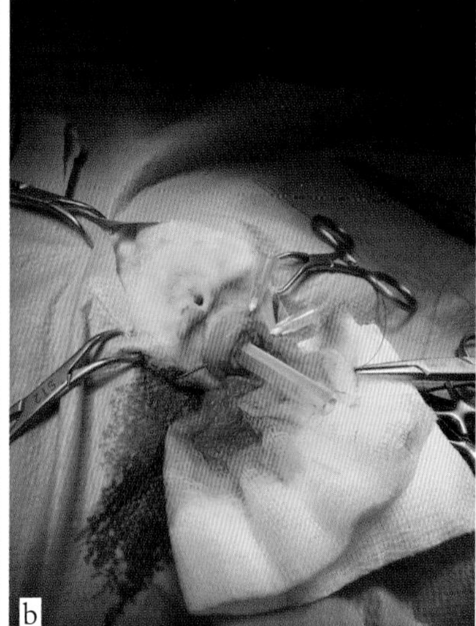
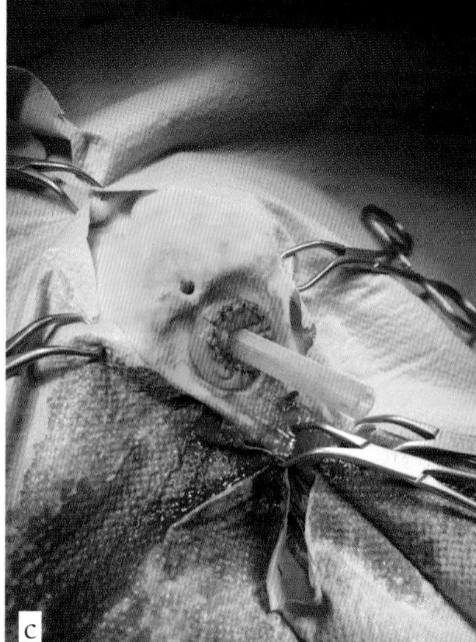

Fig. 3.49a–c Resection of a necrotic rectal prolapse. (Images courtesy of Jon Hall.) a. The necrotic rectum is identified and a probe has been placed through the lumen. Hypodermic needles have been placed through the healthy rectum and probe to minimise tissue retraction. b. The necrotic tissue has been excised caudal to the hypodermic needles. c. The resected areas have been apposed with simple interrupted sutures.

3.6.5 Anal sacs

The anal sacs are situated between the internal and external anal sphincters at the 4 and 8 o'clock positions. The ducts empty at the level of the mucocutaneous junction (Rutherford and Lee, 2015).

In the dog, the anal sacs comprise apocrine sudoriparous glands (fundic portion) and a few sebaceous glands (duct epithelium). In the cat, both types of glands are present in the fundic portion. The low incidence of feline anal sac disease has been attributed to decreased fluid viscosity of the anal gland secretions (high lipid content), minimising duct occlusion.

The most common disorders of the anal sacs are impaction, sacculitis and abscessation (Hill et al., 2006). In impaction, obstruction occurs without any associated inflammation. Sacculitis and abscessation are more commonly seen in small-breed dogs such as Chihuahuas and poodles. German shepherds have their anal sacs located much more deeply along the wall of the rectum and for this reason are also predisposed for anal sac disease (Aronson, 2012). The colour and consistency of the anal sac contents are variable in healthy dogs and there are no pathognomonic signs of anal sac impaction or sacculitis (Pappalardo et al., 2002; Van Duijkeren, 1995).

Clinical signs include scooting, licking, biting of the affected area, discomfort in sitting, painful defaecation and tenesmus. Yeast and bacterial cultures from normal and diseased anal sacs are similar and include streptococci, staphylococci, micrococci, *E. coli*, *Proteus*, *Clostridium*, *Pseudomonas*, *Malassezia* and others (Pappalardo et al., 2002; Robson et al., 2003). Purulent discharge or fistulation may be present in cases of abscessation.

Impaction can be treated by either manual expression or cannulation of the affected duct and irrigation with sterile saline. Sacculitis is best treated with topical infusion of antibiotics and corticosteroids after irrigation with antiseptic solution (0.05% chlorhexidine or 1% povidone-iodine) (Aronson, 2012). Systemic antibiotics may be required if cellulitis is present around the anal sac. Abscesses are treated by incision, drainage and lavage with warm saline and mild antiseptic solution. Antibiotics can be locally infused and the wound left open to granulate (Aronson, 2012). Recurrence of any of the above conditions is an indication for anal sac removal (Charlesworth, 2014).

Anal sacculectomy can be performed through either a closed or open approach. In both techniques, excessive trauma to the external anal sphincter may result in incontinence. The closed technique is associated with the least number of complications (Hill and Smeak, 2002) and is the one preferred by the author. Better delineation of the anal sacs can be achieved by filling them with gel or melted paraffin, or by inserting a Foley catheter (Aronson, 2012; Downs and Stampley, 1998).

Handy hints

The author prefers using a pair of straight haemostats placed through the duct, because gel or paraffin can migrate and a Foley catheter can become dislodged during manipulation.

Step by step: closed anal sacculectomy

- The animal is placed in dorsal recumbency.
- The faeces are manually evacuated from the rectum and a purse-string string is placed cranial to the anal sac opening.
- A pair of small haemostats or a probe is inserted through the anal sac duct.
- A curvilinear incision is made over the anal sac (Fig. 3.50a).
- The anal sac is dissected from the internal and external anal sphincter fibres using Metzenbaum scissors.
- The dissection is continued until the duct is visualised and the sac and duct are free (Fig. 3.50b).

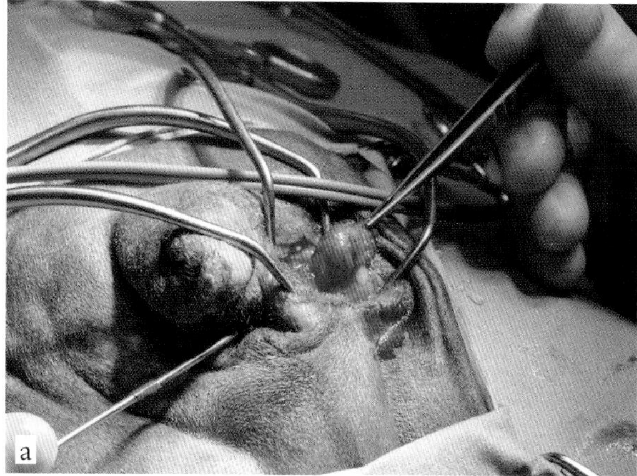

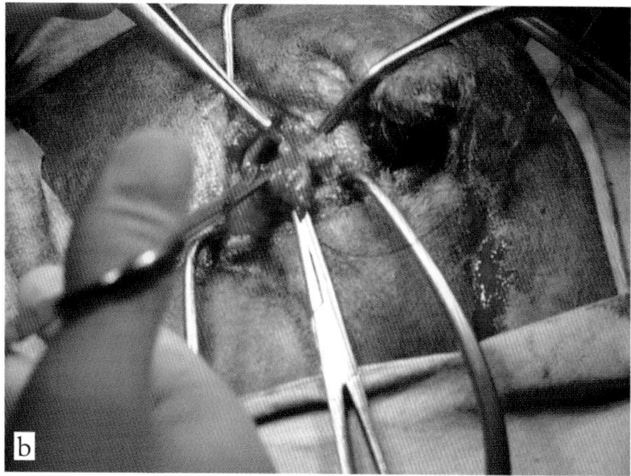

Fig. 3.50a,b Right closed anal sacculectomy. (Images courtesy of Karen Perry.) a. A probe has been inserted through the anal sac duct and a curvilinear incision made over the anal sac; blunt dissection has been initiated. b. The anal sac has been fully dissected and the duct identified and ready for ligation.

- Care must be taken not to damage the muscles or the cranial rectal artery medial to the anal sac duct.
- The duct is ligated at the mucocutaneous junction using 1.5 metric polydioxanone or polyglecaprone-25.
- The duct, distal to the suture, is transected and the anal sac is inspected to confirm complete resection.
- The wound is lavaged and routinely closed in two layers.

Step by step: open anal sacculectomy

- The animal is placed in dorsal recumbency.
- The faeces are manually evacuated from the rectum, and a purse-string suture is placed cranial to the anal sac opening.
- A pair of small haemostats or a probe is inserted in the anal sac duct.
- An oblique incision is made from the external anal sphincter to the lateral-most end of the anal sac (Fig. 3.51a).
- The incision is deepened with Metzenbaum scissors and the duct and anal sac are opened.
- The cut edge of the anal sac and duct are elevated and bluntly dissected from their muscular attachments and surrounding tissue (Fig. 3.51b).
- Care must be taken not to damage the muscles or the cranial rectal artery medial to the anal sac duct.
- The duct is ligated at the mucocutaneous junction, using 1.5 metric polydioxanone or polyglecaprone-25.
- The duct, distal to the suture, is transected and the anal sac is inspected to confirm complete resection.
- The wound is lavaged and routinely closed in two layers (Fig. 3.51c.

The overall complication rate is low (MacPhail, 2008). Immediate postoperative complications include scooting, inflammation, excessive drainage from the surgical site and seroma. Long-term complications include incontinence, fistulation and stricture formation. Infection is reported in association with incomplete resection of the glandular tissue, and revision surgery is advisable (Hill and Smeak, 2002).

Apocrine gland anal sac adenocarcinoma (ASA) is the most common neoplasm of the anal sac, even though adenomas, melanomas and squamous cell carcinomas have also been reported (Esplin et al., 2003; Vinayak et al., 2017). ASAs are typically small but locally invasive, and highly metastatic to the sacral, hypogastric and medial iliac lymph nodes (Bennett et al., 2002; Turek and Withrow, 2012). Distant metastasis has also been reported (Rutherford and Lee, 2015). The majority of ASAs are unilateral, but bilateral masses have been reported in up to 10% of cases (Ross et al., 1991; Rutherford and Lee, 2015). These tumours are commonly found incidentally during a perineal or rectal examination. In the case of metastatis, clinical signs associated with pelvic canal narrowing are observed, such as constipation, tenesmus and ribbon-like faeces. ASAs

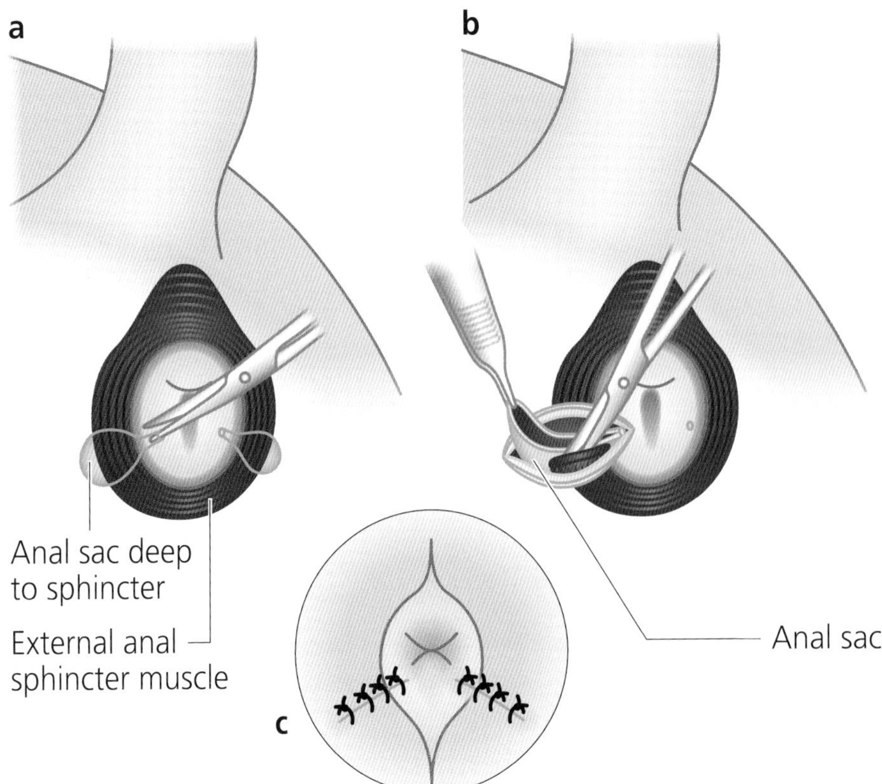

Fig. 3.51a–c Open anal sacculectomy. *Illustrator: Elaine Leggett*

can produce a parathyroid hormone-related protein and cause pseudo-hyperparathyroidism (Bergman, 2012; Messinger et al., 2009). Associated clinical signs include hypercalcaemia, polyuria, polydipsia, anorexia, vomiting and lethargy (Rutherford and Lee, 2015).

Diagnosis can be made by fine needle aspiration of the anal sac mass. Full animal staging with thoracic radiographs, abdominal ultrasonography and blood work should be performed. CT when available may be advantageous.

The treatment of choice is mass removal through anal sacculectomy (unilateral or bilateral), and metastectomy of the abnormal regional lymph nodes (Bennett et al., 2002; Emms, 2005). Resection of the abnormal lymph nodes is performed through a ventral midline approach. Typically, these lymph nodes are well adherent to the spinal musculature and careful dissection is required to minimise potentially severe haemorrhage. Radiation with or without chemotherapy can be used either adjunctively or as a sole treatment, but the role of these modalities has not yet been fully determined (Rutherford and Lee, 2015; Turek and Withrow, 2012).

3.7 The liver

Key points

- The liver is a parenchymatous organ. It plays a role in the metabolism of protein, fat and carbohydrates and is the primary site for detoxification of many substances.
- Surgery is often required in animals with severe diffuse or focal hepatic disease.
- Stabilisation, oncotic support and administration of blood products may be imperative.
- Advanced imaging may facilitate surgical planning.
- Access to surgical staplers and vessel-sealing devices is advantageous but, ultimately, skills and experience directly influence outcome.

3.7.1 Anatomy

The liver is larger on the right side than on the left. The dog and cat both have hepatic fissures that subdivide the liver into different lobes: left lateral, left medial, quadrate, right medial, right lateral and caudate (Fig. 3.52).

The vena cava runs through the right side of the liver and is firmly attached to it. The coronary ligament attaches the liver to the diaphragm and is a continuation of the hepatic peritoneal covering, which is present over the entire surface of the organ with the exception

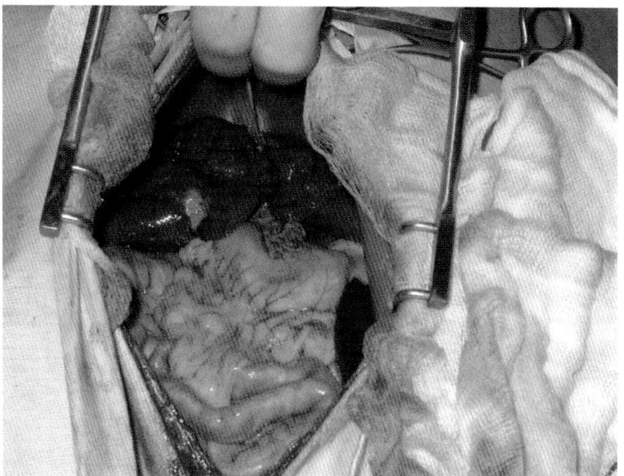

Fig. 3.52 Liver lobes of a dog during an exploratory coeliotomy. Nodular lesions are present in the left lateral, left medial, quadrate and right medial hepatic lobes.

of the porta hepatis region. Emanating from the coronary ligament are two right-sided triangular ligaments and one left-sided. The hepato-renal ligament attaches the caudate lobe to the right kidney.

The liver receives its blood supply from the hepatic artery (branch of the coeliac artery) and the portal vein. The hepatic artery provides 20% of blood volume and 50% of the oxygen while the portal vein supplies 80% of the volume and 50% of the oxygen.

At the level of the porta hepatis, the hepatic artery usually branches to supply different lobes of the liver. The right lateral branch supplies the caudate and right lateral lobe; the right middle branch supplies the right medial lobe, the dorsal part of the quadrate and part of the left medial lobe; the left branch supplies the left lateral, part of the quadrate and the left medial lobe.

The portal vein divides into right and left branches when entering the liver. The right branch supplies the caudate process and right lateral lobe; the left branch gives off a central branch that supplies the right medial lobe and papillary process and then divides into left lateral, left medial and quadrate branches that supply the respective lobes.

In the cat there are usually three main branches – right, left and central – that supply the respective lobes of each division. Six to eight hepatic veins drain the blood flow through the liver.

The epiploic foramen is a natural opening in the omental bursa and is bordered dorsally by the caudal vena cava and ventrally by the portal vein and lies medial to the caudate liver lobe and to the right of midline (Fig. 3.53). Pressure on the epiploic foramen, also known as the 'Pringle manoeuvre', can be used to cause occlusion of the caudal vena cava, hepatic artery and portal vein, stopping inflow to the liver. This can be performed for around 20 minutes in the dog before

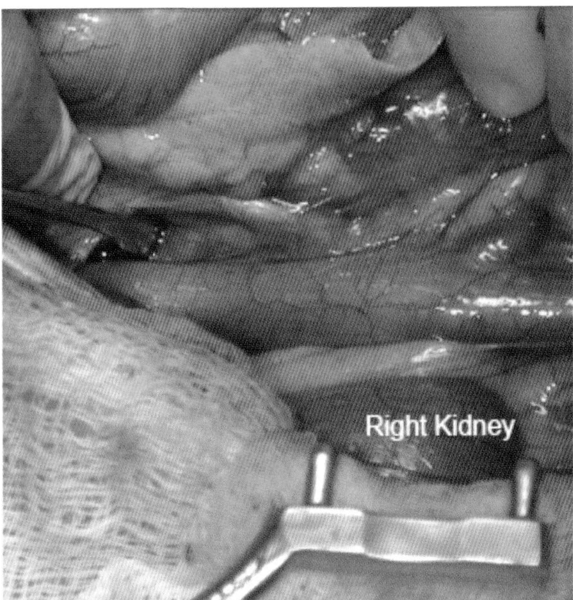

Fig. 3.53 Epiploic foramen visible during an exploratory coeliotomy. The vena cava can be seen dorsally and the coeliac artery is visualised ventrally to the foramen.

causing necrosis of the liver (Evans and de Lahunta, 2013; Mayhew and Weisse, 2012).

3.7.2 Surgical principles

The liver has a crucial function in maintenance of body system homeostasis, including synthesis and clearance of plasma proteins and the production of coagulation factors and anticoagulants. Animals suffering from liver pathology can have any, or most, of these functions compromised. Extensive perioperative support may be required, and the risk of intra-operative complications such as severe haemorrhage may be high. Careful evaluation, preoperative management, knowledge of the anatomy and physiology, and flexibility to change plans intra-operatively are required.

Hepatic surgery carries a risk of haemorrhage which, in some instances, can be life-threatening. Evaluation of coagulation profile, blood type and cross-matching should be performed prior to surgery.

Hypoglycaemia may be present in animals with end-stage liver disease or in those undergoing extensive hepatectomy (up to 70%). For this reason, glucose levels should be carefully monitored and supplementation administered when indicated (Mayhew and Weisse, 2012).

Bacteria from the intestine and endotoxins delivered through the portal system are removed by the liver's mononuclear phagocytic system, primarily the Kupffer cells. However, some controversy remains regarding flora remaining in the liver. In one study, 60% of liver samples had a positive culture for a variety of organisms including strict anaerobes, strict aerobes and facultative anaerobes. The most common isolate was *Clostridium perfringens* followed by *Staphylococcus* spp. For this reason, perioperative antibiosis should be considered.

3.7.3 Liver biopsy

Liver biopsy is commonly performed in small animals. Histopathological assessment allows a histomorphological and sometimes a causal diagnosis to be made, as well as collection of samples for the quantification of copper, zinc and iron as well as for bacterial and fungal culture (Lidbury, 2016). Several methods are reported, including fine needle aspiration biopsy (FNAB, ultrasound-guided), Tru-Cut biopsy, open liver biopsy and laparoscopic liver biopsy.

The technique of FNAB, although safe, has a poor diagnostic accuracy and a single needle biopsy is estimated to represent 0.002% of the entire hepatic parenchyma (Fox et al., 2012). In one study the morphological diagnosis from FNAB, by individual examiners, was in agreement with the morphological diagnosis from larger wedge biopsy specimens for 56 and 67% of the specimens (Cole et al., 2002). Larger and multiple samples are therefore preferable, as pathology variation can occur even within the same liver lobe.

Larger samples can be collected through open surgery or laparoscopically. In the former technique, a ventral midline coeliotomy is performed and a liver sample is collected using single or multiple overlapping guillotine sutures. Vessel-sealing devices, such as Ligasure™ or Harmonic Scalpel™, and pre-tied ligating loops, such as Endoloop®, can also be used. For more central lesions, a Baker biopsy punch (6 mm) is available.

Step by step: open liver biopsy using guillotine method

- A ventral midline coeliotomy is performed.
- An area in the periphery of a liver lobe is identified and packed with sterile laparotomy swabs soaked in warm, sterile saline (Fig. 3.54a).
- A loop of 1.5 or 2.0 metric polydioxanone is placed around the periphery of the isolated liver lobe (Fig. 3.54b).
- The suture is tied, crushing through the parenchyma and securing the blood vessels and biliary ducts (Fig.
- The liver distal to the suture is removed sharply using a fresh scalpel blade or sharp scissors (Fig. 3.54c).
- Alternatively, several overlapping guillotine sutures can be placed in the margin of a liver lobe, allowing a larger sample to be removed.

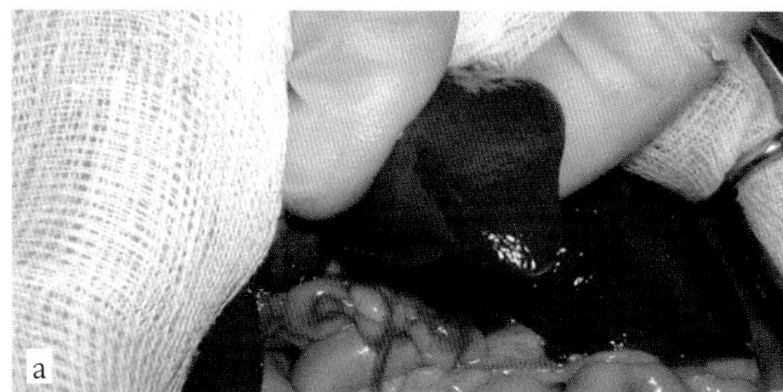

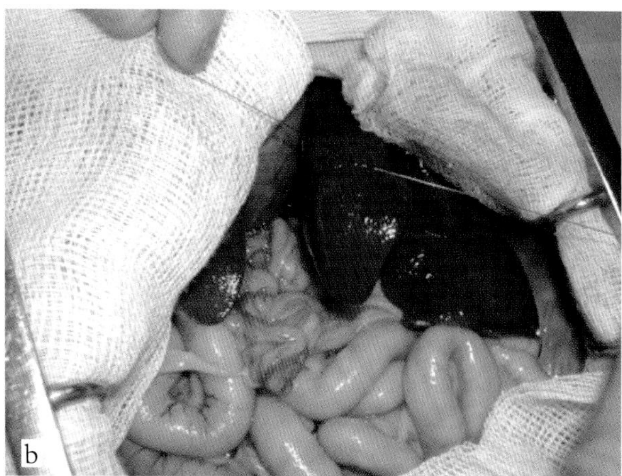

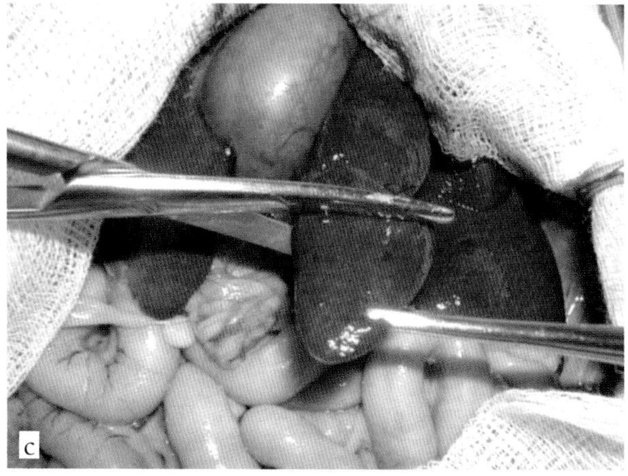

Fig. 3.54a–c Liver biopsy using the guillotine method. (Images courtesy of University of Edinburgh.) a. An area on the periphery of a liver lobe is identified and packed with sterile laparotomy swabs. b. A loop of suture has been placed around the periphery of the liver lobe. c. The suture has been tied, crushing through the parenchyma and securing the blood vessels and biliary ducts. Sharp scissors are used to remove liver tissue distal to the suture line.

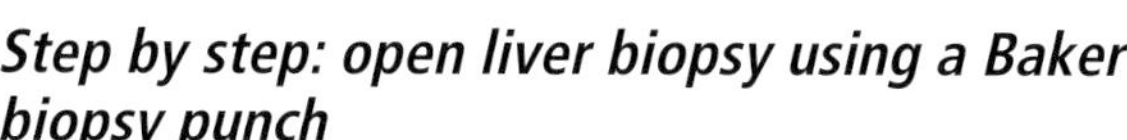

Step by step: open liver biopsy using a Baker biopsy punch

- A ventral midline coeliotomy is performed.
- The area to be sampled (central liver) is identified.
- The biopsy punch is pushed against the parenchyma and advanced with short, rotatory movements in both the clockwise and anticlockwise direction (Fig. 3.55).
- The deeper margin of the sample is separated from the remaining parenchyma using Metzenbaum scissors.
- A synthetic haemostatic agent can be placed into the hepatic defect to control haemorrhage.

Handy hints

The author uses a collagen sponge of bovine origin (Lyostyp®) to lay over areas with mild haemorrhage. The same agent can be cut into shape to fill the small defect created by the Baker biopsy punch.

Laparoscopy provides a minimally invasive method to collect a liver biopsy. It allows optimal visualisation of the liver and a safe biopsy technique. The author uses a two- or three-portal technique, with the first port being placed subumbilical and the second instrument port being placed paramedian in the right or left cranial quadrant (Fig. 3.56). A third port can be placed in the contralateral side for a haemostatic device. Tissue can be collected using cup biopsy forceps, a vessel-sealing device or a pre-tied ligating loop. A recent study showed that samples obtained with a pre-tied ligating loop were significantly heavier, larger in volume and contained more portal tracts and less crush and fragmentation artefacts than those obtained with cup biopsy forceps (Fernandez et al., 2017).

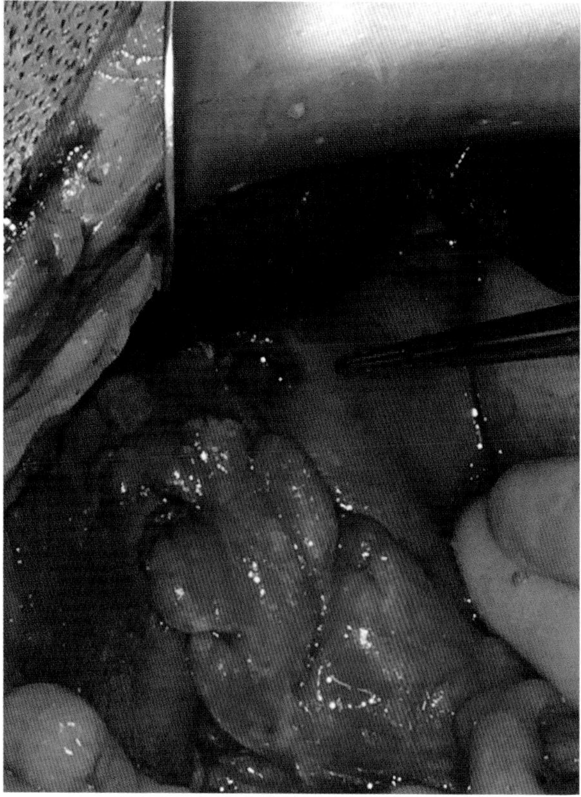

Fig. 3.55 Open liver biopsy using a biopsy punch. (Image courtesy of Samantha Woods.)

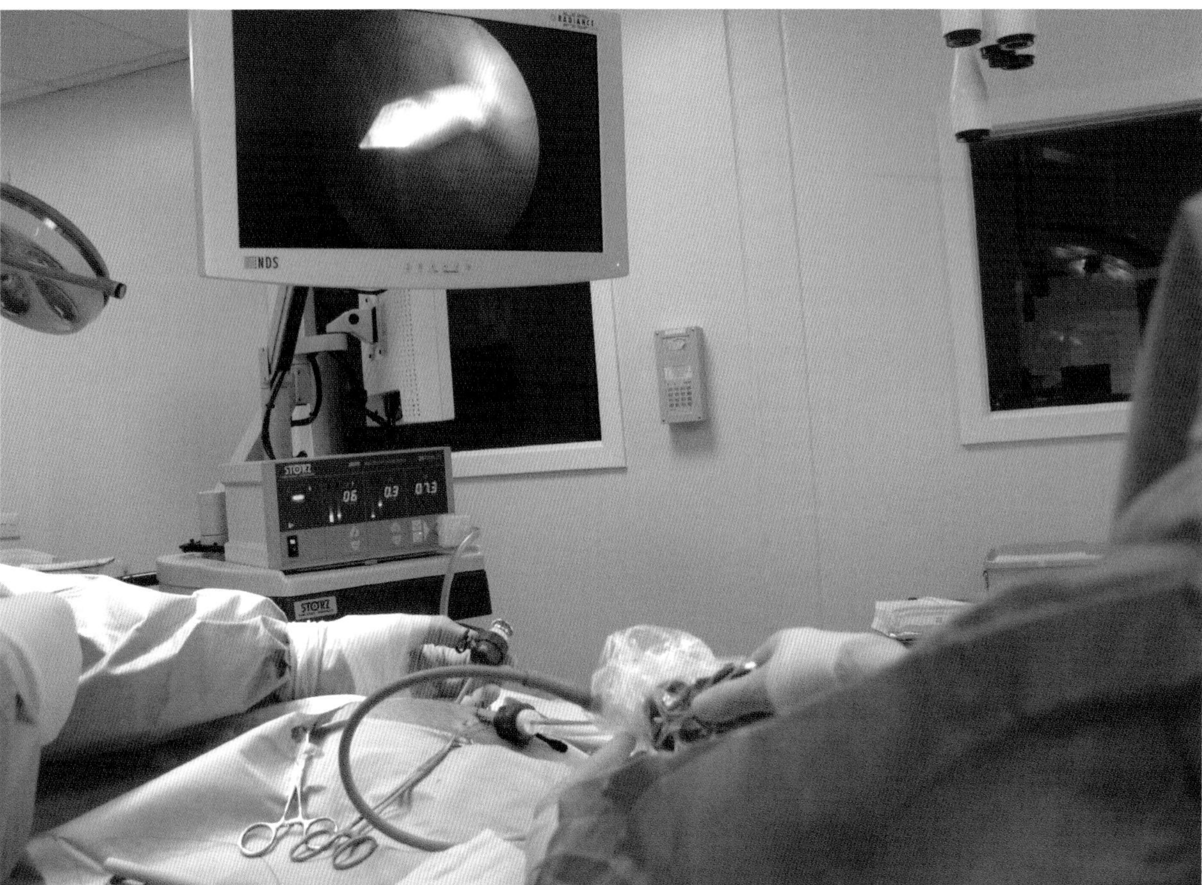

Fig. 3.56 Laparoscopic liver biopsy. A subumbilical camera port has been placed, and a second instrument port is being inserted in a paramedian position under direct visualisation.

3.7.4 Liver lobectomy

Liver lobectomy is often indicated in the management of abscess, tumour and torsed or fractured lobe. Partial liver lobectomy can be performed using a finger fracture or blunt dissection technique, or by using mattress sutures in a similar manner to the biopsy technique. Vessel-sealing devices and surgical staplers can also be used. Complete liver lobectomy should be performed by an experienced surgeon with good knowledge of the local anatomy. If total lobectomy is required, the hilus can be identified and ligated or a similar technique to partial lobectomy followed. Surgical stapling devices (e.g. TA™ stapler) can be also used for complete lobectomy. The left lateral and left medial liver lobes maintain their separation near the hilus. For this reason, these lobes can be removed by placing an encircling suture at the base of the lobe. For resection of the right lateral and caudate lobes, careful dissection around the hepatic caudal vena cava is usually required (Fossum, 2013). Complete liver lobectomy is beyond the scope of this chapter. For further understanding of this technique, the author advises consulting additional literature (Covey et al., 2009; Mayhew and Weisse, 2012). Complications following liver lobectomy include perioperative haemorrhage, impairment of blood supply to the adjacent liver lobe, transient hypoglycaemia, portal hypertension and liver dysfunction (Kinsey et al., 2015; May and Mehler, 2011; Selmic, 2017).

Step by step: partial liver lobectomy

- A ventral midline exploratory coeliotomy is performed.
- Increased exposure to the cranial quadrant is achieved with either a caudal median sternotomy or a diaphragmatic myotomy.
- The liver capsule is transected with a scalpel blade.
- The parenchyma is bluntly dissected using the flat, blunt end of a scalpel handle or the inner cannula of a Poole suction tip.
- Alternatively, a finger fracture technique can be used where digital pressure is applied to fracture the liver parenchyma.
- Small vessels are ligated with electrocautery, suture or vascular staplers (Surgiclips™ or Haemoclips™).
- Alternatively, a pre-tied suture can be placed cranial to the area to be removed, fracturing through the parenchyma and securing the vessels and biliary tracts (Fig. 3.57a,b). Larger vessels are ligated with either suturing or a vessel-sealing device (Fig. 3.57c).

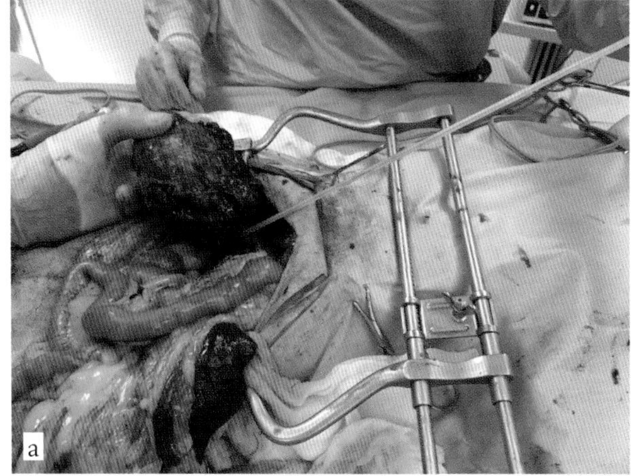

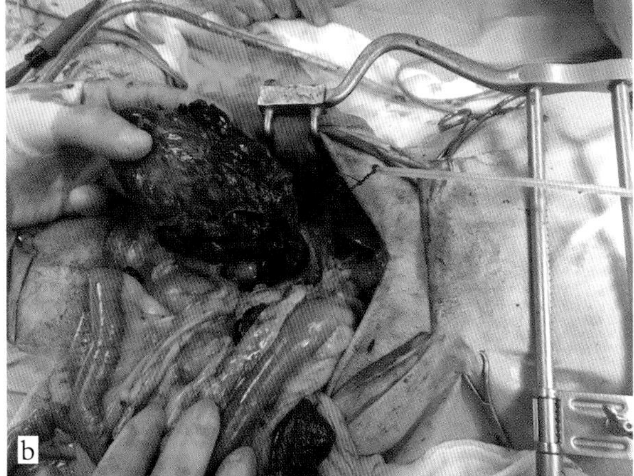

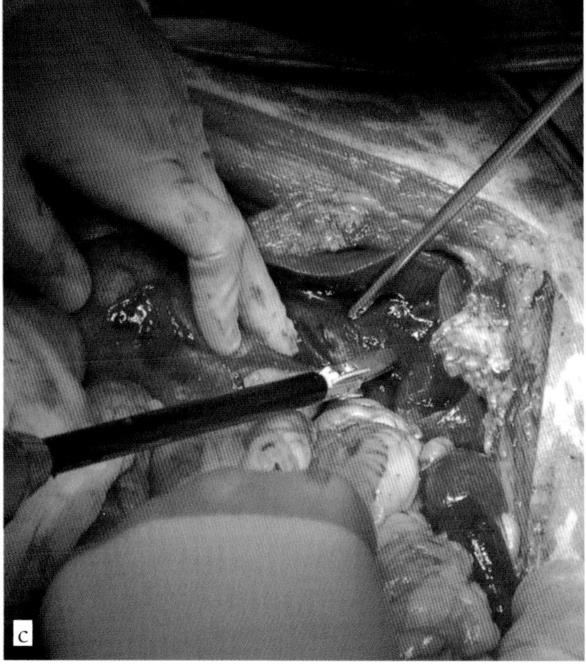

Fig. 3.57a–c Partial liver lobectomy for resection of a hepatocellular carcinoma affecting the caudate lobe. (Images courtesy of Samantha Woods.) a. The affected liver lobe has been identified and initial dissection performed using the finger fracture technique. b. A pre-tied loop of suture has been placed just cranial to the tumour. The suture has been tied, crushing through the parenchyma and securing the blood vessels and biliary tracts. c. Vessel-sealing device controlling haemorrhage during partial liver lobectomy.

3.7.5 Abscess

Hepatic abscessation is a rare condition typically affecting older animals. The clinicopathologic findings are similar to those of other inflammatory hepatic diseases and include anorexia, lethargy, vomiting, diarrhoea, fever, dehydration, abdominal pain, hepatomegaly and mucosal bleeding. Blood work may show leucocytosis with neutrophilia, mild to moderate thrombocytopenia, mild anaemia, high alkaline phosphatase, high alanine aminotransferase, high bilirubin, hypoalbuminaemia and prolonged coagulation values (Farrar et al., 1996).

Diagnosis is most commonly made by ultrasound, where hypoechoic, heteroechoic or hyperechoic masses are identified (Farrar et al., 1996). In one study, solitary lesions >3 cm were more commonly present and the abscesses were mainly poorly echogenic, with central cavitation (Schwarz et al., 1998). *Escherichia coli*, *Clostridium* spp., *Klebsiella pneumoniae*, *Enterococcus* spp., *Staphylococcus epidermidis* and *Staphylococcus intermedius* are the most commonly isolated bacteria. Concurrent infections have been identified in the biliary tract, spleen, blood, endocardium, lung, prostate gland, peritoneum, lymph nodes, salivary gland or brain of several dogs (Farrar et al., 1996). In the cat, cultures yielded polymicrobial growth in 66% of the cases with *E. coli* being the most commonly cultured organism (Sergeeff et al., 2004).

Treatment involves the use of broad-spectrum antibiotics and addressing any predisposing diseases such as diabetes mellitus, urinary tract infection, pancreatitis, glucocorticoid administration, gall bladder rupture and pneumonia (Mayhew and Weisse, 2012). Drainage of the abscess (ultrasound-guided) and surgical excision, through partial hepatectomy, have been reported with good results (Farrar et al., 1996). The indications for surgical resection are unclear from the literature, and a decision must be made on a case-to-case basis. Percutaneous ultrasound-assisted drainage and alcoholisation using 95% ethanol have been described successfully in a cohort of six animals (Zatelli et al., 2005). The prognosis in the dog is good when the disease is diagnosed early. Cats have a worse prognosis, with a reported overall mortality rate of 79% (Sergeeff et al., 2004).

3.7.6 Neoplasia

Primary hepatic tumours are seen in the dog and cat, although most commonly hepatic nodules are metastatic lesions (Strombeck, 1978). Hepatocellular carcinoma is the most common primary liver tumour in the dog, representing 50–70% of all non-haematopoietic

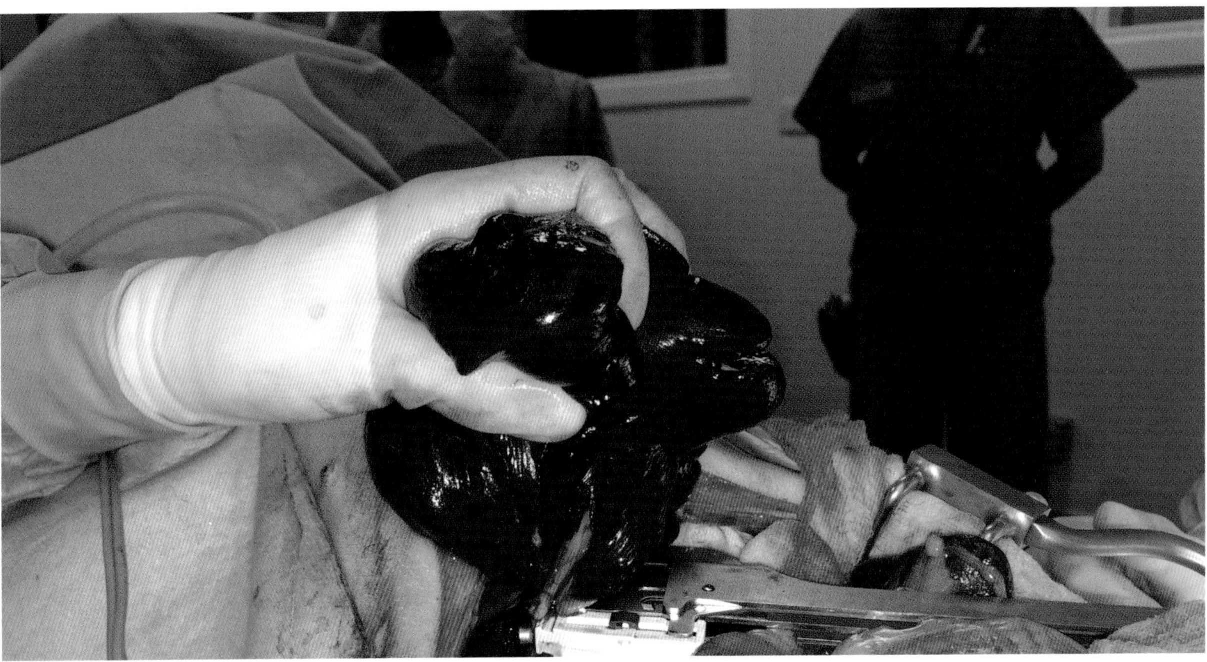

Fig. 3.58 Hilar resection of a massive hepatocellular carcinoma using a TA™ surgical stapler. (Image courtesy of Samantha Woods.)

neoplasms (Mayhew and Weisse, 2012). These can present in one of three forms: (1) massive, where a single large tumour involves only one liver lobe; (2) nodular, where multiple tumours are located in different liver lobes; and (3) diffuse, where either multifocal nodular changes are present in different liver lobes or diffuse changes are present throughout the liver (Selmic, 2017). The massive form is the most commonly seen and is associated with a lower metastatic rate (Patnaik et al., 1981). In the cat, the most common hepatocellular tumour is hepatic adenoma (Patnaik et al., 1980).

Surgery is indicated and is the treatment of choice for massive hepatocellular carcinoma (Fig. 3.58). Masses located in the right hepatic lobes can present a surgical challenge due to their close proximity to vital structures such as the caudal vena cava, portal vein and hepatic artery. Advanced imaging, including CT angiography and MRI, can help with surgical planning and feasibility for surgical resection.

Overall, the prognosis for dogs with massive hepatocellular carcinoma is good with low recurrence rates reported (0–13%; Patnaik et al., 1980; Selmic, 2017). Median survival times >1460 days were documented in a cohort of 42 dogs treated surgically (Mayhew and Weisse, 2012).

Non-resectable massive primary liver tumours have been treated with chemoembolisation, aiming to separate the tumour from its arterial blood supply causing necrosis and ideally tumour shrinkage. The results of this technique are variable, and further studies are required (Weisse, 2009; Weisse et al., 2002). Radiation therapy and chemotherapy have also been reported in the treatment of non-surgical cases (Elpiner et al., 2011; Mori et al., 2015).

3.7.7 Portosystemic shunt

Portosystemic shunt is a disturbance of blood flow that leads to bypassing of the liver circulation and direct flow from the portal to systemic circulation (Connolly, 2016). Congenital shunts are more commonly identified in veterinary medicine, but acquired shunts have also been reported (Leeman et al., 2013). Predisposed breeds, for a single congenital portosystemic shunt, include the miniature schnauzer, Irish wolfhound, Havanese, Yorkshire terrier, Maltese, Dandie Dinmont terrier, pug, Australian cattle dog and Old English sheepdog (Center and Magne, 1990; Connolly, 2016; Maddison, 1988; Tobias and Rohrbach, 2003; Ubbink et al., 1998).

Clinical signs are non-specific and include gastrointestinal and neurological (such as dull mentation and quiet behaviour after meals), failure to thrive and urinary signs including dysuria, stranguria and pollakiuria. Dogs with splenocaval shunts may have more clinical abnormalities in comparison to those with other shunt morphologies (Kraun et al., 2014).

Laboratory testing and diagnostic imaging is crucial to achieving a diagnosis. A complete blood count (CBC), serum biochemistry profile, urinalysis and preprandial and postprandial serum bile acids, and ammonia levels, are recommended. Recently, some veterinarians have begun testing protein-C activity (Mankin, 2015). Changes in CBC may include leucocytosis, microcytosis, and normocytic, normochromic, non-regenerative anaemia. Changes in biochemistry profile may include decreased blood urea nitrogen, hypoalbuminaemia, hypoglycaemia and hypocholesterolaemia. Mild to moderate increases in serum liver enzyme activities may also be present.

Increased fasting ammonia and serum bile acid concentrations are accurate indicators of portosystemic shunts in the dog and cat (Ruland et al, 2010; van Straten et al., 2015). Elevated postprandial serum bile acid concentration is also suggestive of a portosystemic shunt. Male dogs, older dogs and those having received medical management prior to initial evaluation should be considered at increased risk for the development of urolithiasis (Caporali et al., 2015).

Historically, intra-operative mesenteric portography has been performed to diagnose congenital portosystemic shunt. The technique involves placing a catheter in a mesenteric vessel and injecting iodine-based contrast agent followed by radiography or fluoroscopy (Fig. 3.59a–c). Findings of intra-operative mesenteric portography may be predictive of outcome (after attenuation), and the degree of intra-hepatic portal vessel opacification correlates with the ability to completely ligate the shunting vessel (Lee et al., 2006). Less invasive methods are now readily available and used as a first line of diagnosis. These include ultrasound, CT angiography and MRI angiography.

Handy hints

The author uses mesenteric portography as an intra-operative tool when the shunting vessel is not easily identified during an exploratory coeliotomy. This is particularly useful when an intra-hepatic shunt has been misdiagnosed as extra-hepatic during the initial ultrasound. Portovenography is also useful to confirm correct vessel attenuation intra-operatively.

Abdominal ultrasound is an excellent tool in the diagnosis of congenital single portosystemic shunt. Experience of the operator influences the accuracy of diagnosis. Reported sensitivity and specificity range from 80 to 95% and 67 to 100%, respectively (D'Anjou, 2004; Lamb, 1996; Winkler et al., 2003).

Nuclear scintigraphy has been reported as having high sensitivity and specificity in the diagnosis of congenital portosystemic shunt. The technique involves injection of a radionuclide, either into the spleen or per rectum. The requirement for safety measures and association with potential complications makes this a less appealing alternative.

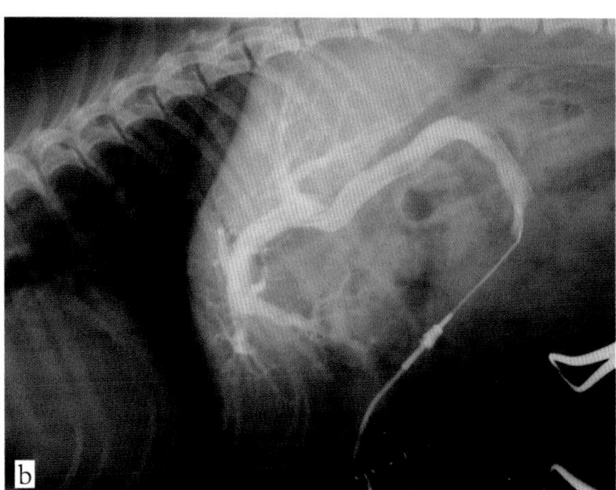

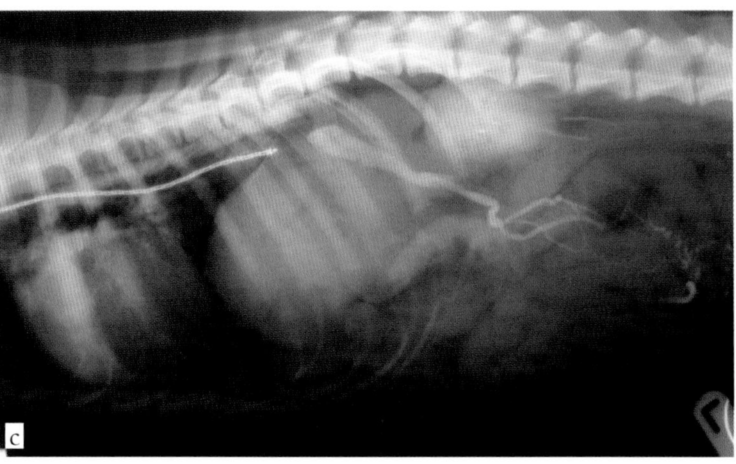

Fig. 3.59a–c Mesenteric portovenography. (Images courtesy of University of Edinburgh.) a. Mesenteric vein catheterised during exploratory coeliotomy and iodine-based contrast agent injected. b. Lateral abdominal radiograph showing a normal portovenogram with contrast uptake and branching of the hepatic portal vessel. c. Portovenograph showing a portoazygus portosystemic shunt.

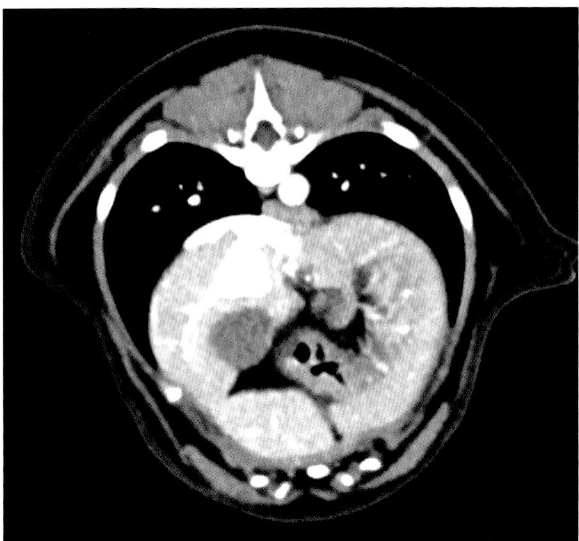

Fig. 3.60 CT angiograph showing a left divisional intra-hepatic shunt.

CT angiography has a high diagnostic sensitivity and specificity in the dog (Fig. 3.60).

This technique is minimally invasive (anaesthetic and intravenous contrast required), rapid and can provide a three-dimensional (3D) reconstruction of the shunting vessel, helping to plan surgical intervention (Kim et al., 2013). MRI with angiography provides good vessel detailing and 3D imaging similar to CT angiography. The technique is more expensive and takes longer, and is therefore less popular.

Once a diagnosis is established, medical treatment must be initiated to ameliorate the clinical signs associated with hepatic encephalopathy. Medical treatment may provide good medium-term outcome and it represents an option for owners that decline surgical intervention. However, surgery has been associated with a better chance of long-term survival (Greenhalgh et al., 2010). Preoperative medical management often consists of administration of oral lactulose, ampicillin and a low-protein diet. Levetiracetam, started 24 hours preoperatively and continued postoperatively, can decrease the rate of post-attenuation neurological syndrome (Fryer et al., 2011; Table 3.4).

Table 3.4 Medical management used by the author to stabilise congenital single portosystemic shunt preoperatively.

Drug	Dose, frequency	Period started preoperatively
Ampicillin	20 mg/kg, q8–12 h	Three weeks
Lactulose	1 ml/kg, q12 h	Three weeks
Levetiracetam	20 mg/kg, q8 h	24 h

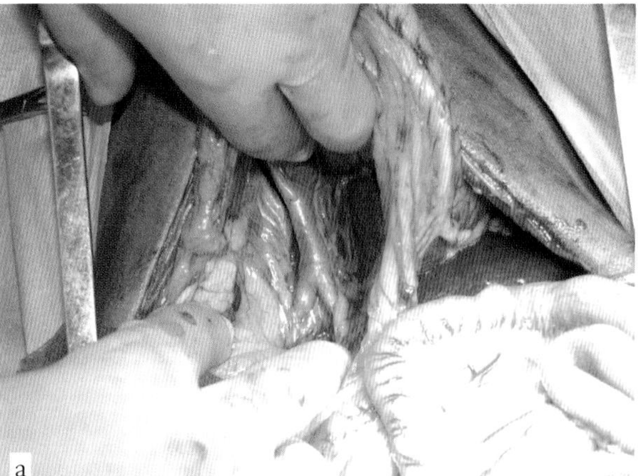

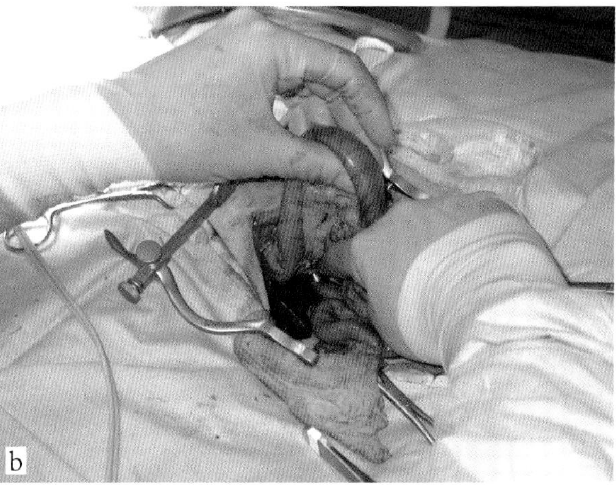

Fig. 3.61a,b Portosystemic shunt attenuation. a. Omental window showing an extra-hepatic portosystemic shunt. b. Attenuation of a portosystemic shunt with an ameroid constrictor.

Surgery is aimed at providing a slow closure of the anomalous vessel (attenuation) to gradually accustom the liver to increased blood flow and prevent the development of portal hypertension. This goal is often accomplished through open surgical techniques, including ameroid constrictor or cellophane band placement (Fig. 3.61a,b; Mankin, 2015; Nelson and Nelson, 2016). These devices are both effective for the attenuation of congenital extra-hepatic portosystemic shunts and result in good to excellent outcomes with low morbidity and mortality. Residual shunting was suspected in a higher proportion of dogs treated with cellophane banding on the basis of abdominal ultrasonography results (Traverson et al., 2018). One- or two-staged suture attenuation for complete closure of intra-hepatic congenital portosystemic shunts has also been reported, with good outcome (Tivers et al., 2017).

Attenuation of intra-hepatic shunts through a standard open approach can be challenging, and is associated with a higher morbidity and mortality rate. Percutaneous trans-jugular coil embolisation (PTCE; stent-supported coil embolisation) is a minimally invasive technique

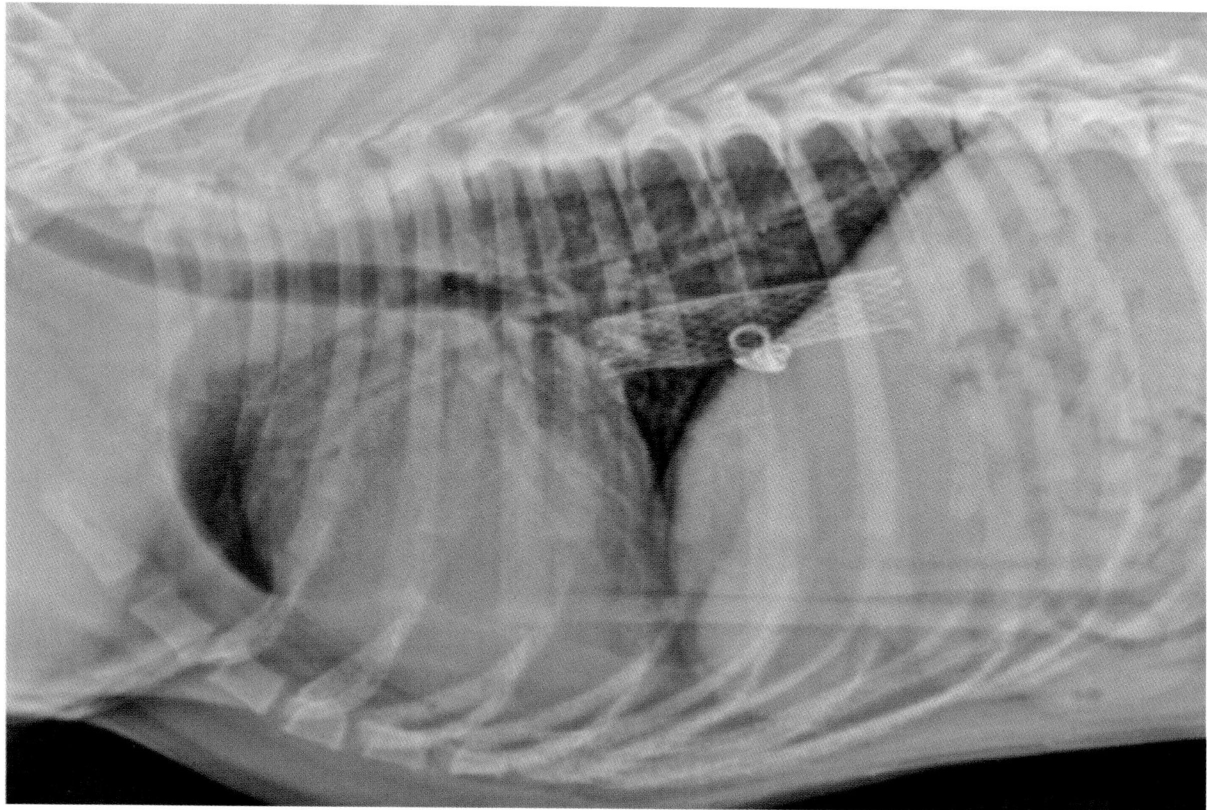

Fig. 3.62 Lateral thoracic radiograph following PTCE of an intra-hepatic portosystemic shunt. A caval stent has been placed, centred at the mouth of the shunt, and is preventing coil migration.

where trans-jugular catheters are used to deploy coils in the shunting vessel while measuring the pressure gradient between the portal vein and caudal vena cava. A vascular caval stent, centred at the mouth of the shunt, prevents coil migration. Fluoroscopy is essential to complete the procedure (Fig. 3.62). PTCE is associated with a good short- and intermediate-term survival (Case et al., 2017; Culp et al., 2018). This subset of animals has been identified as being at risk of gastrointestinal ulceration, and lifelong gastro-protectant medications are now recommended (Weisse et al., 2014).

Postoperative complications following surgical attenuation of a single congenital portosystemic shunt include fatal portal hypertension, post-attenuation neurological syndrome, ascites, residual shunting and development of multiple acquired portosystemic shunts. The pug breed may be at an increased risk of developing fatal neurological complications following surgical attenuation (Wallace et al., 2018). Gradual vessel occlusion and measurement of intra-operative portal pressures decrease the rate of fatal portal hypertension. Residual shunting may or may not be clinically significant, and it is the author's opinion that it is currently under-diagnosed.

Several questions remain regarding the long-term management and outcome following surgical attenuation of a single congenital portosystemic shunt. Predictors of a good long-term outcome are yet to be identified. Postoperative bile acid stimulation tests, residual shunt fraction, liver perfusion and hepatic regeneration are among the parameters that have been studied (Bristow et al., 2017; Tivers et al., 2014; Zwingenberger et al., 2014). Currently, clinical progression, once the medical management has been stopped, is the most reliable outcome measurement and the one used by the author.

3.8 Pancreas

Key points

- The pancreas is situated caudal to the stomach. Visualisation of the right limb is facilitated by the mesoduodenal manoeuvre, and visualisation of the left limb is facilitated by manipulation of the greater omentum.
- The central body is closely associated with the proximal duodenum, and shares its blood supply from the cranial pancreatico-duodenal artery (Fig. 3.63a,b).
- Surgical dissection of this area can be extremely challenging, and may result in necrosis of the pancreas or local duodenum.

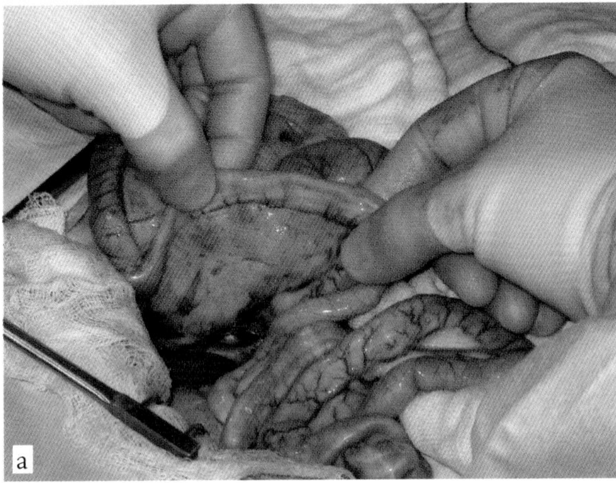

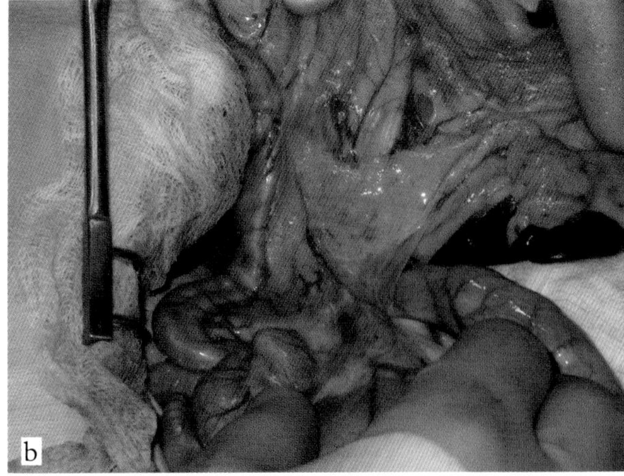

Fig. 3.63a,b Visualisation of the pancreas during an exploratory coeliotomy. a. Mesoduodenal sling allowing visualisation of the right pancreatic limb. b. Omental manipulation showing the central body and left pancreatic limb.

3.8.1 Anatomy

The pancreas comprises right and left lobes and a small central body, which is closely associated with the proximal duodenum. The majority of the pancreas is formed by its exocrine portion (98%) and associated vessels, nerves and ducts. This portion (lobules) is composed of acinar cells, which are responsible for synthesising digestive enzymes and cells that make up the duct system. The endocrine portion is composed of islets of polygonal cells (islets of Langerhans) that contain four distinct polypeptide-secreting cell types: α-cells (produce glucagon), β-cells (produce insulin), δ-cells (produce somatostatin) and F or PP cells (produce pancreatic polypeptide) (Cornell, 2012b).

The splenic artery is the primary blood supply to the left limb of the pancreas, and the hepatic artery terminates as the cranial pancreatico-duodenal artery, which enters the body of the pancreas and supplies the proximal portion of the right limb. Branches from the cranial pancreatico-duodenal artery also supply the closely associated duodenum. The distal right pancreatic limb is supplied by the caudal pancreatico-duodenal artery (Evans and de Lahunta, 2013).

In the majority of dogs, transport of pancreatic secretions to the duodenum is achieved through a single duct from each limb of the pancreas, which join to form a 'Y'. The tail of the 'Y' forms the accessory pancreatic duct (duct of Santorini), which empties into the duodenum at the minor duodenal papilla. A second duct, the pancreatic duct (duct of Wirsung), emerges from the main duct of either lobe and enters the duodenum adjacent to the bile duct as the major duodenal papilla. The majority of cats have a single pancreatic duct that fuses with the bile duct before entering the duodenum at the major duodenal papilla.

3.8.2 Biopsy

Pancreatic biopsy is performed regularly. The distal aspect of the right pancreatic limb is the most easily accessible and should be preferentially biopsied in cases with diffused disease. For focal lesions within the parenchyma, a biopsy can be collected using a Tru-Cut needle or by shaving off a portion of the lesion (Fossum, 2013). If no macroscopic disease is obvious, multiple samples from different pancreatic areas should be collected. Pancreatic duct ligation should be performed with non-absorbable polypropylene suture. The exception is in septic conditions where absorbable monofilament suture material can be used. Postoperative complications are low and mostly include pancreatitis (Pratschke et al., 2015).

Step by step: pancreatic biopsy/pancreatectomy by suture fracture technique

- A ventral midline coeliotomy is performed.
- The mesoduodenum or omentum is incised on each side of the pancreas.
- A suture is passed from one side of the pancreas to the other, through the incisions so that it is placed just proximal to the lesion to be excised.
- The suture is tightened, crushing through the parenchyma and ligating the vessels and ducts (Fig. 3.64).
- The biopsy is excised distally to the suture.
- The mesoduonenum is closed.

Step by step: pancreatic biopsy/pancreatectomy by blunt separation technique

- A ventral midline coeliotomy is performed.
- The mesoduodenum or omentum is incised on each side of the pancreas (Fig. 3.65a).

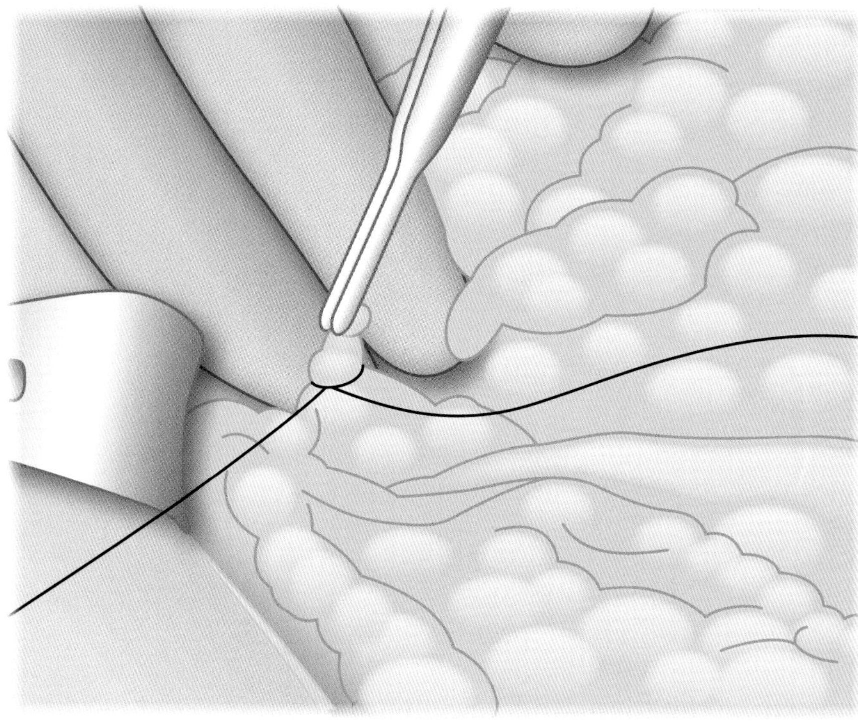

Fig. 3.64 Pancreatic biopsy by suture fracture. *Illustrator: Elaine Leggett*

- For a lesion present in the body of the pancreas, wet sterile Q-tips can be used to gently dissect the parenchyma from the pancreatico-duodenal vessels (Fig. 3.65b).
- For lesions in other locations, the pancreatic parenchyma is bluntly separated using mosquito haemostats.
- The blood vessels and ducts supplying the area to be removed are identified and ligated.
- The biopsy is excised (Fig. 3.65c).
- The mesoduodenum is closed.

3.8.3 Partial pancreatectomy

Partial pancreatectomy is indicated in the management of many conditions including abscess, tumour (e.g. insulinoma) and necrotising pancreatitis. Partial pancreatectomy is performed using the same techniques described for taking biopsies. A linear stapler or vessel-sealing device can also be used, with good results (Biel et al., 2011; Wouters et al., 2011). Provided that the duct to the remaining portion of the pancreas is left intact, 75–90% of the pancreas can be resected without compromising its exocrine and endocrine portions (Cornell, 2012b).

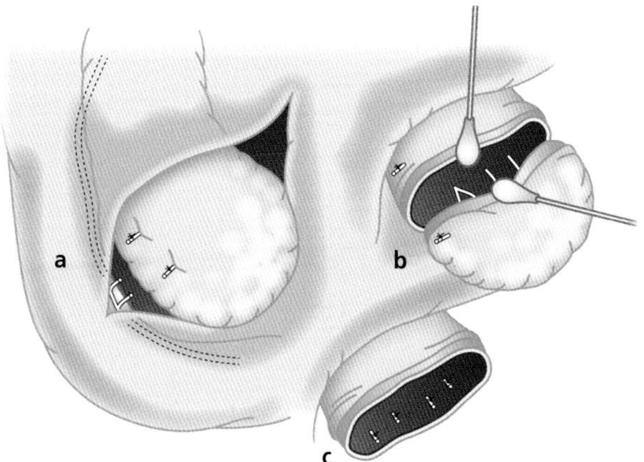

Fig. 3.65a–c Pancreatic biopsy/pancreatectomy by blunt separation technique. *Illustrator: Elaine Leggett*

3.8.4 Abscess

Pancreatic abscesses are usually sterile (negative bacterial cultures) and most commonly secondary to pancreatitis. Reported associated clinical signs include acute onset of lethargy, anorexia, vomiting and diarrhoea (Salisbury et al., 1988).

Diagnosis is made with ultrasound, CT or exploratory surgery. Loss of serosal detail in the cranial abdomen on a plain radiograph may also indicate severe inflammation (Cornell, 2012b).

Surgical management depends on the location and extent of the disease. Drainage, biopsy, resection and omentalisation have been reported (Fig. 3.66). Open peritoneal drainage has become less popular over the years, and omentalisation offers a shorter hospitalisation and better outcomes (Johnson and Mann, 2006). Despite frequent negative cultures being reported, several samples should be collected and submitted for bacteriology to try to identify the causative organism and initiate appropriate antibiotic therapy (Cornell, 2012b).

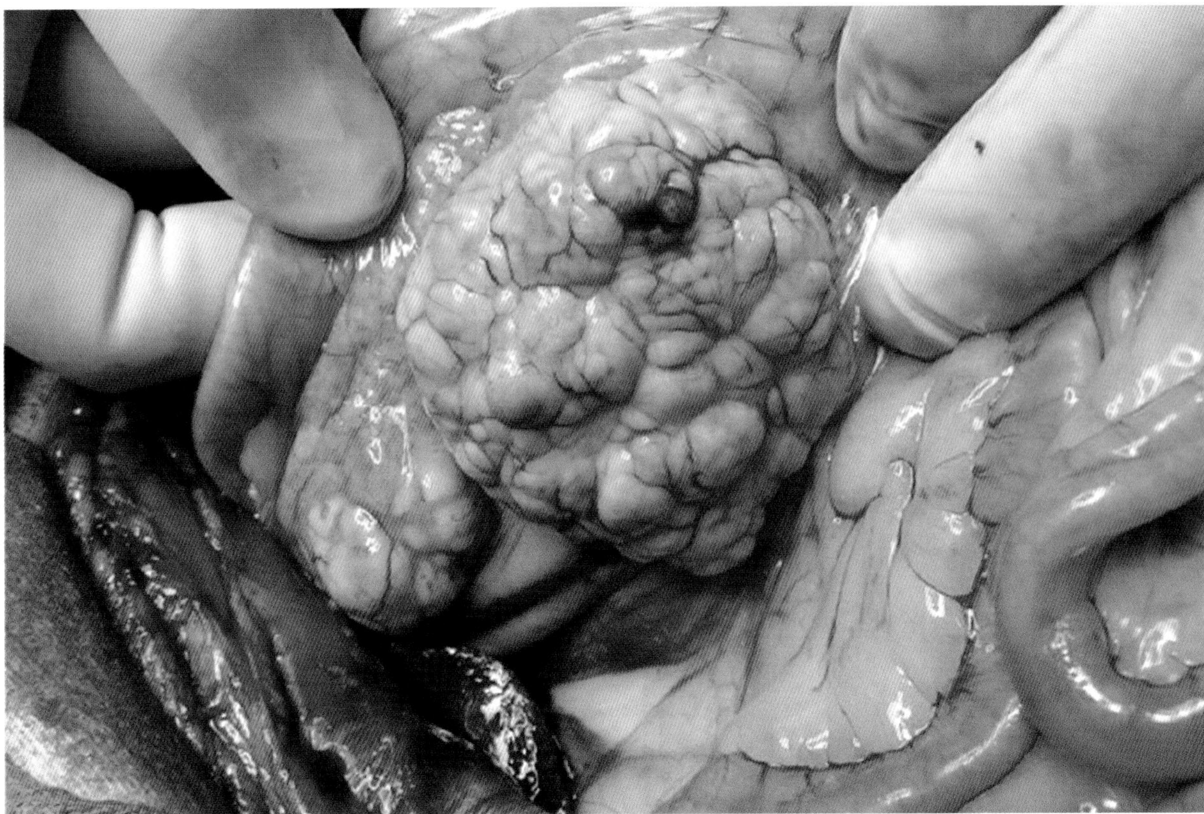

Fig. 3.66 Pancreatic abscess in the body of the pancreas; the lesion was drained and omentalised.

Postoperatively, management is targeted at treating pancreatitis, including nutritional support (enteral or parenteral), fluid support, analgesia and H2 antagonists or proton inhibitors (Fossum, 2013). Reported survival rates for dogs with pancreatic abscess are low (14–55%) (Johnson and Mann, 2006; Salisbury et al., 1988). In one study, elevated blood urea nitrogen, serum alkaline phosphatase activity and rising bicarbonate ion concentration were each found to have statistically significant influence on survival to discharge (Anderson et al., 2008).

3.8.5 Neoplasia

Carcinomas are the most commonly reported tumours of the exocrine pancreas in the dog and cat. Clinical signs are vague and at times mimic pancreatitis (Bennett et al., 2001). Paraneoplastic alopecia has been reported in the cat. Cytopathology of ultrasound or fluoroscopically guided biopsy or fine needle aspirate and impression from surgical biopsy have all been found useful in reaching a diagnosis (Bennett et al., 2001). Metastatic disease to local lymph nodes and liver is common. The prognosis in the dog and cat is extremely poor due to the aggressive nature of this tumour and, for this reason, further surgical intervention is rarely indicated (Cornell, 2012b).

Insulinoma is a malignant functional pancreatic tumour of the β-cells that retains the ability to produce and secrete insulin in excessive amounts independently of the glucose concentration (Goutal et al., 2012).

Clinical signs are typically related to hypoglycaemia and may include tremors, seizures, collapse, ataxia and mental dullness. Laboratory confirmation of hypoglycaemia in association with an inappropriately high serum insulin concentration helps establish a tentative diagnosis (Meleo, 1990). Decreased fructosamine concentration may also be supportive.

Ultrasound is often the most used diagnostic method and helps in assessing for the presence of metastasis. Contrast-enhanced ultrasound may help increase the rate of tumour detection (Iseri et al., 2007; Nakamura et al., 2015). CT has been shown to have a higher sensitivity for lesion detection (Fukushima et al., 2016). Ultimately, intra-operative inspection and palpation of the pancreas has been reported as superior (Robben et al., 2005).

Stabilisation of the animals prior to surgery is required. Frequent meals with high protein and complex carbohydrates are advisable. In severe cases intravenous fluid administration with 5% dextrose may be required, but care must be taken not to stimulate insulin production and exacerbation of the hypoglycaemia. Glucocorticoid administration increases glucose production and decreases its cellular uptake, and may be helpful perioperatively (Cornell, 2012b).

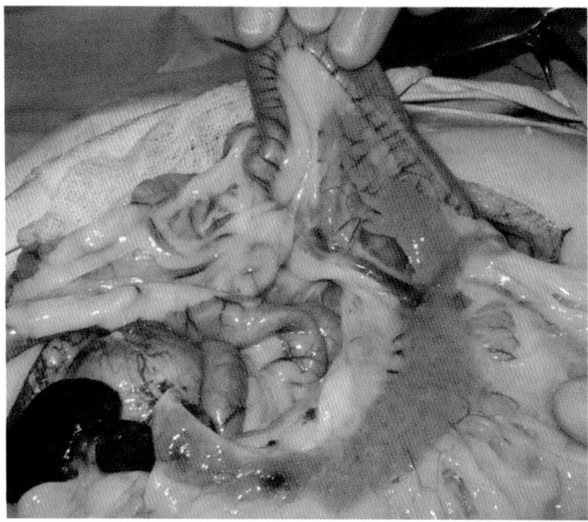

Fig. 3.67 Insulinoma visible in the left pancreatic limb during an exploratory coeliotomy.

Pre-anaesthetic administration of medetomidine significantly suppressed insulin secretion and increased plasma glucose concentration in dogs with insulinoma undergoing surgical management (Guedes and Rude, 2013).

Surgery entails full exploration of the abdomen and the pancreas. Most dogs have a solitary nodule identified on pancreatic palpation (Fig. 3.67). If a nodule cannot be identified, a diluted solution of sterile methylene blue can be given intravenously (3 mg/kg of 1% methylene blue in 250 ml of 9% saline, over 30 min; Cornell, 2012b). Alternatively, biopsies from different pancreatic areas can be collected or, if the ultrasound or CT results suggest that the disease is located in a particular lobe, a partial pancreatectomy of that lobe can be performed. Biopsies of the local lymph nodes and liver should also be collected.

Postoperatively, blood glucose concentrations must be monitored closely. Hyperglycaemia may occur postoperatively and is usually a good prognostic sign; however, insulin administration may be required. The presence of hypoglycaemia postoperatively suggests incomplete tumour excision or the presence of functional micrometastasis (Buishand et al., 2012). The prognosis depends on the extent of the disease and the associated clinical signs. Median survival time is significantly longer in dogs treated surgically than in those treated medically (Tobin et al., 1999). The reported median survival time for dogs in the absence of metastasis is 18 months, and with metastasis is 7–9 months (Cornell, 2012b).

3.9 Spleen

Key points

- The spleen has a role in haematopoiesis and immunosurveillance, filtering microorganisms and antigenic particles from the blood, synthetising immunoglobulins (IgG), cytokines and maturing new red blood cells.
- The spleen also stores red blood cells, platelets and removes aged red blood cells.
- Surgery of the spleen is commonly performed. Removing the whole organ carries a much lesser risk of haemorrhage compared to removing part of it. For this reason, splenectomy is most commonly performed.

3.9.1 Anatomy

The spleen comprises a head (attached to the stomach by the gastro-splenic ligament) and a tail (mobile). It receives its arterial blood supply from the splenic artery, the short gastric arteries and the left gastroepiploic artery. The splenic vein drains into the portal vein (Fig. 3.68).

The splenic parenchyma comprises a red pulp, a white pulp, a capsule and a network of trabeculae. The red pulp stores erythrocytes, traps antigens and is the site of fetal erythropoiesis. The white pulp consists of lymphoid tissue and is involved in immune response. In the dog the spleen is sinusoidal, having a combination of direct arteriovenous endothelial connection and some areas where red blood cells must traverse a region of the red pulp before entering the venous side. In the cat, the spleen is non-sinusoidal with open-ended venous channels and perforated endothelial channels allowing direct contact between arterial and venous vasculature (Evans and de Lahunta, 2013).

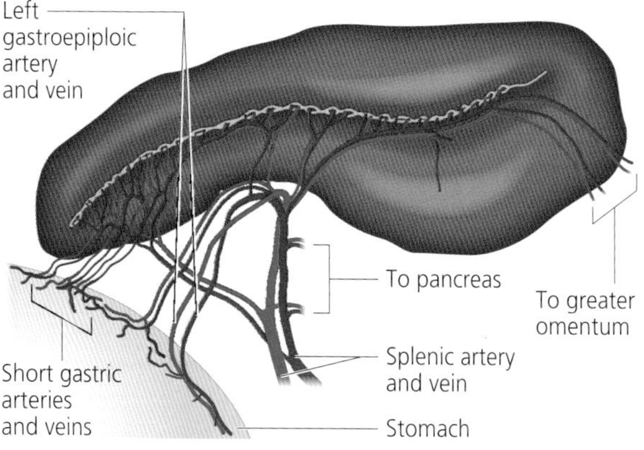

Fig. 3.68 Splenic blood supply. *Illustrator: Elaine Leggett*

3.9.2 Surgical principles

Most animals with splenic disease present with splenomegaly. However, this can be a physiological response following administration of certain drugs including acepromazine, thiopentone and propofol. Distinguishing between these two entities is crucial.

Perioperative antibiotic use is dictated by the nature of the underlying pathology and the length of surgery. Severely debilitated or immunosuppressed dogs may benefit from postoperative antibiotic therapy (Fossum, 2013).

Complications of splenic surgery include haemorrhage; vascular compromise of the pancreatic artery (first branch of the splenic artery) requiring a partial pancreatectomy; cardiac arrhythmias (ventricular premature complexes or ventricular tachycardia); disseminated intravascular coagulation; gastric dilatation and volvulus; infection (due to decreased removal of old or infected red blood cells); and compromised oxygen transport (due to potential haemorrhage decreasing circulatory concentration of red blood cells and loss of splenic reservoir capacity). Perioperative stabilisation and close postoperative monitoring and support may be required.

3.9.3 Splenorrhaphy

Splenorrhaphy entails suturing of the splenic capsule and superficial parenchyma, and is indicated when small lacerations can be controlled by direct pressure. An interrupted suture pattern should be used with fine, absorbable suture material (1.0 or 1.5 metric). After repairing the traumatised portion, a synthetic haemostatic agent can be used to further reduce haemorrhage (Richter, 2012). A polyglycolic acid mesh has been used effectively to control haemorrhage in trauma patients (Rogers et al., 1999).

3.9.4 Partial splenectomy

Partial splenectomy can be considered in animals with focal abscess or traumatic lesions limited to one area of the spleen. It should never be considered in cases of neoplasia, and is technically more challenging than a complete splenectomy due to a higher risk of haemorrhage. The technique can be performed manually or with the aid of a stapling device (TA™).

Step by step: partial splenectomy

- The spleen is exteriorised from the abdominal cavity and isolated from the remaining abdominal contents with moistened laparotomy swabs (Fig. 3.69a).

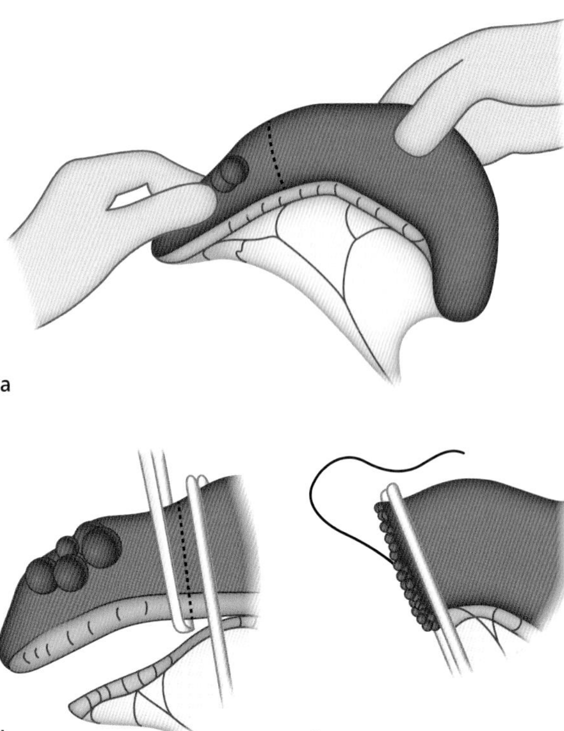

Fig. 3.69a–c Partial splenectomy. *Illustrator: Elaine Leggett*

- The hilar vessels supplying the affected area are double-ligated, creating a line of necrosis clearly visible on the splenic parenchyma.
- Digital pressure is applied along this line without rupturing the capsule and separating the parenchyma.
- A pair of clamps is applied along this line and another pair distally (Fig. 3.69b).
- The spleen is transected between both clamps.
- The capsule is apposed distally to the remaining clamp with a continuous pattern using absorbable sutures (Fig. 3.69c).
- A mattress pattern can also be added to aid haemostasis.

3.9.5 Total splenectomy

Total splenectomy is indicated for most cases of splenic pathology including trauma, torsion and neoplasia. A full exploratory coeliotomy is advisable to look for concomitant injuries or evidence of metastatic disease. The procedure can be performed either manually or by using a surgical stapler or a vessel-sealing device. Surgical staplers and vessel-sealing devices are expensive but significantly shorten the surgical time. Their use may be particularly advantageous in emergency presentations such as haemoabdomen. Laparoscopically assisted splenectomy has been reported effectively in 18 dogs (Wright et al., 2016).

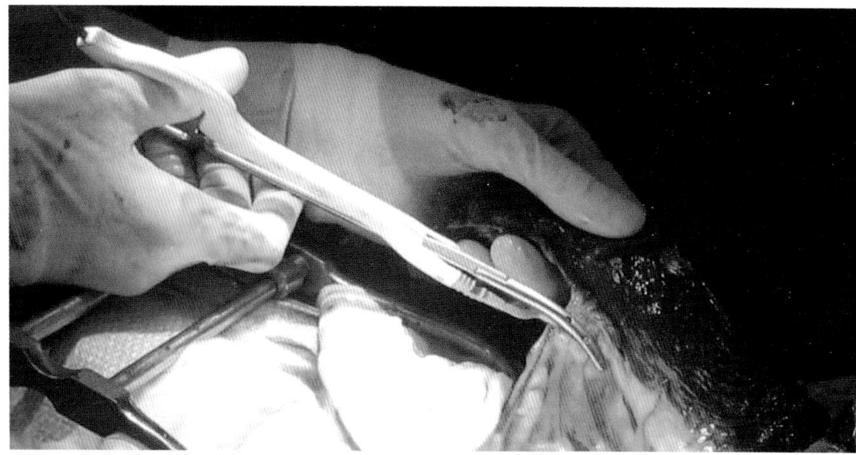

Fig. 3.70 Total splenectomy using a vessel-sealing device. (Image courtesy of Jonathan Bell.)

Step by step: total splenectomy (Fig. 3.70)

- The spleen is exteriorised from the abdominal cavity and isolated from the remaining abdominal contents with moistened laparotomy swabs.
- The hilar vessels are double ligated as close to the parenchyma as possible.

3.9.6 Torsion

Splenic torsion occurs when the spleen rotates on itself, preventing blood drainage and causing subsequent enlargement. The condition most commonly affects larger breeds of dog, with great Danes and German shepherds potentially being at increased risk (Neath et al., 1997). Small breeds have also been reported (Ohta et al., 2009). Acute torsion is most commonly seen, but chronic cases have been reported (Reinhart et al., 2015).

The clinical signs are non-specific and may include intermittent signs of gastrointestinal disease, abdominal discomfort and hypovolaemic or toxic shock (Neath et al., 1997; Richter, 2012). Diagnosis is typically made by ultrasound. Abdominal radiographs may aid diagnosis where a mid-abdominal mass with a C-shape can be appreciated on a lateral view (Stickle, 1989). On ultrasound, the splenic parenchyma can be normal, hypo-echoic or anechoic with interspersed linear echoes (coarse, 'lacy' appearance). Spectral and colour Doppler imaging of the splenic veins may confirm absent measurable flow velocity (Saunders et al., 1998). The presence of a triangular hyperechoic area at the hilus between the veins and the splenic parenchyma, and that is continuous with the hyperechoic mesentery, can be used to more accurately diagnose splenic torsion (Mai, 2006). CT may show lack of contrast uptake and the presence of a twisted soft tissue mass in the location of the splenic pedicle (Patsikas et al., 2001).

Treatment of splenic torsion involves surgery (Fig. 3.71), even though a case of spontaneous resolution has been reported (Szatmári et al., 2000). Stabilisation and a total splenectomy without any attempt to de-rotate the spleen (to avoid releasing any thrombi or toxic factors) are indicated. A prophylactic gastropexy should be considered.

The prognosis for dogs undergoing splenectomy due to acute splenic torsion is favourable. Several risk factors for death prior to discharge were identified, including pre-existing septic peritonitis, intra-operative haemorrhage and postoperative development of respiratory distress (DeGroot et al., 2016).

3.9.7 Neoplasia

Splenic neoplasia is common in the dog, with haemangiosarcoma being mostly diagnosed. Splenic masses can be found incidentally, or present as an acute abdomen (haemoabdomen). Macroscopically, it is impossible to distinguish a benign from a malignant mass, and therefore total splenectomy is always indicated. In one study, incidentally found, non-ruptured splenic masses or nodules without associated haemoperitoneum were most commonly benign (Cleveland and Casale, 2016).

Haemangiosarcoma is an aggressive tumour with a high metastatic rate, and full staging of the animal with

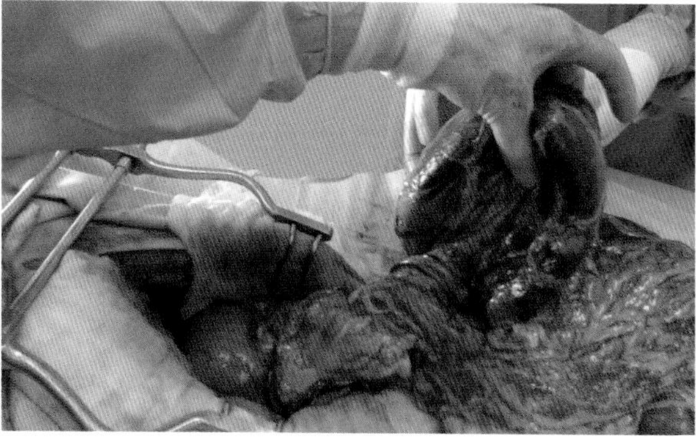

Fig. 3.71 Splenic torsion confirmed during an exploratory coeliotomy. (Image courtesy of Jon Hall.)

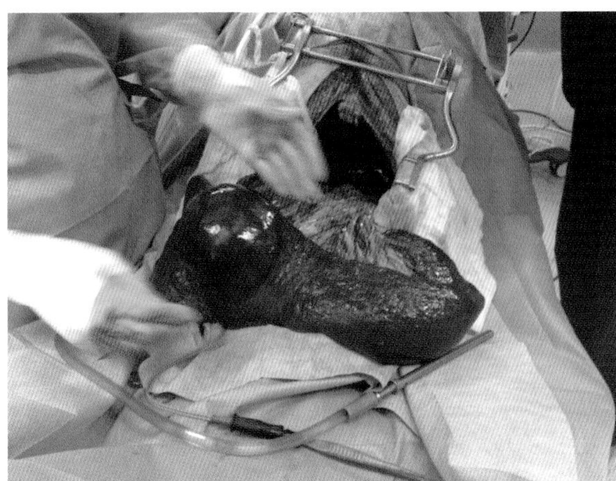

Fig. 3.72 Large splenic mass confirmed during an exploratory coeliotomy. (Image courtesy of Jon Hall.)

thoracic radiographs and echocardiography (check right atrium) should be performed when surgical intervention is not urgent (Richter, 2012). During surgery, a liver biopsy is also indicated to check for metastasis. Marked preoperative thrombocytopenia or anaemia and the development of intra-operative ventricular arrhythmias were identified as risk factors for perioperative death in dogs with splenic masses (Wendelburg et al., 2014).

The prognosis for haemangiosarcoma is poor, and depends on the stage of the disease.

The presence of haemoabdomen significantly worsens the prognosis, and dogs undergoing transfusion more commonly had malignant disease, and increased odds of poor long-term outcome, compared with those that did not undergo transfusion (Lynch et al., 2015; Fig. 3.72). In one study, only the histologically determined mitotic score was significantly associated with survival time (Moore et al., 2017).

Chemotherapy is indicated and most effective when no visible gross metastatic disease is present (Göritz et al., 2013). Reported survival time for various protocols is 140–202 days. Combinations of doxorubicin-based conventional protocols and cyclophosphamide-based metronomic protocols appeared to be more effective than either type of chemotherapy alone, but prolongations in survival time resulting from current protocols were modest (Wendelburg et al., 2015). Treatment using thalidomide may improve survival (Bray et al., 2018).

Bibliography

Adami, C., Di Palma, S., Gendron, K. and Sigrist, N. (2011) Severe esophageal injuries occurring after general anesthesia in two cats: case report and literature review. *Journal of the American Animal Hospital Association* 47, 436–442.

Adamik, K.N., Burgener, I.A., Kovacevic, A., Schulze, S.P. and Kohn, B. (2009) Myoglobin as a prognostic indicator for outcome in dogs with gastric dilatation-volvulus. *Journal of Veterinary Emergency and Critical Care* 19, 247–253.

Adams, P., Halfacree, Z.J., Lamb, C.R., Smith, K.C. and Baines, S.J. (2011) Zygomatic salivary mucocoele in a Lhasa apso following maxillary tooth extraction. *Veterinary Record* 168, 458.

Adams, R.J., Doyle, R.S., Bray, J.P. and Burton, C.A. (2014) Closed suction drainage for treatment of septic peritonitis of confirmed gastrointestinal origin in 20 dogs. *Veterinary Surgery* 43, 843–851.

Aertsens, A., Hernandez, J., Ragetly, G. R. and Poncet, C.M. (2016) Surgical extraction of canine oesophageal foreign bodies through a gastrotomy approach: 12 cases. *Journal of Small Animal Practice* 57, 354–359.

Alcoverro, E., Tabar, M. D., Lloret, A., Roura, X., Pastor, J. and Planellas, M. (2014) Phenobarbital-responsive sialadenosis in dogs: case series. *Topics in Companion Animal Medicine* 29, 109–112.

Alkukhun, A., Caturegli, G., Munoz-Abraham, A.S., Judeeba, S., Patron-Lozano, R., Morotti, R., Rodriguez-Davalos, M.I. and Geibel, J.P. (2017) Use of fluorescein isothiocyanate-inulin as a marker for intestinal ischemic injury. *Journal of Surgical Research* 224, 1066–1073.

Allen, P. and Paul, A. (2014) Gastropexy for prevention of gastric dilatation-volvulus in dogs: history and techniques. *Topics in Companion Animal Medicine* 29, 77–80.

Anagnostou, T.L., Kazakos, G.M., Savvas, I., Kostakis, C. and Papadopoulou, P. (2017) Gastro-oesophageal reflux in large-sized, deep-chested versus small-sized, barrel-chested dogs undergoing spinal surgery in sternal recumbency. *Veterinary Anaesthesia and Analgesia* 44, 35–41.

Anderson, J.R., Cornell, K.K., Parnell, N.K. and Salisbury, S.K. (2008) Pancreatic abscess in 36 dogs: a retrospective analysis of prognostic indicators. *Journal of the American Animal Hospital Association* 44, 171–179.

Anderson, S., Lippincott, C.L. and Gill, P.J. (1992) Single enterotomy removal of gastrointestinal linear foreign bodies. *Journal of the American Animal Hospital Association* 28, 487–490.

Aona, B.D., Rush, J.E., Rozanski, E.A., Cunningham, S.M., Sharp, C.R. and Freeman, L.M. (2017) Evaluation of echocardiography and cardiac biomarker concentrations in dogs with gastric dilatation volvulus. *Journal of Veterinary Emergency and Critical Care* 27, 631–637.

Applewhite, A.A., Hawthorne, J.C. and Cornell, K.K. (2001) Complications of enteroplication for the prevention of intussusception recurrence in dogs: 35 cases (1989–1999). *Journal of the American Veterinary Medical Association* 219, 1415–1418.

Arnell, K., Hill, S., Hart, J. and Richter, K. (2013) Persistent regurgitation in four dogs with caudal esophageal neoplasia. *Journal of the American Animal Hospital Association* 49, 58-63.

Aronson, L.R. (2012) Rectum, anus, and perineum. In: Tobias, K.M. and Johnston, S.A. (eds) *Veterinary Surgery: Small Animal.* Elsevier Saunders, St. Louis, Missouri.

Aslanian, M.E., Sharp, C.R. and Garneau, M.S. (2014) Gastric dilatation and volvulus in a brachycephalic dog with hiatal hernia. *Journal of Small Animal Practice* 55, 535–537.

Atray, M., Raghunath, M., Singh, T. and Saini, N.S. (2012)

Ultrasonographic diagnosis and surgical management of double intestinal intussusception in 3 dogs. *Canadian Veterinary Journal* 53, 860–864

Balsa, I.M., Culp, W.T.N., Drobatz, K.J., Johnston, E.G., Mayhew, P.D. and Marks, S.L. (2017) Effect of laparoscopic-assisted gastropexy on gastrointestinal transit time in dogs. *Journal of Veterinary Internal Medicine* 31, 1680–1685.

Bartfield, D.M., Tivers, M.S., Holahan, M., Welch, K., House, A. and Adamantos, S.E. (2016) Retrospective evaluation of recurrent secondary septic peritonitis in dogs (2000–2011): 41 cases. *Journal of Veterinary Emergency and Critical Care* 26, 281–287.

Bartoe, J.T., Brightman, A.H. and Davidson, H.J. (2007) Modified lateral orbitotomy for vision-sparing excision of a zygomatic mucocele in a dog. *Veterinary Ophthalmology* 10, 127–131.

Bebchuck, T.N. (2002) Feline gastrointestinal foreign bodies. *Veterinary Clinics of North America: Small Animal Practice* 32, 861–880.

Beck, J.J., Staatz, A.J., Pelsue, D.H., Kusnig, S.T., MacPhail, C.M., Seim, H.B. and Monnet, E. (2006) Risk factors associated with short-term outcome and development of perioperative complications in dogs undergoing surgery because of gastric dilatation-volvulus: 166 cases (1992–2003). *Journal of the American Veterinary Medical Association* 229, 1934–1939.

Beer, K.A., Syring, R.S. and Drobatz, K.J. (2013) Evaluation of plasma lactate concentration and base excess at the time of hospital admission as predictors of gastric necrosis and outcome and correlation between those variables in dogs with gastric dilatation-volvulus: 78 cases (2004–2009). *Journal of the American Veterinary Medical Association* 242, 54–58.

Belch, A., Rubinos, C., Barnes, D.C. and Nelissen, P. (2017) Modified tube gastropexy using a mushroom-tipped silicone catheter for management of gastric dilatation-volvulus in dogs. *Journal of Small Animal Practice* 58, 79–88.

Bell, J.S. (2014) Inherited and predisposing factors in the development of gastric dilatation volvulus in dogs. *Topics in Companion Animal Medicine* 29, 60–63.

Bellenger, C.R., Maddison, J.E., MacPherson, G.C. and Ilkiw, J.E. (1990) Chronic hypertrophic pyloric gastropathy in 14 dogs. *Australian Veterinary Journal* 67, 317–320.

Bellezza, E., Bianchini, E., Pettinelli, S., Angeli, G. and Leonardi, L. (2016) Intestinal plasmacytoma causing colocolic double intussusception in an adult dog. *Journal of Small Animal Practice* 57, 718.

Benitez, M.E., Schmiedt, C.W., Radlinsky, M.G. and Cornell, K.K. (2013) Efficacy of incisional gastropexy for prevention of GDV in dogs. *Journal of the American Animal Hospital Association* 49, 185–189.

Benjamino, K.P., Birchard, S.J., Niles, J.D. and Penrod, K.D. (2012) Pharyngeal mucoceles in dogs: 14 cases. *Journal of the American Animal Hospital Association* 48, 31–35.

Bennett, P.F., Hahn, K.A., Toal, R.L. and Legendre, A.M. (2001) Ultrasonographic and cytopathological diagnosis of exocrine pancreatic carcinoma in the dog and cat. *Journal of the American Animal Hospital Association* 37, 466–473.

Bennett, P.F., Denicola, D.B., Bonney, P., Glickman, N.W. and Knapp, D.W. (2002) Canine anal sac adenocarcinomas: clinical presentation and response to therapy. *Journal of Veterinary Internal Medicine* 16, 100–104.

Bergman, P.J. (2012) Paraneoplastic hypercalcemia. *Topics in Companion Animal Medicine* 27, 156–158.

Bertoy, R.W. (2001) Megacolon in the cat. *Veterinary Clinics of North America: Small Animal Practice* 32, 901–915.

Bertoy, R.W., MacCoy, D.M., Wheaton, L.G. and Gelbeng, H.B. (1989) Total colectomy with ileorectal anastomosis in the cat. *Veterinary Surgery* 18, 204–210.

Besalti, O. and Ergin I. (2012) Cystocele and rectal prolapse in a female dog. *Canadian Veterinary Journal* 53, 1314–1316.

Biel, M., Klumpp, S., Peppler, C., Kramer, M. and Thiel, C. (2011) Partial pancreatectomy using a linear stapler device for the treatment of pancreatic neoplasias in three dogs. *Tieraerztliche Praxis Ausgabe K Kleintiere Heimtiere* 39, 441–447.

Binvel, M., Poujol, L., Peyron, C., Dunie-Merigot, A. and Bernardin, F. (2017) Endoscopic and surgical removal of oesophageal and gastric fishhook foreign bodies in 33 animals. *Journal of Small Animal Practice* 59, 45–49.

Bissett, S.A., Davis, J., Subler, K. and Degernes, L.A. (2009) Risk factors and outcome of bougienage for treatment of benign esophageal strictures in dogs and cats: 28 cases (1995–2004). *Journal of the American Veterinary Medical Association* 235, 844–850.

Boag, A.K., Coe, R.J., Martinez, T.A. and Hughes, D. (2005) Acid-base and electrolyte abnormalities in dogs with gastrointestinal foreign bodies. *Journal of Veterinary Internal Medicine* 19, 826–821.

Böhm, B., Milsom, J.W., Kitago, K., Brand, M. and Fazio, V.W. (1994) Laparoscopic oncologic total abdominal colectomy with intra-peritoneal stapled anastomosis in a canine model. *Journal of Laparoendoscopic Surgery* 4, 23–30.

Boland, L., Gomes, E., Payen, G., Bouvy, B. and Poncet, C. (2013) Zygomatic salivary gland diseases in the dog: three cases diagnosed by MRI. *Journal of the American Animal Hospital Association* 49, 333–337.

Boland, L., Lindsay, S., Brunel, L., Podadera, J. and Bennett, P. (2017) Caecocolic intussusception associated with a caecal polyp and concurrent hepatocellular carcinoma in a cat. *Journal of Feline Medicine and Surgery* 3, 1–6.

Bowlt, K.L., Friend, E.J., Delisser, P., Murphy, S. and Polton, G. (2013) Temporally separated bilateral anal sac gland carcinomas in four dogs. *Journal of Small Animal Practice* 54, 432–436.

Boydell, P., Pike, R., Crossley, D. and Whitbread, T. (2000) Sialadenosis in dogs. *Journal of the American Veterinary Medical Association* 216, 872–874.

Boysen, S.R., Tidwell, A.S. and Penninck, D.G. (2003) Ultrasonographic findings in dogs and cats with gastrointestinal perforation. *Veterinary Radiology & Ultrasound* 44, 556–564.

Bray, J.P., Orbell, G., Cave, N. and Munday, J.S. (2018) Does thalidomide prolong survival in dogs with splenic haemangiosarcoma? *Journal of Small Animal Practice* 59, 85–91.

Bristow, P., Tivers. M., Packer, R., Brockman, D., Ortiz, V., Newson, K. and Lipscomb, V.J. (2017) Long-term serum bile acid concentrations in 51 dogs after complete extrahepatic congenital portosystemic shunt ligation. *Journal of Small Animal Practice* 58, 454–460.

Broux, O., Clercx, C., Etienne, A.L., Busoni, V., Claeys, S., Hamaide, A. and Billen, F. (2017) Effects of manipulations to detect sliding hiatal hernia in dogs with brachycephalic airway obstructive syndrome. *Veterinary Surgery* 47, 243–251.

Brown, D.C. (2012). Small intestine. In: Tobias, K.M. and Johnston, S.A. (eds) *Veterinary Surgery: Small Animal*. Elsevier Saunders, St. Louis, Missouri.

Bruchim, Y., Itay, S., Shira, B.H., Kelmer, E., Sigal, Y., Itamar, A. and Gilad, S. (2012) Evaluation of lidocaine treatment on frequency of cardiac arrhythmias, acute kidney injury, and hospitalization time in dogs with gastric dilatation volvulus. *Journal of Veterinary Emergency and Critical Care* 22, 419–427.

Bruchim, Y. and Kelmer, E. (2014) Postoperative management of dogs with gastric dilatation and volvulus. *Topics in Companion Animal Medicine* 29, 81–85.

Buber, T., Saragusty, J., Ranen, E., Epstein, A., Bdolah-Abram, T. and Bruchim, Y. (2007) Evaluation of lidocaine treatment and risk factors for death associated with gastric dilatation and volvulus in dogs: 112 cases (1997–2005). *Journal of the American Veterinary Medical Association* 230, 1334–1339.

Buishand, F.O., van Erp, M.G., Groenveld, H.A., Mol, J.A., Kik, M., Robben, J.H., Kooistr, H.S. and Kirpensteijn, J. (2012) Expression of insulin-like growth factor-1 by canine insulinomas and their metastases. *Veterinary Journal* 191, 334–340.

Burton, A.G., Talbot, C.T. and Kent, M.S. (2017) Risk factors for death in dogs treated for esophageal foreign body obstruction: a retrospective cohort study of 222 cases (1998–2017). *Journal of Veterinary Internal Medicine* 31, 1686–1690.

Bush, M., Carno, M.A., Germaine, L. and Hoffmann, D.E. (2016) The effect of time until surgical intervention on survival in dogs with secondary septic peritonitis. *Canadian Veterinary Journal* 57, 1267–1273.

Cannon, M.S., Paglia, D., Zwingenberger, A.L., Boroffka, S.A., Hollingsworth, S.R. and Wisner, E.R. (2011) Clinical and diagnostic imaging findings in dogs with zygomatic sialadenitis: 11 cases (1999-2009). *Journal of the American Veterinary Medical Association* 239, 1211-1218.

Caporali, E.H., Phillips, H., Underwood, L. and Selmic, L.E. (2015) Risk factors for urolithiasis in dogs with congenital extrahepatic portosystemic shunts: 95 cases (1999–2013). *Journal of the American Veterinary Medical Association* 246, 530–536.

Cariou, M.P. and Lipscomb, V.J. (2011) Successful surgical management of a perforating oesophageal foreign body in a cat. *Journal of Feline Medicine and Surgery* 13, 50-55.

Case, J.B., Marvel, S.J., Stiles, M.C., Maisenbacher, H.W., Toskich, B.B., Smeak, D.D. and Monnet, E.L. (2017) Outcomes of cellophane banding or percutaneous transvenous coil embolization of canine intra-hepatic portosystemic shunts. doi: 10.1111/vsu.12750. [Epub ahead of print].

Cattai, A., Levorato, S. and Franci, P. (2017) A case of acute postoperative transitory sialadenosis of the submandibular glands in a healthy dog. *Journal of Veterinary Medical Science* 78, 1907–1910.

Center, S.A. and Magne, M.L. (1990) Historical, physical examination, and clinicopathologic features of portosystemic vascular anomalies in the dog and cat. *Seminars in Veterinary Medicine and Surgery (Small Animal)* 5, 83–93.

Cerny, J.H. (1996) Alternative method for retrieving fishhooks from dogs and cats. *Journal of the American Veterinary Medical Association* 208, 184.

Charlesworth, T.M. (2014) Risk factors for postoperative complications following bilateral closed anal sacculectomy in the dog. *Journal of Small Animal Practice* 55, 350–354.

Ciasca, T.C., David, F.H. and Lamb, C.R. (2013) Does measurement of small intestinal diameter increase diagnostic accuracy of radiography in dogs with suspected intestinal obstruction? *Veterinary Radiology & Ultrasound* 54, 207–211.

Clark, G.N. and Wise, L.A. (1994) Stapled typhlectomy via colotomy for treatment of cecal inversion in a dog. *Journal of the American Veterinary Medical Association* 204, 1641–1643.

Clarke, B.S. and L'Eplattenier, H.F. (2010) Zygomatic salivary mucocoele as a postoperative complication following caudal hemimaxillectomy in a dog. *Journal of Small Animal Practice* 51, 495–498.

Cleveland, M.J. and Casale, S. (2016) Incidence of malignancy and outcomes for dogs undergoing splenectomy for incidentally detected nonruptured splenic nodules or masses: 105 cases (2009–2013). *Journal of the American Veterinary Medical Association* 248, 1267–1273.

Cole, T.L., Center, S.A. and Flood, S.N. (2002) Diagnostic comparison of needle and wedge biopsy specimens of the liver in dogs and cats. *Journal of the American Veterinary Medical Association* 220, 1483–1490.

Connolly, S.L (2016) Canine portosystemic shunts: Single or multiple tests to make the correct diagnosis? *Veterinary Journal* 207, 6–7.

Coolman, B.R., Ehrhart, N. and Marretta, S.M. (2000) Use of skin staples for rapid closure of gastrointestinal incisions in the treatment of canine linear foreign bodies. *Journal of the American Animal Hospital Association* 36, 542–547.

Cornell, K. (2012a) Stomach. In: Tobias K.M. and Johnston S.A. (eds) *Veterinary Surgery: Small Animal*. Elsevier Saunders, St. Louis, Missouri.

Cornell, K. (2012b) Pancreas. In: Tobias K.M. and Johnston S.A. (eds) *Veterinary Surgery: Small Animal*. Elsevier Saunders, St. Louis, Missouri.

Covey, J.L., Degner, D.A., Jackson, A.H., Hofeling, A.D. and Walshaw, R. (2009) Hilar liver resection in dogs. *Veterinary Surgery* 38, 104–111.

Crawshaw J., Berg, J., Sardinas, J.C., Engler, S.J., Rand, W.M., Ogilvie, G.K., Spodnick, G.J., Keefe, D.A., Vail, D.M. and Henderson, R.A. (1998) Prognosis for dogs with nonlymphomatous, small intestinal tumours treated by surgical excision. *Journal of the American Animal Hospital Association* 34, 451–456.

Crouse, Z., Phillips, B., Flory, A., Mahoney, J., Richter, K. and Kidd, L. (2017) Post-chemotherapy perforation in cats with discrete intermediate- or large-cell gastrointestinal lymphoma. *Journal of Feline Medicine and Surgery*. [Epub ahead of print.]

Culp, W.T., Zwingenberger, A.L., Giuffrida, M.A., Wisner, E.R., Hunt, G.B., Steffey, M.A., Mayhew, P.D. and Marks, S.L. (2018) Prospective evaluation of outcome of dogs with intra-hepatic portosystemic shunts treated via percutaneous transvenous coil embolization. *Veterinary Surgery* 47, 74–85.

Cuthbertson, E.M., Gilfillan, R.S., Burhenne, H.J. and Mackby, M.J. (1970) Massive small bowel resection in the beagle, including laboratory data in severe undernutrition. *Surgery* 68, 698–705.

D'Anjou, M.A., Penninck, D., Cornejo, L. and Pibarot, P. (2004) Ultrasonographic diagnosis of portosystemic shunting in dogs and cats. *Veterinary Radiology & Ultrasound* 45, 424–437.

Danova, N.A., Robles-Emanuelli, J.C. and Bjorling, D.E. (2006) Surgical excision of primary canine rectal tumours by an anal approach in twenty-three dogs. *Veterinary Surgery* 35, 337–340.

Davis, D.J., Demianiuk, R.M., Musser, J., Podsiedlik, M. and Hauptman, J. (2018) Influence of preoperative septic peritonitis and anastomotic technique on the dehiscence of enterectomy sites in dogs: A retrospective review of 210 anastomoses. *Veterinary Surgery* 47, 125–129.

Dayer, T., Howard, J. and Spreng, D. (2013) Septic peritonitis from pyloric and non-pyloric gastrointestinal perforation: prognostic factors in 44 dogs and 11 cats. *Journal of Small Animal Practice* 54, 625–629.

De Battisti, A., Harran, N., Chanoit, G. and Warren-Smith C. (2013) Use of negative contrast computed tomography for diagnosis of a colonic duplication in a dog. *Journal of Small Animal Practice* 54, 547–550.

De Battisti, A., Toscano, M.J. and Formaggini, L. (2012) Gastric foreign body as a risk factor for gastric dilatation and volvulus in dogs. *Journal of the American Veterinary Medical Association* 241, 1190–1193.

De Papp, E., Drobatz, K.J. and Hughes, D. (2002) Plasma lactate concentration as a predictor of gastric necrosis and survival among dogs with gastric dilatation-volvulus: 102 cases (1995–1998). *Journal of the American Veterinary Medical Association* 215, 49–52.

DeGroot, W., Giuffrida, M.A., Rubin, J., Runge, J.J., Zide, A., Mayhew, P.D., Culp, W.T., Mankin, K.T., Amsellem, P.M., Petrukovich, B., Ringwood, P.B., Case, J.B. and Singh A. (2016) Primary splenic torsion in dogs: 102 cases (1992–2014). *Journal of the American Veterinary Medical Association* 248, 661–668.

Della Ripa, M.A., Gaschen, F., Gaschen, L. and Cho, D.Y. (2010) Canine bronchoesophageal fistulas: case report and literature review. *Compendium on Continuing Education for the Practising Veterinarian*, 32: E1.

Deroy, C., Corcuff, J.B., Billen, F. and Hamaide, A. (2015) Removal of oesophageal foreign bodies: comparison between oesophagoscopy and oesophagotomy in 39 dogs. *Journal of Small Animal Practice* 56, 613–617.

Desmas, I., Burton, J.H., Post, G., Kristal, O., Gauthier, M., Borrego, J.F., Di Bella, A. and Lara-Garcia, A. (2017) Clinical presentation, treatment and outcome in 31 dogs with presumed primary colorectal lymphoma (2001–2013). *Veterinary and Comparative Oncology* 15, 504–517.

Dickinson, A.E., Summers, J.F., Wignal, J., Boag, A.K. and Keir, I. (2015) Impact of appropriate empirical antimicrobial therapy on outcome of dogs with septic peritonitis. *Journal of Veterinary Emergency and Critical Care* 25, 152–159.

Downs, M.O. and Stampley, A.R. (1998) Use of a Foley catheter to facilitate anal sac removal in the dog. *Journal of the American Animal Hospital Association* 34, 395–397.

Duell, J.R., Thieman Mankin, K.M., Rochat, M.C., Regier, P.J., Singh, A., Luther, J.K., Mison, M.B., Leeman, J.J. and Budke, C.M. (2016) Frequency of dehiscence in hand-sutured and stapled intestinal anastomoses in dogs. *Veterinary Surgery* 4, 100–103.

Dujowich, M., Keller, M.E. and Reimer, S.B. (2010) Evaluation of short- and long-term complications after endoscopically assisted gastropexy in dogs. *Journal of the American Veterinary Medical Association* 236, 177–182.

Durand, A., Finck, M., Sullivan, M. and Hammond, G. (2016) Computed tomography and magnetic resonance diagnosis of variations in the anatomical location of the major salivary glands in 1680 dogs and 187 cats. *Veterinary Journal* 209, 156–162.

Eastwood, J.M., McInnes, E.F., White, R.N., Elwood, C.M. and Stock, G. (2005) Caecal impaction and chronic intestinal pseudo-obstruction in a dog. *Journal of Veterinary Medicine. A, Physiology, Pathology, Clinical Medicine.* 52, 43–44.

Ellison, G.W. (2011) Complications of gastrointestinal surgery in companion animals. *Veterinary Clinics of North America: Small Animal Practice* 41, 915–934.

Elpiner, A.K, Brodsky, E.M. and Hazzah, T.N. (2011) Single-agent gemcitabine chemotherapy in dogs with hepatocellular carcinomas. *Veterinary and Comparative Oncology* 9, 260–268.

Emms, S.G. (2005) Anal sac tumours of the dog and their response to cytoreductive surgery and chemotherapy. *Australian Veterinary Journal* 83, 340–343.

Esplin, D.G., Wilson, S.T. and Hillinger, G.A. (2003) Squamous cell carcinoma of the anal sac in five dogs. *Veterinary Pathology* 40, 332–334.

Evans, H.E. and de Lahunta, A. (2013). The digestive apparatus and abdomen. In: *Miller's Anatomy of the Dog*, 4th edn., Elsevier Saunders, St Louis, Missouri.

Farrar, E.T., Washabau, R.J. and Saunders, H.M. (1996) Hepatic abscesses in dogs: 14 cases (1982–1994). *Journal of the American Veterinary Medical Association* 208, 243–247.

Fernandez, Y., Seth, M., Murgia, D. and Puig, J. (2017) Ileocolic junction resection in dogs and cats: 18 cases. *Journal of the American Veterinary Medical Association* 37, 175–181.

Formaggini, L. (2016) Unanswered questions on gastric dilatation/volvulus and gastropexy. *Veterinary Record* 179, 624–625.

Fossum, T.W., (2013) Surgery of the digestive system. In: *Small Animal Surgery*, 4th edn. Elsevier Saunders, St Louis, Missouri.

Fossum, T.W. and Hedlund, C.S. (2003) Gastric and intestinal surgery. *Veterinary Clinics of North America: Small Animal Practice* 33, 1117–1145.

Fox, A.N., Jeffers, L.J. and Rajender, R.K. (2012) Liver biopsy and laparoscopy. In: Schiff, E.R., Maddrey, W.C. and Sorrell M.F. (eds) *Schiff's Diseases of the Liver.* Wiley, Chichester, UK, pp. 44–57.

Fraune, C., Gaschen, F. and Ryan, K. (2009) Intralesional corticosteroid injection in addition to endoscopic balloon dilation in a dog with benign oesophageal strictures. *Journal of Small Animal Practice* 50, 550–553.

Fryer, K.J., Levine, J.M., Peycke, L.E., Thompson, J.A. and Cohen, N.D. (2011) Incidence of postoperative seizures with and without levetiracetam pretreatment in dogs undergoing portosystemic shunt attenuation. *Journal of Veterinary Internal Medicine* 25, 1379–1384.

Fukushima. K., Fujiwara, R., Yamamoto, K., Kanemoto, H., Ohno, K., Tsuboi, M., Uchida, K., Matsuki, N., Nishimura, R. and Tsujimoto, H. (2016) Characterization of triple-phase computed tomography in dogs with pancreatic insulinoma. *Journal of Veterinary Medical Science* 77, 1549–1553.

Garcia, R.S., Belafsky, P.C., Della Maggiore, A., Osborn, J.M.,

Pypendop, B.H., Pierce, T., Walker, V.J., Fulton, A. and Marks, S.L. (2017) Prevalence of gastroesophageal reflux in cats during anesthesia and effect of omeprazole on gastric pH. *Journal of Veterinary Internal Medicine* 31, 734–742.

García-Osogobio, S.M., Takahashi-Monroy, T., Velasco, L., Gaxiola, M., Sotres-Vega, A. and Santillán-Doherty, P. (2006) Single-layer colonic anastomoses using polyglyconate (Maxon) vs. two-layer anastomoses using chromic catgut and silk. *Revista de investigacion clinica, organo del hospital de enfermedales de la nuticion* 58, 198–203.

Garneau, M.S. and McCarthy, R.J. (2015) Multiple magnetic gastrointestinal foreign bodies in a dog. *Journal of the American Veterinary Medical Association* 246, 537–539.

Gazzola, K.M. and Nelson, L.L. (2014) The relationship between gastrointestinal motility and gastric dilatation-volvulus in dogs. *Topics in Companion Animal Medicine* 29, 64–66.

Gianella, P., Pfammatter, N.S. and Burgener, I.A. (2009) Oesophageal and gastric endoscopic foreign body removal: complications and follow-up of 102 dogs. *Journal of Small Animal Practice* 50, 649–654.

Gieger, T. (2011) Alimentary lymphoma in cats and dogs. *Veterinary Clinics of North America: Small Animal Practice* 41, 419–432.

Gilor, C., Gilor, S. and Graves, T. K. (2010) Phenobarbital-responsive sialadenosis associated with an esophageal foreign body in a dog. *Journal of the American Animal Hospital Association* 46, 115–120.

Glazer, A. and Walters, P. (2008) Esophagitis and esophageal strictures. *Compendium on Continuing Education for the Practising Veterinarian* 30, 281–292.

Glen, J.B. (1972) Canine salivary mucocoeles. Results of sialographic examination and surgical treatment of fifty cases. *Journal of Small Animal Practice* 13, 515–526.

Glickman, L.T., Glickman, N.W., Schellenberg, D.B., Raghavan, M. and Lee, T.L. (2000a) Incidence of and breed-related risk factors for gastric dilatation-volvulus in dogs. *Journal of the American Veterinary Medical Association* 216, 40–45.

Glickman, L.T., Glickman, N.W., Schellenberg, D.B., Raghavan, M. and Lee, T. (2000b) Non-dietary risk factors for gastric dilatation-volvulus in large and giant breed dogs. *Journal of the American Veterinary Medical Association* 217, 1492–1499.

Goldhammer, M.A., Haining, H., Milne, E.M., Shaw, D.J. and Yool, D.A. (2010) Assessment of the incidence of GDV following splenectomy in dogs. *Journal of Small Animal Practice* 51, 23–28.

Goldsworthy, S. J., Burton, C. and Guilherme, S. (2013) Parotid duct foreign body in a dog diagnosed with CT. *Journal of the American Animal Hospital Association* 49, 250–254.

Goodrich, Z.J., Powell, L.L. and Hulting, K.J. (2013) Assessment of two methods of gastric decompression for the initial management of gastric dilatation-volvulus. *Journal of Small Animal Practice* 54, 75–79.

Gordon, L.C., Friend, E.J. and Hamilton, M.H. (2010) Hemorrhagic pleural effusion secondary to an unusual type III hiatal hernia in a 4-year-old great Dane. *Journal of the American Animal Hospital Association* 46, 336–340.

Göritz, M., Müller, K., Krastel, D., Staudacher, G., Schmidt, P., Kühn, M., Nickel, R. and Schoon, H.A. (2013) Canine splenic haemangiosarcoma: influence of metastases, chemotherapy and growth pattern on post-splenectomy survival and expression of angiogenic factors. *Journal of Comparative Pathology* 149, 30–39.

Goutal, C.M., Brugmann, B.L. and Ryan, K.A. (2012) Insulinoma in dogs: a review. *Journal of the American Animal Hospital Association* 48, 151–163.

Grange, A.M., Clough, W. and Casale, S.A. (2012) Evaluation of splenectomy as a risk factor for gastric dilatation-volvulus. *Journal of the American Veterinary Medical Association* 241, 461–466.

Green, J.L., Cimino Brown, D. and Agnello, K.A. (2012) Preoperative thoracic radiographic findings in dogs presenting for gastric dilatation-volvulus (2000–2010): 101 cases. *Journal of Veterinary Emergency and Critical Care* 22, 595–600.

Green, T.I., Tonozzi, C.C., Kirby, R. and Rudloff, E. (2010) Evaluation of initial plasma lactate values as a predictor of gastric necrosis and initial and subsequent plasma lactate values as a predictor of survival in dogs with gastric dilatation-volvulus: 84 dogs (2003–2007). *Journal of Veterinary Emergency and Critical Care* 21, 36–44.

Greenhalgh, S.N., Dunning, M.D., McKinley, T.J., Goodfellow, M.R., Kelman, K.R., Freitag, T., O'Neill, E.J., Hall, E.J., Watson, P.J. and Jeffery, N.D. (2010) Comparison of survival after surgical or medical treatment in dogs with a congenital portosystemic shunt. *Journal of the American Veterinary Medical Association* 236, 1215–1220.

Grimes, J.A., Schmiedt, C.W., Cornell, K.K. and Radlinksy, M.A. (2011) Identification of risk factors for septic peritonitis and failure to survive following gastrointestinal surgery in dogs. *Journal of the American Veterinary Medical Association* 238, 486–494.

Grimes, J., Schmiedt, C., Milovancev, M., Radlinsky, M. and Cornell, K. (2013) Efficacy of serosal patching in dogs with septic peritonitis. *Journal of the American Animal Hospital Association* 49, 246–249.

Gualtieri, M., Monzeglio, M.G. and Scanziani, E. (1999) *Gastric Neoplasia* 29, 415–440.

Guedes, A.G. and Rude, E.P. (2013) Effects of preoperative administration of medetomidine on plasma insulin and glucose concentrations in healthy dogs and dogs with insulinoma. *Veterinary Anaesthesia and Analgesia* 40, 472–481.

Guffy, M.M., Wallace, L. and Anderson, N.V. (1970) Inversion of the caecum into the colon of a dog. *Journal of the American Veterinary Medical Association* 156, 183–186.

Guieu, L.V., Bersenas, A.M., Holowaychuk, M.K., Brisson, B.A. and Weese, J.S. (2015) Serial evaluation of abdominal fluid and serum amino-terminal pro-C-type natriuretic peptide in dogs with septic peritonitis. *Journal of Veterinary Internal Medicine* 29, 1300–1306.

Guieu, L.V., Bersenas, A.M., Brisson, B.A., Holowaychuk, M.K., Ammersbach, M.A., Beaufrère, H., Fugita, H. and Weese, J.S. (2016) Evaluation of peripheral blood and abdominal fluid variables as predictors of intestinal surgical site failure in dogs with septic peritonitis following celiotomy and the placement of closed-suction abdominal drains. *Journal of the American Veterinary Medical Association* 249, 515–525.

Guilford, W.G. and Strombeck, D.R. (1996) Neoplasms of

the gastrointestinal tract, APUD tumors, endocrinopathies and the gastrointestinal tract. In: Guilford, W.G., Center, S.A., Strombeck, D.R., Williams, D.A. and Meyer, D.J. (eds) *Strombeck Small Animal Gastroenterology*. Saunders, Philadelphia, Pennsylvania, pp. 519–539.

Guiot, L.P., Landsdowne, J.L., Rouppert, P. and Stanley, B.J. (2008) Hiatal hernia in the dog: a clinical report of four Chinese shar peis. *Journal of the American Animal Hospital Association* 44, 335–341.

Gustafson, T.L., Villamil, A., Taylor, B.E. and Flory, A. (2014) A retrospective study of feline gastric lymphoma in 16 chemotherapy-treated cats. *Journal of the American Animal Hospital Association* 50, 46–52.

Guthrie, K.M. and Hardie, R.J. (2014) Surgical excision of the parotid salivary gland for treatment of a traumatic mucocele in a dog. *Journal of the American Animal Hospital Association* 50, 216–220.

Hammer, A., Getzy, D., Ogilvie, G., Upton, M., Klausner, J. and Kisseberth, W.C. (2001) Salivary gland neoplasia in the dog and cat: survival times and prognostic factors. *Journal of the American Animal Hospital Association* 37, 478–482.

Han, H., Mann, F.A. and Park, J.Y. (2016) Canine sialolithiasis: Two case reports with breed, gender, and age distribution of 29 cases (1964–2010). *Journal of the American Animal Hospital Association* 52, 22–26.

Haraguchi, T., Kimura, S., Itoh, H., Nishikawa, S., Hiyama, M., Tani, K., Iseri, T., Itoh, Y., Nakaichi, M., Taura, Y. and Itamoto, K. (2017) Comparison of postoperative pain and inflammation reaction in dogs undergoing preventive laparoscopic-assisted and incisional gastropexy. *Journal of Veterinary Medical Science* 79, 1524–1531.

Harai, B.H., Johnson, S.E. and Sherding, R.G. (1995) Endoscopically guided balloon dilation of benign esophageal strictures in 6 cats and 7 dogs. *Journal of Veterinary Internal Medicine* 9, 332–335.

Harkey, M.A., Villagran, A.M., Venkataraman, G.M., Leisenring, W.M., Hullar, M.A.J. and Torok-Storb, B.J. (2017) Associations between gastric dilatation-volvulus in Great Danes and specific alleles of the canine immune-system genes DLA88, DRB1, and TLR5. *American Journal of Veterinary Research* 78, 934–954.

Hayes, G. (2009) Gastrointestinal foreign bodies in dogs and cats: a retrospective study of 208 cases. *Journal of Small Animal Practice* 50, 576–583.

Hill, L.N. and Smeak, D.D. (2002) Open versus closed bilateral anal sacculectomy for treatment of non-neoplastic anal sac disease in dogs: 95 cases (1969–1994). *Journal of the American Veterinary Medical Association* 221, 662–665.

Hill, P.B., Lo, A., Eden, C.A., Huntley, S., Morey, V., Ramsey, S., Richardson, C., Smith, D.J., Sutton, C., Taylor, M.D., Thorpe, E., Tidmarsh, R. and Williams, V. (2006) Survey of the prevalence, diagnosis and treatment of dermatological conditions in small animals in general practice. *Veterinary Record* 158, 533–539.

Hobday, M.M., Pachtinger, G.E., Drobatz, K.J. and Syring, R.S. (2014) Linear versus non-linear gastrointestinal foreign bodies in 499 dogs: clinical presentation, management and short-term outcome. *Journal of Small Animal Practice* 55, 560–565.

Hoffberg, J.E. and Koenigshof, A. (2017) Evaluation of the safety of early compared to late enteral nutrition in canine septic peritonitis. *Journal of the American Animal Hospital Association* 53, 90–95.

Holt, D., Callan, M.B., Washabau, R.J. and Saunders, H.M. (1998) Medical treatment versus surgery for hiatal hernias. *Journal of the American Veterinary Medical Association* 213, 800.

Hugen, S., Thomas, R.E., German, A.J., Burgener, I.A. and Mandigers, P.J. (2017) Gastric carcinoma in canines and humans, a review. *Veterinary and Comparative Oncology* 15, 692–705.

Humm, K. and Bartfield, D. (2017) Differentiating between food bloat and gastric dilatation and volvulus in dogs. *Veterinary Record* 181, 561–562.

Hunt, G.B., Worth, A. and Marchevsky, A. (2004) Migration of wooden skewer foreign bodies from the gastrointestinal tract in eight dogs. *Journal of Small Animal Practice* 45, 362–367.

Hyun-Jung, S., Dai Jung, C., A-Jin, L., Hyo-Jin, C., Dae-Hyun, K., Ki-Dong, E., Sun Hee, D. and Hwi-Yool, K. (2015) Abnormal changes in both mandibular salivary glands in a dog: Non-mineral radiopaque sialoliths. *Canadian Veterinary Journal* 56, 1025–1028.

Iseri. T., Yamada, K., Chijiwa, K., Nishimura, R., Matsunaga, S., Fujiwara, R. and Sasaki, N. (2007) Dynamic computed tomography of the pancreas in normal dogs and in a dog with pancreatic insulinoma. *Veterinary Radiology & Ultrasound* 48, 328–331.

Jankowski, M., Spuzak, J., Kubiak, K., Glińska-Suchocka, K. and Nicpoń, J. (2013) Oesophageal foreign bodies in dogs. *Polish Journal of Veterinary Sciences* 16, 571–572.

Johnson, M.D. and Mann, F.A. (2006) Treatment for pancreatic abscesses via omentalization with abdominal closure versus open peritoneal drainage in dogs: 15 cases (1994–2004). *Journal of the American Veterinary Medical Association* 228, 397–402.

Julian, T.B., Kolachalam, R.B. and Wolmark, N. (1989) The triple-stapled colonic anastomosis. *Diseases of the Colon & Rectum* 32, 989–995.

Juvet, F., Pinilla, M., Shiel, R.E. and Mooney, C.T. (2010) Oesophageal foreign bodies in dogs: factors affecting success of endoscopic retrieval. *Irish Veterinary Journal* 63, 163–168.

Kaiser, S., Thiel, C., Kramer, M. and Peppler, C. (2016) Complications and prognosis of cervical sialoceles in the dog using the lateral surgical approach. *Tieraerztliche Praxis Ausgabe K Kleintiere Heimtiere* 44, 323–331.

Kapatkin, A.S., Mullen, H.S., Matthiesen, D.T. and Patnaik, A.K. (1992) Leiomyosarcoma in dogs: 44 cases (1983–1988). *Journal of the American Veterinary Medical Association* 201, 1077–1079.

Katsikas, D., Sechas, M., Antypas, G., Floudas, P., Moshovos, K., Gogas, J., Rigas, A., Papacharalambous, N. and Skalkeas, G. (1977) Beneficial effect of omental wrapping of unsafe intestinal anastomoses. An experimental study in dogs. *International Surgery* 62, 435–437.

Keir, I., Woolford, L., Hirst, C. and Adamantos, S. (2010) Fatal aortic oesophageal fistula following oesophageal foreign body removal in a dog. *Journal of Small Animal Practice* 51, 657–660.

Kim, S.E., Giglio, R.F., Reese, D.J., Reese, S.L., Bacon, N.J. and Ellison, G.W. (2013) Comparison of computed tomographic angiography and ultrasonography for the detection and characterization of portosystemic shunts in dogs. *Veterinary Radiology & Ultrasound* 54, 569–574.

King, J.M. (2001) Esophageal foreign body and aortic perforation in a dog. *Veterinary Medicine* 96, 828.

Kinsey, J.R., Gilson, S.D., Hauptman, J. and Mehler S.J. (2015) Factors associated with long-term survival in dogs undergoing liver lobectomy as treatment for liver tumors. *Canadian Veterinary Journal* 56, 598–604.

Kishimoto, T.E., Yoshimura, H., Saito, N., Michishita, M., Kanno, N., Ohkusu-Tsukada, K. and Takahashi, K. (2015) Salivary gland epithelial-myoepithelial carcinoma with high-grade transformation in a dog. *Journal of Comparative Pathology* 153, 111–115.

Kneissl, S., Weidner, S. and Probst, A. (2011) CT sialography in the dog – a cadaver study. *Anatomia, Histologia, Embryologia* 40, 397–401.

Koenig, A. and Verlander, L.L. (2015) Usefulness of whole blood, plasma, peritoneal fluid, and peritoneal fluid supernatant glucose concentrations obtained by a veterinary point-of-care glucometer to identify septic peritonitis in dogs with peritoneal effusion. *Journal of the American Veterinary Medical Association* 247, 1027–1032.

Kraun, M.B., Nelson, L.L., Hauptman, J.G. and Nelson, N.C. (2014) Analysis of the relationship of extra-hepatic portosystemic shunt morphology with clinical variables in dogs: 53 cases (2009–2012). *Journal of the American Veterinary Medical Association* 245, 540–549.

Kyles, A.E. (2012) Esophagus. In: Tobias K.M. and Johnston S.A. (eds) *Veterinary Surgery: Small Animal.* Elsevier Saunders, St. Louis, Missouri.

Lakatos, L. and Ruckstuhl, B. (1977) Hypertrophic pyloric stenosis in the dog. *Schweizer Archiv fuer Tierheilkunde* 119, 155–160.

Lam, N., Weisse, C., Berent, A., Kaae, J., Murphy, S., Radlinsky, M., Ritcher, K., Dunn, M. and Gingerich, K. (2013) Esophageal stenting for treatment of refractory benign strictures in dogs. *Journal of Veterinary Internal Medicine* 27, 1064–1070.

Lamb, C.R. (1996) Ultrasonographic diagnosis of congenital portosystemic shunts in dogs: results of a prospective study. *Veterinary Radiology & Ultrasound* 37, 281–288.

Lamoureux, A., Maurey, C. and Freiche, V. (2017) Treatment of inflammatory rectal strictures by digital bougienage: a retrospective study of nine cases. *Journal of Small Animal Practice* 58, 293–297.

Landon, B.P., Abraham, L.A., Charles, J.A. and Edwards, G.A. (2007) Recurrent rectal prolapse caused by colonic duplication in a dog. *Australian Veterinary Journal* 85, 381–385.

Lee, K. C., Lipscomb, V. J., Lamb, C. R., Gregory, S. P., Guitian, J. and Brockman, D. J. (2006) Association of portovenographic findings with outcome in dogs receiving surgical treatment for single congenital portosystemic shunts: 45 cases (2000–2004). *Journal of the American Veterinary Medical Association* 229, 1122–1129.

Lee, N., Choi, M., Keh, S., Kim, T., Kim, H. and Yoon, J. (2014) Zygomatic sialolithiasis diagnosed with computed tomography in a dog. *Journal of Veterinary Medical Science* 76, 1389–1391.

Leeman, J.J., Kim, S.E. and Reese, D.J. (2013) Multiple congenital PSS in a dog: case report and literature review. *Journal of the American Animal Hospital Association* 49, 281–285.

Leib, M.S., Saunders, G.K., Moon, M.L., Mann, M.A., Martin, R.A., Matz, M.E., Nix, B., Smith, M.M. and Waldron, D.R. (1993) Endoscopic diagnosis of chronic hypertrophic pyloric gastropathy in dogs. *Journal of Veterinary Internal Medicine* 7, 335–341.

Leib, M.S., Dinnel, H., Ward, D.L., Reimer, M.E., Towell, T.L. and Monroe, W.E. (2001) Endoscopic balloon dilation of benign esophageal strictures in dogs and cats. *Journal of Veterinary Internal Medicine* 15, 547–552.

Leib, M.S. and Sartor, L.L. (2008) Esophageal foreign body obstruction caused by a dental chew treat in 31 dogs (2000–2006). *Journal of the American Veterinary Medical Association* 232, 1021–1025.

Lenoci, D. and Ricciardi, M. (2015) Ultrasound and multidetector computed tomography of mandibular salivary gland adenocarcinoma in two dogs. *Open Veterinary Journal* 5, 173–178.

Levien, A.S. and Baines, S.J. (2011) Histological examination of the intestine from dogs and cats with intussusception. *Journal of Small Animal Practice* 52, 599–606.

Levine, J.S., Pollard, R.E. and Marks, S.L. (2014) Contrast videofluoroscopic assessment of dysphagic cats. *Veterinary Radiology & Ultrasound* 55, 465–471.

Lidbury, J.A. (2016) Getting the most out of liver biopsy. *Veterinary Clinics of North America: Small Animal Practice* 47, 569–583.

Liu, D.T., Brown, D.C. and Silverstein, D.C. (2012) Early nutritional support is associated with decreased length of hospitalization in dogs with septic peritonitis: A retrospective study of 45 cases (2000–2009). *Journal of Veterinary Emergency and Critical Care* 22, 453–459.

Lorinson, D. and Bright, R.M. (1998) Long-term outcome of medical and surgical treatment of hiatal hernias in dogs and cats: 27 cases (1978–1996). *Journal of the American Veterinary Medical Association* 213, 381–384.

Loy Son, N.K., Singh, A., Amsellem, P., Kilkwnny, J., Brisson, B.A., Oblak, M.L. and Ogilvie, A.T. (2016) Long-term outcome and complications following prophylactic laparoscopic-assisted gastropexy in dogs. *Veterinary Surgery* 45, 77–83.

Lynch, A.M., O'Toole, T.E. and Hamilton, J. (2015) Transfusion practices for treatment of dogs undergoing splenectomy for splenic masses: 542 cases (2001–2012). *Journal of the American Veterinary Medical Association* 247, 636–642.

Maas, C.P., ter Haar, G., van der Gaag, I. and Kirpensteijn, J. (2007) Reclassification of small intestinal and cecal smooth muscle tumors in 72 dogs: clinical, histologic, and immunohistochemical evaluation. *Veterinary Surgery* 36, 302–313.

MacDonald, P.H., Dinda, P.K., Beck, I.T. and Mercer, C.D. (1993) The use of oximetry in determining intestinal blood flow. *Surgery, Gynecology & Obstetrics* 176, 451–458.

Mackenzie, G., Barnhart, M., Kennedy, S., DeHoff, W. and Schertel, E. (2010) A retrospective study of factors influencing survival following surgery for gastric dilatation-volvulus syndrome in 306 dogs. *Journal of the American Animal Hospital Association* 46, 97–102.

MacPhail, C. (2008) Anal sacculectomy. *Compendium on Continuing Education for the Practising Veterinarian* 30 530–535.

Maddison, J.E. (1988) Canine congenital portosystemic encephalopathy. *Australian Veterinary Journal* 65, 245–249.

Mai, W. (2006) The hilar perivenous hyperechoic triangle as a sign of acute splenic torsion in dogs. *Veterinary Radiology & Ultrasound* 47, 487–491.

Maki, L.C., Males, K.N., Byrnes, M.J., El-Saad, A.A. and Coronado, G.S. (2017) Incidence of gastric dilatation-volvulus following a splenectomy in 238 dogs. *Canadian Veterinary Journal* 58, 1275–1280.

Mankin, K.M. (2015) Current concepts in congenital portosystemic shunts. *Veterinary Clinics of North America: Small Animal Practice* 45, 47–487.

Marques, A.I., Munro, E. and Welsh, E.M. (2008) Migrating foreign body in the parotid duct of a boxer dog. *Veterinary Record* 163, 691–692.

Marsh, A. and Adin, C. (2013) Tunneling under the digastricus muscle increases salivary duct exposure and completeness of excision in mandibular and sublingual sialoadenectomy in dogs. *Veterinary Surgery* 42, 238–242.

Mason, D.R., Lamb, C.R. and McLellan, G.J. (2001) Ultrasonographic findings in 50 dogs with retrobulbar disease. *Journal of the American Animal Hospital Association* 37, 557–562.

May, L.R. and Mehler., S.J. (2011) Complications of hepatic surgery in companion animals. *Veterinary Clinics of North America: Small Animal Practice* 41, 935–948.

Mayhew, P.D. and Brown, D.C. (2009) Prospective evaluation of two intracorporeally sutured prophylactic laparoscopic gastropexy techniques compared with laparoscopic-assisted gastropexy in dogs. *Veterinary Surgery* 38, 738–746.

Mayhew, P.D., Marks, S.L., Pollard, R., Culp, W.T.N. and Kass, P.H. (2017) Prospective evaluation of surgical management of sliding hiatal hernia and gastroesophageal reflux in dogs. *Veterinary Surgery* 46, 1098–1109.

Mayhew, P.D. and Weisse, C. (2012) Liver and biliary system. In: Tobias, K.M. and Johnston, S.A. (eds) *Veterinary Surgery: Small Animal.* Elsevier Saunders, St. Louis, Missouri.

McCready, R.A. and Beart, R.W. (1979) The surgical treatment of incapacitating constipation associated with idiopathic megacolon. *Mayo Clinic Proceedings* 54, 779–783.

Meleo, K. (1990) Management of insuloma patients with refractory hypoglycemia. *Problems in Veterinary Medicine* 2, 602–609.

Messinger, J.S., Windham, W.R. and Ward, C.R. (2009) Ionised hypercalcaemia in dogs: a retrospective study of 109 cases (1998–2003). *Journal of Veterinary Internal Medicine* 23, 514–519.

Militerno, G., Bazzo, R. and Marcato, P.S. (2005) Cytological diagnosis of mandibular salivary gland adenocarcinoma in a dog. *Journal of Veterinary Medicine. A, Physiology, Pathology, Clinical Medicine* 52, 514–516.

Monnet, E. and Culp, W.T. (2013) Anal sac disease. In: Monnet, E. (ed.) *Small Animal Soft Tissue Surgery.* Wiley-Blackwell, Chichester, UK, pp. 399–405.

Mooney, E., Raw, C. and Hughes, D. (2014) Plasma lactate concentration as a prognostic biomarker in dogs with gastric dilation and volvulus. *Topics in Companion Animal Medicine* 29, 71–76.

Moore, A.H. (2001) Removal of oesophageal foreign bodies in dogs: use of the fluoroscopic method and outcome. *Journal of Small Animal Practice* 42, 227–230.

Moore, A.S., Rassnick, K.M. and Frimberger, A.E. (2017) Evaluation of clinical and histologic factors associated with survival time in dogs with stage II splenic hemangiosarcoma treated by splenectomy and adjuvant chemotherapy: 30 cases (2011–2014). *Journal of the American Veterinary Medical Association* 251, 559–565.

Morello, E., Martano, M., Squassino, C., Iussich, S., Caccamo, R., Sammartano, F., Zabarino, S., Bellino, C., Pisani, G. and Buracco, P. (2008) Trans-anal pull-through rectal amputation for treatment of colorectal carcinoma in 11 dogs. *Veterinary Surgery* 37, 420–426.

Mori, T., Ito, Y. and Kawabe, M. (2015) Three-dimensional conformal radiation therapy for inoperable massive hepatocellular carcinoma in six dogs. *Journal of Small Animal Practice* 56, 441–445.

Muir, P. and Rosin, E. (1995) Failure of the single enterotomy technique to remove a linear intestinal foreign body from a cat. *Veterinary Record* 136, 75.

Mukaratirwa, S., Petterino, C. and Bradley, A. (2015) Spontaneous necrotizing sialometaplasia of the submandibular salivary gland in a Beagle dog. *Journal of Toxicologic Pathology* 28, 177–180.

Nakamura, K., Lim, S.Y., Ochiai, K., Yamasaki, M., Ohta, H., Morishita, K., Takagi, S. and Takiguchi, M. (2015) Contrast-enhanced ultrasonographic findings in three dogs with pancreatic insulinoma. *Veterinary Radiology & Ultrasound* 56, 55–62.

Neath, P.J., Brockman, D.J. and Saunders, H.M. (1997) Retrospective analysis of 19 cases of isolated torsion of the splenic pedicle in dogs. *Journal of Small Animal Practice* 38, 387–392.

Nelson, N.C. and Nelson, L.L. (2016) Imaging and clinical outcomes in 20 dogs treated with thin film banding for extrahepatic portosystemic shunts. *Veterinary Surgery* 45, 736–745.

Nivy, R., Caldin, M., Lavy, E., Shaabon, K., Segev, G. and Aroch, I. (2014) Serum acute phase protein concentrations in dogs with spirocercosis and their association with esophageal neoplasia – a prospective cohort study. *Veterinary Parasitology* 203, 153–159.

Nucci, D.J., Liptak, J.M., Selmic, L.E., Culp, W.T., Durant, A.M., Worley, D., Maritato K.C., Thomson, M., Annoni, M., Singh, A., Matz, B., Benson, J. and Buracco, P.J. (2014) Complications and outcomes following rectal pull-through surgery in dogs with rectal masses: 74 cases (2000–2013). *Journal of the American Veterinary Medical Association* 15, 684–695.

Ober, C.A., Peştean, C.P., Bel, L.V., Taulescu, M., Cătoi, C., Bogdan, S., Milgram, J., Schwarz, G. and Oana, L.I. (2016) Vaginal prolapse with urinary bladder incarceration and consecutive irreducible rectal prolapse in a dog. *Acta Veterinaria Scandinavica* 58, 54.

Odendaal, J.S. and Cronje, J.D. (1983) Lymphosarcoma as a rare cause of rectal prolapse in a dog. *Journal of the South African Veterinary Association* 54, 61–62.

Ohta, H., Takagi, S., Murakami, M., Sasaki, N., Yoshikawa, M., Nakamura, D.K., Hwang, S.J., Yamasaki, M. and Takiguchi, M. (2009) Primary splenic torsion in a Boston terrier. *Journal of Veterinary Medical Science* 71, 1533–1535.

O'Neill, D.G., Church, D.B., McGreevy, P.D., Thomson, P.C. and Brodbelt, D.C. (2014) Prevalence of disorders recorded in dogs attending primary-care veterinary practices in England. *PLoS ONE* 9, e90501.

Panti, A., Bennett, R.C., Corletto, F., Brearley, J., Jeffery, N. and Mellanby, R.J. (2009) The effect of omeprazole on oesophageal pH in dogs during anaesthesia. *Journal of Small Animal Practice* 50, 540–544.

Papazoglou, L.G., Tzimtzimis, E., Rampidi, S. and Tzimitris, N. (2015) Ventral approach for surgical management of feline sublingual sialocele. *Journal of Veterinary Dentistry* 32, 201–203.

Pappalardo, E., Martino, P.A. and Noli, C. (2002) Macroscopic, cytological and bacteriological evaluation of anal sac content in normal dogs and in dogs with selected dermatological diseases. *Veterinary Dermatology* 13, 315–322.

Paris, J.K., Yool, D.A., Reed, N., Ridyard, A.E., Chandler, M.L. and Simpson, J.W. (2011) Chronic gastric instability and presumed incomplete volvulus in dogs. *Journal of Small Animal Practice* 52, 651–655.

Park, H.A., Kim, J.W. and Park, H.M. (2012) Characteristics of esophageal diverticula using computed tomography and three-dimensional reconstruction in a Maltese dog. *Journal of Veterinary Medical Science* 74, 1233–1236.

Patnaik, A.K., Hurvitz, A.I. and Lieberman, P.H. (1980) Canine hepatic neoplasms: a clinicopathologic study. *Veterinary Pathology* 17, 553–564.

Patnaik, A.K., Hurvitz, A.I. and Lieberman, P.H. (1981) Canine hepatocellular carcinoma. *Veterinary Pathology* 18, 427–438.

Patsikas, M.N., Rallis, T., Kladakis, S.E. and Dessiris, A.K. (2001) Computed tomography diagnosis of isolated splenic torsion in a dog. *Veterinary Radiology & Ultrasound* 42, 235–237.

Patsikas, M.N., Papazoglou, L.G., Papaioannou, N.G. and Dessiris, A.K. (2004) Normal and abnormal ultrasonographic findings that mimic small intestinal intussusception in the dog. *Journal of the American Animal Hospital Association* 40, 147–151.

Patsikas, M.N., Papazoglou, L.G. and Adamama-Moraitou, K.K. (2008) Spontaneous reduction of intestinal intussusception in five young dogs. *Journal of the American Animal Hospital Association* 44, 41–47.

Pavletic, M.M. (1994) Stapling in esophageal surgery. *Veterinary Clinics of North America: Small Animal Practice* 24, 395–412.

Penninck, D. and Mitchell, S.L. (2003) Ultrasonographic detection of ingested and perforating wooden foreign bodies in four dogs. *Journal of the American Veterinary Medical Association* 15, 206–209.

Philp, H.S., Rhodes, M., Parry, A. and Baines, S.J. (2012) Canine zygomatic salivary mucocoele following suspected oropharyngeal penetrating stick injury. *Veterinary Record* 171, 402.

Pohlman, L.M., Higginbotham, M.L. and Welles, E.G. (2009) Immunophenotypic and histologic classification of 50 cases of feline gastrointestinal lymphoma. *Veterinary Pathology* 46, 259–268.

Poirier, V.J., Mayer-Stankeová, S., Buchholz, J., Vail, D.M. and Kaser Hotz, B. (2017) Efficacy of radiation therapy for the treatment of sialocele in dogs. *Journal of Veterinary Internal Medicine* 32, 107–110.

Pratschke, K.M., Ryan, J., McAlinden, A. and McLauchlan, G. (2015) Pancreatic surgical biopsy in 24 dogs and 19 cats: postoperative complications and clinical relevance of histological findings. *Journal of Small Animal Practice* 56, 60–66.

Pratt, C.L., Reineke, E.L. and Drobatz, K.J. (2014) Sewing needle foreign body ingestion in dogs and cats: 65 cases (2000–2012). *Journal of the American Veterinary Medical Association* 245, 302–308.

Proot, J.L., Nelissen, P., Ladlow, J.F., Bowlt Blacklock, K., Kulendra, N., de la Puerta, B. and Sheahan, D.E. (2016) Parotidectomy for the treatment of parotid sialocoele in 14 dogs. *Journal of Small Animal Practice* 57, 79–83.

Prymak, C., Saunders, H.M. and Washabau, R.J. (1989) Hiatal hernia repair by restoration and stabilization of normal anatomy. An evaluation in four dogs and one cat. *Veterinary Surgery* 18, 386–391.

Przywara, J.F., Abel, S.B., Peacock, J.T. and Shott, S. (2014) Occurrence and recurrence of gastric dilatation with or without volvulus after incisional gastropexy. *Canadian Veterinary Journal* 55, 981–984.

Raghavan, M., Glickman, N., McCabe, G., Lantz, G. and Glickman, L.T. (2004) Diet-related risk factors for gastric dilatation-volvulus in dogs of high-risk breeds. *Journal of the American Animal Hospital Association* 40, 192–203.

Raj, B.R., Subbu, K. and Manoharan, G. (1997) Omental plug closure of large duodenal defects – an experimental study. *Tropical Gastroenterology* 18, 180–182.

Randolph, J.G. (1975) Y–U advancement pyloroplasty. *Annals of Surgery* 181, 586–590.

Ranen, E., Shamir, M.H., Shahar, R. and Johnston, D.E. (2004) Partial esophagectomy with single layer closure for treatment of esophageal sarcomas in 6 dogs. *Veterinary Surgery* 33, 428–434.

Ranen, E., Dank, G., Lavy, E., Perl, S., Lahav, D. and Orgad, U. (2008) Oesophageal sarcomas in dogs: histological and clinical evaluation. *Veterinary Journal* 178, 78–84.

Rawlings, C.A., Mahaffey, M.B., Bement, S. and Canalis, C. (2002) Prospective evaluation of laparoscopic-assisted gastropexy in dogs susceptible to gastric dilatation. *Journal of the American Veterinary Medical Association* 221, 1576–1581.

Reeve, E.J., Sutton, D., Friend, E.J. and Warren-Smith, C.M.R. (2017) Documenting the prevalence of hiatal hernia and oesophageal abnormalities in brachycephalic dogs using fluoroscopy. *Journal of Small Animal Practice* 58, 703–708.

Reinhart, J.M., Sherwood, J.M., KuKanich, K.S., Klocke, E. and Biller, D.S. (2015) Chronic splenic torsion in two dogs. *Journal of the American Animal Hospital Association* 51, 185–190.

Richter, M.C. (2012) Abdomen. In: Tobias, K.M. and Johnston, S.A. (eds) *Veterinary Surgery: Small Animal*. Elsevier Saunders, St. Louis, Missouri.

Ritter, M.J. and Stanley, B.J. (2012) Salivary glands. In: Tobias, K.M. and Johnston, S.A. (eds) *Veterinary Surgery: Small Animal*. Elsevier Saunders, St. Louis, Missouri.

Ritter, M.J., von Pfeil, D.J., Stanley, B.J., Hauptman, J.G. and Walshaw, R. (2006) Mandibular and sublingual sialocoeles in the dog: a retrospective evaluation of 41 cases, using the ventral approach for treatment. *New Zealand Veterinary Journal* 54, 333–337.

Robben, J.H., Pollak, Y.W., Kirpensteijn, J., Boroffka, S.A., van den Ingh, T.S., Teske, E. and Voorhout, G. (2005) Comparison of ultrasonography, computed tomography, and single-photon emission computed tomography for the detection and localization of canine insulinoma. *Journal of Veterinary Internal Medicine* 19, 15–22.

Robson, D.C., Burton, G.G. and Lorimer, M.F. (2003) Cytological examination and physical characteristics of the anal sacs in 17 clinically normal dogs. *Australian Veterinary Journal* 81, 36–41.

Rodríguez-Alarcón, C.A., Usón, J., Beristain, D.M., Rivera, R., Andrés, S. and Pérez, E.M. (2010) Breed as risk factor for oesophageal foreign bodies. *Journal of Small Animal Practice* 51, 357.

Rogers, F.B., Baumgartner, N.E., Robin, A.P. and Barrett, J.A. (1999) Absorbable mesh splenorrhaphy for severe splenic injuries: functional studies in an animal model and an additional patient series. *Journal of Trauma* 31, 200–204.

Ross, J., Scavelli, T., Matthiesen, D. and Patnaik, A.K. (1991) Adenocarcinoma of the apocrine glands of the anal sac in dogs: a review of 32 cases. *Journal of the American Animal Hospital Association* 27, 349–355.

Ruland, K., Fischer, A. and Hartmann, K. (2010) Sensitivity and specificity of fasting ammonia and serum bile acids in the diagnosis of portosystemic shunts in dogs and cats. *Veterinary Clinical Pathology* 39, 57–64.

Rutherford, L. and Lee, K. (2015) Anal sac disease in dogs. *Clinical Practice Companion Animals* 37, 9.

Ryan, T., Welsh., E., McGorum, I. and Yool, D. (2008) Sublingual salivary gland sialolithiasis in a dog. *Journal of Small Animal Practice* 49, 254–256.

Salisbury, S.K., Lantz, G.C., Nelson, R.W. and Kazacos, E.A. (1988) Pancreatic abscess in dogs: six cases (1978–1986). *Journal of the American Veterinary Medical Association* 193, 1104–1108.

Sapierzyński, R. (2006) Gastrointestinal tract tumors in dogs and cats. Part II. Esophageal, gastric, and intestinal tumours. *Życie weterynaryjne* 81, 316–325.

Sartor, A.J., Bentley, A.M. and Brown, D.C. (2013) Association between previous splenectomy and gastric dilatation-volvulus in dogs: 453 cases (2004–2009). *Journal of the American Veterinary Medical Association* 15, 1381–1384.

Saunders, H.M., Neath, P.J. and Brockman, D.J. (1998) B-mode and Doppler ultrasound imaging of the spleen with canine splenic torsion: a retrospective evaluation. *Veterinary Radiology & Ultrasound* 39, 349–353.

Schroeder, H. and Berry, W.L. (1998) Salivary gland necrosis in dogs: a retrospective study of 19 cases. *Journal of Small Animal Practice* 39, 121–125.

Schwandt, C.S. (2008) Low-grade or benign intestinal tumours contribute to intussusception: a report on one feline and two canine cases. *Journal of Small Animal Practice* 49, 651–654.

Schwarz, L.A., Penninck, D.G. and Leveille-Webster, C. (1998) Hepatic abscesses in 13 dogs: a review of the ultrasonographic findings, clinical data and therapeutic options. *Veterinary Radiology & Ultrasound* 39, 357–365.

Seiler, G., Rytz, U. and Gaschen, L. (2001) Radiographic diagnosis – cavitary mediastinal abscess. *Veterinary Radiology & Ultrasound* 42, 431–433.

Seim-Wikse, T., Jörundsson, E., Nødtvedt, A., Grotmol, T., Bjornvad, C.R., Kristensen, A.T. and Skancke, E. (2013) Breed predisposition to canine gastric carcinoma – a study based on the Norwegian canine cancer register. *Acta Veterinaria Scandinavica* 55, 25.

Sellon, R.K. and Willard, M.D. (2003) Esophagitis and esophageal strictures. *Veterinary Clinics of North America: Small Animal Practice* 33, 945–967.

Selmic, L.E. (2017) Hepatobiliary neoplasia. *Veterinary Clinics of North America: Small Animal Practice* 47, 725–735.

Selting, K.A. (2013) Intestinal tumors. In: Withrow, S., Vail, D. and Page, R. (eds) *Withrow & MacEwen's Small Animal Clinical Oncology*. Elsevier Saunders, Philadelphia, Pennsylvania, pp. 412–423.

Sergeeff, J.S., Armstrong, P.J. and Bunch, S.E. (2004) Hepatic abscesses in cats: 14 cases (1985–2002). *Journal of Veterinary Internal Medicine* 18, 295–300.

Sharma, A., Thompson, M.S., Scrivani, P.V., Dykes, N.L., Yeager, A.E., Freer, S.L. and Erb, H.N. (2011) Comparison of radiography and ultrasonography for diagnosing small-intestinal mechanical obstruction in vomiting dogs. *Veterinary Radiology & Ultrasound* 52, 248–255.

Sharp, C.R. and Rozanski, E.A. (2014) Cardiovascular and systemic effects of gastric dilatation and volvulus in dogs. *Topics in Companion Animal Medicine* 29, 67–70.

Shipov, A., Kelmer, G., Lavy, E., Milgram, J., Aroch, I. and Segev, G. (2015) Long-term outcome of transendoscopic oesophageal mass ablation in dogs with *Spirocerca lupi*-associated oesophageal sarcoma. *Veterinary Record* 177, 365.

Sivacolundhu, R.K., Read, R.A. and Marchevsky, A.M. (2002) Hiatal hernia controversies – a review of pathophysiology and treatment options. *Australian Veterinary Journal* 80, 48–53.

Smart, L., Reese, S. and Hosgood, G. (2017) Food engorgement in 35 dogs (2009–2013) compared with 36 dogs with gastric dilation and volvulus. *Veterinary Record* 181, 563.

Snowdon, K.A., Smeak, D.D. and Chiang, S. (2016) Risk factors for dehiscence of stapled functional end-to-end intestinal anastomosis in dogs: 53 cases (2001–2012). *Veterinary Surgery* 45, 91–99.

Sozmen, M., Brown, P.J. and Eveson, J.W. (2003) Salivary gland basal cell adenocarcinoma: a report of cases in a cat and two dogs. *Journal of Veterinary Medicine. A, Physiology, Pathology, Clinical Medicine* 50, 399–401.

Sozmen, M., Brown, P.J. and Whitbread, T.J. (2000) Idiopathic salivary gland enlargement (sialadenosis) in dogs: a microscopic study. *Journal of Small Animal Practice* 41, 243–247.

Spangler, W.L. and Culbertson, M.R. (1991) Salivary gland disease in dogs and cats: 245 cases (1985–1988). *Journal of the American Veterinary Medical Association* 198, 465–469.

Spillebeen, A.L., Robben, J.H., Thomas, R., Kirpensteijn, J. and van Nimwegen, S.A. (2017) Negative pressure therapy versus passive open abdominal drainage for the treatment of septic peritonitis in dogs: A randomized, prospective study. *Veterinary Surgery* 46, 1086–1097.

Spużak, J., Ciaputa, R., Kubiak, K., Jankowski, M., Glińska-Suchocka, K., Poradowski, D. and Nowak, M. (2017) Adenocarcinoma of the posterior segment of the gastrointestinal tract in dogs – clinical, endoscopic, histopathological and immunohistochemical findings. *Polish Journal of Veterinary Sciences* 20, 539–549.

Stanton, M.E., Bright, R.M., Toal, R., DeNovo, R.C., McCracken, M. and McLauren, J.B. (1987) Effects of the Y-U pyloroplasty on gastric emptying and duodenogastric reflux in the dog. *Veterinary Surgery* 16, 392–397.

Steelman-Szymeczek, S.M., Stebbins, M.E. and Hardie, E.M. (2003) Clinical evaluation of a right-sided prophylactic gastropexy via a grid approach. *Journal of the American Animal Hospital Association* 39, 397–402.

Stickle, R.L. (1989) Radiographic signs of isolated splenic torsion in dogs: eight cases (1980–1987) *Journal of the American Veterinary Medical Association* 194, 103–106.

Strombeck, D.R. (1978) Clinicopathologic features of primary and metastatic neoplastic disease of the liver in dogs. *Journal of the American Veterinary Medical Association* 173, 267–269.

Stuckey, J.A., Miller, W.W. and Almond, G.T. (2012) Use of a sclerosing agent (1% polidocanol) to treat an orbital mucocele in a dog. *Veterinary Ophthalmology* 15, 188–193.

Suh, H.J., Chung, D.J., Lee, A.J., Chung, H.J., Kim, D.H., Eom, K.D., Do, S.H., Kim, H.Y., Sullivan, M. and Yool, D.A. (1998) Gastric disease in the dog and cat. *Veterinary Journal* 156, 91–106.

Suh, H.J., Chung, D.J., Lee, A.J., Chung, H.J., Kim, D.H., Eom, K.D., Do, S.H., Kim, H.Y. (2015) Abnormal changes in both mandibular salivary glands in a dog: Non-mineral radiopaque sialoliths. *Canadian Veterinary Journal* 56, 1025–1028.

Sutton, J.S., Culp, W.T., Scotti, K., Seibert, R.L., Lux, C.N., Singh, A., Wormser, C., Runge, J.J., Schmiedt, C.W., Corrie, J., Philips, H., Selimic, L.E., Nucci, D.J., Mayhew, P.D. and Kass, P.H. (2016) Perioperative morbidity and outcome of esophageal surgery in dogs and cats: 72 cases (1993–2013). *Journal of the American Veterinary Medical Association* 249, 787–793.

Swann, H.M. and Holt, D.E. (2002) Canine gastric adenocarcinoma and leiomyosarcoma: a retrospective study of 21 cases (1986–1999) and literature review. *Journal of the American Animal Hospital Association* 38, 157–164.

Szabo, S.D., Jermyn, K., Neel, J. and Mathews, K.G. (2011) Evaluation of postceliotomy peritoneal drain fluid volume, cytology, and blood-to-peritoneal fluid lactate and glucose differences in normal dogs. *Veterinary Surgery* 40, 444–449.

Szatmári, V., Péntek, G. and Vörös, K. (2000) Spontaneous resolution of splenic torsion in a dog. *Veterinary Record* 147, 247–248.

Termote, S. (2003) Parotid salivary duct mucocoele and sialolithiasis following parotid duct transposition. *Journal of Small Animal Practice* 44, 21–23.

Terragni, R., Vignoli, M., Rossi, F. and Tassoni, M. (2006) Colorectal neoplasia in dogs and cats: experiences of a five year. *Veterinaria* 20, 19–25.

Tivers, M.S., Lipscomb, V.J., Smith, K.C., Wheeler-Jones, C.P. and House, A.K. (2014) Markers of hepatic regeneration associated with surgical attenuation of congenital portosystemic shunts in dogs. *Veterinary Journal* 200, 305–311.

Tivers, M.S., Lipscomb, V.J. and Brockman, D.J. (2017) Treatment of intra-hepatic congenital portosystemic shunts in dogs: a systematic review. *Journal of Small Animal Practice* 58, 485–494.

Tivers, M.S., Lipscomb, V.J., Bristow, P. and Brockman, D.J. (2018) Intra-hepatic congenital portosystemic shunts in dogs: short- and long-term outcome of suture attenuation. *Journal of Small Animal Practice* 59, 201–210.

Tobias, K.M. and Rohrbach, B.W. (2003) Association of breed with the diagnosis of congenital portosystemic shunts in dogs: 2,400 cases (1980–2002). *Journal of the American Veterinary Medical Association* 223, 1636–1639.

Tobin, R.L., Nelson, R.W., Lucroy, M.D., Wooldridge, J.D. and Feldman, E.C. (1999) Outcome of surgical versus medical treatment of dogs with beta cell neoplasia: 39 cases (1990–1997). *Journal of the American Veterinary Medical Association* 215, 226–230.

Tollefson, D.F., Wright, D.J., Reddy, D.J. and Kintanar, E.B. (1995) Intra-operative determination of intestinal viability by pulse oximetry. *Annals of Vascular Surgery* 9, 357–360.

Torad, F.A. and Hassan, E.A. (2013) Clinical and ultrasonographic characteristics of salivary mucoceles in 13 dogs. *Veterinary Radiology & Ultrasound* 54, 293–298.

Traverson, M., Lussier, B., Huneault, L. and Gatineau M. (2018) Comparative outcomes between ameroid ring constrictor and cellophane banding for treatment of single congenital extra-hepatic portosystemic shunts in 49 dogs (1998–2012). *Veterinary Surgery* 47, 179–187.

Trevail, T., Gunn-Moore, D., Carrera, I., Courcier, E. and Sullivan, M. (2011) Radiographic diameter of the colon in normal and constipated cats and in cats with megacolon. *Veterinary Radiology & Ultrasound* 52, 516–520.

Tsioli, V., Papazoglou, L.G., Basdani, E., Kosmas, P., Brellou, G., Poutahidis, T. and Bagias, S. (2013) Surgical management of recurrent cervical sialoceles in four dogs. *Journal of Small Animal Practice* 54, 331–333.

Turek, M.M. and Withrow, S.J. (2012) Perianal tumours. In: Withrow, S.J., Vail, D.M. and Page, R.L. (eds) *Withrow & MacEwen's Small Animal Clinical Oncology*. Elsevier Saunders, Philadelphia, Pennsylvania, pp. 424–430.

Tyrrell, D. and Beck, C. (2006) Survey of the use of radiography vs. ultrasonography in the investigation of gastrointestinal foreign bodies in small animals. *Veterinary Radiology & Ultrasound* 47, 404–408.

Ubbink, G.J., van de Broek, J., Meyer, H.P. and Rothuizen, J. (1998) Prediction of inherited portosystemic shunts in Irish Wolfhounds on the basis of pedigree analysis. *American Journal of Veterinary Research* 59, 1553–1556.

Ullman, S.L. (1994) Surgical stapling of the small intestine. *Veterinary Clinics of North America: Small Animal Practice* 24, 305-322.

Ullmann, B., Seehaus, N., Hungerbühler, S. and Meyer-Lindenberg, A. (2016) Gastric dilatation volvulus: a retrospective study of 203 dogs with ventral midline gastropexy. *Journal of Small Animal Practice* 57, 18–22.

Vallefuoco, R., Jardel, N.E., Mrini, M., Stambouli, F. and Cordonnier, N. (2011) Parotid salivary duct sialocele associated with glandular duct stenosis in a cat. *Journal of Feline Medicine and Surgery* 13, 781–783.

Valli, V.E., Jacobs, R.M. and Norris, A. (2000) The histological classification of 602 cases of feline lymphoproliferative disease using the National Cancer Institute working formulation. *Journal of Veterinary Diagnostic Investigation* 12, 295–306.

Van Duijkeren, E. (1995) Disease conditions of canine anal sacs. *Journal of Small Animal Practice* 36, 12–16.

Van Kruiningen, H.J., Gargamelli, C., Havier, J., Frueh, S., Jin, L. and Suib, S. (2013) Stomach gas analyses in canine acute gastric dilatation with volvulus. *Journal of Veterinary Internal Medicine* 27, 1260–1261.

Van Straten, G., Spee, B., Rothuizen, J., van Straten, M. and Favier, R.P. (2015) Diagnostic value of the rectal ammonia tolerance test, fasting plasma ammonia and fasting plasma bile acids for canine portosystemic shunting. *Veterinary Journal* 204, 282–286.

Verschoof, J., Moritz, A., Kramer, M. and Bauer, N. (2015) Hemostatic variables, plasma lactate concentration, and inflammatory biomarkers in dogs with gastric dilatation-volvulus. *Tieraerztliche Praxis Ausgabe K Kleintiere Heimtiere* 43, 389–398.

Vinayak, A., Frank, C.B., Gardiner, D.W., Thieman-Mankin K.M. and Worley, D.R. (2017) Malignant anal sac melanoma in dogs: eleven cases (2000–2015). *Journal of Small Animal Practice* 58, 231–237.

Von Bavo, V., Eberle, N., Mischke, R., Meyer-Lindenberg, A., Hewicker-Trautwein, M., Nolte, I. and Betz, D. (2012) Canine non-hematopoietic gastric neoplasia. Epidemiologic and diagnostic characteristics in 38 dogs with post-surgical outcome of five cases. *Journal of the American Animal Hospital Association* 40, 243–249.

Waldron, D.R. and Smith, M.M. (1991) Salivary mucoceles. *Problems in Veterinary Medicine* 3, 270–276.

Wallace, M.L., MacPhail, C.M. and Monnet, E. (2018) Incidence of postoperative neurologic complications in pugs following portosystemic shunt attenuation surgery. *Journal of the American Animal Hospital Association* 54, 46–49.

Walter, M.C. and Matthiesen, D.T. (1989) Gastric outflow surgical problems. *Problems in Veterinary Medicine* 1, 196–214.

Washabau, R.J. and Holt, D. (1999) Pathogenesis, diagnosis, and therapy of feline idiopathic megacolon. *Veterinary Clinics of North America: Small Animal Practice* 29, 589–603.

Washabau, R.J. and Stalis, I.S. (1996) Alterations in colonic smooth muscle function in cats with idiopathic megacolon. *American Journal of Veterinary Research* 57, 580–587.

Webb, C.B., McCord, K.W. and Twedt, D.C. (2007) Rectal strictures in 19 dogs: 1997–2005. *Journal of the American Animal Hospital Association* 43, 332–336.

Weidner, S., Probst, A. and Kneissl, S. (2012) MR anatomy of salivary glands in the dog. *Anatomia, Histologia, Embryologia* 41, 149–153.

Weisse, C. (2009) Hepatic chemoembolization: a novel regional therapy. *Veterinary Clinics of North America: Small Animal Practice* 39, 627–630.

Weisse, C., Clifford, C.A. and Holt, D. (2002) Percutaneous arterial embolization and chemoembolization for treatment of benign and malignant tumors in three dogs and a goat. *Journal of the American Veterinary Medical Association* 221, 1430–1436.

Weisse, C., Berent, A.C., Todd, K., Solomon, J.A. and Cope, C. (2014) Endovascular evaluation and treatment of intrahepatic portosystemic shunts in dogs: 100 cases (2001–2011). *Journal of the American Veterinary Medical Association* 244, 78–94.

Wendelburg, K.M., O'Toole, T.E., McCobb, E., Price, L.L., Lyons, J.A. and Berg, J. (2014) Risk factors for perioperative death in dogs undergoing splenectomy for splenic masses: 539 cases (2001–2012). *Journal of the American Veterinary Medical Association* 245, 1382–1390.

Wendelburg, K.M., Price, L.L., Burgess, K.E., Lyons, J.A., Lew, F.H. and Berg, J. (2015) Survival time of dogs with splenic hemangiosarcoma treated by splenectomy with or without adjuvant chemotherapy: 208 cases (2001–2012). *Journal of the American Veterinary Medical Association* 247, 393–403.

Westgarth, S., Singh, A. and Vince, A.R. (2013) Subclinical cecal impaction in a dog. *Canadian Veterinary Journal* 54, 171–173.

Willard, M.D. (2005) Digestive system. In: Nelson, R.W. and Couto, C.G. (eds) *Internal Diseases of Small Animals*. Galaktyka, Łódź, pp. 328–329.

Williams, J.M. (2012) Colon. In: Tobias, K.M. and Johnston, S.A. (eds) *Veterinary Surgery: Small Animal*. Elsevier Saunders, St. Louis, Missouri.

Winkler, J.T., Bohling, M.W. and Tillson, D.M. (2003) Portosystemic shunts: diagnosis, prognosis and treatment of 64 cases (1993–2001). *Journal of the American Animal Hospital Association* 39, 169–185.

Wouters, E.G., Buishand, F.O., Kik, M. and Kirpensteijn, J. (2011) Use of a bipolar vessel-sealing device in resection of canine insulinoma. *Journal of Small Animal Practice* 52, 139–145.

Wright, T., Singh, A., Mayhew, P.D., Runge, J.J., Brisson, B.A., Oblak, M.L. and Case, J.B. (2016) Laparoscopic-assisted splenectomy in dogs: 18 cases (2012–2014). *Journal of the American Veterinary Medical Association* 248, 916–922.

Wylie, K.B. and Hosgood, G. (1994) Mortality and morbidity of small and large intestinal surgery in dogs and cats: 74 cases (1980–1992). *Journal of the American Animal Hospital Association* 30, 85-90.

Yanoff, S.R. and Willard, M.D. (1989) Short bowel syndrome in dogs and cats. *Seminars in Veterinary Medicine and Surgery (Small Animal)* 4, 226.

Yas, E., Kelmer, G., Shipov, A., Ben-Oz, J. and Seveg, G. (2013) Successful transendoscopic oesophageal mass ablation in two dogs with *Spirocerca lupi* associated oesophageal sarcoma. *Journal of Small Animal Practice* 54, 495–498.

Yoon, H.Y., Min, B.S., Kim, S.Y., Lee, D.E. and Kim, J.H. (2017) Surgical management of parotid salivary duct rupture secondary to non-iatrogenic trauma in a dog. *Journal of Veterinary Medical Science* 79, 82–85.

Zacher, L.A., Berg, J., Shaw, S.P. and Kudej, R.K. (2010) Association between outcome and changes in plasma lactate concentration during presurgical treatment in dogs with gastric dilatation-volvulus: 64 cases (2002–2008), *Journal of the American Veterinary Medical Association* 236, 892–897.

Zacuto, A.C., Marks, S.L., Osborn, J., Douthitt, K.L., Hollingshead, K.L., Hayashi, K., Kapatkin, A.S., Pypendop, B.H. and Belafsky, P.C. (2012) The influence of esomeprazole and cisapride on gastrooesophageal reflux during anesthesia in dogs. *Journal of Veterinary Internal Medicine* 26, 518–525.

Zatelli, A., Bonfanti, U., Zini, E., D'Ippolito, P. and Bussadori, C. (2005) Percutaneous drainage and alcoholization of hepatic abscesses in five dogs and a cat. *Journal of the American Animal Hospital Association 41*, 34–38.

Zimmer, J.F. (1981) Removal of gastric foreign bodies using flexible fiberoptic endoscopy. *Seminars in Veterinary Medicine and Surgery (Small Animal)* 76, 1611–1619.

Zwingenberger, A.L., Daniel, L., Steffey, M.A., Mayhew, P.D., Mayhew, K.N., Culp, W.T. and Hunt, G.B. (2014) Correlation between liver volume, portal vascular anatomy, and hepatic perfusion in dogs with congenital portosystemic shunt before and after placement of ameroid constrictors. *Veterinary Surgery* 43, 926–934.

Case 3.1

A 10-year-old male neutered Border collie is presented as an emergency for assessment of collapse. No history of trauma is reported.

On presentation, the animal is responsive but collapsed. Major body systems assessment shows:

- Mucous membranes are pale.
- Capillary refill time is more than 2 seconds.
- Heart rate and pulse rate are synchronous; tachycardia (180 bpm); pulse quality is poor; no cardiac arrhythmias or murmurs are detected.
- Heart sounds not muffled.
- Respiratory rate is 40 pm and lung sounds are normal bilaterally.
- The abdomen is dilated with a fluid thrill.

Problem list

- collapse
- pale mucous membranes
- prolonged capillary refill time
- tachycardia
- poor pulse quality
- distended abdomen with fluid thrill
- signs of hypovolaemic shock.

Plan

- Emergency blood panel: PCV/TS, urea, creatinine, electrolyes, coagulation panel, blood typing.
- Cardiovascular stabilisation, including fluid boluses of crystalloids (15–20 ml/kg over 15 minutes initially and reassess clinical examination and monitor blood pressure; shock doses of crystalloids are up to 60–90 ml/kg; consider colloids if required), oxygenation.
- Aim for a minimal mean arterial blood pressure of 60 mmHg or a minimal systolic blood pressure of 100 mmHg.
- Appropriate analgesia (opioids would be suitable, e.g. pethidine IM; methadone IV).
- Short abdominal ultrasound.
- Abdominocentesis and fluid analysis.

Investigation

- Emergency blood panel showed a PCV of 35% (range, 35–55%) and total protein (TP) of 4.0 g/dl (range, 5.2–7.8 g/dl). Coagulation times (prothrombin and partial thromboplastin) were normal.
- IV fluid resuscitation was initiated with two boluses of Hartmann's over 15 minutes (20 ml/kg), following which heart rate was 120 bpm and the pulse quality improved.
- Oxygen 'flow by' was provided.
- Analgesia was provided with methadone 0.2 mg/kg, IV.
- Abdominal ultrasound revealed a large volume of abdominal fluid; abdominocentesis revealed a haemorrhagic effusion with a PCV of 32% and TP of 2.6 g/dl. A recheck revealed peripheral blood PCV of 20% and TP of 2.2 g/dl.
- Transfusion of a unit of packed red blood cells was initiated and crystalloids continued at a rate of 15 ml/kg.

Surgery

The animal was anaesthetised and ventilated. A ventral midline coeliotomy was performed and a haemoabdomen was confirmed. The free blood was suctioned (Fig. 3.73) (and measured) and the spleen was exteriorised (Fig. 3.74). Several splenic nodules were identified, one of which was actively bleeding. The splenic vasculature was clamped to control the haemorrhage and a splenectomy was performed by double-ligating each vessel with 2.0 metric polyglecaprone-25. The abdominal cavity was lavaged and no further abnormalities were found on exploration. An incisional liver biopsy was performed. The abdominal cavity was routinely closed in three layers using 3.5 metric polydioxanone in the linea alba, 3.0 metric polyglecaprone-25 in the subcutaneous layer and 2.0 metric polyglecaprone-25 in the subcuticular layer. Perioperative antibiotics were not provided.

Postoperative care

- A recheck at recovery revealed peripheral blood PCV of 22% and TP of 3.2 g/dl.
- Pain scores and multimodal analgesia (systemic opioids and paracetamol) were provided.
- Vital parameters and blood pressure were monitored every 4 hours for the first 48 hours.
- Intravenous crystalloids were provided (2–4 ml/kg/h) as required according to clinical examination and blood pressure, until the animal was eating.
- Antibiotics were not provided postoperatively.
- The patient recovered uneventfully from his anaesthetic and started eating 24 hours postoperatively.
- He continued to improve and was discharged from the hospital 72 hours postoperatively.
- Histopathological evaluation of the liver biopsy revealed a splenic haemangiosarcoma with hepatic metastasis.
- Retrospective staging and chemotherapy was offered to the client, but were declined.

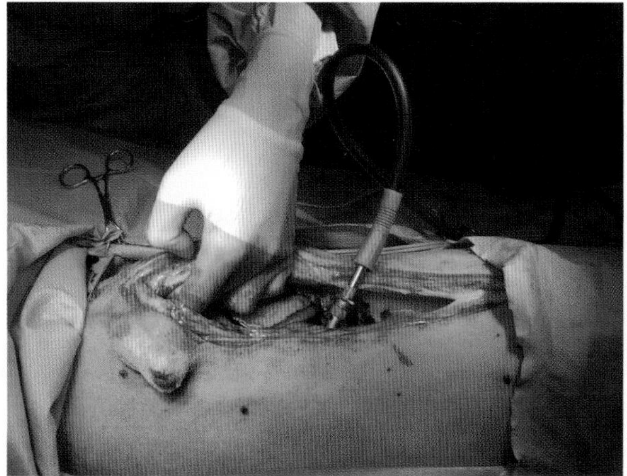

Fig. 3.73 Ventral midline coeliotomy confirming the presence of haemoabdomen. The free peritoneal blood is being suctioned to facilitate exploration. (Image courtesy of Jon Hall.)

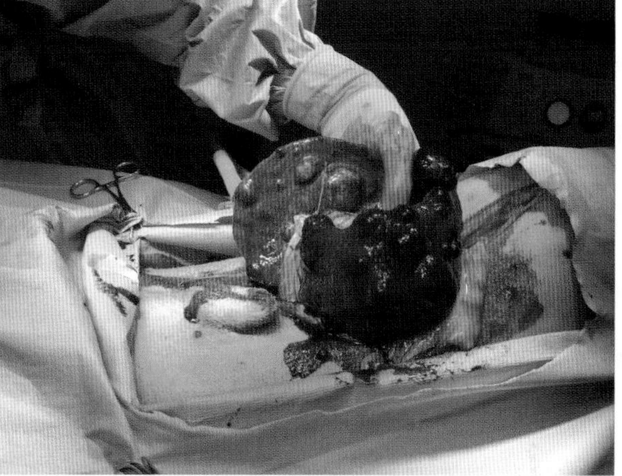

Fig. 3.74 The spleen is exteriorised revealing the presence of several nodular lesions, one of which was actively haemorrhaging. (Image courtesy of Jon Hall.)

Case 3.2

A 2-year-old female neutered Labrador retriever is presented with a history of intermittent vomiting and inappetance of 2 days' duration.

On presentation, the animal is quiet but alert and responsive. Major body systems assessment shows:

- Mucous membranes are pink.
- Capillary refill time is less than 2 seconds.
- Heart rate and pulse rate are synchronous; tachycardia (160 bpm); pulse quality is good; no cardiac arrhythmias or murmurs are detected.
- Respiratory rate is 40 pm and lung sounds are normal bilaterally.
- The abdomen is painful on palpation.

Problem list

- vomiting
- inappetence
- tachycardia
- painful abdomen.

Plan

- Survey blood panel: PCV/TS, urea, creatinine, electrolytes, blood gas analysis.
- Determine source of tachycardia and pain/dehydration, start fluid therapy and provide analgesia accordingly (opioids would be suitable, e.g. pethidine IM; methadone IV).
- Survey abdominal radiographs ± abdominal ultrasound.

Investigation

- Survey blood panel showed a PCV of 36% (range, 35–55%) and total protein (TP) of 7.8 g/dl (range, 5.2–7.8 g/dl). Blood gas analysis showed a mild metabolic acidosis.
- IV fluids were initiated with a bolus of Hartmann's over 15 minutes (10 ml/kg), following which heart rate was 100 bpm.
- Analgesia was provided with IV methadone at 0.2 mg/kg.
- Maropitant (1 mg/kg) was given IV.
- Lateral and ventrodorsal abdominal radiographs showed the presence of a radiopaque intestinal foreign body (Fig. 3.75a,b).

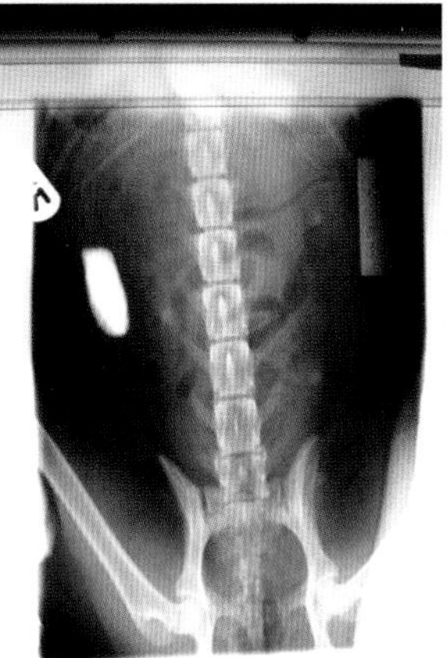

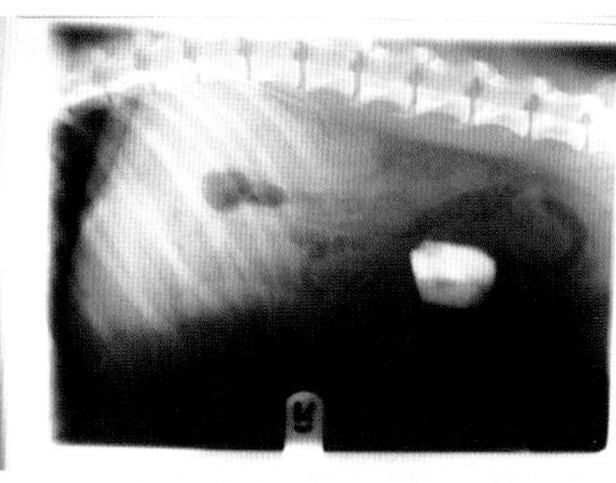

Fig. 3.75a,b Lateral and ventrodorsal abdominal radiographs showing a radiopaque intestinal foreign body. (Images courtesy of Jon Hall.)

Surgery

The animal was anaesthetised and ventilated. A ventral midline exploratory coeliotomy was performed, confirming a jejunal foreign body (stone; Fig. 3.76). The intestinal contents were milked away from the affected intestinal area and non-crushing forceps were applied proximal and distal to the foreign body. An enterotomy distal to the foreign body was performed and closed with a continuous suture pattern using 1.5 metric polydioxanone. The suture line was leak-tested and omentalised. The abdominal cavity was routinely lavaged and closed in three layers, using 3.5 metric polydioxanone in the linea alba, 3.0 metric polyglecaprone-25 in the subcutaneous layer and 2.0 metric polyglecaprone-25 in the subcuticular layer. Perioperative antibiotics were provided with cefuroxime 20 mg/kg at induction and repeated every 2 hours.

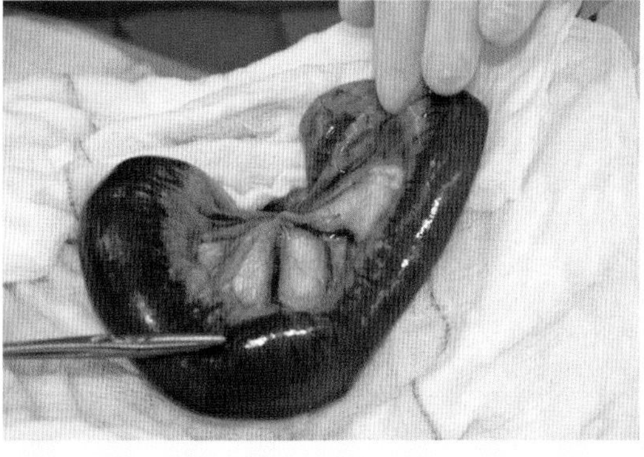

Fig. 3.76 Jejunal foreign body (stone). (Image courtesy of Jon Hall.)

Postoperative care

- Pain scores and multimodal analgesia (systemic opioids, paracetamol and maropitant) were provided.
- Intravenous crystalloids were provided at a maintenance rate (2 ml/kg/h) until the animal was eating.
- Antibiotics were not provided postoperatively.
- The patient recovered uneventfully from her anaesthetic and started eating small amounts of food 24 hours postoperatively.
- She continued to improve and was discharged from the hospital 48 hours postoperatively.
- No postoperative complications were encountered.

Surgery of the urinary tract

4

Anna Nutt and Guillaume Chanoit

Chapter summary

4.1 Renal and ureteral surgical diseases

Surgical treatment of renal disease is usually limited to the management of neoplasia, traumatic injury, obstruction and obtainment of biopsies. Renal transplantation is not available in the UK but is available elsewhere. Surgery of the ureter is usually performed for the treatment of obstruction and ectopic ureter. Thorough preoperative investigation is essential, as patients with renal disease are often high-risk anaesthetic and surgical candidates due to the importance of the kidneys in the removal of waste products, and in the maintenance of blood pressure and normal fluid balance. Such investigations should include a complete blood count, serum biochemistry, coagulation panel, urinalysis, urine culture and blood pressure (BP) measurement. Abnormalities seen may include azotaemia, dehydration and acid–base imbalance. Hyperkalaemia is often seen due to urinary obstruction, uroabdomen or parenchymal dysfunction, whereas hypokalaemia can be present in chronic kidney disease and diuretic therapy. Both can predispose to cardiac abnormalities. The risk of haemorrhage is increased in patients with azotaemia, hypertension (systemic BP >180 mmHg) or thrombocytopenia (Bigge et al., 2001; Vaden et al., 2005a). Renal imaging provides information regarding kidney structure, and can help identify the presence of calculi or primary/metastatic neoplasia. Whilst radiography is useful for determining kidney size and shape, ultrasonography and more advanced imaging (CT/MRI) allow a more detailed assessment of the renal structure. Use of contrast agent during intravenous urography (IVU) provides further detail of the renal vasculature and excretion of urine via the collecting ducts, renal pelvis, ureters, bladder and urethra. Pyelography (injection of contrast directly into the renal pelvis) is sometimes used when there is concern about giving a systemic dose of contrast, or when the renal artery is obstructed. Contrast computed tomography (CT) is thought to be superior to IVU in distinguishing renal vasculature and identifying renal cysts (Bouma et al., 2003; Reichle et al., 2002). Thoracic radiography or CT should be performed in any animal suspected of neoplasia.

4.1.1 Surgical anatomy

The kidneys lie within the retroperitoneal space in the dorsal abdomen, lateral to the aorta and vena cava. The right kidney lies adjacent to the first three lumbar vertebrae and its cranial pole is covered by the caudate process of the caudate liver lobe. The left kidney lies further caudally between the second and fourth lumbar vertebrae. The renal pelvis receives urine from the collecting ducts and directs it to the ureter, which is found medially at the renal hilus and travels caudally to the bladder where it enters on the dorsal surface via a slit-like orifice. The renal vein and renal artery are also found at the renal hilus. The renal vein lies more ventrally and the renal artery more dorsally. Multiple renal arteries (more often on the left side) are reported

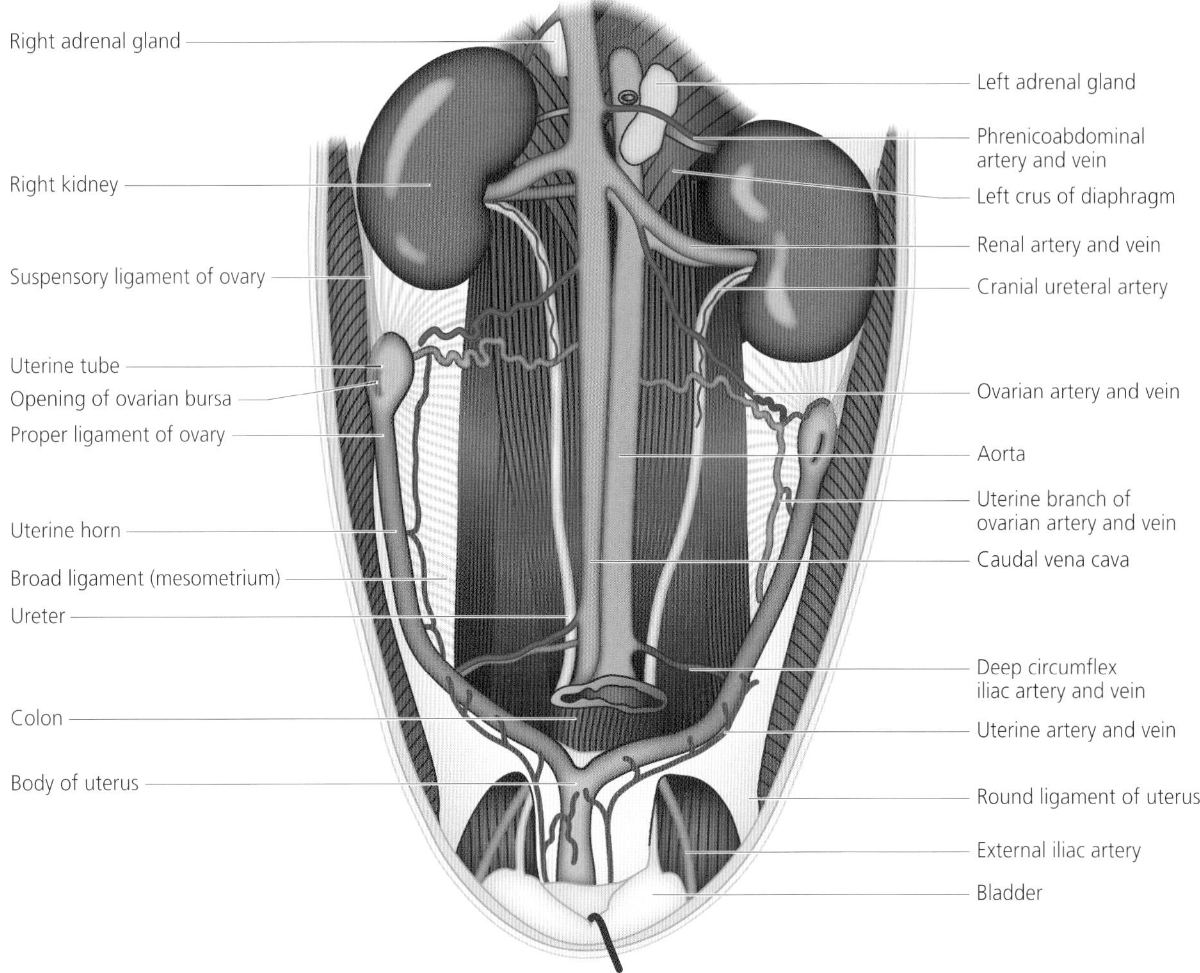

Fig. 4.1 Anatomy of the urogenital system. *Illustrator: Elaine Leggett*

in 13% of canine kidneys and in 10% of feline kidneys (Rawlings et al., 2003a). The kidneys are surrounded by a substantial amount of fat, and the renal parenchyma is covered by a thin fibrous capsule that is readily torn. Both parenchyma and capsule bleed easily when punctured (Fig. 4.1).

4.1.2 Specific diseases

Renal neoplasia

Key points

- Lymphoma is the most common renal neoplasia in the cat.
- In decreasing order of frequency, tumours seen in the dog are carcinomas such as renal tubular carcinoma (85% of all primary renal tumours), sarcomas, lymphomas and nephroblastomas.
- Due to the high rate of bilateral primary renal neoplasia (4–32%), it is important to assess both kidneys.
- Nephrectomy is the most common treatment for unilateral primary renal neoplasia

Types

Primary renal neoplasia is uncommon in the dog and cat, and is most often malignant (Fig. 4.2a,b). Most tumours affect adult dogs with a mean age of 8 years (with the exception of nephroblastomas, which occur in young to middle-aged dogs, and affect males more frequently than females (ratio 1.6:1.0) (Bryan et al., 2006). Lymphoma is the most common renal neoplasia in the cat, and can be primary or secondary to alimentary lymphoma. It is important to obtain a fine needle aspiration biopsy of the kidney in a cat suspected of having renal neoplasia, as chemotherapy is the first-line treatment for lymphoma, not surgery. Ureteral neoplasia is very uncommon, with only 17 cases reported in the literature. Eight of these were benign fibroepithelial polyps, and the remainder were leiomyomas, various sarcomas and transitional cell carcinomas (Mathews, 2017).

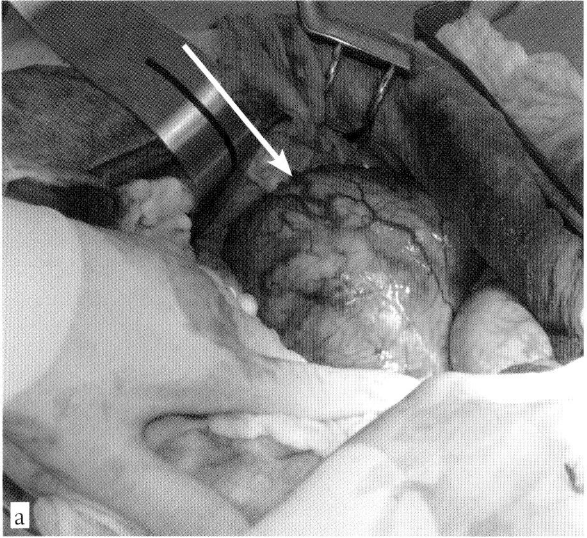

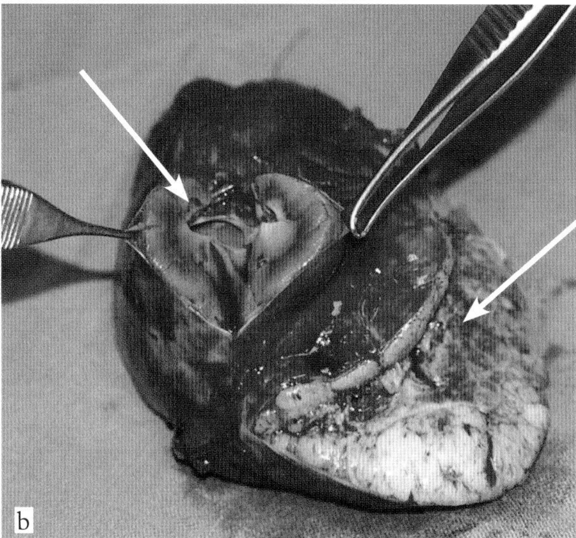

Fig. 4.2a,b a. Renal mass (carcinoma, black arrow) in a dog. The normal renal anatomy is not recognised. b. Renal nephroblastoma in a cat. Normal renal architecture (black arrow) is recognised within the distorted renal capsule and neoplastic tissue (black arrowhead).

Diagnosis

Often the history is vague and non-specific, and includes haematuria, lethargy, inappetence and weight loss. An abdominal mass may be found on abdominal palpation. It is important to assess both kidneys, as bilateral involvement is reported in 4–32% of dogs with primary renal neoplasia.

Clinicopathological findings include anaemia or neutrophilia (seen commonly). Serum biochemistry findings are often non-specific and mild, and azotaemia is not always present. Findings on urinalysis are more common, with haematuria, pyuria and proteinuria seen in approximately 50% of the cases (Bryan et al., 2006).

Diagnostic imaging should include abdominal and thoracic radiography or CT (the latter is useful for assessment of potential vascular involvement), and abdominal ultrasound. Staging is important as renal tumours are reported to metastasise to the lungs in 16–48% of dogs with primary renal tumours (Bryan et al., 2006).

Treatment

Nephrectomy is the most common treatment for unilateral primary renal neoplasia when there is no evidence of metastases. Median survival times for carcinomas, sarcomas and nephroblastomas are reported to be 16, 9 and 6 months, respectively. If nephrectomy is performed before metastasis, long-term survival is possible (Bryan et al., 2006). Nephrectomy is usually curative with benign neoplasia.

Nephrectomy: indications

Indications for complete nephrectomy (more correctly termed uretero-nephrectomy, as the ureter is also removed) include neoplasia, irreparable trauma, pyelonephritis resistant to medical therapy, essential/idiopathic renal haematuria (if sclerotherapy is not available), vascular avulsion (surprisingly, traumatic vascular avulsion does not usually result in fatal bleeding) and hydronephrosis complicated with infection, abdominal pain or ureteral malformation beyond repair. Ideally, renal function of the opposite kidney should be assessed prior to nephrectomy by measurement of glomerular filtration rate, either through administration of an exogenous marker or by nuclear scintigraphy. A complete uretero-nephrectomy includes resection of the kidney and the attached ureter at the level of the uretero-vesicular junction. The ureter should not be left attached to the bladder, as this could predispose the patient to developing urinary tract infection.

Step by step: nephrectomy

- The standard approach is made through a ventral midline incision. The incision should extend from the xiphoid to the pubis in cases of neoplasia, as the whole abdomen should be examined for metastases.
- The area of the left and right kidneys is exposed after a colonic or duodenal manoeuvre is performed. Both kidneys should be visualised to confirm their presence, and to ensure that the one to remain looks grossly normal.
- The affected kidney is detached from its peritoneal attachments using a combination of sharp and blunt dissection and then rotated medially to expose the renal artery (dorsal) and vein (ventral). Separation of the perirenal fat is required for full visualisation of the

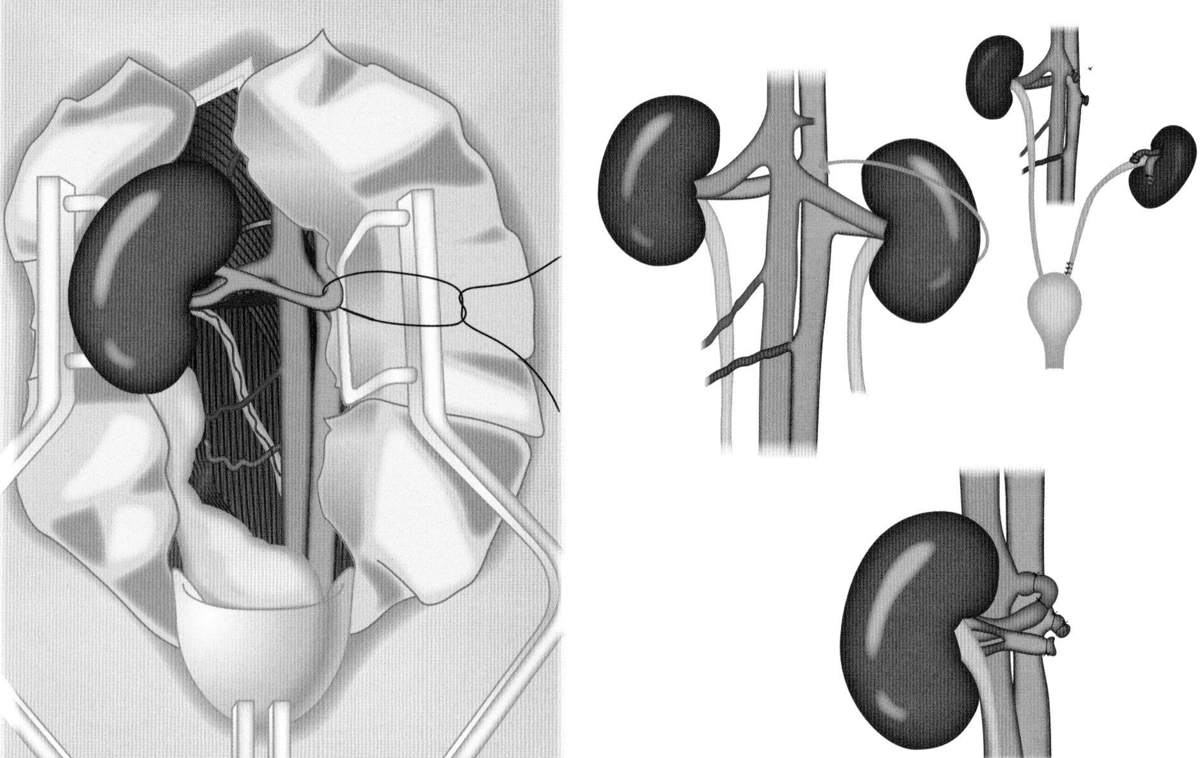

Fig. 4.3 Uretero-nephrectomy. The renal vessels are isolated and ligated; resection of the ureter is performed at the level of the bladder neck. *Illustrator: Elaine Leggett*

vessels at the hilus. This can be accomplished easily using a dry swab.

- The vessels are ligated close to their attachment to the aorta and vena cava, to ensure that all branches have been ligated (Fig 4.3). However, if surgery is performed on an entire dog, it is important to identify the testicular or ovarian vein which drain into the left renal vein, and instead ligate the renal vein distal to the opening of the gonadal vein.
- Ligation is usually performed with a long-lasting absorbable suture such as polydioxanone (PDS) or polyglyconate (Maxon), or a non-absorbable material such as nylon or polypropylene.
- Two ligatures should be placed on the portion of vessel to remain (either two circumferential or one circumferential and one transfixing), or a vascular clip may be used alongside one circumferential ligature. A ligature or haemostat placed on the portion of vessel to be removed will prevent backflow.
- Once the vessels have been ligated and transected, the kidney is freed of any remaining attachments and the renal fossa is inspected for haemorrhage.
- The ureter is then readily dissected from its retroperitoneal position, ligated close to its entrance to the bladder (but externally to the bladder) and is transected, leaving as little ureter remaining as possible.

Partial nephrectomy: indications

There are few indications for partial nephrectomy: very well-circumscribed renal masses (including abscesses), localised infarcts or resection and repair following substantial renal damage. Because significant haemorrhage can occur following this procedure, it is important to ensure absolute haemostasis following resection. Biomechanical studies have shown that horizontal mattress sutures provide the greatest resistance to urine leakage/haemorrhage (Simon et al., 2010). The approach is as described for nephrectomy, and the vascular pedicle is temporarily occluded using a Rumel tourniquet or vascular clamp (Satinsky). The renal capsule is peeled back, if possible, to expose the parenchyma, and horizontal mattress sutures are then pre-placed in an overlapping fashion proximal to the portion to be removed. The sutures are then tightened, the affected area resected and the sutures tied. The capsule is then re-apposed over the resected parenchyma if possible (Fig. 4.4a–d).

Renal biopsy

Renal biopsies are performed for diagnostic purposes and are indicated to evaluate causes of haematuria, proteinuria or acute renal failure, or when a primary renal disease is suspected. Contraindications include uncontrolled coagulopathy or hypertension, severe pyelonephritis, renal cysts or abscesses and severe

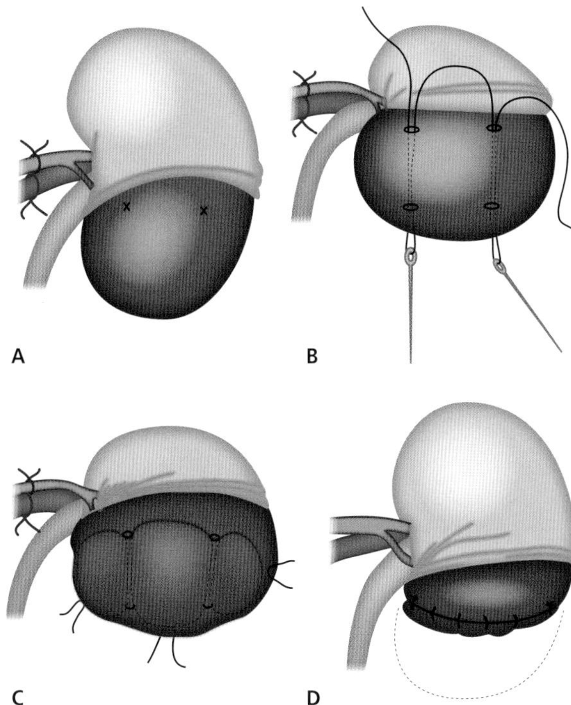

Fig. 4.4a–d Partial nephrectomy. a. Proposed resection sites (crosses). A partial nephrectomy is only possible if the lesion does not extend beyond the renal hilus. b. The sutures are placed (mattress pattern). c. Sutures are tied. Care is taken not to damage the renal hilus. d. If possible, the capsule is sutured to provide better haemostasis on the cut surface of the kidney. It is advisable to perform the entire procedure under inflow occlusion (renal vessels are isolated and temporarily occluded). *Illustrator: Elaine Leggett*

hydronephrosis. Biopsies can be performed percutaneously, laparoscopically or surgically. Surgical biopsies are taken either by biopsy needles/guns, manual devices (such as Tru-Cut) or wedge resection. Percutaneous samples should be taken under ultrasound guidance, and spring-loaded biopsy instruments are the preferred collection tool as these are easier to control and samples are more likely to be of good quality. Deep penetration into the medulla should be avoided, due to the risk of puncture of large blood vessels and the requirement for harvesting glomeruli (which lie within the cortex). Use of a 16- or 18-gauge needle may reduce the risk of medullary penetration (Vaden et al., 2005b). For surgical wedge biopsies, the approach to the kidney is as described previously and the renal vessels are temporarily occluded. Haemostasis following biopsy is critical.

Step by step: renal biopsy

- A no. 11 or 15 scalpel blade is used to make a 5–10 mm-long and 5 mm-deep incision, and a second is made at right angles to the first to remove a wedge of parenchyma.
- Digital pressure should be applied to control haemorrhage – haemostatic sponges can be used to help promote blood clot formation.
- For closure, wide, simple interrupted sutures using 3.0 or 4.0 monofilament absorbable material are placed across the defect to include the capsule and parenchyma (Fig. 4.5a–c).

Handy hints

Care should be taken not to pull the suture upwards, as this will result in tearing through the tissues thus increasing the risk of haemorrhage.

Complications of renal biopsy are reported in up to 21.7% of animals, with haemorrhage being the most common. However, the mortality rate is very rare after renal biopsy (Vaden et al., 2005a).

Renal and ureteral calculi

Key points

- Struvite and calcium oxalate are the most common types of uroliths in the dog, whilst calcium oxalate accounts for the majority of uroliths in the cat.
- Clinical signs may be absent, or they may be typical of a urinary tract infection.
- The presence of renal and ureteral calculi is not necessarily an indication for intervention.
- Surgical options include nephrotomy/pyelolithotomy/ureterotomy, double-pigtail ureteral stent placement, ureteral resection with re-implantation and the more recently reported subcutaneous ureteral bypass (SUB).

Urolithiasis is considered a common cause of lower urinary tract disease in the dog and cat, with incidence rates believed to be between 0.2 and 3% (Bartges et al., 2004). Nephrolithiasis and ureterolithiasis are uncommon forms, comprising less than 5% of canine uroliths (Osborne et al., 2008), though the incidence of feline upper urinary tract uroliths has increased tenfold in recent years (Ross et al., 2007). Struvite (magnesium ammonium phosphate) and calcium oxalate are the most common types in the dog, whilst calcium oxalate accounts for the majority in the cat. Calculi may occur unilaterally or bilaterally, and cystic calculi may be also be found in up to half of dogs (Ling et al., 1998). Concurrent cystic calculi are found much less commonly in cats with ureteroliths (<10%; Kyles et al., 2005).

Diagnosis

Clinical signs may be absent (e.g. with unilateral obstruction where contralateral renal function is normal or

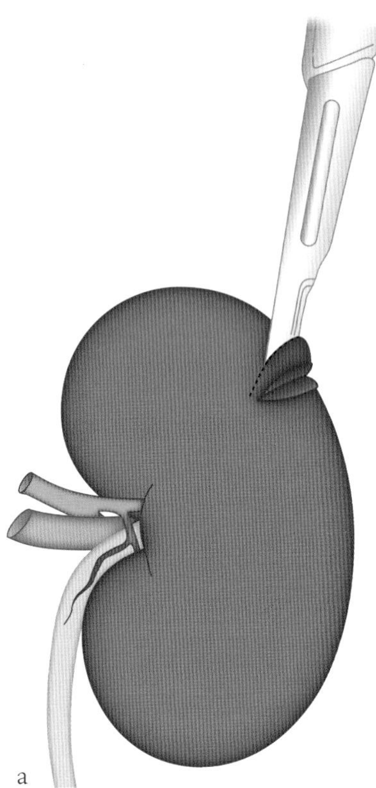

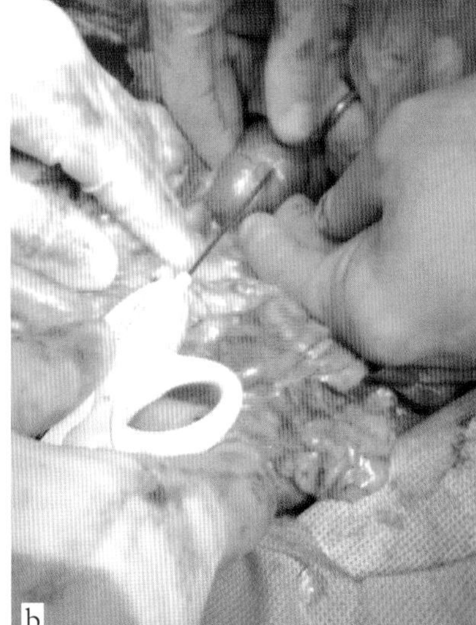

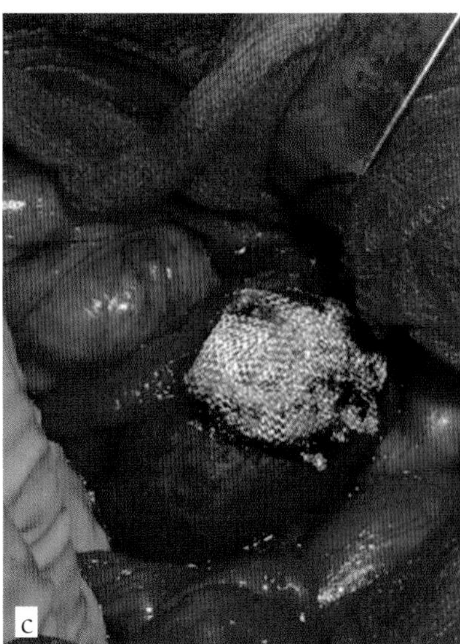

Fig. 4.5a–c Renal biopsy. a. Renal wedge biopsy. b. Open renal Tru-Cut biopsy. Although bleeding is minimised using this technique, the collected samples are smaller compared to those taken using the wedge biopsy technique. c. Renal biopsy site. Haemostasis is achieved by using a combination of sutures and haemostatic agents. *Illustrator: Elaine Leggett*

not sufficiently severe to cause uraemia), or they may be typical of a urinary tract infection (stranguria, pollakiuria, haematuria) or chronic kidney disease / acute kidney injury (lethargy, anorexia, vomiting, polydipsia / polyuria). Other findings may include non-specific abdominal pain, renomegaly or signs relating to an underlying condition (e.g. encephalopathy in animals with aportosystemic shunt). A complete blood count, serum biochemistry, urinalysis and urine culture should be performed. Abnormalities on blood work may only be present if there is bilateral renal disease / obstruction, pyelonephritis or an underlying condition. Findings on urinalysis may include haematuria, pyuria, bacteriuria and / or crystalluria. Radiography is useful for diagnosis, as most renal and ureteral calculi are radio-opaque (Fig. 4.6a,b). However, all types of uroliths can be seen on ultrasound and both diagnostics (radiography and ultrasonography) are recommended. Because the majority of cats with ureteral calculi have ureteral obstruction, dilation of the ureter and / or renal pelvis is detectable on ultrasonography. CT or percutaneous antegrade pyelography may also be useful (Adin et al., 2003).

Treatment

Renal and ureteral calculi may be incidental radiographic or ultrasonographic findings, and their presence is not necessarily an indication for intervention. One study concluded that medical management was reasonable in cats with mild to moderate renal disease and non-obstructive renal calculi, since there was no association between the presence of these calculi and progression of renal disease or mortality rate (Ross et al., 2007). Advanced treatment is, however, recommended when calculi are causing obstruction, or when there is severe haematuria or persistent urinary tract infection resistant to medical therapy. Non-surgical options include the administration of ureteral relaxants such as glucagon or amitriptyline. However, the latter drugs show inconsistent results and are not generally recommended (Forman et al., 2004). Lithotripsy can be used successfully in dogs to fragment ureteroliths to a size that will pass into the bladder. However, the small diameter of the ureter precludes the use of lithotripsy in cats. Surgery may be considered once the animal has been stabilised and it has been determined that diuresis has failed to move the calculus. Surgical options include nephrotomy / pyelolithotomy / ureterotomy, double-pigtail ureteral stent placement, ureteral resection with re-implantation or the more recently reported SUB. Ureteral stent placement, ureteral resection with re-implantation and SUB placement require specialist equipment, and referral is recommended. Placement of a locking-loop pigtail nephrostomy tube prior to the definitive intervention can be considered in cases with severe azotaemia. Prognosis is dependent on the underlying cause of the uroliths and whether recurrence can be prevented (i.e. resolution of infection, dissolution diet), the procedure performed, the degree and

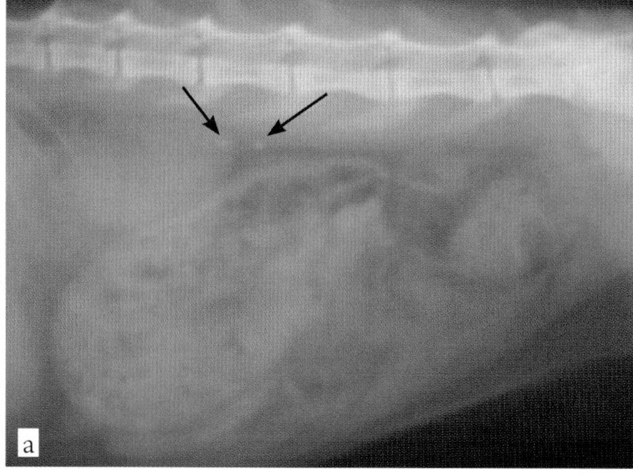

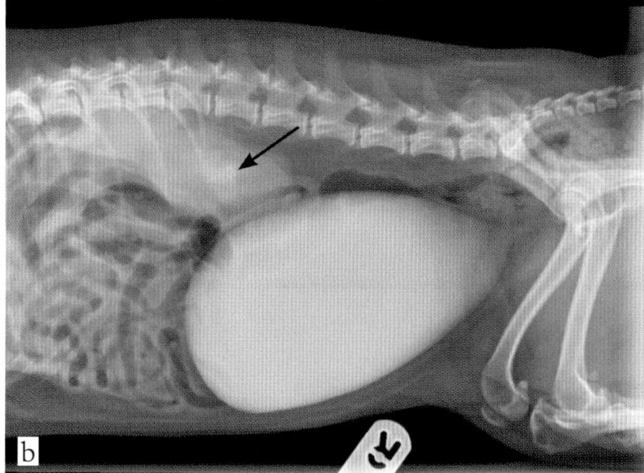

Fig. 4.6a,b Radiographs of uroliths. a. Calcium oxalate stones present in the feline ureter (black arrows). b. Urate stone present in the renal pelvis of a dog with portosystemic shunt (black arrow). (Image courtesy of Hervé Brissot.)

duration of the obstruction and the functionality of the contralateral kidney.

Nephrotomy: indications

Indications for nephrotomy include exploration of the renal pelvis (e.g. for masses or to identify causes of renal haematuria) and retrieval of obstructive calculi. Nephrotomy does not modify glomerular filtration rate and therefore the effects of this procedure on renal function are usually considered minimal (Stone et al., 2002). However, the effects of nephrotomy on renal function are known only in the normal dog and cat and therefore extrapolation of these data to dogs or cats with potential kidney disease is difficult. It is recommended to perform a staged procedure if a bilateral intervention is necessary.

Step by step: nephrotomy

- The renal vessels are isolated and occluded temporarily with vascular clamps, a tourniquet or finger pressure. Safe warm ischaemia time is relatively long (20 minutes) but should be reduced to the minimum time necessary.
- Access into the renal pelvis is achieved by either:
  - Bisection approach: the kidney is incised on its convex surface and parenchyma is bluntly dissected towards the pelvis.
  - Intersegmental approach: a scalpel handle is used to bluntly dissect the renal parenchyma, and the blood vessels are identified and ligated prior to transection. This reduces haemorrhage and parenchymal damage, though glomerular filtration rate studies have found no advantage over the bisection technique (Stone and Barsanti, 1992).
- Once access is gained, the renal pelvis is gently explored using right-angled forceps and the recesses can be flushed using a syringe and small red rubber catheter.
- The patency of the ureter should be assessed by passing a rubber urinary catheter and flushing the ureter normograde.
- Blood flow is restored when closure begins.
- Digital pressure is applied to appose the cut surfaces of the kidney for 1–5 minutes to allow a fibrin seal to form, and then the renal capsule is apposed using a continuous (preferred) or horizontal mattress pattern. Sutures can enter the cortex superficially, but should not penetrate deep into the cortex to avoid excessive tissue damage. The use of pledgeted sutures can be useful as tissues are quite friable.
- Once closure and haemostasis are complete, the renal fossa is lavaged and the kidney replaced.
- Nephropexy (renal capsule to perirenal fat and body wall) is recommended if the kidney is freely movable, to minimise the risk of renal torsion (Fig. 4.7a–e).

Pyelolithotomy

This can be performed to remove calculi if the proximal ureter and renal pelvis are significantly dilated, and avoids the parenchymal damage associated with nephrotomy. However, the procedure carries a high risk of postoperative leakage from the surgery site.

Ureterotomy

Ureterotomy can be performed if obstructive calculi are present, though there is a high risk of urine leakage and postoperative stricture. The incision is made longitudinally over the calculus/obstruction. Closure can be performed longitudinally or, if stricture seems likely, transversally, using 7-0 (large dog) to 10-0 (small cat) absorbable suture material in a simple interrupted fashion. Use of an operating microscope or wearing of loupes for magnification is highly recommended (Fig. 4.8).

Ureteral stent

Ureteral stents are double-pigtail indwelling catheters that allow urine to flow from the kidney (renal pelvis)

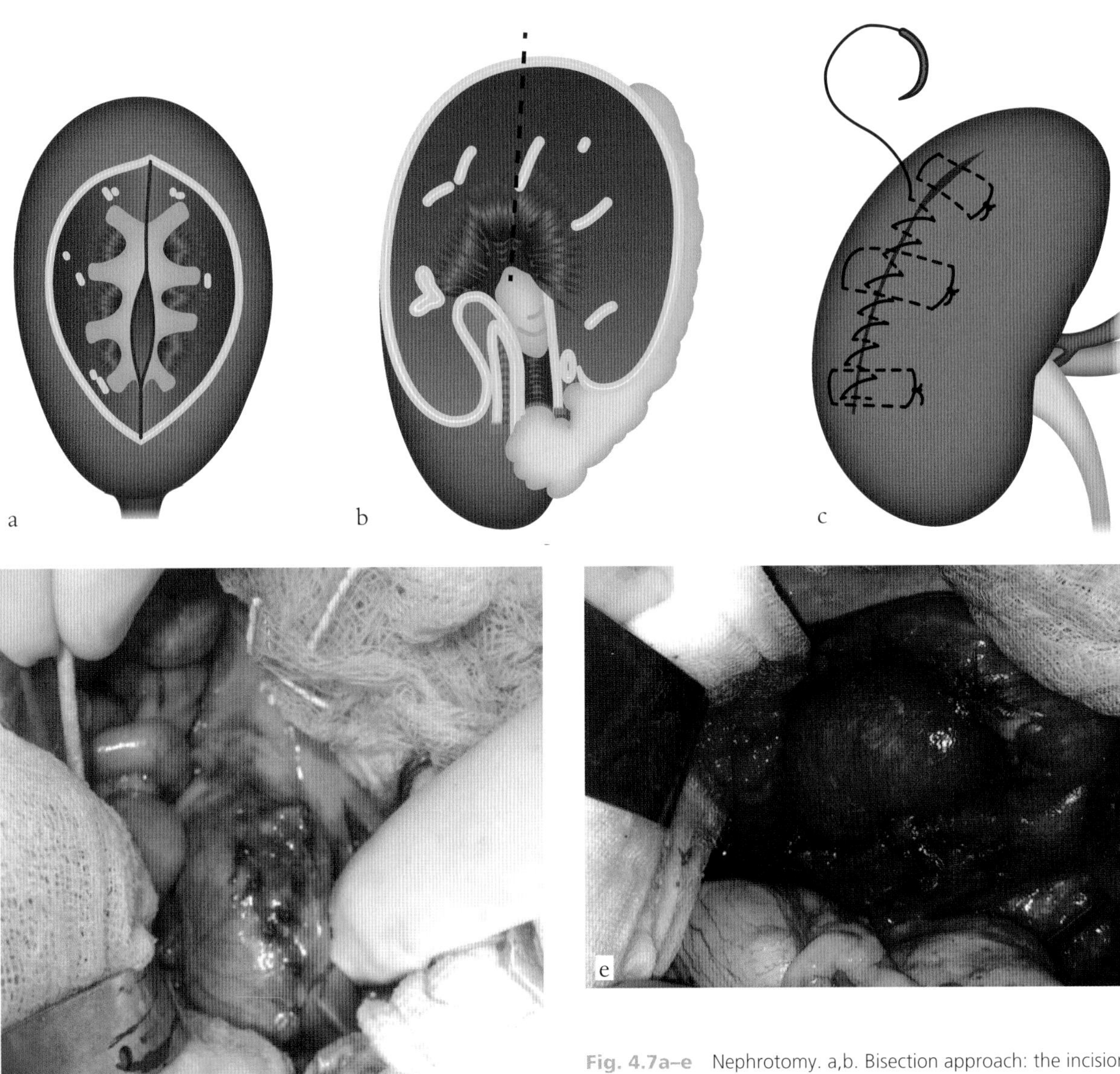

Fig. 4.7a–e Nephrotomy. a,b. Bisection approach: the incision is made on the convex aspect of the kidney after temporary occlusion of the renal vessels. c. Suturing of the capsule using a combination of mattress sutures and simple continuous sutures. d. Closure of nephrotomy using simple interrupted pattern. e. Nephropexy using cruciate sutures in the peri-renal fat and body wall. (Image courtesy of Hervé Brissot.) *Illustrator: Elaine Leggett*

to the bladder. They are completely internal and can remain in place for months to years. Ureteral stents are most commonly performed in the cat and dog in the treatment of benign obstructions with calculi or strictures (Berent et al., 2014; Manassero et al., 2014; Zaid et al., 2011). Placement can be achieved percutaneously, via endoscopy or ventral midline coeliotomy, though in the cat only the latter is recommended (Berent et al., 2011, 2014). The stents are placed either retrograde, from the uretero-vesicular junction, or normograde via an approach to the renal pelvis using fluoroscopic guidance. A guide wire is inserted first. A ureteral dilator is then passed over the top followed by the double-pigtail indwelling catheter. One end of the catheter is situated within the renal pelvis and the other in the bladder lumen. The ureterolith is usually not removed unless it prevents passage of the guide wire, in which case a ureterotomy may be performed (Fig. 4.9a,b). Reported complications include dysuria, haematuria, stranguria, urinary tract infection, stent migration, fracture or obstruction (necessitating replacement) and ureteral trauma during stent placement (Berent et al., 2014; Manassero et al., 2014; Wormser et al., 2016).

Subcutaneous ureteral bypass

The SUB technique (Norfolk Vet Products) involves placement of an internal locking-loop nephrostomy tube and an internal cystostomy tube connected via a specialised port sutured subcutaneously on the outer surface of the body wall to completely bypass the

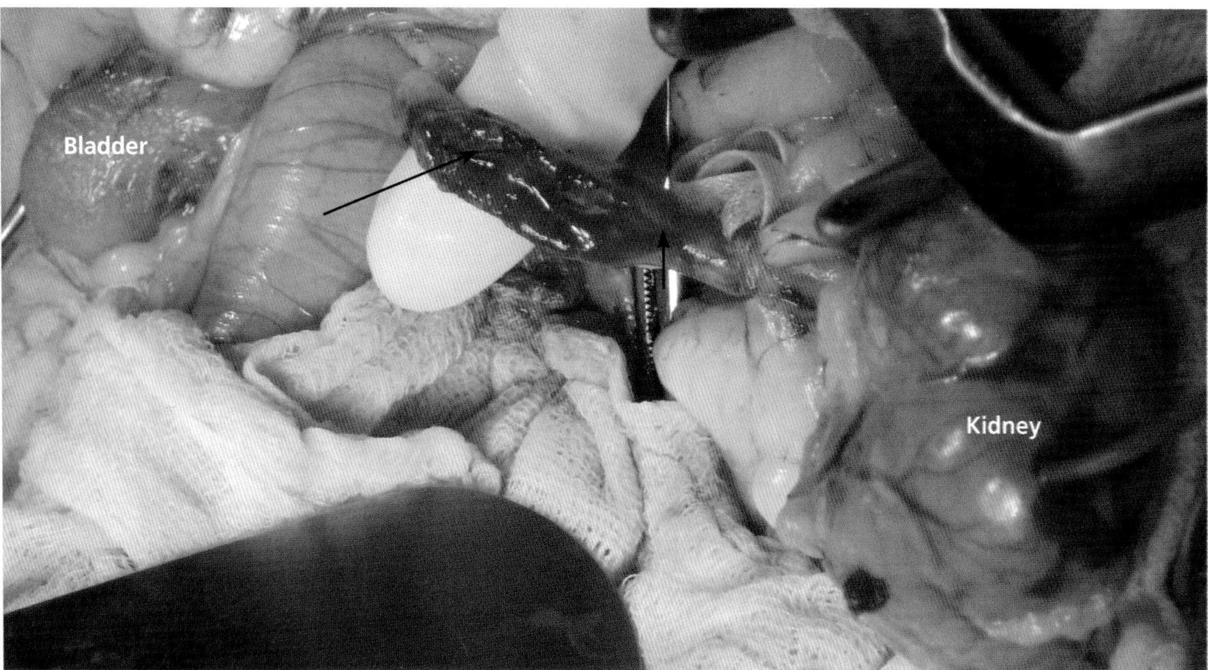

Fig. 4.8 Longitudinal ureterotomy (black arrows) in a dog.

ureter. It is becoming a popular method of treatment for ureteral and pyelic obstruction in the cat, with reports that the outcome for feline patients with ureteral obstruction is better for those treated with a SUB than by other methods (Berent, 2015; Berent and Weisse, 2011). Complications include blockage of the device by urolith material, blood clots or purulent material, device kinking, device leakage, urinary tract infection and non-infectious cystitis (Berent, 2015; Cray et al., 2018; Livet et al., 2017; Runge et al., 2011).

Step by step: SUB technique

- A ventral midline coeliotomy is performed. The nephrostomy catheter is usually placed under fluoroscopic guidance using a modified Seldinger technique. In a recent study, SUB devices were successfully placed without fluoroscopic, radiographic or ultrasonographic guidance (Livet et al., 2017).
- The nephrostomy tube is secured by locking the pigtail and suturing and/or gluing the Dacron cuff to the renal capsule.
- The cystostomy tube is then placed through a purse-string suture in the bladder wall, and the Dacron cuff and overlying silicone ring are secured to the bladder serosa using sutures and sterile tissue glue.
- A subcutaneous pocket is created on the abdominal wall for the port, and the free ends of the two tubes are then tunnelled through the body wall and are connected.

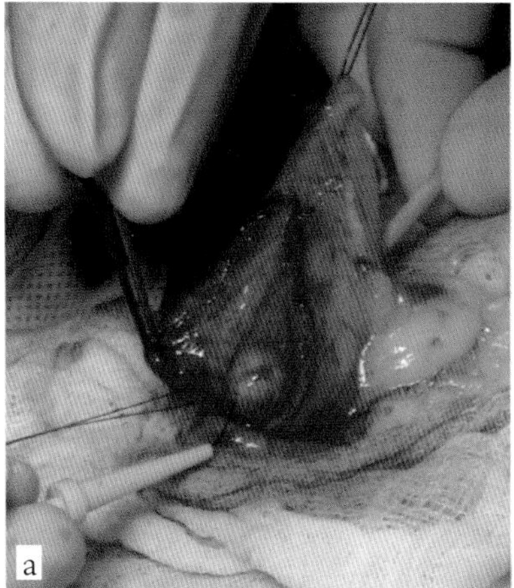

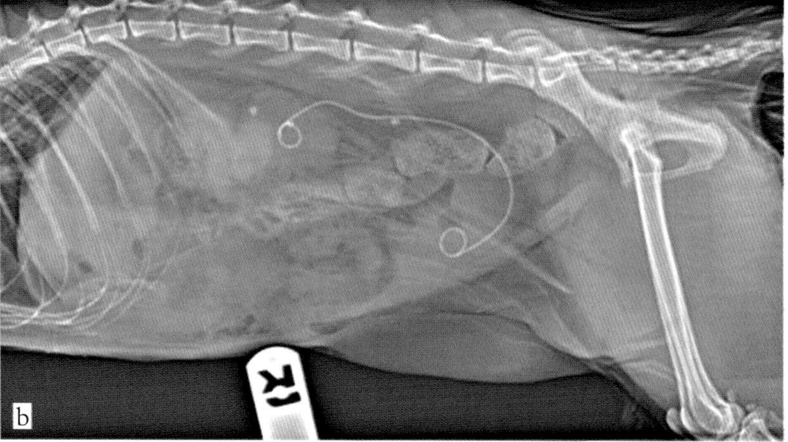

Fig. 4.9a,b Ureteral stent placement. a. Intraoperative view of retrograde (from the uretero-vesicular junction) placement of a ureteral stent. The guide wire is inserted first. b. Postoperative radiograph demonstrating placement of a ureteral stent.

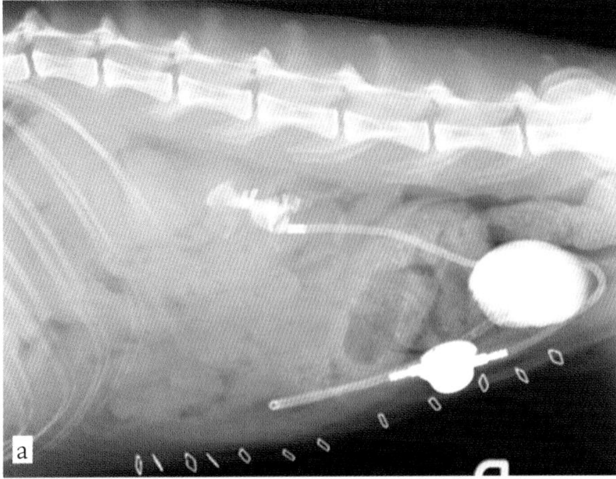

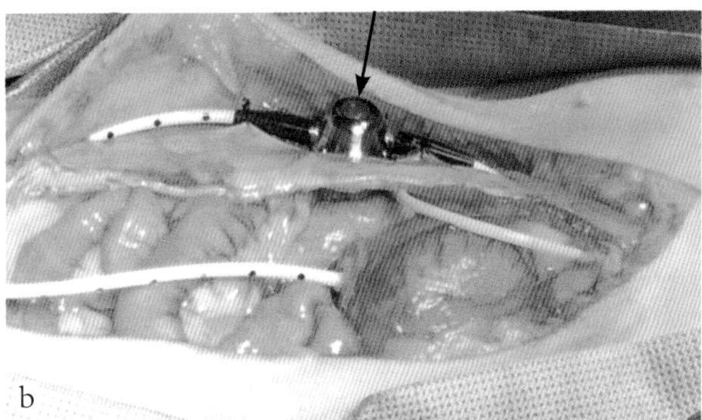

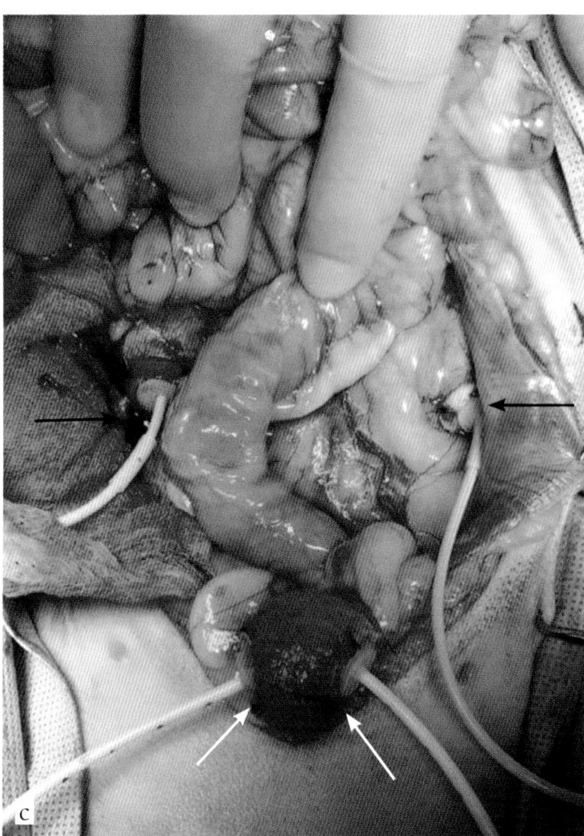

Fig. 4.10a–c SUB placement. a. Radiograph showing the SUB device in place. b. Intra-operative view. The port (black arrow) is sutured to the rectus sheath. c. Bilateral SUB placement. Note the renal catheters (black arrowheads) and the bladder catheters (white arrowheads). Each side is attached to an individual port, which may be useful for troubleshooting any blockages. The alternative is to use a port that can accommodate the two renal catheters.

- The port is sutured to the body wall with non-absorbable monofilament suture (Berent and Weisse, 2011; Fig. 4.10a–c).

Ectopic ureter

Key points

- Ectopic ureter is classed as either intramural or extramural.
- Concomitant urogenital abnormalities such as hydro-ureter, small or absent kidneys and vestibule-vaginal abnormalities are common.
- Urinary incontinence is usually constant but may be intermittent.
- Urinary tract infections are common.
- CT is most useful in assessment of the morphology of ectopic ureter.
- Intramural ectopic ureter can be treated surgically via neo-ureterostomy.
- Extramural ectopic ureter is treated surgically by uretero-neocystostomy.

Ectopic ureter (ureteral ectopia) is a congenital abnormality affecting one or both ureters and causing urinary incontinence. Dogs are more commonly affected than cats, and females more than males (Holt, 1990b). Ectopic ureter is classed as either intramural or extramural. Intramural ectopic ureter is much more common and is distinguished by a normal anatomic entrance into the trigone region of the bladder (Fig. 4.11a–d). However, rather than ending at that site, it continues submucosally and instead opens in the urethra (most often) or vagina. Extramural ectopic ureter is seen more often in the cat, and does not enter the bladder at all; instead it enters directly into the urethral lumen or vagina. The distal segment of ectopic ureter can vary, with some having ureteral troughs or multiple ureteral openings. Concomitant urogenital abnormalities such as hydro-ureter, small or absent kidneys and vestibule-vaginal abnormalities are also common. Presenting animals are usually young (median age is 10 months), though it is possible for clinical signs to develop later in life, especially in males. Golden and Labrador retrievers and Skye terriers are the breeds found to be most at risk (Holt et al., 2000).

Diagnosis

Urinary incontinence is usually constant but may be intermittent, and affected animals usually retain the ability to produce a conscious stream of urine even

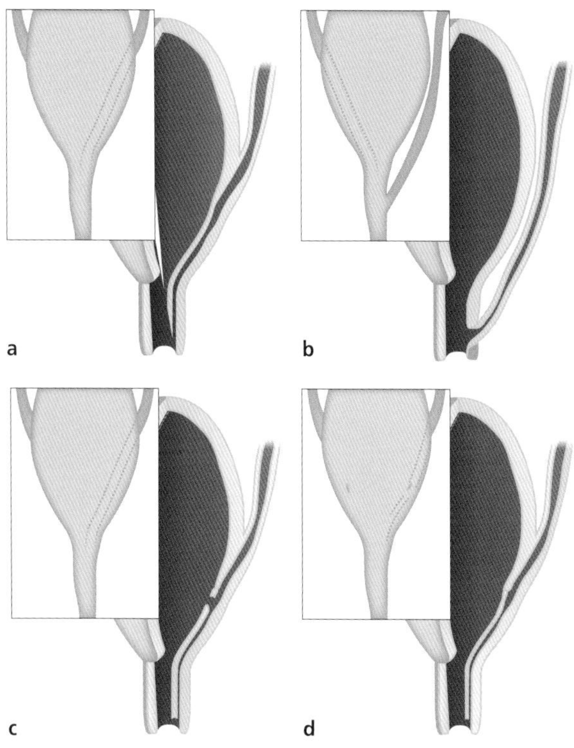

Fig. 4.11a–d Different types of ureteral ectopia. a. Intramural ectopic ureter (most common). b. Extramural ectopic ureter. c. Double ureteral opening. d. Ureteral trough. *Illustrator: Elaine Leggett*

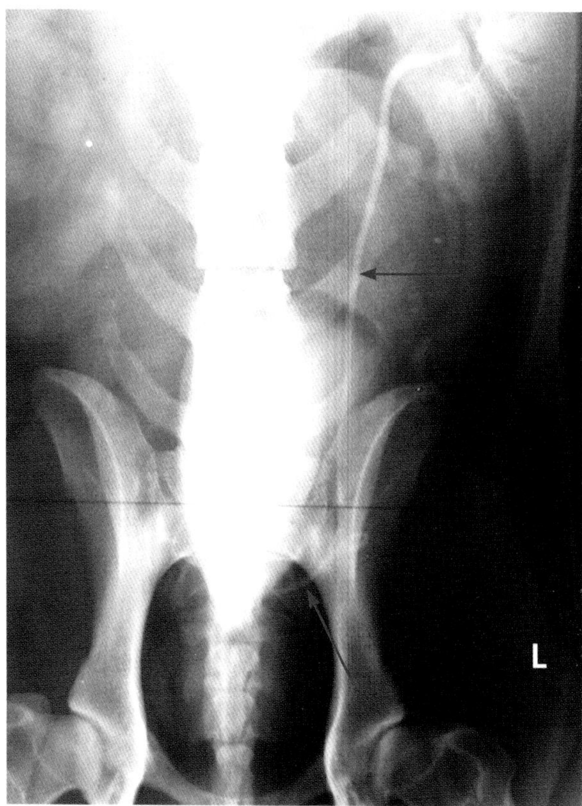

Fig. 4.12 Intravenous urography. The left ureter is ectopic (red arrows) and extramural.

when ureteral ectopia is bilateral. This is most likely due to a retrograde flow of urine into the bladder. Chronic urinary tract infections are common, with consequential haematuria, pollakiuria and dysuria. Affected animals may develop perivulval dermatitis due to chronic urine scalding. Sometimes ectopic ureter is an incidental finding and therefore should be considered in cases of hydronephrosis, even when urinary incontinence has not been reported. Complete blood count, serum biochemistry, urinalysis and urine culture should be performed. Abnormal renal parameters may reflect pyelonephritis or obstructive uropathy, and other abnormalities may be found with concurrent congenital disorders. Diagnostic imaging to confirm ectopic ureter may be undertaken using a variety of contrast-enhanced radiographic techniques. CT is most useful in assessment of the morphology of ectopic ureter, as it allows evaluation of the ureter in multiple planes without surrounding structures obscuring the images. Excretory urography is reported to allow accurate identification of ectopic ureters in up to 76% of cases (Holt et al., 1982; Fig. 4.12), and the use of pneumocystography in combination may improve visualisation of the distal ureter. Fluoroscopy has the added benefit of being able to evaluate ureteral peristalsis and follow urine (contrast) boluses. Retrograde urethrocystography can also be performed with or without fluoroscopy, but has been found to be less reliable (Samii et al., 2004). Ultrasound can also be a valuable imaging modality. Ectopic ureter can be identified at the bladder neck or proximal urethra, and the bladder can be evaluated for the presence of 'jets' of urine, seen due to the turbulence of urine exiting from normally positioned ureters into the bladder. Endoscopy is extremely useful in confirming the presence of ectopic ureter and other urogenital abnormalities, such as paramesonephric remnants or 'vaginal bands' (Fig. 4.13a–c).

Treatment

Whilst surgical or laser correction is required to treat ectopic ureter, if concurrent urethral sphincter mechanism incontinence is present then urine leakage will persist. Medical treatment with alpha-adrenergic agonists (e.g. phenylpropanolamine) may be used to increase urethral sphincter tone. Surgical techniques performed for ureteral ectopia depend on the type. Intramural ectopic ureter can be treated surgically via neo-ureterostomy, whereby the distal ureter is ligated or resected and a new opening for the ureter is created in the correct position, or by cystoscopic laser treatment. Extramural ectopic ureter is treated surgically by uretero-neocystostomy, which involves distal ureteral ligation, transection and re-implantation into the bladder. These procedures all require specialist equipment

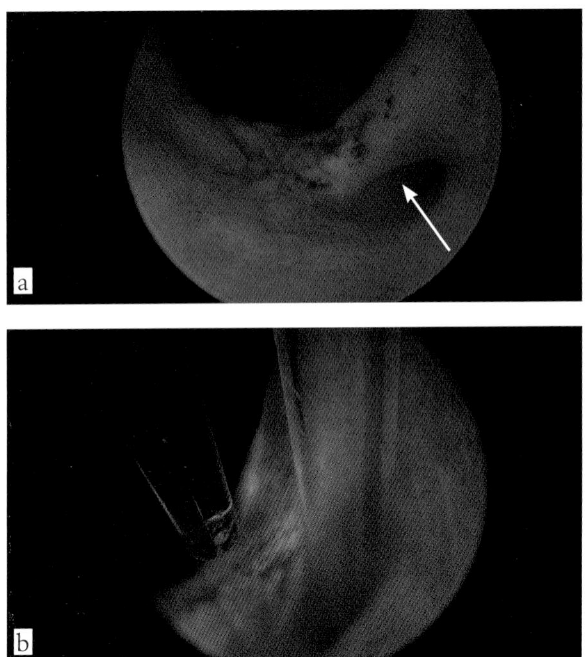

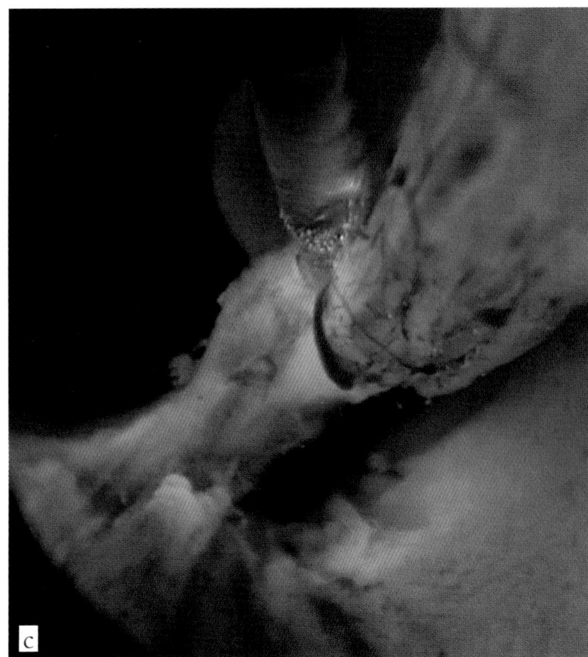

Fig. 4.13a–c Cystoscopic images of an intramural ectopic ureter. a. The ectopic ureter (arrow) is seen within the urethra running alongside the bladder. b. The ectopic ureter is catheterised and the laser applied to the medial wall of the ectopic ureter. c. Lasering is continued to the level of the trigone.

and expertise, and therefore referral should be considered. Uretero-nephrectomy may be required if the condition is unilateral and there is severe, unsalvageable hydronephrosis.

Prognosis

Urinary incontinence persists in between 22 and 72% of patients following surgical repair alone. A further 7–28% of dogs treated both surgically and medically with drugs such as phenylpropanolamine become continent, suggesting that urethral sphincter mechanism incompetence (USMI) is often present (Mayhew et al., 2006; McLaughlin and Miller, 1991). Animals remaining incontinent are likely to have other functional abnormalities of the bladder and urethra.

Neo-ureterostomy: indications

This technique is used for cases of intramural ectopic ureter. Cystoscopic treatment is preferred, but surgery may be indicated in patients that are too small to accept a cystoscope, or if the ectopic ureteral orifice is too narrow for a laser fibre.

Step by step: neo-ureterostomy (Fig. 4.14a–d)

- The bladder is exposed via a ventral midline coeliotomy, and a ventral incision into the bladder is made.
- The intramural ectopic ureter is identified, aided by applying digital pressure to the distal part to cause bulging towards the bladder lumen. Alternatively, a small catheter can be introduced into the ectopic ureter opening though this often requires extension of the bladder incision to the proximal urethra.
- An incision is made through the bladder mucosa and into the ureteral lumen at the trigone, the anatomically correct location of the ureteral orifice.
- The ureteral and bladder mucosae are sutured together using 5-0 to 9-0 monofilament absorbable sutures in a simple interrupted fashion. Magnification is highly recommended.
- A catheter is placed in the distal ureteral segment, and one or two sutures are pre-placed through the dorsal bladder wall and around the catheter within the mucosa / submucosa using 3-0 or 4-0 non-absorbable suture material. The suture(s) should not enter the ureteral lumen.
- The catheter is removed and the sutures are then tightened to close off the ureteral lumen.
- Alternatively, the distal segment of ureter can be excised and the dorsal ureteral mucosa sutured to the bladder mucosa. This prevents possible re-canalisation of the ureter, though it has not been shown to reduce the incidence of postoperative incontinence (Mayhew et al. 2006).

Uretero-neocystostomy: indications

Uretero-neocystostomy is indicated in cases of extramural ureteral ectopia, distal ureteral masses or rupture, and distal ureteral obstructions (stones) whereby significant fibrosis of the ureter is present and patency post-ureterotomy would be questionable. In this latter

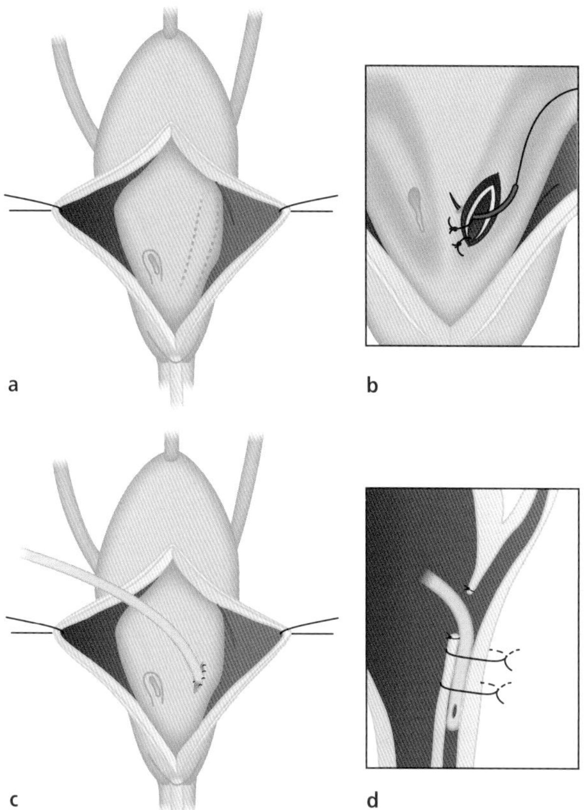

Fig. 4.14a–d Neo-ureterostomy. a. Ventral cystotomy; approach to the trigone. b. Incision in the bladder mucosa into the ureter; the ureteral mucosa is sutured to the bladder. c. A catheter is placed in the distal ureter. d. Non-absorbable sutures are placed distal to the new ureterostomy site; the suture is tied on the bladder side. Care is taken to avoid placing sutures through the bladder mucosa. *Illustrator: Elaine Leggett*

indication, the ureter length is reduced and it is advisable to combine uretero-neocystostomy with a procedure to caudally relocate the kidney (renal descensus) and cystopexy.

Step by step: uretero-neocystostomy

- The bladder is exposed via a ventral midline coeliotomy, and a ventral incision into the bladder is made.
- The ureter is transected where it joins the urethra (ectopic ureters) or the bladder (ureteral obstruction/mass), and the defect in the urethra/bladder is sutured closed.
- An incision in the dorsal bladder wall is made in a position that ensures no tension on the ureter.
- The distal end of the ureter is resected if diseased, and is spatulated.
- A small pair of haemostats is passed through the bladder incision from the mucosal surface, and the ureter is grasped and pulled back through.
- The ureteral and vesicular mucosae are sutured together in a simple interrupted pattern using 5-0 to 9-0 monofilament absorbable sutures. A three-suture technique has been described (Pratschke, 2015). Magnification is highly recommended.
- Alternatively, the ureter can be fed through an intramural tunnel in the bladder wall before it is sutured.
- An extravesicular technique can also be employed whereby a ventral cystotomy is not made, and instead an incision in the dorsal bladder wall is made from the serosal surface. The transected and spatulated ureter is then fed through and sutured to the bladder mucosa with knots external to the lumen (Fig. 4.15a–d).

4.2 Surgical diseases of the urinary bladder and urethra

Surgical conditions of the bladder and urethra are seen more frequently than upper urinary tract diseases, with cystolithiasis/urethrolithiasis, neoplasia and rupture being the most common. Urethral trauma (e.g. rupture caused by road traffic accident, urolith obstruction, bite/gunshot wound) and uroperitoneum are medical emergencies, and patients should be stabilised appropriately before surgical intervention.

Initial investigations should include a complete blood count, serum biochemistry including electrolytes and acid–base status, blood pressure and electrocardiogram (ECG). Azotaemia, metabolic acidosis and hyperkalaemia are frequently present in these animals. Hyperkalaemia can cause life-threatening alterations in myocardial conduction, seen as bradycardia and ECG changes (increased P–R interval, decreased R-wave amplitude and increased T-wave amplitude). Generally, this responds well to crystalloid fluid therapy, abdominal or bladder drainage (for uroabdomen or urethral rupture, respectively) and elimination of the obstruction. However, emergency treatment of hyperkalaemia is required whenever the patient has high serum potassium and is showing consistent clinical or ECG changes. Specific treatment includes intravenous calcium gluconate (which counteracts the effects of high potassium on myocardial conduction), IV soluble insulin and dextrose (which promotes potassium uptake into cells along with glucose) or (rarely) sodium bicarbonate. Stabilisation for 6–12 hours is often adequate to normalise serum electroytes and decrease azotaemia and metabolic acidosis, making the patient a better surgical candidate. Diagnostic imaging should include ultrasonography and radiography.

Ultrasound is the most sensitive method for evaluating bladder size and location, identifying calculi and bladder wall lesions and thickening. It can also be used to guide cystocentesis or abdominocentesis when uroabdomen is suspected.

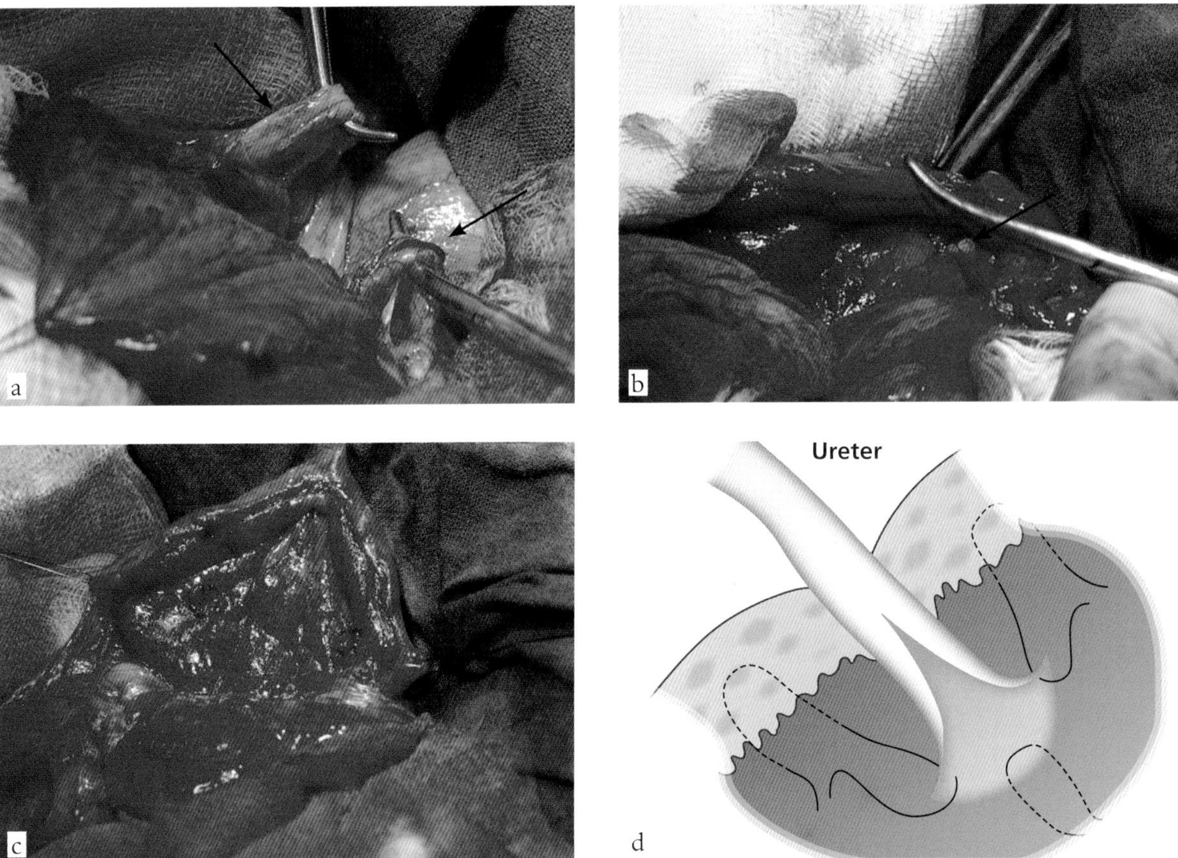

Fig. 4.15a–d Uretero-neocystostomy. a. The extramural ectopic ureter is isolated and transected. b. The transected ureter is advanced to an intravesicular position following an incision in the dorsal wall of the bladder. c. Intravesical uretero-neocystostomy arrows. d. The 3-stitches technique: the ureter is sutured to the mucosa of the bladder by three separate stiches at approximately 120° intervals around the spatulation, so that they will help to maintain spatulation once tied. (Images courtesy of K.M. Pratschke.) *Illustrator: Elaine Leggett*

Radiography is useful for identification of the bladder, though free abdominal fluid may obscure its outline. Pelvic fractures and radio-opaque calculi will be visible radiographically, and contrast radiography should be performed if either of these is seen. Retrograde urethrocystography with or without fluoroscopy is used to identify the location of urethral or bladder trauma, calculi and masses. An IV urogram may be required to evaluate extension to the ureters in cases of neoplasia. Thoracic radiography or CT should be performed in any animal suspected of neoplasia.

Cystoscopy can be performed in dogs and cats using either a rigid cystoscope (prepubic percutaneous in males) or a flexible cystoscope. This provides direct visualisation of the urethral and bladder mucosa and is useful in the identification of many conditions such as urethral stricture, urolithiasis, neoplasia and rupture. Interventional procedures may also be performed, such as biopsy, calculus retrieval and lithotripsy.

4.2.1 Surgical anatomy

The bladder lies in the caudal peritoneal cavity, and is attached to the abdominal wall via lateral ligaments and the ventral median ligament. In the dog it lies just cranial to or within the pelvic cavity when empty, and extends ventrocranially into the abdomen as it distends (Fig. 4.16). In the cat the bladder is always intra-abdominal, even when empty. The body of the bladder ends caudally at the trigone, which connects to the urethra. The urethra in the male dog is long (10–35 cm) and is divided into prostatic, pelvic (membranous) and penile portions. The urethra passes through the prostate in the prostatic section, where the ampullae of the ductus deferens enter on either side of the dorsally located colliculus seminalis. The penile segment is the longest and is surrounded by the corpus spongiosum for its entire length. The size of the urethra increases proximally. The male feline urethra measures 8.5–10.5 cm and includes a pre-prostatic portion (not present in the dog) that forms a distinct urethral sphincter. The average diameter at the level of the bulbourethral glands is 1.3 mm, twice that of the penile urethra. The female canine urethra is shorter (7–10 cm) and wider (0.5 cm), and is proportionally similar in cats. Urethral mucosa heals rapidly and can completely regenerate in seven days.

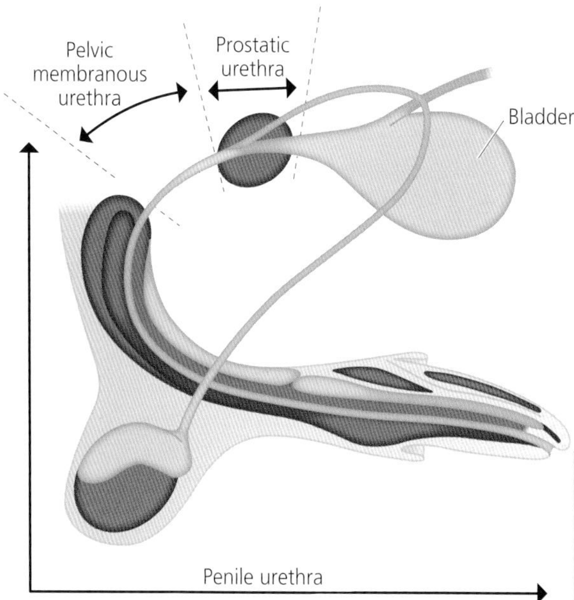

Fig. 4.16 Anatomy of the bladder and urethra in the male dog. *Illustrator: Elaine Leggett*

Vascular supply

The blood supply to the bladder is via the cranial and caudal vesical arteries, which branch from the umbilical and urogenital arteries, respectively. The urogenital artery is a branch of the internal pudendal artery. Venous drainage is into the internal pudendal veins. The urethra is a highly vascular structure that will bleed profusely when traumatised and will swell dramatically with excessive manipulation. The blood supply to the urethra is from branches of the internal pudendal arteries and veins (urethral, prostatic, penile; Fig. 4.17).

Innervation

The bladder and urethra are innervated by the hypogastric, pelvic and pudendal nerves. The hypogastric nerve stimulates β-adrenergic receptors in the bladder wall, resulting in detrusor muscle relaxation to allow storage of urine. It also stimulates α-adrenergic receptors in the bladder neck and proximal urethra, causing smooth muscle contraction and prevention of urine flow. The pelvic nerve is stimulated by stretch receptors in the detrusor muscle when the bladder nears capacity, and initiates detrusor contraction. The stretch receptors also depress sympathetic outflow to relax smooth and striated urethral musculature. The pudendal nerve provides somatic innervation to the peri-urethral striated muscle at the bladder neck (the external urethral sphincter). The muscle is normally in a steady state of contraction, and is inhibited during urination (Evans and de Lahunta, 2013; Wang et al., 1999; Fig. 4.18).

4.2.2 Specific diseases

Urinary bladder and urethral calculi

Key points

- The majority of canine and feline uroliths are struvite or calcium oxalate.
- Common clinical findings are stranguria, pollakiuria, haematuria, dysuria and abdominal pain.
- Urinary tract infection is also common.
- In females with unknown composition of the calculi, medical treatment such as dissolution diets and antibiosis for urinary tract infections may be successful.
- Dissolution is not appropriate in the male.
- Urethrotomy should be avoided if possible due to the high risk of complications.

The bladder is the most common location for urolithiasis in the dog and cat. Calculi form when dissolved salts in the urine precipitate to form crystals, which, if not excreted, may aggregate to form solid concretions. This is particularly likely around a nidus (e.g. a plug of cell debris, suture material or a mass). The majority of canine and feline uroliths are struvite (magnesium ammonium phosphate) or calcium oxalate, and the most recent reports suggest a similar proportion of both types in both species (around 40–50%; Cannon et al., 2007; Houston and Moore, 2010; Low et al., 2010; Osborne et al., 2008). Other less common uroliths include urate, cystine, silica and mixed types. Various factors can predispose to certain urolith composition types: pH (struvite forms in alkaline urine, calcium oxalate in acidic urine); presence of UTI with urease-producing bacteria which increase the urine pH (struvite); age (struvite in dogs under 1 year due to UTI); breed (e.g. cystine in English bulldog, urate in Dalmatian); sex (struvite more common in female dogs, calcium oxalate more common in male dogs); and underlying conditions (urate uroliths with portosystemic shunt, calcium oxalate with hypercalcaemia).

Diagnosis

Common clinical findings are stranguria, pollakiuria, haematuria, dysuria and abdominal pain. If there is concurrent obstruction, bladder distension and signs of post-renal azotaemia develop such as progressive lethargy, vomiting and collapse. Investigations should include a complete blood count, serum biochemistry (including electrolytes, especially if obstruction is suspected), urinalysis and urine culture. Azotaemia may be present with pyelonephritis or obstruction, electrolyte abnormalities are common with obstructions, whilst

Male

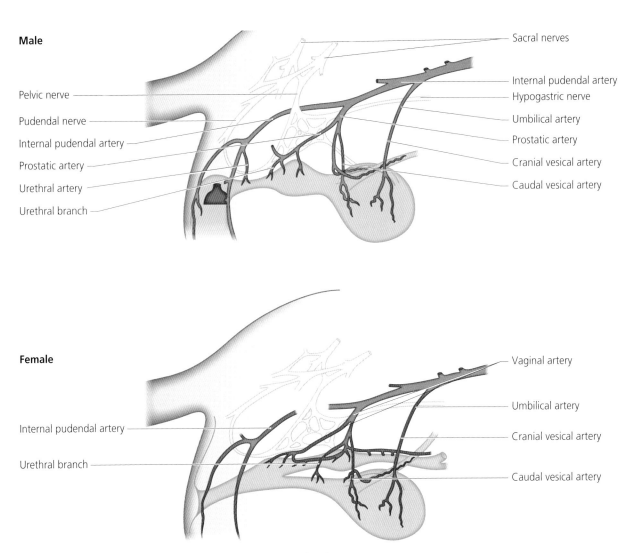

Sacral nerves
Internal pudendal artery
Hypogastric nerve
Umbilical artery
Prostatic artery
Cranial vesical artery
Caudal vesical artery
Pelvic nerve
Pudendal nerve
Internal pudendal artery
Prostatic artery
Urethral artery
Urethral branch

Female

Vaginal artery
Umbilical artery
Cranial vesical artery
Caudal vesical artery
Internal pudendal artery
Urethral branch

Fig. 4.17 Vascular and nervous supply in the canine male and female. *Illustrator: Elaine Leggett*

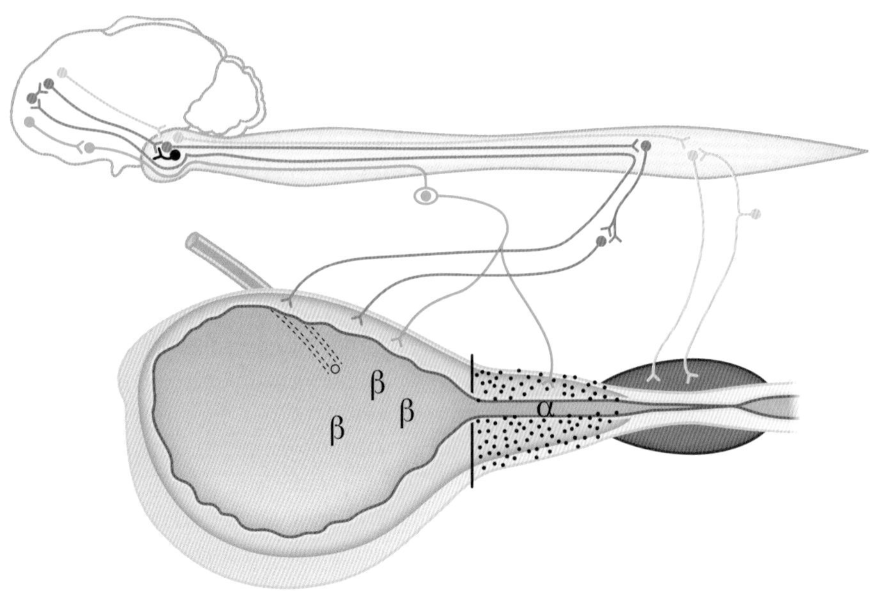

Fig. 4.18 Distribution of the autonomous (α- and ß-receptors of the sympathetic [hypogastric nerve: green] nerve and acetylcholine receptors of the parasympathetic [pelvic nerve: orange] nervous system) and somatic (acetylcholine receptors, pudendal nerve: yellow) nervous systems in the bladder and proximal urethra. Muscles: detrusor (pink); internal urethral sphincter (stippled black); external urethral sphincter (solid red/brown). *Illustrator: Elaine Leggett*

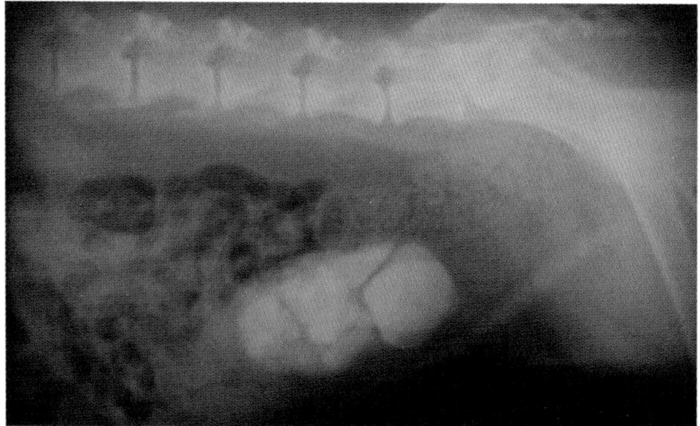

Fig. 4.19 Plain lateral radiographs of a dog showing multiple large cystic calculi outlining the shape of the bladder.

hepatic insufficiency may be present in animals with urate calculi. Urinary tract infection is common, even in the absence of pyuria, bacteriuria, haematuria or proteinuria. Urine sediment examination often shows crystals in normal animals, though these may give a clue to the type of calculus. It may be possible to retrieve small uroliths via catheter or voiding hydropropulsion. Though struvite and calcium oxalate calculi should be seen on plain radiography (Fig. 4.19), pneumocystography, double-contrast cystography and ultrasonography are much more sensitive techniques for the detection of all types of calculi, and are especially useful in the identification of non-radio-opaque uroliths such as urate. If bladder calculi are found, it is important to image the remainder of the urinary tract for uroliths in other locations.

Treatment

In the female without obstruction (obstruction is very rare in females due to the wide urethra) and known composition of the calculi, medical treatment such as dissolution diets and antibiosis for urinary tract infections may be successful for removal of cystoliths. Only struvite, urate and cysteine are amenable to dissolution, though diets generally are better at preventing other stones from forming following removal, rather than dissolving them. Dissolution is not appropriate in the male due to the risk of life-threatening obstruction. Regular radiographs should be taken if dissolution is tried to monitor the uroliths. Other methods of non-surgical cystolith removal include voiding urohydropropulsion, transurethral cystoscopic retrieval and lithotripsy. Urethral obstruction is occasionally chronic, but more often is acute and life-threatening and requires emergency treatment. This initially involves stabilisation – for example, IV fluid therapy and correction of acid–base and electrolyte abnormalities (hyperkalaemia commonly). Once the patient is fit for general anaesthesia, attempts can then be made to dislodge the obstructive material by means of retrohydropropulsion. If successful, the calculi should then be removed via cystotomy.

Alternatively, laparoscopically assisted cystotomy (Fig. 4.20a,b) or percutaneous cystotomy may be performed (Pinel et al., 2013; Rawlings et al., 2003b; Runge et al., 2011).

If it is not possible to dislodge the urethrolith, a

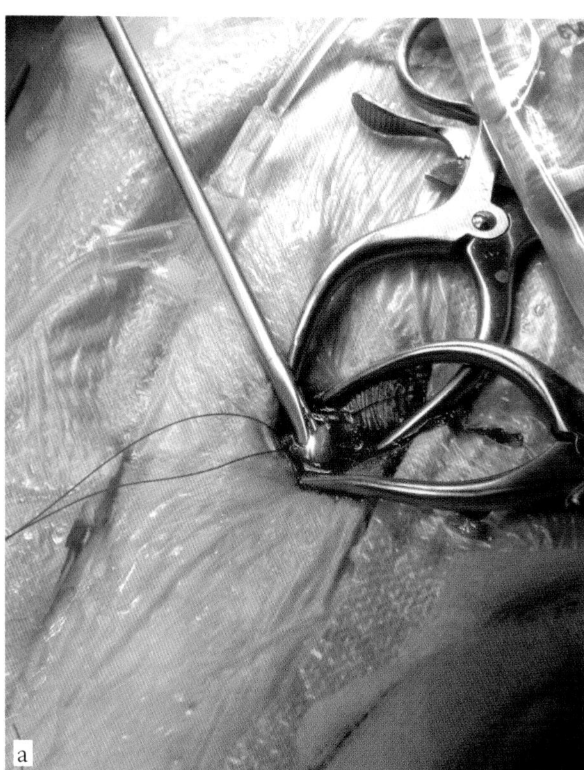

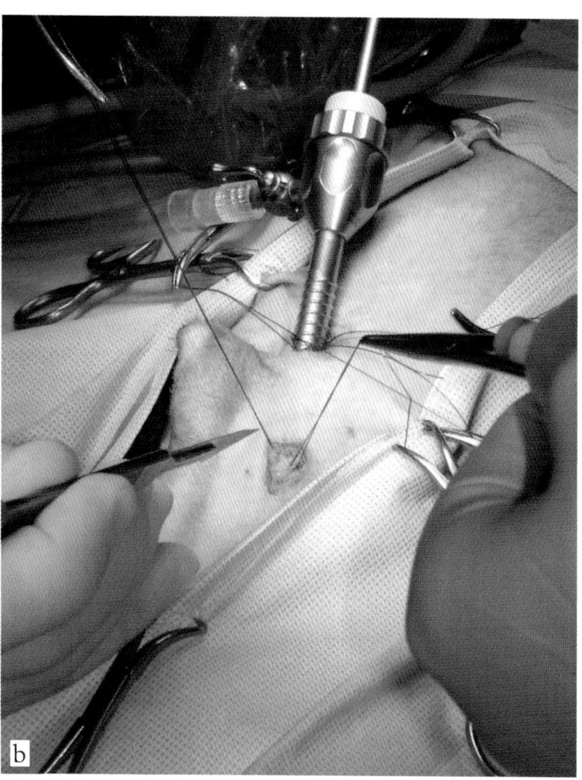

Fig. 4.20a,b Laparoscopically assisted cystotomy.

urethrotomy must be performed. This should be avoided if possible due to the high risk of complications, such as haemorrhage and urethral stricture. It is important to submit the uroliths for chemical analysis so that dietary management can be initiated. For recurrent obstructions, a urethrostomy should be considered. This procedure involves creating a permanent stoma in a wider part of the urethra to allow stones to pass during urination. Scrotal urethrostomy is preferred in the male dog as the urethra is relatively superficial and wide at the level of the scrotum, and less haemorrhage occurs at this site than at other locations. Other possible sites are prescrotal, perineal and prepubic, but complications are much more likely. Perineal urethrostomy is preferred in the male cat, though transpelvic, prepubic or subpubic locations are possible and may be warranted in certain cases.

All permanent urethrostomy techniques are associated with similar complications. Short-term complications include haematuria, haemorrhage from surrounding tissue, dysuria, pollakiuria, partial wound dehiscence and stricture formation. Stricture formation is the most common and most difficult complication to manage. It is predisposed by inflammation, indwelling urinary catheter, suture tension, self-trauma, inadequate mucosa to skin apposition, wound infection, failure to mobilise the pelvic and penile urethra, and granulation tissue formation after urine leakage. The risk can be reduced by avoiding misuse of indwelling catheters, preventing self-trauma and good surgical technique. Long-term complications include urinary incontinence, recurring urinary tract infections and urine scalding, the complication rates of which are dependent on the technique used.

Prognosis

Recurrence of urolithiasis is reportedly higher in the dog than in the cat. Calcium oxalate has the highest rate of recurrence in the dog of up to 50% within three years, compared to only 7% in the cat (Albasan et al., 2009; Lulich et al., 1992). Periodic radiographic screening should be performed in dogs with recurrent non-dissolvable cystoliths so that these can be removed non-surgically before they are too large. Struvite has been reported to recur in 21% of dogs and 2.7% of cats (Albasan et al., 2009; Brown et al., 1977). Complete resolution is possible with long courses of antibiotics in cases where calculi form due to urinary tract infection, though sometimes prophylactic antibiotics are required when recurrence occurs despite appropriate investigations and management. Urate calculi reportedly recur in 33% of dogs and 13% of cats, and cystine uroliths recurred in 47% of dogs in one study (Albasan et al., 2009; Brown et al., 1977; Lulich et al., 1992). In the cat, urethral obstruction recurs in 22–51% of cases although it is uncommon if perineal urethrostomy is performed (Gerber et al., 2008; Segev et al., 2011).

Retrohydropropulsion: indications

Retrohydropropulsion is indicated in cases of urethral obstruction, in order to advance obstructive material back into the bladder.

Step by step: retrohydropropulsion

- A catheter coated with sterile aqueous lubricant is introduced into the urethra distal to the obstruction.
- Sterile saline is injected firmly into the catheter with a 50 ml syringe (dog) or 10 or 20 ml syringe (cat or small dog), while simultaneously compressing the pelvic per urethra rectum. This allows the urethra distal to the compression to distend, and frees up stones from the crevices of the collapsed urethral wall.
- The digital pressure should then be suddenly released while flushing is still maintained, in order to propel the material into the bladder (Fig. 4.21a–c).

If it is not possible to relieve the obstruction, cystocentesis may be performed and retrohydropropulsion tried again 12 hours later, or a temporary urethral diversion can be placed i.e. tube cystostomy (surgical or minimally invasive using a pigtail catheter).

Cystotomy: indications

Indications for cystotomy are wide-ranging and include the removal of calculi, biopsy or mass removal, repair of trauma, surgical treatment of ectopic ureter and as part of the investigation of idiopathic renal haematuria.

Step by step: cystotomy

- A caudal midline laparotomy incision is made, from the umbilicus to the pubis.
- The bladder is identified and packed off from the remainder of the abdomen with moistened laparotomy swabs.
- A stay suture is placed in the apex of the bladder.
- A ventral cystotomy is easier to perform than a dorsal cystotomy, and there is less risk of damaging the ureteral openings.
- A stab incision is made into approximately the midline of the ventral bladder using a scalpel, in the area of least vascularity. Residual urine is removed using suction.
- The incision is extended as needed, and further stay sutures are placed at the edges of the cystotomy incision to allow the relevant procedure to be performed (e.g. calculus/mass removal).

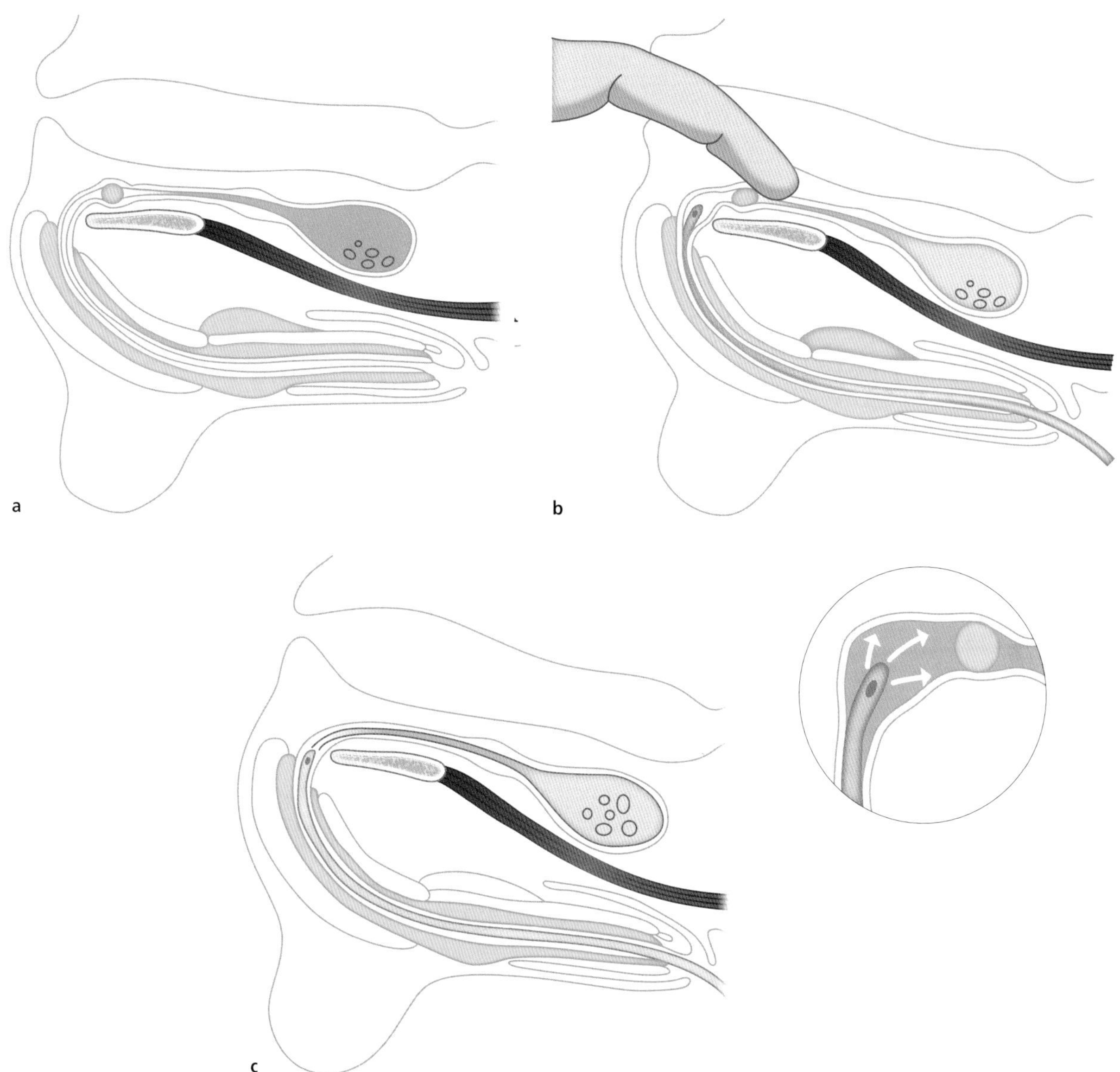

Fig. 4.21a–c Retrohydropropulsion in the dog. *Illustrator: Elaine Leggett*

- The cystotomy incision is closed in one layer using a monofilament, absorbable suture material in a simple continuous pattern (Fig. 4.22a–d).

Scrotal urethrostomy: indications

Urethrostomy is indicated for cases where it has not been possible to dislodge the calculi by retrohydropropulsion, or when recurrence of the stone formation is very likely. Other indications for urethrostomy include penile amputation. A scrotal urethrostomy is most often performed in the male dog as the urethra is wider in this area than in the prescrotal region. This location is also optimal as the urethra is more superficial than the prescrotal location.

Step by step: scrotal urethrostomy

- The dog is positioned in dorsal recumbency and a canine urinary catheter placed in the penile urethra up to the obstruction, to facilitate identification of the urethra.
- An elliptical incision is made in the scrotal region (if the dog is entire, castration and scrotal ablation are needed), and the subcutaneous tissues are dissected until the penile shaft is identified.
- The retractor penis muscles are retracted laterally to expose the purple urethra surrounded by corpus spongiosum.
- An incision is made over the urinary catheter (if possible) using a no. 15 blade. Bleeding will occur when the corpus spongiosum is incised, which can be controlled with direct pressure.
- The obstructive material is removed (if possible), and the catheter advanced into the urinary bladder to confirm patency.
- The urethral mucosa is sutured to the skin. Bites

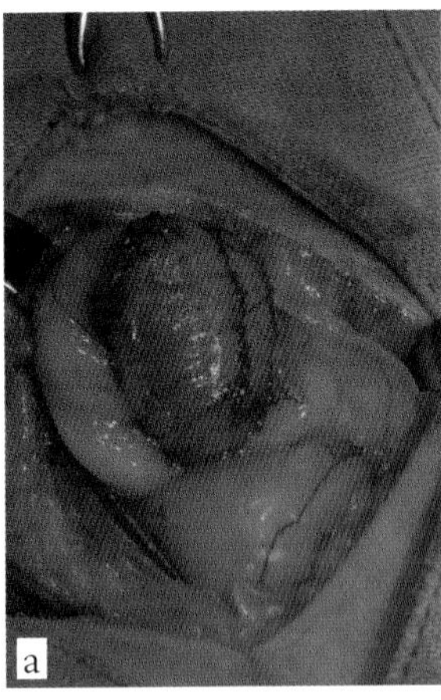
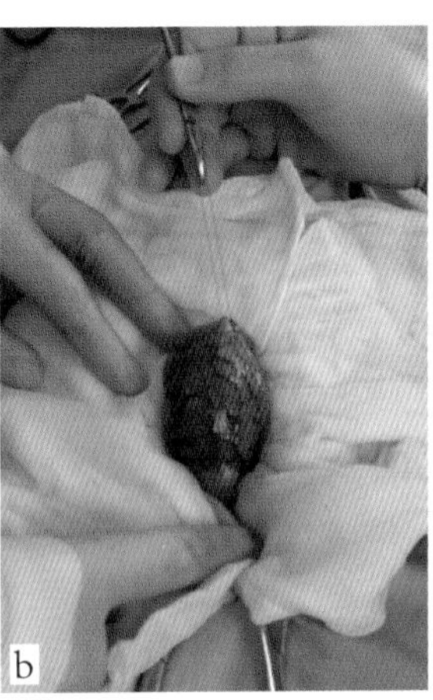
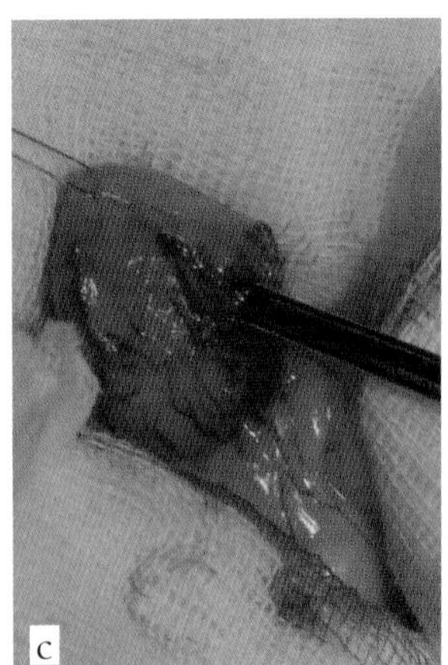
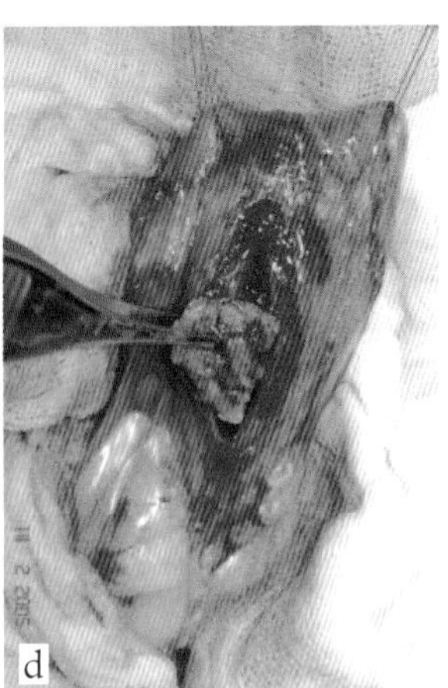

Fig. 4.22a–d Cystotomy. a. Exposure of the urinary bladder. b. Stay suture placed to facilitate manipulation of the bladder. c. Opening of the bladder on its ventral surface. d. Retrieval of uroliths.

can include the tunica albuginea but not the corpus spongiosum. A simple interrupted or simple continuous pattern can be used (absorbable or non-absorbable monofilament).

- A cystotomy may then be performed to remove any other calculi, and the urethra flushed retrograde and antegrade to ensure that no more remain (Fig. 4.23a–d).

If a urethrotomy needs to be performed, the prescrotal region is usually preferred. The urethra is approached following an incision between the os penis and the scrotal region. The urethra is incised longitudinally after subcutaneous dissection and incision of the tunica albuginea. The urethrotomy may be left to heal by secondary intension, but profuse haemorrhage can occur from the site for up to 14 days postoperatively. Urethral stricture following primary closure is possible but rare, and it is preferable to close the incision using 4-0 or 5-0 monofilament absorbable suture in a simple interrupted or continuous pattern, incorporating the urethral mucosa and tunica albuginea.

Partial cystectomy: indications

The indications for partial cystectomy include discrete bladder neoplasia/polyp, bladder necrosis (e.g. following prolonged obstruction), excision of a patent urachus and bladder diverticulum.

Technique. When neoplasia is suspected, a full exploratory laparotomy should be performed to examine the abdomen for metastatic lesions. A midline coeliotomy, extending from xiphoid to pubis, is therefore performed and the abdomen is explored, paying particular attention to the sublumbar lymph nodes. The bladder is exposed and the tumour identified. If possible, the lesion is excised, being careful to identify and spare the ureters as they enter the dorsal trigone. The bladder is sutured using a simple continuous pattern with 3-0 monofilament absorbable suture material (Fig. 4.24a,b). If the ureteral orifices are involved, it is possible to transect and re-implant these into a different area of the bladder wall (Stone et al., 1996). However, because the nerve supply to the bladder enters the dorsal aspect of the trigone, the risk of postoperative incontinence is much higher if this region is excised. Urinary diversion

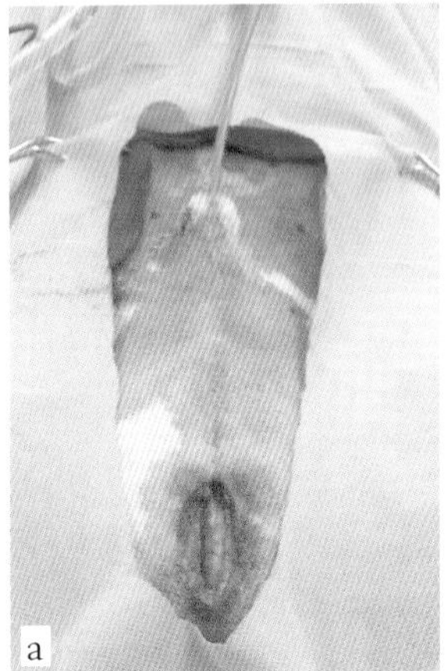
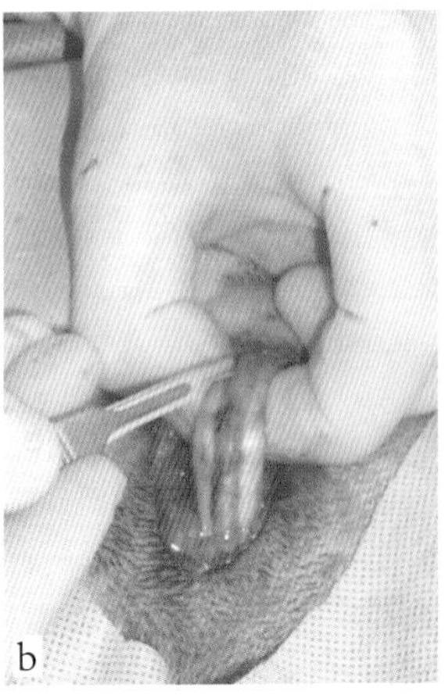
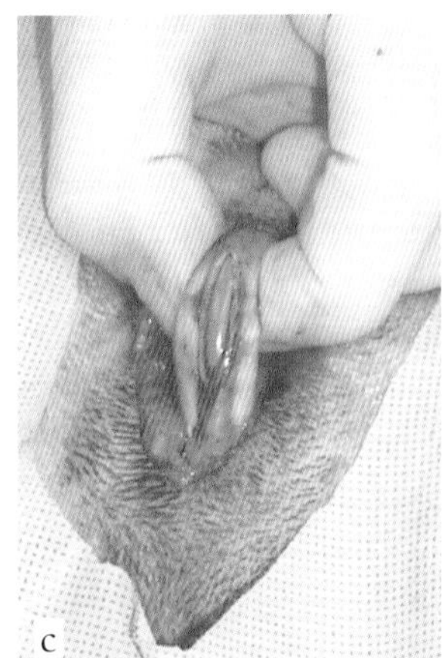
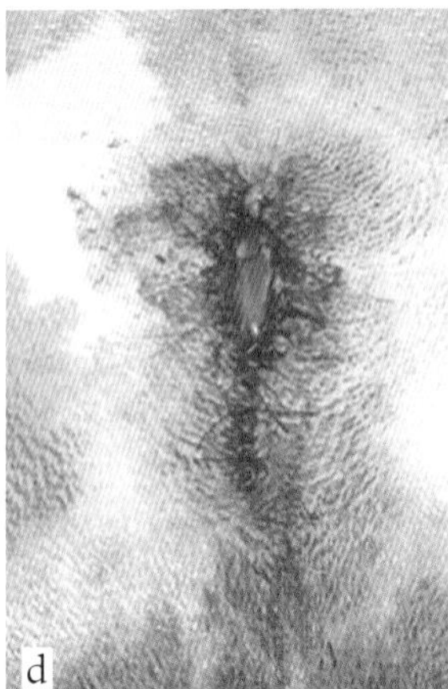

Fig. 4.23a–d Scrotal urethrostomy. a. Elliptical incision in the scrotal region. b. The shaft of the penis is held in the non-dominant hand and the retractor penis muscle is retracted to the side. c. The urethra is incised longitudinally. d. Urethrostomy completed.

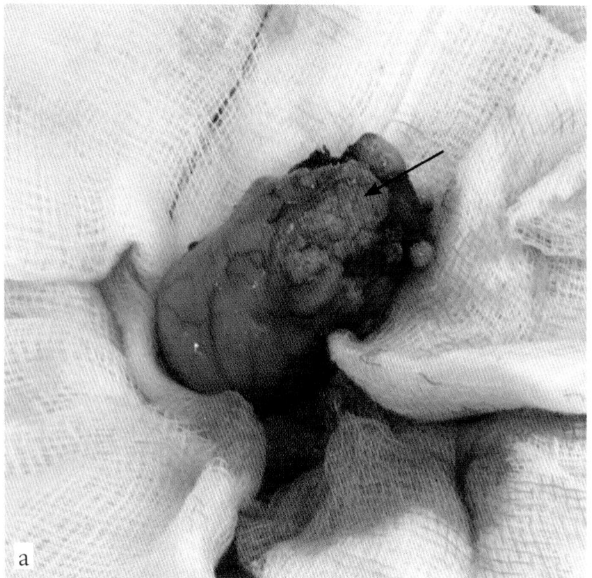

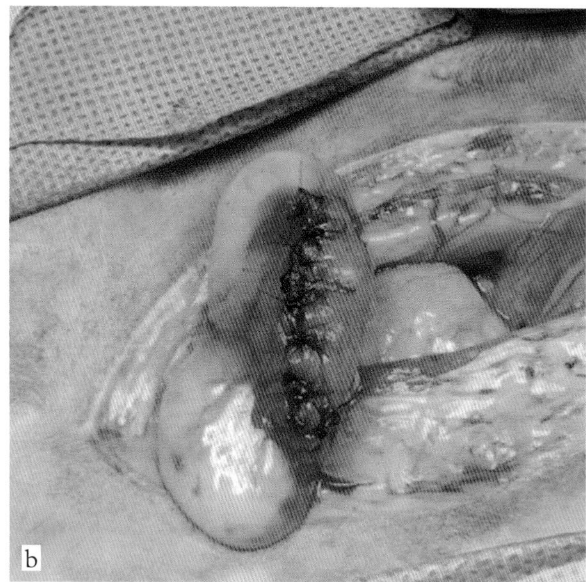

Fig. 4.24a,b Partial cystectomy in a 3-year-old cat with a bladder tumour (transitional cell carcinoma). a. Tumour *in situ* at the level of the apex of the bladder (black arrow). b. Closure of the remnant of the bladder following tumour excision. The bladder is closed in two layers. This patient went on to live for an additional 4 months following surgery, with no adjuvant treatment.

by uretero-colonic anastomosis carries unacceptable morbidity and is not recommended (Stone et al., 1988), though diversion to the vagina or prepuce may result in fewer complications (Saeki et al., 2015).

Urinary tract rupture

Key points

- Clinical signs of urinary bladder rupture include abdominal pain and bruising, haematuria, anuria, dysuria, progressive lethargy and vomiting.
- Ultrasonography may identify free fluid and can be used to guide sample collection.
- Urinary diversion can be achieved by placement of an indwelling urinary catheter or cystostomy tube for urethral rupture.
- Abdominal drainage can be performed in cases of uroabdomen, by placement of a pigtail cystostomy tube or other soft tube drain.
- Primary repair of ureteral ruptures may not be possible, and carries a considerable risk of ureteral stricture.
- When ureteral rupture is very distal, transection and re-implantation may be possible.
- In urinary bladder rupture, the edges should be debrided and the defect sutured.

Any area of the urinary tract can be ruptured, though the bladder (usually the apex) is most commonly affected usually as a result of external trauma. Rupture may also occur due to neoplasia or urethral obstruction, or following iatrogenic damage when placing a urinary catheter, performing cystocentesis or during manual expression.

Diagnosis

Bladder rupture causes leakage of urine into the abdomen, but rupture of the kidney or ureter does not always result in uroabdomen as these are retroperitoneal structures. However, clinical signs are similar regardless of the location and include abdominal pain and bruising (if urinary tract rupture is due to trauma), haematuria, anuria, dysuria, progressive lethargy and vomiting. Hallmark metabolic abnormalities that develop are azotaemia, metabolic acidosis and hyperkalaemia. Diagnosis is confirmed by diagnostic imaging and abdominocentesis or paracentesis of the retroperitoneal space. Ultrasonography may identify free fluid (peritoneal or retroperitoneal) and can be used to guide sample collection. Radiography will show loss of serosal detail when free abdominal fluid is present. Definitive diagnosis requires testing of the fluid to confirm that it is urine. The creatinine content will be higher than that of a serum sample if the fluid is urine, because the creatinine molecule is large and cannot pass across the peritoneum. Potassium will similarly be elevated compared to serum. Haematocrit and total protein estimation should be performed to rule out haemoabdomen and to help classify an effusion. Cytology may show intracellular bacteria in the sediment, thus indicating septic peritonitis. In this case, the fluid should be submitted for culture and sensitivity whilst starting empirical intravenous antibiosis. Once the fluid has been confirmed to be urine, further imaging is required to locate the source of leakage. This can be achieved

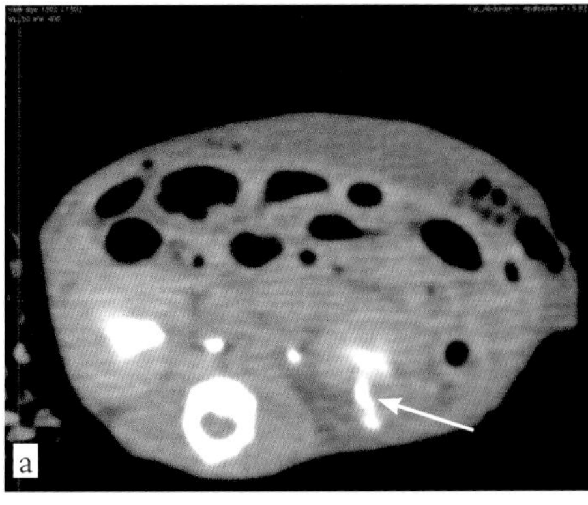

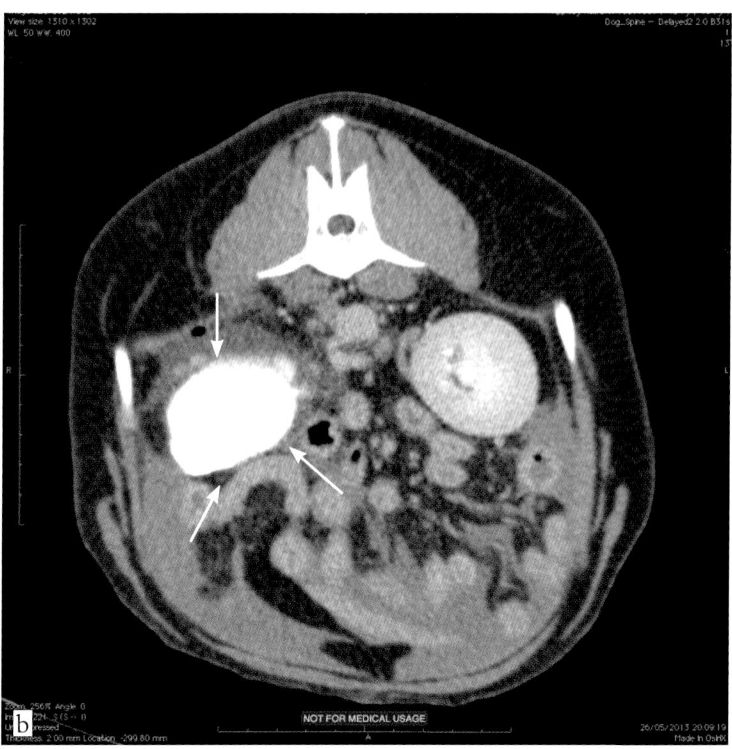

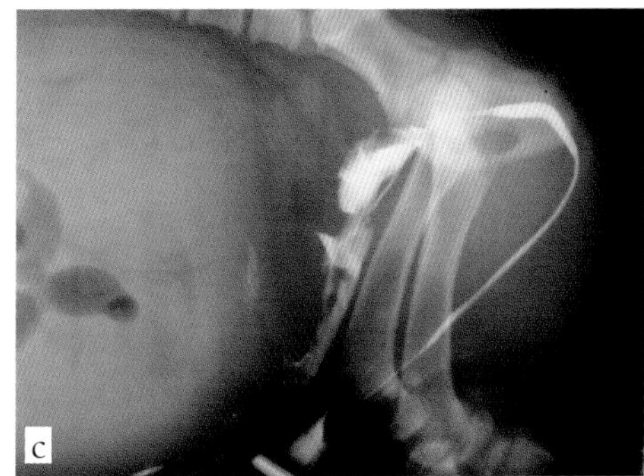

Fig. 4.25a–c Imaging techniques used to identify urinary tract ruptures. a. CT scan demonstrating a leak of contrast material through the renal parenchyma and ruptured capsule (red arrow) following a dog bite. b. CT scan demonstrating a complete rupture of the proximal ureter with pooling of contrast agent in the retroperitoneal space (red arrows). c. Retrograde urethrocystogram showing a complete rupture at the level of the neck of the bladder with extravasation of contrast material into the abdomen.

by retrograde contrast urethrocystography, which will highlight the intestinal loops with bladder or cranial urethral rupture and will show leakage of contrast in the pelvic region with more caudal urethral rupture. Negative contrast should be avoided due to the risk of causing an air embolus in trauma cases. Fluoroscopy can make identification of the rupture location more apparent. IV urography or IV CT is required for identification of ureteral and renal ruptures (Fig. 4.25a–c).

Treatment

Treatment initially involves stabilisation (e.g. IV fluid therapy and correction of acid–base and electrolyte abnormalities – usually hyperkalaemia). Urinary diversion can be achieved by placement of an indwelling urinary catheter or cystostomy tube for urethral rupture. In cases of uroabdomen, abdominal drainage can be performed by placement of a pig-tail cystostomy tube or other soft tube drain. Once the patient is sufficiently stable to undergo general anaesthesia, a full exploratory laparotomy should be performed. In cases of trauma, all abdominal organs should be examined. It may be possible to suture a renal rupture (as described for nephrotomy), but uretero-nephrectomy may be required if the kidney is not salvageable. Primary repair of ureteral rupture may not be possible, and carries a considerable risk of ureteral stricture. When ureteral rupture is very distal, transection and re-implantation may be possible (see uretero-neocystostomy). Alternatively, a ureteral stent may be placed or a SUB can be performed. In cases of bladder rupture (Fig. 4.26), the edges should be debrided and the defect sutured. If the trauma is in the region of the bladder neck and is difficult to suture, a urethral catheter or tube cystostomy can be placed before reconstruction and maintained post-operatively to allow decompression whilst healing occurs. The ventral midline incision may need to be extended into the pubic region and a pubic osteotomy carried out if there is urethral damage. The three treatment options for managing a urethral rupture are temporary urinary diversion to bypass the injured segment, primary repair and a permanent diversion by urethrostomy proximal to the urethral lesion. Temporary urinary diversion can be achieved by urethral or cystostomy catheterisation. This allows healing by secondary intention and/or enables delayed primary repair. Primary repair is challenging due to the size of the urethra and associated complications, including urethral dehiscence and stricture formation. It is performed by anastomosing the transected segments of the urethra over a catheter. An indwelling catheter should be left in place post-operatively for 10 days to act as a stent allowing soft tissue healing. A vagino-urethroplasty has also been reported as a urinary diversion salvage procedure after failure of primary repair in a female cat (Halfacree et

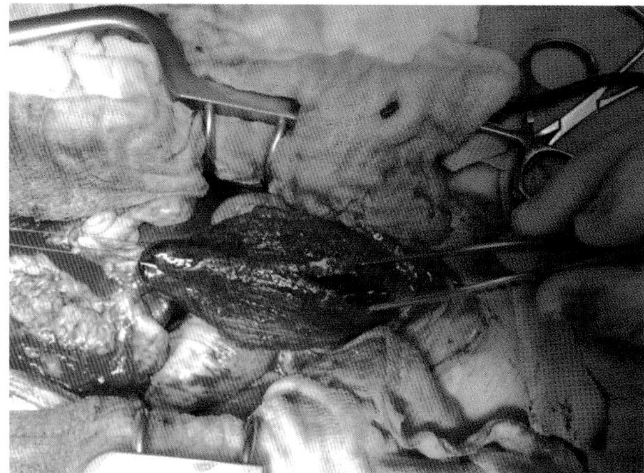

Fig. 4.26 Bladder rupture in a dog following a road traffic accident.

al., 2011). More extensive techniques, such as uretero-colonic and trigone-colonic anastomosis, have also been reported, but these are associated with high complication rates.

Tube cystostomy: indications

Tube cystostomy is performed when urinary diversion or prevention of bladder distension is required. Several types of catheter may be used, including Foley, mushroom-tip (de Pezzer) and percutaneous. Low-profile cystostomy tubes are also available; these were designed by modification of gastrostomy tubes and are designed for longer-term use (Stevenson et al., 2001). Tube cystostomy can be performed open or can be placed laparoscopically (Fig. 4.28).

Step by step: tube cystostomy

- A caudal laparotomy is performed and the cystostomy tube is pulled through a stab incision in the body wall adjacent to the bladder (Fig. 4.27a).
- A purse-string suture is then placed in the bladder adjacent to the abdominal incision using monofilament absorbable suture material (Fig. 4.27b).
- A stab incision is made into the bladder in the centre of the purse-string, and the tip of the catheter is placed through this. If a Foley is used it should be inflated with the appropriate volume of saline to secure the tube within the bladder.
- The purse-string suture is tied, and three or four non-penetrating interrupted sutures are placed between the bladder and the body wall (an omental flap can also be wrapped around the tube) (Fig. 4.27c–e).
- The laparotomy incision is closed routinely, and the cystostomy tube is secured to the skin via a Roman sandal suture (Fig. 4.27f).
- A dressing is placed over the tube's exit point, and a string vest is applied.
- A minimally invasive technique using a pig-tail catheter can be performed rapidly if surgical laparotomy is not possible/required. The catheter contains a stylet, which is used to penetrate the abdominal wall and bladder and guide the catheter inside. The stylet is removed and the distal end of the catheter is coiled by pulling and securing the incorporated string, which then prevents catheter removal (Fig. 4.29a–d).

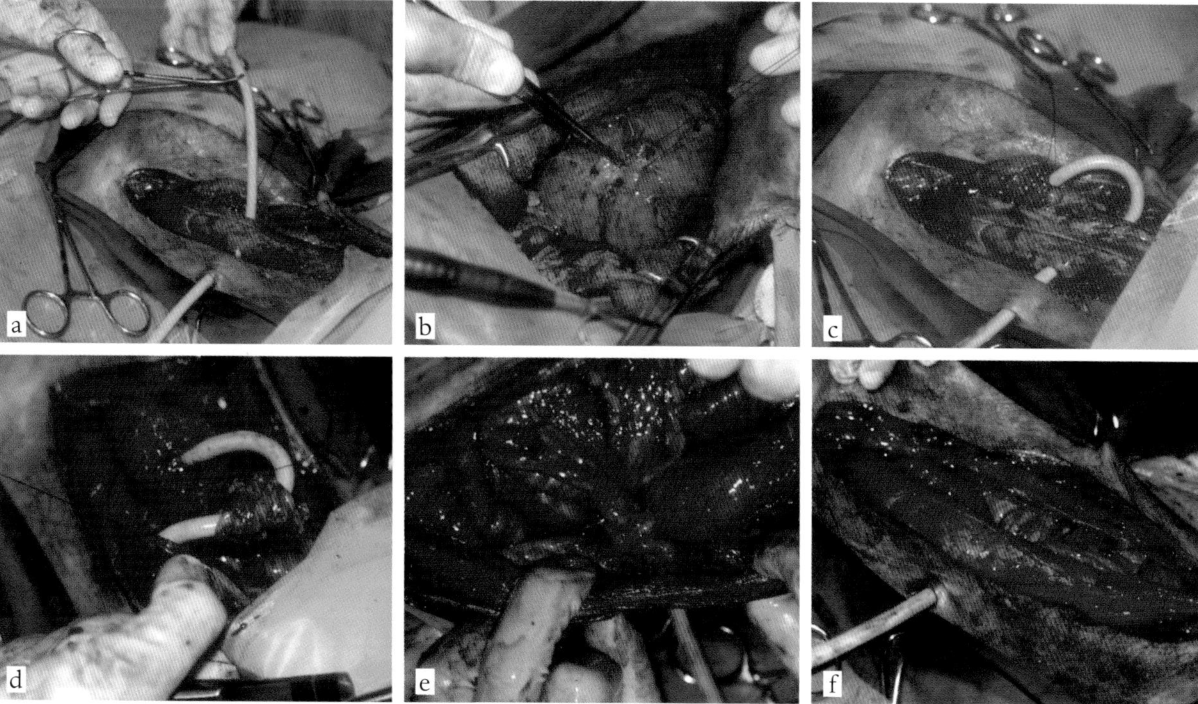

Fig. 4.27a–f Open cystostomy tube placement.

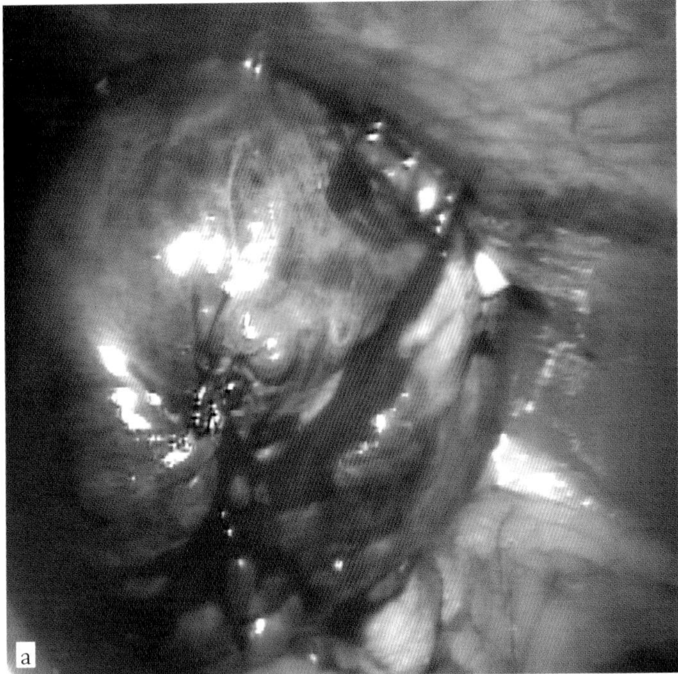
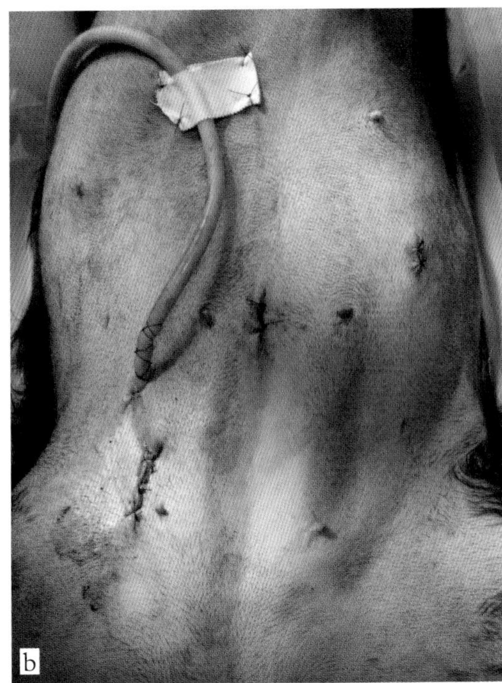

Fig. 4.28a,b Laparoscopically guided cystostomy tube placement.

Urethral sphincter mechanism incompetence (USMI)

Key points

- Contributing factors for USMI include bladder position, urethral tone and length, body size and breed, gonadectomy and hormones.
- USMI-related incontinence is unlikely to be cured by a single type of therapy.
- Medical treatment with oestrogens or sympathomimetics should be tried before recommending surgery.
- Surgical treatments include colposuspension, techniques to reposition the bladder (urethropexy/ cystourethropexy), intra-urethral injections of

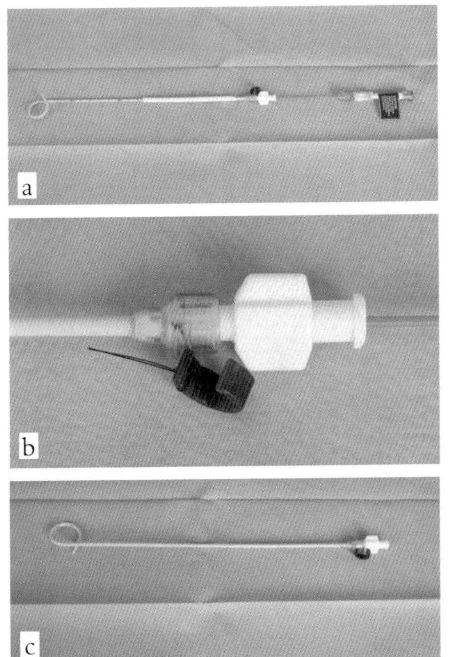
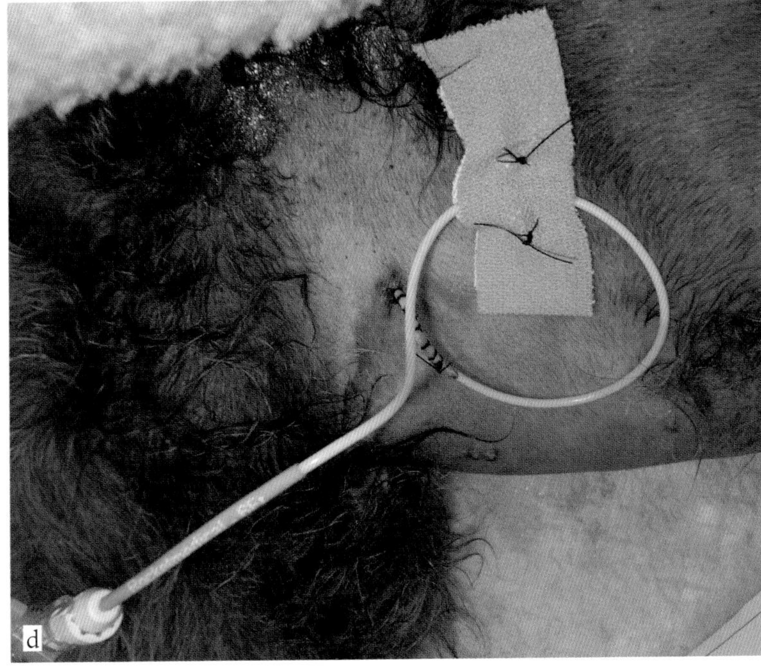

Fig. 4.29a–d Placement of a pigtail catheter. a. The entire pigtail is presented here alongside the delivery system. b. Close-up view of the locking system. c. The pigtail catheter is shown without the trocar. The loop is maintained in place by the locking mechanism located at the hub of the catheter. d. Pigtail catheter in place.

collagen, transvaginal tape-obturator (TVT-O) and artificial urethral sphincter placement (AUS).
- Medical and surgical treatments in the male dog tend to be less successful than in the female.

USMI is the most common cause of urinary incontinence in the adult dog, and is second only to ureteral ectopia in the juvenile dog. It is rarely seen in the cat. The condition may be congenital or acquired, with congenital conditions including absence of the urethra, diverticulum and urethral dilation. Acquired USMI in the dog usually follows neutering, and is seen in up to 20% of female spayed dogs. The precise cause of USMI is unknown, but contributing factors are thought to be related to bladder position ('intra-pelvic bladder'), urethral tone and length (less tone and short urethra), body size and breed (larger breeds predisposed), gonadectomy and hormones (Adams and DiBartola, 1983; Applegate et al., 2017; Hamaide et al., 2005; Holt and Thrusfield, 1993; Krawiec, 1989). Although rare, USMI can also affect male dogs and may be congenital or acquired. Congenital causes include urethral dilatation or prostatic diverticulum, and the acquired form is associated with neutering, larger breeds and an intra-pelvic bladder (Aaron et al., 1996; Power et al., 1998).

Investigations

Diagnosis is made by exclusion of other causes of incontinence (anatomical, neurogenic, calculi, infection) and investigations should include a complete blood count, serum biochemistry, urinalysis, urine culture and digital rectal and vestibular examination. Blood tests and urinalysis are usually unremarkable unless a UTI is present. Advanced imaging such as retrograde urethrocystography and/or IV urography should be performed when incontinence is suspected to be congenital.

Treatment

Whilst there are many treatment options available, USMI-related incontinence is unlikely to be cured by a single type of therapy: single-therapy treatment provides a cure in only around 50% of patients.

Medical treatment with oestrogens or sympathomimetic agents, which increase urethral sphincter tone, is often trialled initially, with diethylstilboestrol (DES) and phenylpropanolamine (PPA) being the most commonly used drugs, respectively. When used in high doses, DES can cause side effects such as bone marrow toxicity and alopecia, and so dosages greater than 1 mg/day should be avoided. The main disadvantage of PPA is that it has to be administered two to three times daily. A combination of both drugs may allow lower dosages to be used, and therefore with fewer side effects.

Surgical treatments include colposuspension, techniques to reposition the bladder (urethropexy/cystourethropexy), intra-urethral injections of collagen, transvaginal tape-obturator (TVT-O) and artificial urethral sphincter placement (AUS).

Both medical and surgical treatments in the male dog tend to be less successful than in the female (Holt, 2012). Medical management with PPA, oestrogens and anticholinergic drugs has been reported, but the reported response to these agents is poor (Aaron et al., 1996). Treatment with methyl-testosterone has also been previously reported, with poor results (Aaron et al., 1996). However, a recent study found a response to treatment with testosterone cypionate in 50% (4/8) of dogs, and no adverse effects (e.g. prostatic hyperplasia and behavioural aggression due to androgenic stimulation) were encountered (Palerme et al., 2017).

Colposuspension

This technique involves anchoring the vaginal wall on either side of the urethra to the prepubic tendon, with the aim of increasing the functional urethral length and relocating the bladder neck to an intra-abdominal position (Fig. 4.30a–c). The short-term outcome is often excellent, though the success rate for long-term complete continence is only around 50% (Holt, 1985, 1990a). Complications include recurrent UTIs, tenesmus, pain during first defaecation and increased frequency of urination.

Cystourethropexy and urethropexy

These techniques also result in relocation of the bladder neck into an intra-abdominal position, and involve placing anchoring sutures through the seromuscular layer of the bladder and/or urethra and the prepubic tendon. Urethropexy is reported to result in continence in 56% of dogs (White, 2001), whereas only 20% of dogs were cured in a study describing cystourethropexy (Massat et al., 1993). A more recent study reported complete continence in 70% of bitches following a combination of colposuspension and urethropexy (Martinoli et al., 2013).

Intra-urethral injection of collagen

Bovine cross-linked collagen is the recommended material for submucosal circumferential urethral injection, but recurrence of incontinence generally occurs within a year and the procedure has been associated with lymphoplasmacytic reactions (Sumner et al., 2012).

Transvaginal tape-obturator

TVT-O involves placement of a tape which is placed around the dorsal urethra, through the obturator foraminae and is tied on the ventral aspect of the pubic

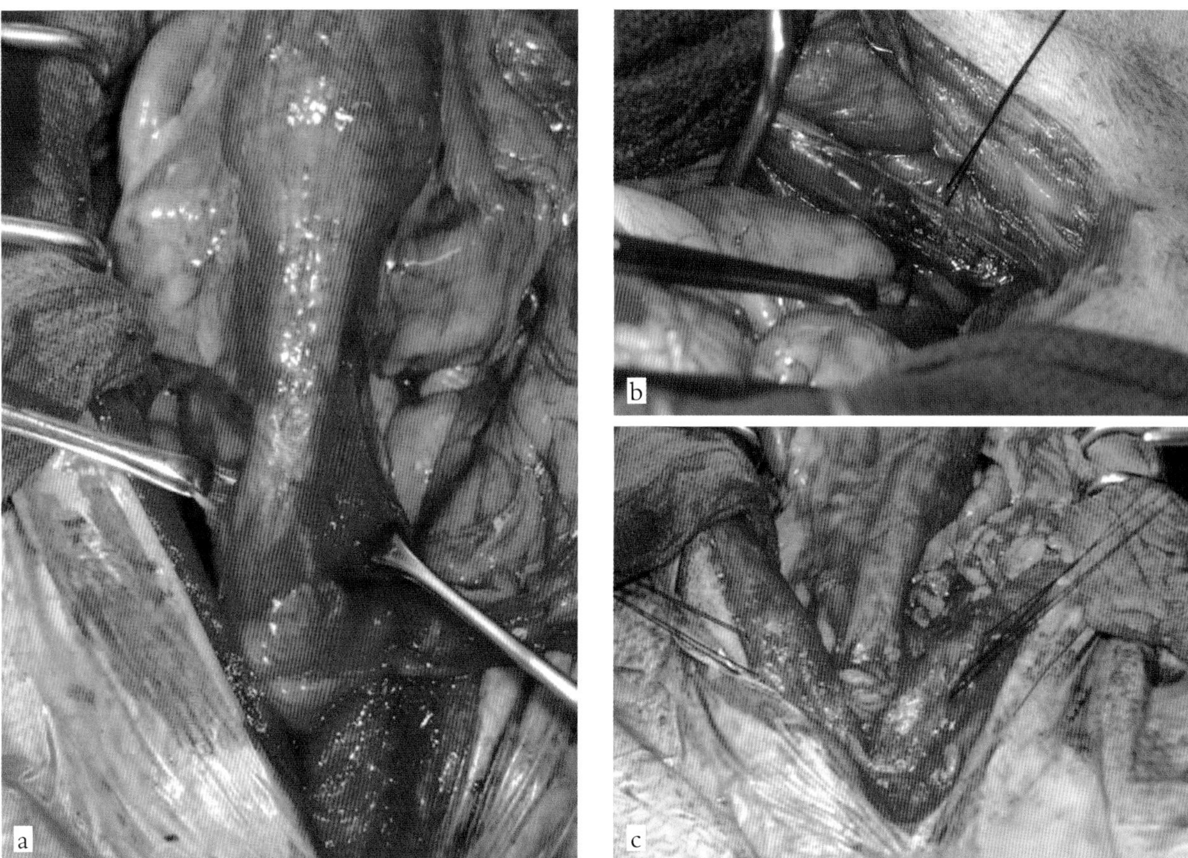

Fig. 4.30a–c Colposuspension. a. The Allis tissue forceps are holding the vaginal wall on each side of the bladder neck. b. Non-absorbable sutures are placed through the vaginal wall and into the prepubic tendon. c. Sutures in position before tying. It is important not to over- or under-tie these sutures. It is recommended to tie them with either a urinary catheter in place or an instrument positioned between the pubic bone and urethra, to avoid over-tying. Conversely, it is recommended to tie the sutures after the caudal part of the linea alba has been sutured to avoid under-tying.

symphysis. In one study, six out of seven dogs were continent at the mean follow-up (11.3 months). Urethral pressure profiles showed significantly increased maximal urethral closure pressure and integrated pressure, and no postoperative complications were encountered (Claeys et al. 2010).

Artificial urethral sphincter

This more recent procedure is aimed at maintaining a constant low level of urethral compression, and is gaining popularity. Its uses include management of USMI, pelvic bladder, ectopic ureter when incontinence continues despite other treatments, and urethral hypoplasia. The device has recently been used in cats with USMI, with resolution of incontinence in two of three cases in one report (Wilson et al., 2016). The silicone hydraulic occluder is placed around the proximal urethra and is connected via tubing to a subcutaneous port located on the caudal abdomen, where it can be inflated with saline as necessary until continence is achieved. Cuffs are available in diameters (named according to that of the closed cuff) ranging from 6 to 16 mm and in widths of either 11 or 14 mm. For dogs, a 14 mm width is usually suitable, and 8, 10 and 12 mm are the diameters most often used (Currao et al., 2013; Reeves et al., 2012).

Step by step: artificial urethral sphincter (AUS)

- A caudal ventral midline coeliotomy is performed and extended to the pubic brim for maximal exposure of the cranial urethra.
- In the female, the bladder is retracted with a stay suture, and a 2 cm area of urethra is exposed from the peri-urethral adipose tissue using blunt dissection, approximately 3–4 cm caudal to the trigone (Fig. 4.31a).
- In the male, a 2 cm area of urethra is exposed just caudal to the prostate. Alternatively, the AUS can be placed around the urethra in the perineal region (Fig. 4.32).
- A piece of suture or a Penrose drain is used to measure the circumference of the isolated urethra. The required AUS cuff diameter size is chosen by dividing the circumference by two (e.g. a 20 mm circumference would require a 10 mm cuff). The next size up is

always chosen if the measured circumference is between sizes.

- The AUS is primed with fluid to flush out the air – this is done by inserting a catheter into the actuating tubing and injecting saline.
- The access port is also primed with saline – this is done using a 22-gauge Huber needle which prevents removal of a core of the silicone.
- The tubing is connected to the access port, and inflation of the cuff is trialled.
- The AUS is deflated and placed around the exposed urethra, ensuring that the actuating tubing is directed cranially (Fig. 4.31b,c).
- A length of polypropylene or nylon suture is passed through the eyelets of the cuff ends and tied to encircle the urethra.
- An area of skin on the caudal abdomen is undermined to expose the external rectus sheath for placement of the access port. The port location should be easily accessible for cuff inflation (i.e. lateral to the rectus abdominis muscle).
- The tubing is disconnected from the port and is tunnelled through the caudal abdominal wall musculature to the desired port location (Fig. 4.31d).
- The port is reattached to the tubing, the boot cuff advanced over the male adaptor-tubing connection and the port sutured to the external rectus fascia with polypropylene suture. The port should be sutured so as not to kink the actuating tubing (Fig. 4.31e).
- The abdominal incision is closed, ensuring that the elevated subcutaneous tissue is reapposed to the external rectus sheath.

Often placement of the deflated cuff is enough for continence to be achieved (in the female dog). In cases where incontinence remains, cuff inflation should be delayed for six weeks post-surgery to allow for resolution of inflammation and re-vascularisation of the periurethral tissue. After this time, the author prefers to inject 0.1 ml of saline with a Huber needle every two weeks until continence is gained. This should be performed under aseptic conditions, and before injection the AUS should be aspirated to confirm prior volume placement. Following inflation, the animal should be observed as being able to urinate and the owner should be instructed to monitor for stranguria/dysuria at home.

Long-term outcome is excellent due to the ability to inflate the cuff (and therefore partially occlude the urethra) as needed. Complete continence in the medium term was reported to be 36–56% (Currao et al., 2013; Delisser et al., 2012), but a recent study of 20 female dogs found a long-term (mean 3.5 years) complete continence of 90% (Gomes et al., 2018). Minor complications include dysuria, bacterial cystitis, urinary retention, incisional seroma, haematuria and pain when urinating. A reported major complication is urethral stricture (Currao et al., 2013), and the authors have

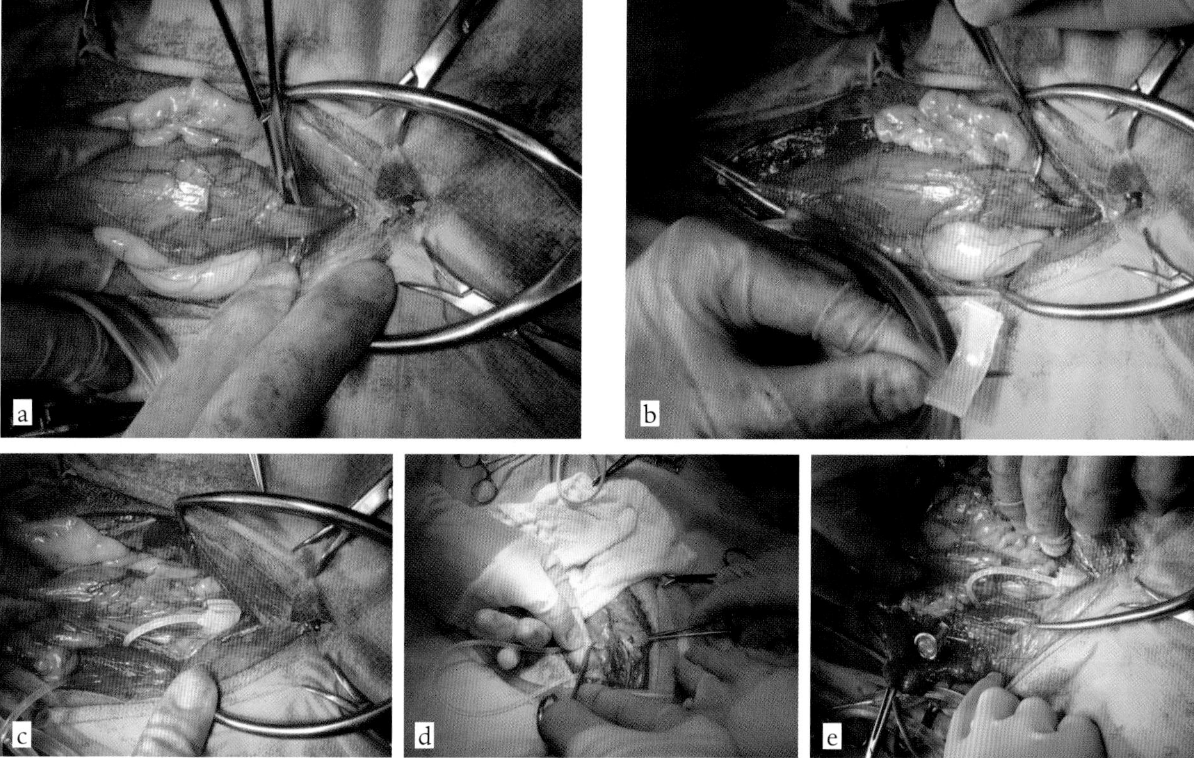

Fig. 4.31a–e Artificial sphincter placement in a female dog (intra-abdominal approach). See details in the step-by-step procedure.

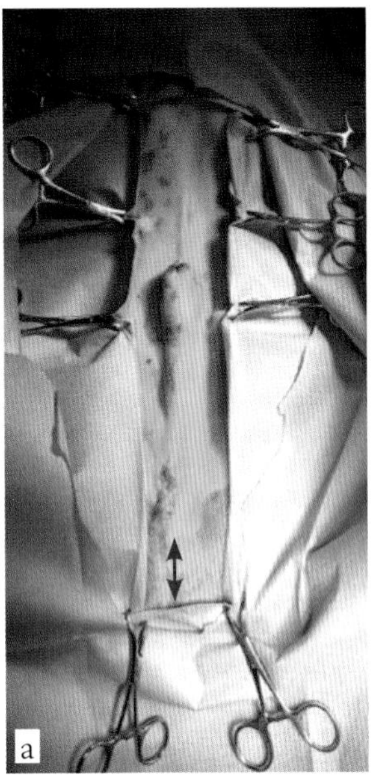

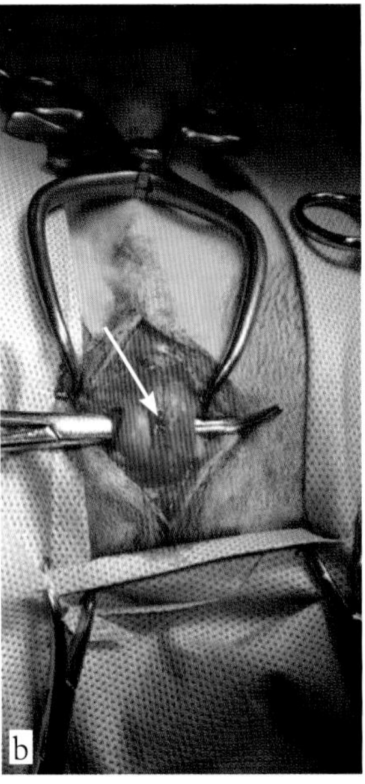

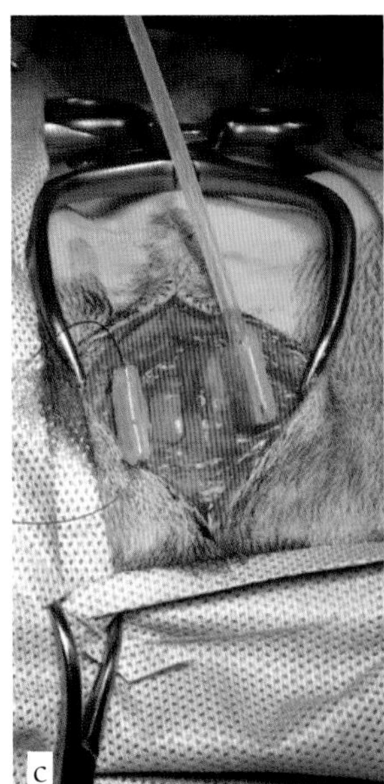

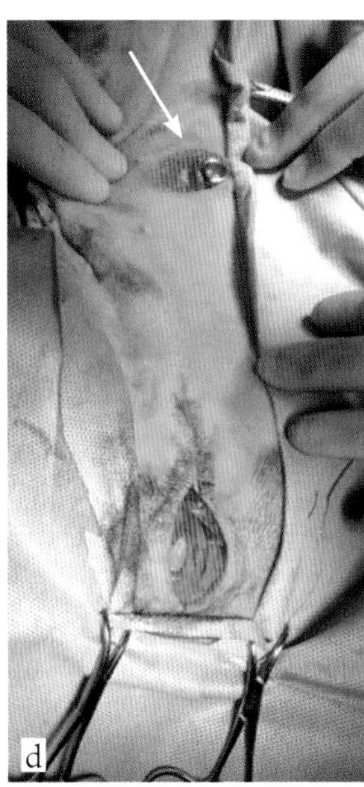

Fig. 4.32a–d Artificial sphincter placement in a male dog (perineal approach). a. Surgical site. The urethra needs to be catheterised retrograde; the incision site is shown (red double arrow).b. A tunnel is created dorsal to the penile corpus spongiosum and bulbospongiosus muscle. The retractor penis muscle is visible ventral to the urethra (white arrow). c. The cuff of the AUS is inserted around the corpus spongiosum and bulbospongiosus muscle. d. The tubing is tunnelled cranially and the port is inserted on the side of the prepuce (white arrow).

observed infection of the port/cuff site and accidental puncture of the device, necessitating implant removal and replacement respectively.

References

Aaron, A., Eggleton, K., Power, C. and Holt, P.E. (1996) Urethral sphincter mechanism incompetence in male dogs: a retrospective analysis of 54 cases. *Veterinary Record* 139, 542–546.

Adams, W.M. and DiBartola, S.P. (1983) Radiographic and clinical features of pelvic bladder in the dog. *Journal of the American Veterinary Medical Association* 182, 1212–1217.

Adin, C.A., Herrgesell, E.J., Nyland, T.G., Hughes, J.M., Gregory, C.R., Kyles, A.E., Cowgill, L.D. and Ling, G.V. (2003) Antegrade pyelography for suspected ureteral obstruction in cats: 11 cases (1995–2001). *Journal of the American Veterinary Medical Association* 222, 1576–1581.

Albasan, H., Osborne, C.A., Lulich, J.P., Lekcharoensuk, C., Koehler, L.A., Ulrich, L.K. and Swanson, L.L. (2009) Rate and frequency of recurrence of uroliths after an initial ammonium urate, calcium oxalate, or struvite urolith in cats. *Journal of the American Veterinary Medical Association* 235, 1450–1455.

Applegate, R., Olin, S. and Sabatino, B. (2017) Urethral sphincter mechanism incompetence in dogs: an update. *Journal of the American Animal Hospital Association* 54, 22–29.

Bartges, J.W., Kirk, C. and Lane, I.F. (2004) Update: management of calcium oxalate uroliths in dogs and cats. *Veterinary Clinics of North America: Small Animal Practice* 34, 969–987.

Berent, A.C. (2015) Interventional urology: endourology in small animal veterinary medicine. *Veterinary Clinics of North America: Small Animal Practice* 45, 825–855.

Berent, A.C. and Weisse, C. (2011) The SUB: a subcutaneous ureteral bypass system, a surgical guide. Available at: www.norfolkvetproducts.com (accessed 1 December 2017).

Berent, A.C., Weisse, C., Beal, M.W., Brown, D.C., Todd, K. and Bagley D. (2011) Use of indwelling, double-pigtail stents for treatment of malignant ureteral obstruction in dogs: 12 cases (2006–2009). *Journal of the American Veterinary Medical Association* 238, 1017–1025.

Berent, A.C., Weisse, C.W., Todd, K. and Bagley, D.H. (2014) Technical and clinical outcomes of ureteral stenting in cats with benign ureteral obstruction: 69 cases (2006–2010). *Journal of the American Veterinary Medical Association* 244, 559–576.

Bigge, L.A., Brown, D.J. and Penninck, D.G. (2001) Correlation between coagulation profile findings and bleeding complications after ultrasound-guided biopsies: 434 cases (1993–1996). *Journal of the American Animal Hospital Association* 37, 228–233.

Bouma, J.L., Aronson, L.R., Keith, D.G. and Saunders, H.M. (2003) Use of computed tomography renal angiography for screening feline renal transplant donors. *Veterinary Radiology & Ultrasound* 44, 636–641.

Brown, N.O., Parks, J.L. and Greene, R.W. (1977) Recurrence of canine urolithiasis. *Journal of the American Veterinary Medical Association* 170, 419–422.

Bryan, J.N., Henry, C.J., Turnquist, S.E., Tyler, J.W., Liptak, J.M., Rizzo, S.A., Sfiligoi, G., Steinberg, S.J., Smith, A.N. and Jackson, T. (2006) Primary renal neoplasia of dogs. *Journal of Veterinary Internal Medicine* 20, 1155–1160.

Cannon, A.B., Westropp, J.L., Ruby, A.L. and Kass, P.H. (2007) Evaluation of trends in urolith composition in cats: 5,230 cases (1985–2004). *Journal of the American Veterinary Medical Association* 231, 570–576.

Claeys, S., De Leval, J. and Hamaide, A. (2010) Transobturator vaginal tape inside out for treatment of urethral sphincter mechanism incompetence: preliminary results in 7 female dogs. *Veterinary Surgery* 39, 969–979.

Cray, M., Berent, A.C., Weisse, C.W. and Bagley, D. (2018) Treatment of pyonephrosis with a subcutaneous ureteral bypass device in four cats. *Journal of the American Veterinary Medical Association* 252, 744–753.

Currao, R.L., Berent, A.C., Weisse, C. and Fox, P. (2013) Use of a percutaneously controlled urethral hydraulic occluder for treatment of refractory urinary incontinence in 18 female dogs. *Veterinary Surgery* 42, 440–447.

Delisser, P.J., Friend, E.J., Chanoit, G.P. and Parsons K.J. (2012) Static hydraulic urethral sphincter for treatment of urethral sphincter mechanism incompetence in 11 dogs. *Journal of Small Animal Practice* 53, 338–343.

Evans, H.E. and de Lahunta, A. (2013) *Miller's Anatomy of the Dog*, 4th edn. Elsevier Saunders, St. Louis, Missouri.

Forman, M.A., Francey, T. and Cowgill, L.D. (2004) Use of glucagon in the management of acute ureteral obstruction in 25 cats. *Journal of Veterinary Internal Medicine* 18, 417 (A).

Gerber, B., Eichenberger, S. and Reusch, C.E. (2008) Guarded long-term prognosis in male cats with urethral obstruction. *Journal of Feline Medicine and Surgery* 10, 16–23.

Gomes, C., Doran, I., Friend, E., Tivers, M.S. and Chanoit, G.P.A. (2018) Long-term outcome of female dogs treated with static hydraulic urethral sphincter for urethral sphincter mechanism incompetence. *Journal of the American Animal Hospital Association* (in press).

Halfacree, Z.J., Tivers, M.S. and Brockman, D.J. (2011) Vaginourethroplasty as a salvage procedure for management of traumatic urethral rupture in a cat. *Journal of Feline Medicine and Surgery* 13, 768–771.

Hamaide, A.J., Verstegen, J.P., Snaps, F.R., Onclin, K.J. and Balligand, M.H. (2005) Influence of the estrous cycle on urodynamic and morphometric measurements of the lower portion of the urogenital tract in dogs. *American Journal of Veterinary Research* 66, 1075–1083.

Holt, P.E. (1985) Urinary incontinence in the bitch due to sphincter mechanism incompetence: surgical treatment. *Journal of Small Animal Practice* 26, 237–246.

Holt, P.E. (1990a) Long-term evaluation of colposuspension in the treatment of urinary incontinence due to incompetence of the urethral sphincter mechanism in the bitch. *Veterinary Record* 127, 537–542.

Holt, P.E. (1990b) Urinary incontinence in dogs and cats. *Veterinary Record* 127, 347–350.

Holt, P.E. (2012) Sphincter mechanism incompetence. In: Johnston, S.A. and Tobias, K.M. (eds) *Veterinary Surgery: Small Animal*. Elsevier Saunders, St. Louis, Missouri, pp. 2011–2018.

Holt, P.E. and Thrusfield, M.V. (1993) Association in bitches between breed, size, neutering and docking, and acquired urinary incontinence due to incompetence of the urethral sphincter mechanism. *Veterinary Record* 133, 177–180.

Holt, P.E., Gibbs, C. and Pearson, H. (1982) Canine ectopic ureter – a review of twenty-nine cases. *Journal of Small Animal Practice* 23, 195–208.

Holt, P.E., Thrusfield, M.V. and Moore, A.H. (2000) Breed predisposition to ureteral ectopia in bitches in the UK. *Veterinary Record* 146, 561.

Houston, D.M. and Moore, A.E.P. (2010) Canine and feline urolithiasis: examination of over 50 000 urolith submissions to the Canadian veterinary urolith centre from 1998 to 2008. *Canadian Veterinary Journal* 50, 1263–1268.

Krawiec, D.R. (1989) Diagnosis and treatment of acquired canine urinary incontinence. *European Journal of Companion Animal Practice*, 19, 12–20.

Kyles, A.E., Hardie, E.M., Wooden, B.G., Adin, C.A., Stone, E.A., Gregory, C.R., Mathews, K.G., Cowgill, L.D., Vaden, S., Nyland, T.G. and Ling, G.V. (2005) Clinical, clinicopathologic, radiographic, and ultrasonographic abnormalities in cats with ureteral calculi: 163 cases (1984–2002). *Journal of the American Veterinary Medical Association* 226, 932–936.

Ling, G.V., Franti, C.E., Ruby, A.L., Johnson, D.L. and Thurmond, M. (1998) Urolithiasis in dogs. I: Mineral prevalence and interrelations of mineral composition, age, and sex. *American Journal of Veterinary Research* 59, 624–629.

Livet, V., Pillard, P., Goy-Thollot, I., Maleca, D., Cabon, Q., Remy, D., Fau, D., Viguier, É., Pouzot, C., Carozzo, C. and Cachon, T. (2017) Placement of subcutaneous ureteral bypasses without fluoroscopic guidance in cats with ureteral obstruction: 19 cases (2014–2016). *Journal of Feline Medicine and Surgery* 19, 1030–1039.

Low, W.W., Uhl, J.M., Kass, P.H., Ruby, A.L. and Westropp, J.L. (2010) Evaluation of trends in urolith composition and characteristics of dogs with urolithiasis: 25,499 cases (1985–2006). *Journal of the American Veterinary Medical Association* 236, 193–200.

Lulich, J.P., Perrine, L., Osborne, C.A. and Unger, L. (1992) Postsurgical recurrence of calcium oxalate uroliths in dogs. *Journal of Veterinary Internal Medicine* 6, 119 (A).

Manassero, M., Decambron, A., Viateau, V., Bedu, A., Vallefuoco, R., Benchekroun, G., Moissonnier, P. and Maurey, C. (2014) Indwelling double pigtail ureteral stent combined or not with surgery for feline ureterolithiasis: complications and outcome in 15 cases. *Journal of Feline Medicine and Surgery* 16, 623–630.

Martinoli, S., Nelissen, P. and White, R.A.S. (2013) The outcome of combined urethropexy and colposuspension for management of bitches with urinary incontinence associated with urethral sphincter mechanism incompetence. *Veterinary Surgery* 43, 52–57.

Massat, B.J., Gregory, C.R., Ling, G.V., Cardinet, G.H. and Lewis EL. (1993) Cystourethropexy to correct refractory urinary incontinence due to urethral sphincter mechanism incompetence. Preliminary results in ten bitches. *Veterinary Surgery* 22, 260–268.

Mathews, K. (2017) Ureters. In: Johnston, S.A. and Tobias, K.M. (eds) *Veterinary Surgery: Small Animal*. Elsevier Saunders, St. Louis, Missouri, pp. 2202–2217.

Mayhew, P.D., Lee, K.C., Gregory, S.P. and Brockman, D.J. (2006) Comparison of two surgical techniques for management of intramural ureteral ectopia in dogs: 36 cases (1994–2004). *Journal of the American Veterinary Medical Association* 229, 389–393.

McLaughlin, R. and Miller, C.W. (1991) Urinary incontinence after surgical repair of ureteral ectopia in dogs. *Veterinary Surgery* 20, 100–103.

Osborne, C.A., Lulich, J.P., Kruger, J.M., Ulrich, L.K. and

Koehler, L.A. (2008) Analysis of 451,891 canine uroliths, feline uroliths, and feline urethral plugs from 1981 to 2007: perspectives from the Minnesota Urolith Center. *The Veterinary Clinics of North America: Small Animal Practice* 39, 183–197.

Palerme, J.S., Mazepa, A., Hutchins, R.G., Ziglioli, V. and Vaden, S.L. (2017) Clinical response and side effects associated with testosterone cypionate for urinary incontinence in male dogs. *Journal of the American Animal Hospital Association* 53, 285–290.

Pinel, C.B., Monnet, E. and Reems, M.R. (2013) Laparoscopic-assisted cystotomy for urolith removal in dogs and cats – 23 cases. *The Canadian Veterinary Journal* 54, 36–41.

Power, S.C., Eggleton, K.E., Aaron, A.J., Holt, P.E. and Cripps, P.J. (1998) Urethral sphincter mechanism incompetence in the male dog: importance of bladder neck position, proximal urethral length and castration. *Journal of Small Animal Practice* 39, 69–72.

Pratschke, K.M. (2015) Ureteral implantation using a three-stitch ureteroneocystostomy: description of technique and outcome in nine dogs. *Journal of Small Animal Practice* 56, 566–571.

Rawlings, C.A., Bjorling, D.E. and Christie, B.A. (2003a) Principles of urinary tract surgery. In: Slatter, D.H. (ed.) *Textbook of Small Animal Surgery*. Elsevier Saunders, Philadelphia, Pennsylvania, pp. 1594–1628.

Rawlings, C.A., Mahaffey, M.B., Barsanti, J.A. and Canalis, C. (2003b) Use of laparoscopic-assisted cystoscopy for removal of urinary calculi in dogs. *Journal of the American Veterinary Medical Association* 222, 759–761.

Reeves, L., Adin, C., McLoughlin, M., Ham, K. and Chew, D. (2012) Outcome after placement of an artificial urethral sphincter in 27 dogs. *Veterinary Surgery* 42, 12–18.

Reichle, J.K., DiBartola, S.P. and Léveillé, R. (2002) Renal ultrasonographic and computed tomographic appearance, volume, and function of cats with autosomal dominant polycystic kidney disease. *Veterinary Radiology & Ultrasound* 43, 368–373.

Ross, S.J., Osborne, C.A., Lekcharoensuk, C., Koehler, L.A. and Polzin, D.J. (2007) A case-control study of the effects of nephrolithiasis in cats with chronic kidney disease. *Journal of the American Veterinary Medical Association* 230, 1854–1859.

Runge, J.J., Berent, A.C., Mayhew, P.D. and Weisse, C. (2011) Transvesicular percutaneous cystolithotomy for the retrieval of cystic and urethral calculi in dogs and cats: 27 cases (2006–2008). *Journal of the American Veterinary Medical Association* 239, 344–349.

Saeki, K., Fujita, A., Fujita, N., Nakagawa, T. and Nishimura, R. (2015) Total cystectomy and subsequent urinary diversion to the prepuce or vagina in dogs with transitional cell carcinoma of the trigone area: a report of 10 cases (2005–2011). *Canadian Veterinary Journal* 56, 73–80.

Samii, V.F., McLoughlin, M.A., Mattoon, J.S., Drost, W.T., Chew, D.J., DiBartola, S.P. and Hoshaw-Woodard, S. (2004) Digital fluoroscopic excretory urography, digital fluoroscopic urethrography, helical computed tomography, and cystoscopy in 24 dogs with suspected ureteral ectopia. *Journal of Veterinary Internal Medicine* 18, 271–281.

Segev, G., Livne, H., Ranen, E. and Lavy, E. (2011) Urethral obstruction in cats: predisposing factors, clinical, clinicopathological characteristics and prognosis. *Journal of Feline Medicine and Surgery* 13, 101–108.

Simon, J., Finter, F., Ignatius, A., Meilinger, M. and Dürselen, L. (2010) Maximum tensile force of different suture techniques in reconstruction of the renal remnant after nephron-sparing surgery. *Surgical Endoscopy* 25, 503–507.

Stevenson, M.A., Miller, N.A., Cornell, K.K., Glerum, L.E. and Rawlings, C.A. (2001) Low-profile cystostomy tubes in 2 dogs and a cat. *Veterinary Surgery* 30, 507.

Stone, E.A. and Barsanti, J.A. (1992) Surgical therapy for urinary tract trauma. In: Stone, E.A. *Urologic Surgery of the Dog and Cat*. Lea and Febiger, Philadelphia, Pennsylvania, p. 107.

Stone, E.A., Withrow, S.J., Page, R.L., Schwarz, P.D., Wheeler, S.L. and Seim, H.B. (1988) Ureterocolonic anastomosis in ten dogs with transitional cell carcinoma. *Veterinary Surgery* 17, 147–153.

Stone, E.A., George, T.F., Gilson, S.D. and Page, R.L. (1996) Partial cystectomy for urinary bladder neoplasia: surgical technique and outcome in 11 dogs. *Journal of Small Animal Practice* 37, 480–485.

Stone, E.A., Robertson, J.L. and Metcalf, M.R. (2002) The effect of nephrotomy on renal function and morphology in dogs. *Veterinary Surgery* 31, 391–397.

Sumner, J.P., Hardie, R.J., Henningson, J.N., Drees, R. and Bjorling, D. (2012) Evaluation of submucosally injected polyethylene glycol-based hydrogel and bovine cross-linked collagen in the canine urethra using cystoscopy, magnetic resonance imaging and histopathology. *Veterinary Surgery* 41, 655–663.

Vaden, S.L., Levine, J.F., Lees, G.E., Groman, R.P., Grauer, G.F. and Forrester, S.D. (2005a) Renal biopsy: a retrospective study of methods and complications in 283 dogs and 65 cats. *Journal of Veterinary Internal Medicine* 19, 794–801.

Vaden, S.L., Levine, J.F., Lees, G.E., Groman, R.P., Grauer, G.F. and Forrester, S.D. (2005b) Renal biopsy: a retrospective study of methods and complications in 283 dogs and 65 cats. *Journal of Veterinary Internal Medicine* 19, 794–801.

Wang, B., Bhadra, N. and Grill, W.M. (1999) Functional anatomy of the male feline urethra: morphological and physiological correlations. *Journal of Urology* 161, 654–659.

White, R.N. (2001) Urethropexy for the management of urethral sphincter mechanism incompetence in the bitch. *Journal of Small Animal Practice* 42, 481–486.

Wilson, K.E., Berent, A.C. and Weisse, C.W. (2016) Use of a percutaneously controlled hydraulic occluder for treatment of refractory urinary incontinence in three female cats. *Journal of the American Veterinary Medical Association* 248, 544–551.

Wormser, C., Clarke, D.L. and Aronson, L.R. (2016) Outcomes of ureteral surgery and ureteral stenting in cats: 117 cases (2006–2014). *Journal of the American Veterinary Medical Association* 248, 518–525.

Zaid, M.S., Berent, A.C., Weisse, C. and Caceres A. (2011) Feline ureteral strictures: 10 cases (2007–2009). *Journal of Veterinary Internal Medicine* 25, 222–229.

Case 4.1

A 3-year-old male neutered English bulldog presents with vomiting, abdominal pain and lethargy. The owner has noted stranguria for the past 48 hours.

- What further clinical history is important in reaching a diagnosis?
- What further clinical examination do you wish to perform?

On further discussion with the owner, you discover that the dog had been frequently passing small amounts of urine over the past 2 days, but in the past 12 hours had not been able to pass any at all despite straining. The dog had a history of two previous episodes of urethral obstruction in the past, which were treated by urethral flushing and cystotomy. The uroliths were not submitted for analysis. On examination, the dog is tachycardic (128 bpm) and panting. The mucous membranes are pale and tacky, with a capillary refill time of two seconds. On rectal examination the prostate feels normal, and on abdominal palpation the bladder is found to be enlarged and hard.

- What are your differentials at this stage?
- What diagnostic procedures would you like to perform?

The owner was informed that urethral obstruction due to uroliths was the most likely diagnosis. Due to the dog's young age and previous history of obstruction due to uroliths, other causes of urethral obstruction such as neoplasia were less likely.

Biochemistry revealed a moderate azotaemia (BUN 14 mmol/l and creatinine 212 μmol/l) and moderate hyperkalaemia (6.8 mmol/l). The dog was mildly hypotensive (mean blood pressure 56 mmHg). The dog received fluid resuscitation and a dose of calcium gluconate, and within one hour the heart rate had normalised and the potassium had reduced to 6.0 mmol/l. The dog was then sedated for a retrograde urethrogram with fluoroscopy (Fig. 4.33).

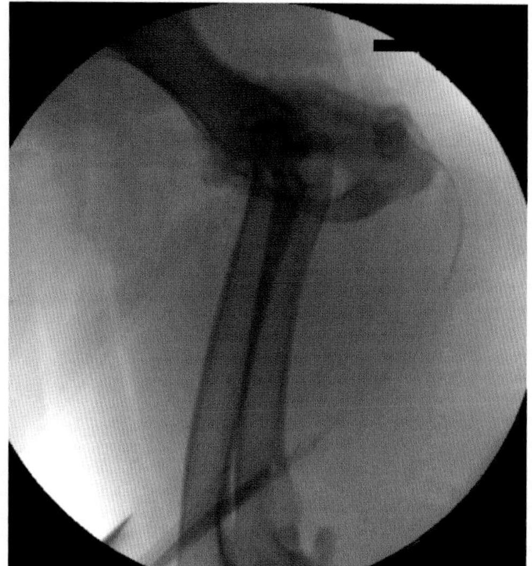

Fig. 4.33 Fluoroscopic image of the pelvis and urethra showing two filling defects in the penile urethra.

- What is the most likely diagnosis based from the image presented?
- What is the next step in management of this case?

Retrograde hydropropulsion was attempted, but it was not possible to dislodge the urethroliths. During sedation the dog developed a cardiac arrhythmia, and further biochemical analysis showed that the serum potassium had increased again to 7.0 mmol/l.

- What are the treatment options available now?
- What procedure does the radiograph (Fig. 4.34) show has been performed?

As the dog was not fit for general anaesthesia, a pigtail cystostomy tube was placed to bypass the obstruction and help resolve the hyperkalaemia (Fig. 4.34). Urine was collected and submitted for urinalysis and culture and sensitivity. The dog received further calcium gluconate and was maintained on fluid therapy overnight.

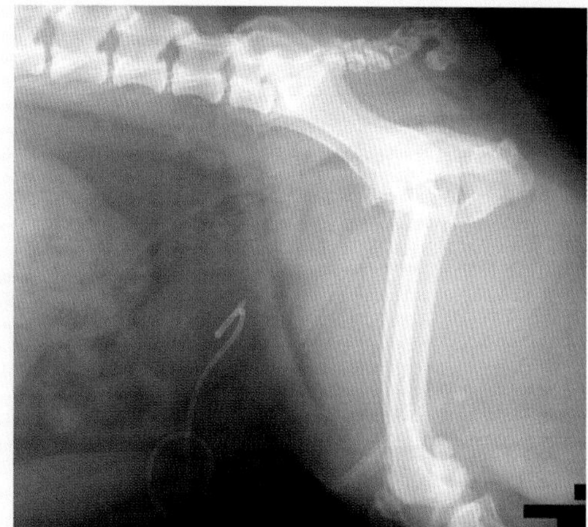

Fig. 4.34 Pigtail cystostomy tube in place.

- What surgical treatment options are available to the owner?
- What are the reported complications for each procedure?
- What long-term management may be required?

The following day the blood parameters had all normalised. The dog then underwent a scrotal ablation and scrotal urethrostomy, and a cystotomy was performed to enable flushing of the bladder and urethra until there were no remaining stones. The uroliths were submitted for compound analysis, and were confirmed to be cystine. Urine bacterial culture was negative. The dog was started on a therapeutic urine-alkalinising diet to help prevent future stone production.

Case 4.2

A 14-week-old female entire golden retriever presents with a lifelong history of urine leakage. In the past week the urine had been red-tinged according to the owner. Otherwise the dog has been well.

- What further clinical history is important in reaching a diagnosis?
- What further clinical examination do you wish to perform?

On further discussion with the owner, you discover that the dog does posture to urinate on walks, but in-between times has constant dripping of urine from the vulva. The dog has been treated twice for perivulval dermatitis and urinary tract infection. In the past week the dog has been polydipsic and spends longer posturing to urinate when outside.

On clinical examination the hair around the vulva is wet, but no other abnormalities are noted.

- What are your differentials at this stage?
- What diagnostic procedures would you like to perform?

Differential diagnoses of persistent urinary incontinence include recurrent urinary tract infection, ureteral ectopia, urethral sphincter mechanism incompetence and congenital malformations such as bladder hypoplasia or agenesis.

Urinalysis shows haematuria, proteinuria and bacteriuria, indicating bacterial cystitis.

The dog then undergoes diagnostic imaging followed by cystoscopy (Fig. 4.35).

- What is the diagnosis based on the image presented?
- What other imaging modalities can be used to make the diagnosis?

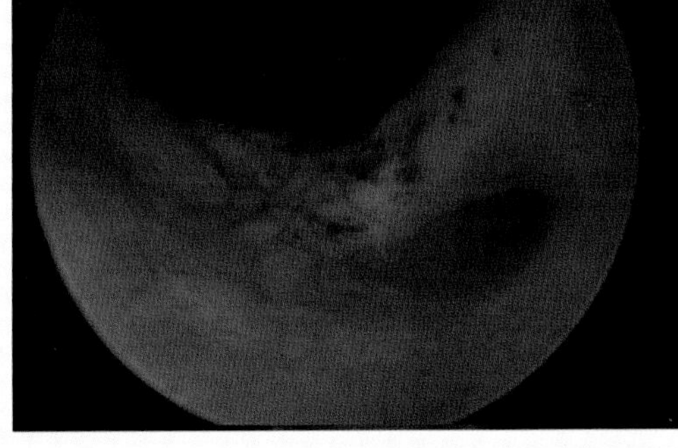

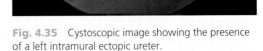

Fig. 4.35 Cystoscopic image showing the presence of a left intramural ectopic ureter.

The cystoscopic image shows the presence of a left intramural ectopic ureter. The bladder entrance at the top of the image, and the ureter opening, can be seen just distal to this, coursing alongside the bladder within the wall. The right ureter is also ectopic. A diagnosis of bilateral intramural ectopic ureter is made.

An intravenous urogram using computed tomography (CT IVU) is often performed prior to cystoscopy to help identify the ureters and classify them as intra- or extramural. A retrograde urethrocystogram (±fluoroscopy) is also useful in identifying ectopic ureter or any concurrent congenital urogenital abnormalities.

- What is the next step in management of this case?
- What surgical treatment options are available to the owner?
- What are the reported complications for each procedure?

Antibiosis was initiated on the basis of urine culture and sensitivity.

The dog underwent laser ablation of the ectopic ureters using cystoscopy. The alternative treatment for intramural ectopic ureters is open surgery and neo-ureterostomy.

Complications of laser ablation include urethritis, urethral obstruction due to post-laser inflammation, uroabdomen if lasering is performed too far cranially and the ureter is perforated and persistence of urinary incontinence.

Complications of neo-ureterostomy include ureteral obstruction causing hydro-ureter/hydronephritis due to postoperative swelling, recanalisation of the distal segment and persistence of urinary incontinence.

Surgery of the reproductive tract

5

Anna Nutt and Guillaume Chanoit

Chapter summary

Surgical procedures of the small animal reproductive tract are divided into two categories: those which *prevent* reproduction, reproductive diseases or diseases/conditions related to the presence of the reproductive organs and those which *treat* pathological conditions of the reproductive tract. Neutering (ovariectomy or ovariohysterectomy in females, and castration in males) is the most common surgical procedure. It may be performed to limit breeding, but also to prevent or treat tumours controlled by hormones, such as mammary, testicular and perianal tumours; prevent or treat diseases such as pyometra, metritis, prostatic abscessation; treat dystocia; and stabilise systemic conditions such as diabetes and epilepsy.

Diagnostic work-up of reproductive tract disease should start with a thorough physical examination. In females, this should include palpation of the mammary glands for masses/discharge/asymmetry; vaginal/vestibular examination or rectal exam for palpation of the vagina when it is too small for a digital evaluation; abdominal palpation for the presence of an enlarged uterus, a mass or pain; and examination of the vulva and perivulval skin for abnormal conformation or skin folds. In males, a rectal examination should be performed to evaluate the prostate for enlargement, abnormal texture, pain and mobility; and abdominal palpation should be performed for evidence of pain or enlarged sublumbar lymph nodes. The testicles should be palpated for size, asymmetry, texture and sensitivity, and the scrotum examined for thickenings, masses, sensitivity and scrotal adhesions. The penis and prepuce should be evaluated for abnormalities such as trauma, masses and congenital abnormalities, and this examination should include full extrusion of the penis.

Depending on the condition suspected, further investigations of reproductive tract disorders may include a complete blood count, serum biochemistry, hormonal assay, urinalysis, cytology (of masses, discharge, prostatic fluid and urine), culture (if infection is suspected), vaginal endoscopy and diagnostic imaging (radiography, ultrasonography, computed tomography).

5.1 Female reproductive tract

5.1.1 Surgical anatomy

The female reproductive tract is made up of the ovaries, oviduct, uterus, vagina, vulva and mammary glands (Fig. 5.1).

The ovaries are around 15 mm long in a medium-sized dog and 8 mm long in the cat. They are located

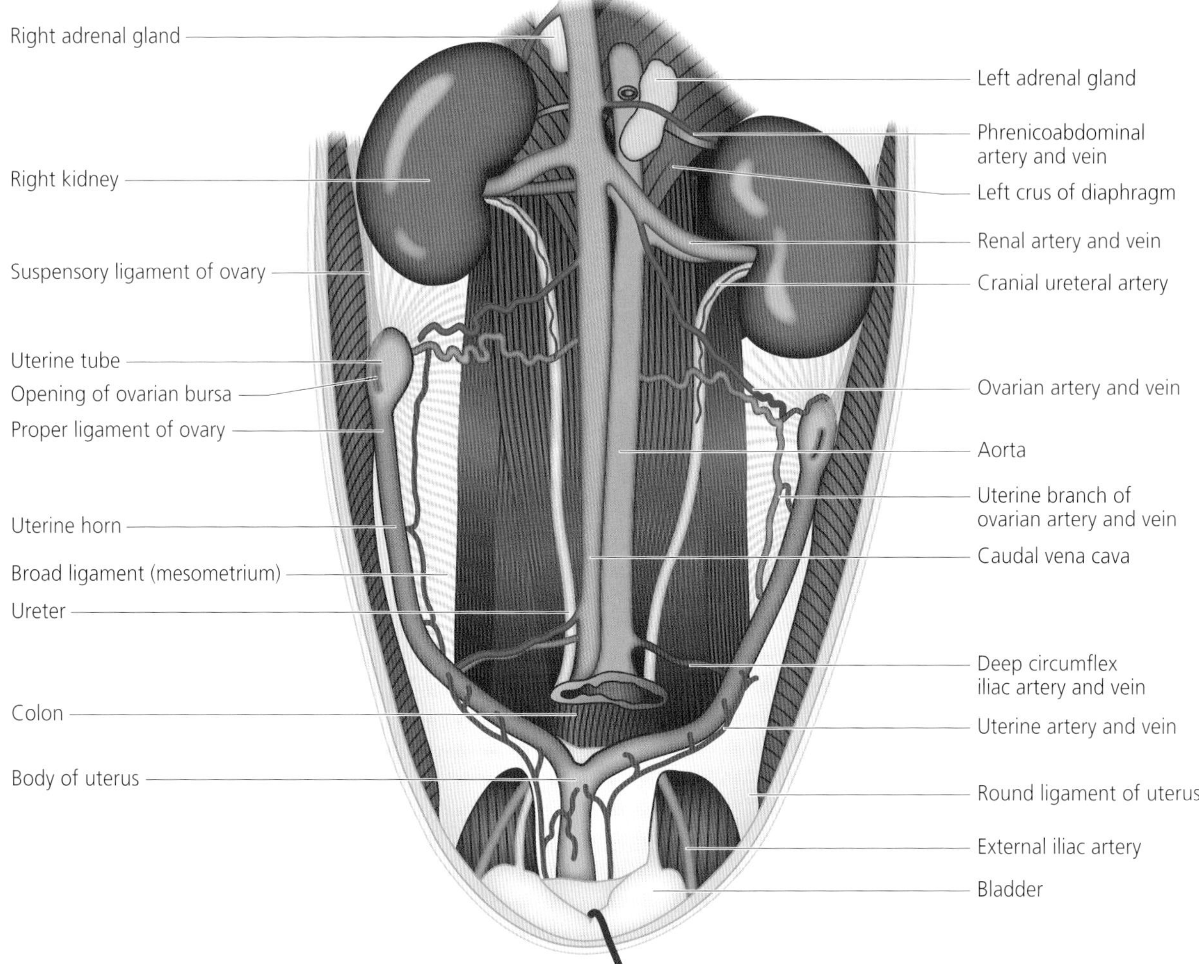

Fig. 5.1 Anatomy of the female reproductive tract. *Illustrator: Elaine Leggett*

at the caudal pole of the kidneys, and lie within a peritoneal sac called the ovarian bursa, which has a slit-like opening medially. The oviduct (uterine tube) connects the peritoneal and uterine cavities, and at the ovarian end is enclosed within the ovarian bursa. At the entrance near the opening of the ovarian bursa, it has a wide, funnel-shaped infundibulum which is fringed with fimbriae to prevent loss of oocytes into the peritoneal cavity. The exit of the oviduct is called the uterine osteum and, as its name suggests, opens into the uterine horn. The ovary is held in position by the suspensory ligament, which attaches to the last rib, and the proper ligament, which connects to the uterine horn. The blood supply to the ovaries is via paired ovarian arteries, which branch from the aorta. Venous drainage is by the ovarian veins; the right ovarian vein drains into the caudal vena cava and the left ovarian vein drains into the left renal vein. The ovarian arteries and veins anastomose with the uterine arteries and veins. Lymphatic drainage is to the lumbar lymph nodes.

The mesovarium is the cranial portion of the broad ligament and attaches the ovary to the dorsolateral body wall. It contains the suspensory ligament and the utero-ovarian vessels, and is continuous with the mesometrium – the caudal part of the broad ligament that attaches the uterus to the body wall. The round ligament is continuous with the proper ligament, runs in the free edge of the broad ligament and passes through the inguinal canal with the vaginal tunic.

The uterus is made up of a neck, body and two horns, and is suspended from the abdomen by the broad ligament. The cervix is found at the caudal part of the uterus, and lies diagonally in dogs and horizontally in the cat. The blood supply to the uterus is via paired uterine arteries (which branch from the vaginal arteries) and anastomosing ovarian arteries. The uterine veins follow the course of the arteries. Lymphatic drainage is to the hypogastric and lumbar lymph nodes.

The vagina is long and extends from the cervix to the vestibule. It has prominent longitudinal folds in the mucosa, and at the vestibulovaginal junction there is a transverse, palpable mucosal ridge. The vestibular mucosa is smooth. The urethral tubercle lies 1 cm caudal to the vestibulovaginal junction on the ventral surface, and the clitoris (within the clitoral fossa) is found further caudal, again on the ventral aspect. The labia of the vulva meet on the midline to cover the clitoris and are thick and pointed. The blood supply to the vagina, urethra and vestibule is provided by branches of the vaginal artery, which arises from the internal pudendal artery. The vulva is supplied by branches of the external pudendal artery. Venous drainage mirrors arterial supply. Lymphatic drainage of the vagina and vestibule is into the internal iliac lymph nodes, and the external genitalia drain into the superficial iliac lmph nodes.

The dog has five pairs of mammary glands: the cranial and caudal thoracic glands (pairs 1 and 2), the cranial and caudal abdominal glands (pairs 3 and 4) and the inguinal glands (pair 5). The cat has four pairs, though a rudimentary fifth (inguinal) pair is sometimes present. Each mamma comprises a glandular network and associated papilla (teat). Vascular supply to the thoracic mammary glands is via the internal thoracic, intercostal and lateral thoracic arteries (Fig. 5.2). The caudal thoracic mammae are also supplied by mammary branches of the cranial superficial epigastric arteries, as are the cranial abdominal mammae, and the caudal abdominal and inguinal mammae are supplied by mammary branches of the caudal superficial epigastric arteries. The cranial and caudal superficial epigastric arteries anastomose with each other, and veins are satellite to the arteries. The axillary and inguinal lymph nodes are the primary drainage sites for the mammary glands. In the dog, the thoracic mammae drain to the axillary lymph nodes, though sometimes also to the sternal lymph nodes. The abdominal mammae drain to both the axillary and inguinal lymph nodes, and the inguinal mammae drain to the inguinal and medial iliac lymph nodes. In addition, the popliteal lymph nodes occasionally drain the fourth and fifth mammary glands. Lymphatic drainage in cats is similar, but the caudal thoracic and cranial abdominal mammae may drain caudally to the inguinal lymph nodes or cranially to the axillary lymph nodes. Some studies have shown that the lymphatic drainage of mammary tissue is altered in the presence of neoplasia. For example, the thoracic gland is normally drained by the axillary lymph centre, but in mammary neoplasia either the superficial cervical or ventral thoracic lymph centres can be involved. Cranial and caudal abdominal glands may be drained by the axillary, inguinofemoral and popliteal lymph centres. However, the popliteal drainage is specific for the healthy caudal abdominal mammary gland. The inguinal gland can be drained by both inguinofemoral and popliteal lymph centres in both neoplastic and healthy conditions. Mammary lymphatic communications are more developed in neoplastic glands (40.9%) compared to healthy glands (33.33%), with increased contralateral anastomosis (50%) compared to healthy ones (33%) (Pereira et al., 2003).

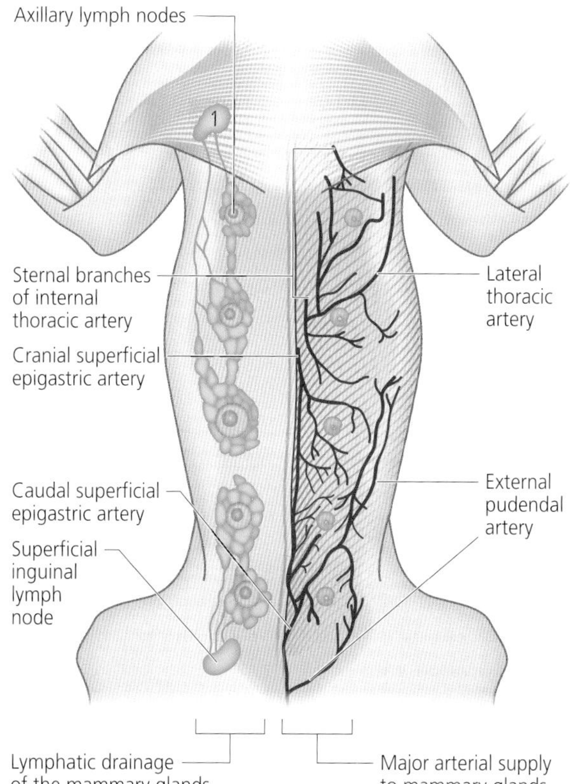

Fig. 5.2 Arterial and lymphatic supply to the mammary glands. The mammary lymphatic drainage is altered and contralateral communications are increased by the presence of neoplasia. *Illustrator: Elaine Leggett*

5.1.2 Ovaries and uterus

Key points

- An increased plasma oestrogen concentration is suggestive of ovarian remnants or adrenocortical problems.
- The prognosis for all types of ovarian tumour is good provided there has been no metastasis.
- Canine uterine tumours are most often benign, with leiomyoma accounting for 90% and leiomyosarcoma representing the remaining 10%.
- Unlike vaginal prolapse, uterine prolapse is not under the influence of the hormonal cycle.
- Clinical signs of uterine torsion may include abdominal pain, tenesmus and vaginal discharge, and may progress to lethargy, collapse and signs of toxic shock.

Ovarian remnant syndrome

Ovarian remnant syndrome in the dog and cat is usually the result of improper surgical technique, whereby a segment of ovarian tissue is left behind. Clinical signs mirror those of recurrent oestrus, and include vulvar enlargement in dogs and attraction of males and willingness to breed in both species. Vaginal discharge is not commonly seen unless uterine tissue remains.

Diagnosis

Diagnosis is based on a history of ovariohysterectomy/ ovariectomy, and tests such as vaginal cytology (presence of superficial ('cornified') cells indicating oestrus) and hormonal assays. In the dog, serum oestradiol and progesterone concentrations exceeding 15 pg/ml and 2 ng/ml, respectively, are suggestive of remnant ovarian tissue (Feldman and Nelson, 2004). Cats are more challenging to diagnose; changes on cytology are more subtle, and prior luteinisation is required by administration of HCG or GnRH to detect elevated progesterone concentrations (>2.5 ng/ml 5–7 days after luteinisation). An increased plasma oestrogen concentration is suggestive of ovarian remnants or adrenocortical disease.

Treatment

Treatment is via surgical exploration, either by laparotomy or laparoscopy, to locate and remove remaining ovarian tissue. The author finds laparoscopic exploration superior due to enhanced visualisation through the use of gas insufflation, abdominal tilting and magnification.

Handy hints

It is preferable to perform surgery when the animal is in oestrus or dioestrus, as the presence of corpora lutea or follicles can make remnants easier to identify.

Ovarian tumours

Ovarian tumours in the dog are almost exclusively epithelial or sex cord stromal in origin, though germ cell tumours (dysgerminoma, teratoma, teratocarcinoma) occasionally occur. Epithelial tumours may be benign (papillary adenoma and cystadenoma) or malignant (papillary adenocarcinoma (Fig. 5.3) and undifferentiated carcinoma). Metastasis of malignant tumours is not common, but trans-coelomic seeding may occur, causing abdominal or pleural effusion. Granulosa cell tumours are the most common sex cord stromal tumour and up to 20% are malignant. These tumours are functional and may produce oestrogen and/or progesterone, causing signs of persistent proestrus or oestrus, cystic endometrial hyperplasia or pyometra. In the cat, sex cord stromal cell tumours are the most common, followed by dysgerminomas, whilst epithelial tumours are rare. Diagnostic work-up should include comprehensive blood tests and thoracic and abdominal imaging. Bone marrow aplasia and pancytopenia may

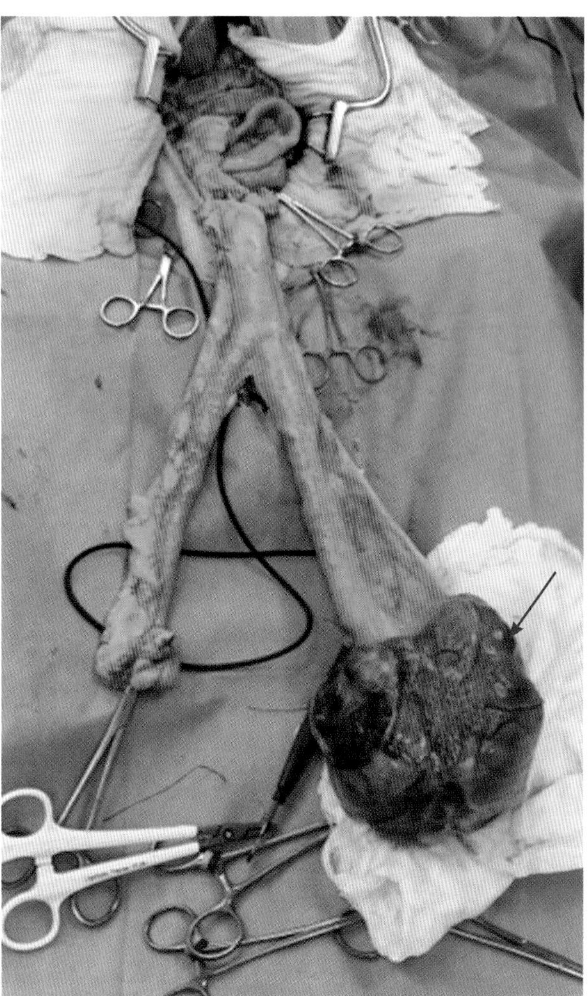

Fig. 5.3 Unilateral ovarian adenocarcinoma (bottom right).

be identified in dogs and cats with oestrogen-secreting granulosa cell tumours. Treatment of ovarian tumours when metastasis is not present is by ovariectomy or ovariohysterectomy. The prognosis for all types of ovarian tumours is good provided there has been no metastasis.

Uterine tumours

Canine uterine tumours are most often benign, with leiomyoma accounting for 90% and leiomyosarcoma representing the remaining 10%. They are usually incidental findings on abdominal palpation unless they cause compression of the uterus or surrounding structures, in which case dyschezia, stranguria and signs associated with pyometra may be seen. A mass is seen during abdominal imaging, and diagnosis usually confirmed following excisional biopsy (ovariohysterectomy [OHE]). Treatment by OHE is curative unless the tumour is malignant, and the prognosis is still good in these cases unless there is already metastatic spread.

Feline uterine tumours are usually adenocarcinomas. Clinical signs often include vaginal discharge and

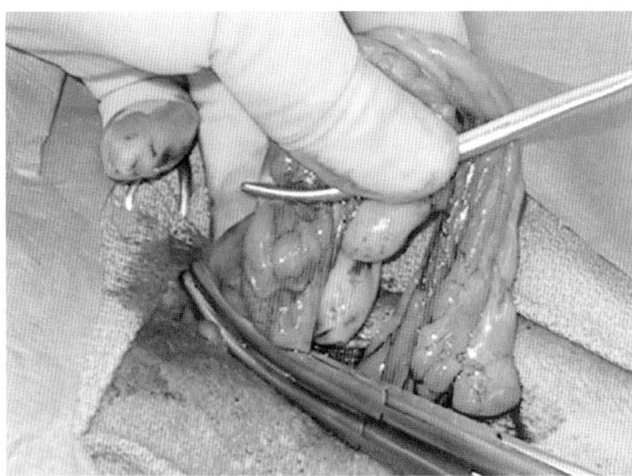

Fig. 5.6 Ovariohysterectomy/ovariectomy. Three-clamp technique on the ovarian pedicle. Two pairs of artery forceps are placed on the ovarian pedicle and one on the proper ligament of the ovary. (Image courtesy of Kyle Mathews.)

- The ovaries are identified by means of an index finger or spay hook. It can be easier to locate the bladder first to identify the uterine body, which lies immediately dorsal, and then follow the uterine horns cranially to the ovary.
- The ovary is then held between thumb and middle finger, and the suspensory ligament is torn or stretched using the index finger to allow exteriorisation.
- A defect is created in the broad ligament adjacent to the ovarian vessels and two pairs of haemostatic forceps are applied across the ovarian vessels, leaving enough space between the ovary and proximal pair to enable transection without risking leaving ovarian tissue behind. A third pair is applied across the mesosalpinx and ovarian-uterine vessels immediately caudal to the ovary.
- A circumferential ligature using 0 to 3-0 braided or monofilament absorbable suture (depending on pedicle size) is loosely placed distal to the most proximal pair of forceps, and is then tightened into the crush mark as they are removed. Use of catgut is not recommended because of its poor knot security and potential inflammatory reaction/granuloma formation resulting from its use.
- Either a circumferential (if the pedicle is small) or transfixing-encircling ligature is placed distal to the first ligature (proximal to the second haemostat). Use of surgeon knots or Miller knots is recommended.
- The pedicle is then transected along the distal aspect of the second haemostat, and then lowered gently to the dorsal abdomen before removing the haemostat and observing for haemorrhage.
- This is repeated for the second ovary, and then any remaining suspensory ligament, the round ligament and the broad ligament, are transected or gently torn to the level of the cervix, ligating any large blood vessels encountered.
- A circumferential ligature is placed around the uterine body just cranial to the cervix, and a transfixing-encircling ligature is placed cranial to the first. This is performed by passing the needle through the edge of the uterus, placing two square knots and then passing the suture to the opposite side of the uterus and finishing the knot. When the blood vessels are large (e.g. in pregnant animals or those with pyometra), a transfixing-encircling ligature may be needed on both sides.
- Two pairs of haemostatic forceps are then placed cranial to the most cranial knot, and the uterus is transected in-between. This ensures that any uterine contents or blood within the uterine vessels are contained, and allows a controlled release of the stump whilst observing for haemorrhage.
- Once the ovaries and uterus have been removed, each gutter is inspected for haemorrhage before closure of the abdomen in three layers. A long-lasting absorbable suture material should be used to close the rectus sheath (e.g. polydioxanone). Generally size USP 2-0 (3.0 metric) is suitable for dogs up to 20 kg, USP 0 (3.5 metric) for dogs between 20 and 30 kg and USP 1 (4.0 metric) for dogs over 30 kg.

The technique in the queen is often performed via a flank incision (Fig. 5.7). The surgical field should be clipped from just cranial to the last rib to the iliac crest in a craniocaudal direction, and from the transverse process of the lumbar vertebrae to the flank fold in a dorsoventral direction.

Handy hints

- A flank spay can be performed on either side, but may be easier on the left flank for right-handed surgeons, as the suspensory ligament will be orientated in the correct direction for stretching with the right hand.
- The landmark for incision is found by creating a triangle with the thumb, index finger and middle finger. The last rib and iliac crest is palpated with the index and middle finger, and the thumb is placed so as to create an equilateral triangle. A 2–3 cm incision in the skin is made in the centre of this triangle, and this is extended through the subcutaneous tissue, abdominal musculature and peritoneum.

The three-clamp technique is not possible in the cat due to the size and fragility of the pedicle. The authors prefer to place one haemostat distal to the second pedicle ligature and one caudal to the ovary prior to transection. Similarly with the uterine body, two haemostats

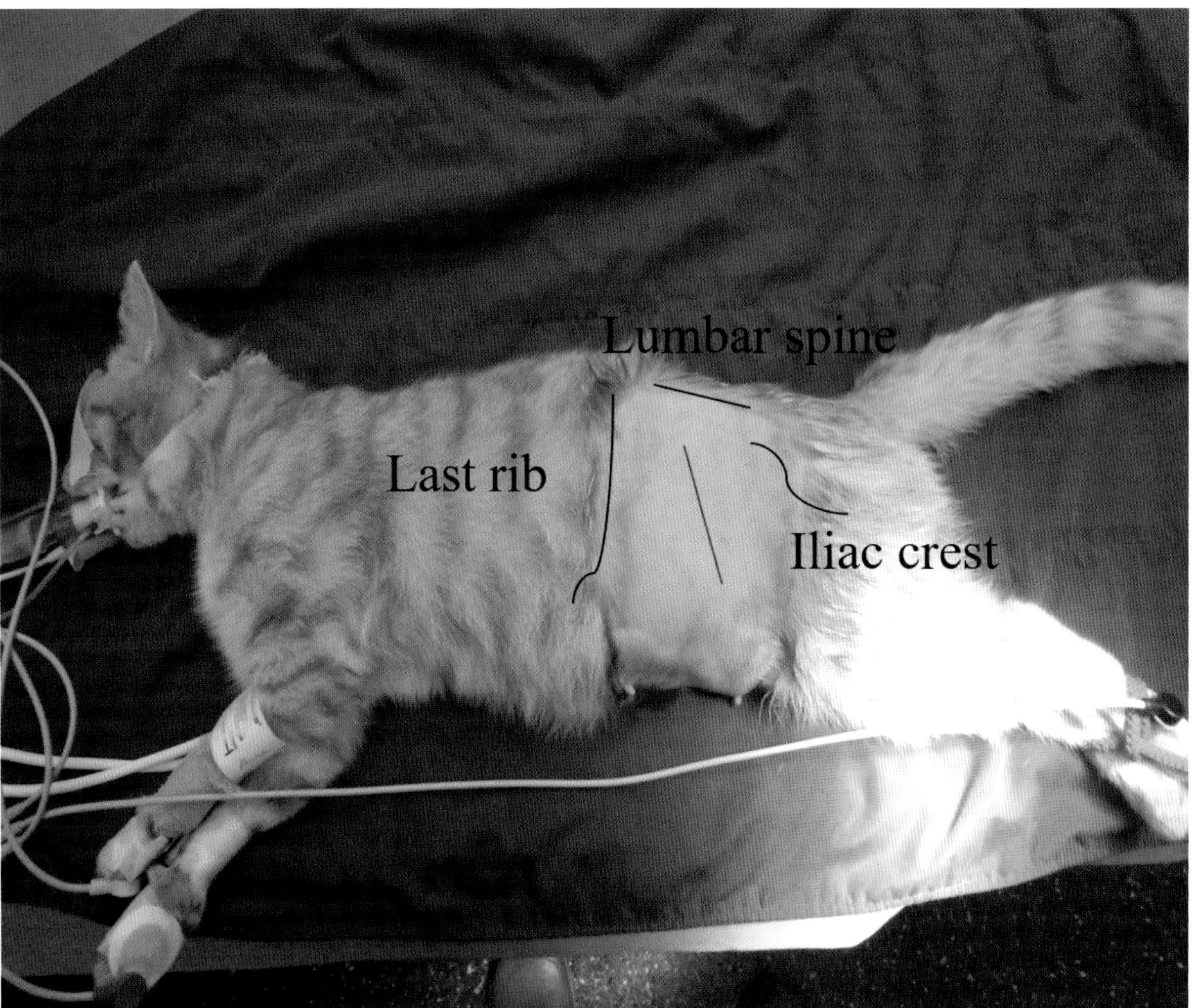

Fig. 5.7 Landmarks for flank approach. Incision (red line) in a dorsoventral direction, starting from just caudal to the midpoint between the last rib and iliac crest; length = 2–3 cm.

are placed once the two ligatures are in place, and the uterus is transected in-between. Closure is routine, although the external and internal abdominal oblique muscles should be closed separately if possible.

Ovariectomy (OVE)

This technique involves removing the ovaries while leaving the uterus *in situ*. It can be safely performed in bitches and queens and constitutes an appropriate spaying method in both species, provided no ovarian remnant remains and there is no future treatment with progestogens (which could lead to cystic endometrial hyperplasia and pyometra). OVE can be performed through a midline or flank approach in both bitch and queen, though the latter approach in the bitch requires that the animal be repositioned during surgery. During ovariectomy the pedicle is ligated as for OHE, but in addition the uterine artery and vein are ligated and transected at the level of the proper ligament, immediately cranial to the uterine horn.

Laparoscopic spay

In this technique, OHE or OVE is performed with the aid of a laparoscope (i.e. rigid camera introduced into the abdomen; Fig. 5.8a,b). Special surgical instruments are used to enable handling of the ovaries and sealing of the vessels. Surgical time is longer for beginners than with the standard (i.e. open) procedure. Studies have shown faster recovery of bitches undergoing laparoscopic spay in comparison to standard spay (Davidson et al., 2003; Devitt et al., 2005). The benefit of laparoscopic spay in queens remains unconfirmed.

There are variations in the number and location of the ports (including the use of a single-port laparoscopic surgery (SILS) device), but the authors' preference for OVE is to create a camera portal just caudal to the umbilicus, and two instrument portals, one a few centimetres cranial to the first portal and the other one a few centimetres caudal to the first portal (for a 15 kg dog). The patient is tilted 15–30 degrees to the opposite

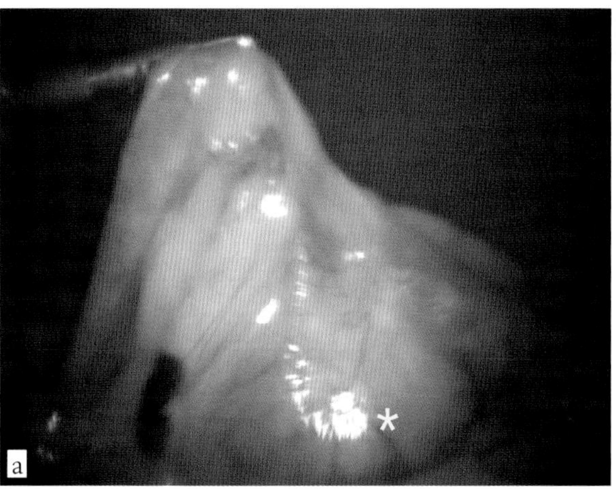

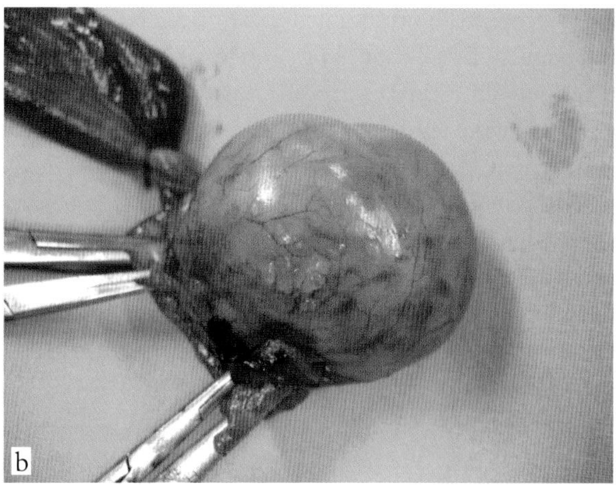

Fig. 5.8a,b Laparoscopic spay for a suspected cystic ovary. a. The proper ligament of the ovary is grasped with endoscopic forceps, revealing the distended ovarian bursa (yellow asterisk). b. Surgical specimen following excision. The fluid contained within the ovarian bursa was pus.

side of the ovary to facilitate ovary identification, and laparoscopic Allis tissue forceps are used to grasp and elevate the ovary. Through the other instrument portal, a vessel-sealing device is used to seal and transect the suspensory ligament, mesovarium and mesometrium. Once the ovary is free of its attachments, the pedicle is inspected for bleeding and the ovary is removed through the instrument cannula. The cannula may be too narrow, in which case it is removed and the ovary is withdrawn through the incision. Occasionally the ovary is still too large, in which case the incision must be widened to allow removal and then a temporary purse-string suture placed through the external rectus sheath and around the replaced cannula to maintain an airtight seal. The dog is then tilted to the other side, the abdomen re-insufflated and the process repeated for the remaining ovary.

Complications

Complications of OHE most frequently encountered include pain, inflammation/infection of the incision site, intra- or postoperative haemorrhage, urinary incontinence and gastrointestinal upset. Less common complications include ureteral damage, granuloma

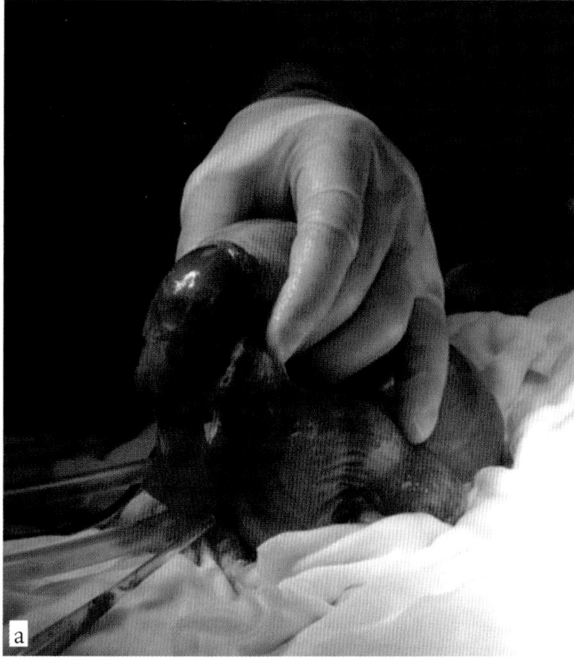

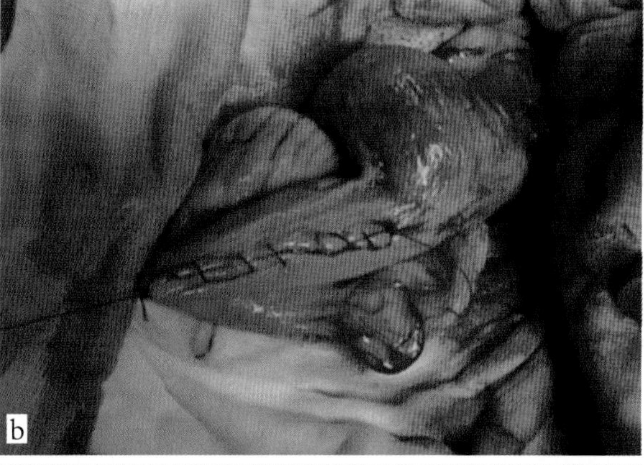

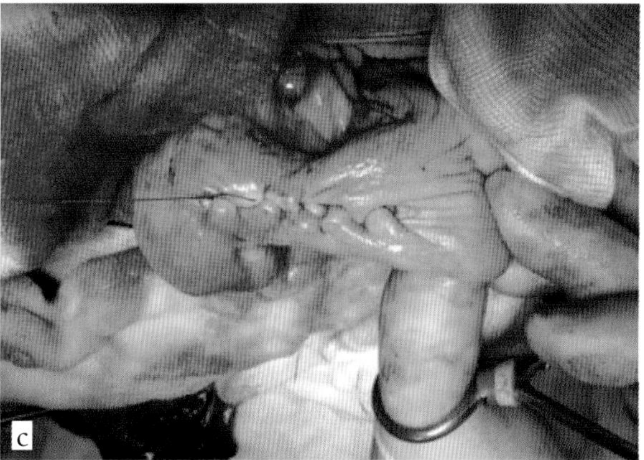

Fig. 5.9a–c Caesarean section. a. An incision is made at the level of the uterine horn. b. Hysterosynthesis: the first layer is a simple continuous appositional layer. c. Hysterosynthesis: the second layer is an inverting pattern (Cushing).

formation at the uterine or ovarian pedicle remnants, retained swab foreign body, ovarian remnant syndrome and intestinal or urethral obstruction from adhesions or inappropriate ligature placement, respectively. Inadvertent ligation of a ureter may occur with inadequate visualisation of the caudal pole of the kidney or the uterine body, especially when the pedicle has been dropped and there is haemorrhage (Forster et al., 2011; Okkens et al., 1981). Complications of ovariectomy are the same, though with laparoscopic OVE there is no risk of swab foreign body.

Step by step: Caesarean section (C-section)

Handy hints

Indications for Caesarean section in the bitch (Fig. 5.9a–c) include dystocia, fetal distress and systemic signs of disease, or it may be planned for high-risk pregnancies. The key element is that extraction of fetuses needs to be performed as rapidly as possible post-induction of anaesthesia. Special anaesthetic agents and modalities (e.g. epidural) can be used to minimise anaesthetic-related neonatal depression. Clipping and the first surgical scrub should be done on a non-anaesthetised animal to minimise time under anaesthesia.

- The abdominal incision is made more caudal than in a regular spay, and the body of the uterus is exteriorised gently as uterine vessels are quite friable at this stage of the pregnancy and can rupture easily.
- Stay sutures are placed on each side of the area of the incision, which are used to tent up the uterus by an assistant. This avoids damage of the fetuses while the uterine incision is made.
- Once the uterine body is open, the fetuses are gently milked towards this incision. The amniotic sac is opened, the umbilical cord is clamped and the newborn is handed to a sterile assistant for neonate support.
- The hysterotomy incision is sutured in two layers using a monofilament absorbable suture (size 3-0 or 4-0) material with one simple continuous and one inverting suture (Cushing pattern).

5.1.3 Vagina, vestibule and vulva

Key points

- Obesity is considered a risk factor for development of a recessed vulva.
- Vaginal oedema is distinguished from true (and rare) vaginal prolapse, which presents as a circumferential 'doughnut' of vaginal mucosa protruding from the vulva.
- Reported malignancies include transmissible venereal tumour (TVT), transitional cell tumours and neuroendocrine tumours.

Recessed vulva

This condition historically was thought to be a consequence of early OHE, with subsequent low oestrogen levels causing abnormal vulvar development. However, a more recent study found no direct link between juvenile OHE and recessed vulva but suggested that breed and bodyweight (medium and large breeds) may be a factor (Hammel and Bjorling, 2002). Obesity is considered a risk factor for development of a skin fold, though there are no reliable data to support this. Clinical signs relate to perivulval dermatitis or vaginitis in around half of patients (vulval pruritus, discharge and licking), whilst signs relating to urinary tract infection or apparent urinary incontinence are evident in the other half. Physical examination reveals a skin fold that covers the most dorsal aspect of the vulvar labia (sometimes the whole vulva), which is responsible for skin fold dermatitis and vulvar urine scalding. Diagnosis is apparent on physical examination, but urinalysis and urine culture should be performed due to the high risk of urinary tract infections.

Treatment

The dog should be treated with a course of antibiotics suitable for pyoderma prior to surgery. Weight loss may help to reduce the size of the skin flap and expose the vulva, but treatment generally consists of an episioplasty, whereby a crescent-shaped skin fold dorsal to the vulva is removed. For this procedure the dog is positioned in ventral recumbency with the pelvic limbs placed over a padded end of the operating table. The tail is wrapped and held dorsocranially using tape, the perineal skin is prepped and a purse-string suture is placed in the anal orifice.

Step by step: surgical correction of a recessed vulva (Fig. 5.10a–e)

- The area of skin to be removed is established by pinching it with finger and thumb until the vulva is no longer covered.
- A sterile surgical marker pen is used to mark the area of skin to be removed in a crescent shape.
- The crescent-shaped section of skin is excised, and the defect closed in two layers (subcutaneous and skin) using a simple interrupted pattern.
- Sutures should be placed at 12 o'clock, 3 o'clock and 9 o'clock first to assess effectiveness of the resection and to prevent the formation of a dog ear at one end.

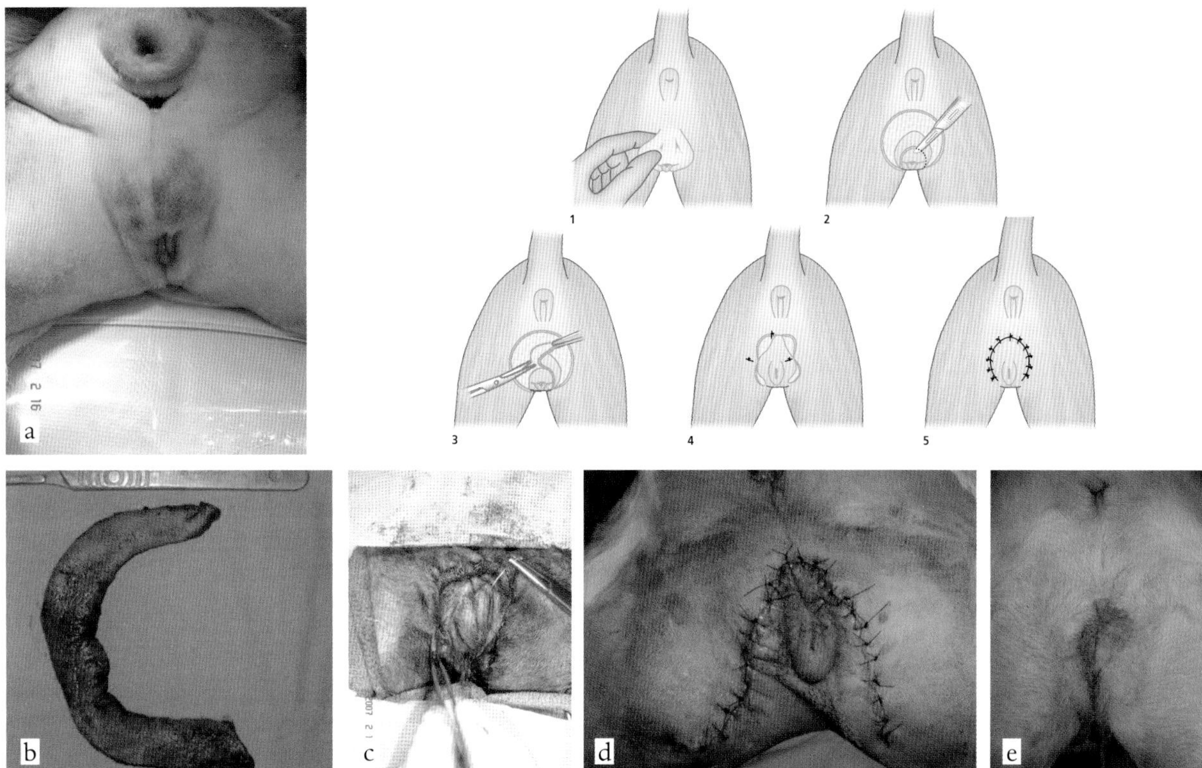

Fig. 5.10a–e Treatment of a recessed vulva. a. The dorsal vulvar fold is almost entirely covering the vulvar commissure. 1 and 2. A crescent-shaped incision is made at the level of the vulvar fold, engaging the subcutaneous/fat tissue. b. Excised tissue. c and 3–5. The edges are then re-approximated using subcutaneous sutures (simple continuous) or a series of cruciate sutures (especially at the most dorsal edge of the incision and on the lateral edges). d. Skin sutures are sometimes placed to perfect cutaneous apposition. e. Postoperative result at suture removal – the dorsal commissure of the vulva is visible. *Illustrator: Elaine Leggett*

Outcome

Complications are rare, but include surgical site infection due to the proximity to the anus, or wound dehiscence due to extensive skin resection and tension. The prognosis for resolution of clinical signs is very good.

Vaginal oedema and vaginal prolapse

Vaginal oedema occurs in young female dogs in proestrus or oestrus, due to the influence of oestrogen. A mass of oedematous tissue develops on the ventral floor of the vagina, just cranial to the urethral orifice, and protrudes from the vulva when large enough. The condition is distinguished from true (and rare) vaginal prolapse, which presents as a circumferential 'doughnut' of vaginal mucosa protruding from the vulva. Clinical signs are usually noticed only once the tissue is protruding, and it may appear traumatised from abrasion, licking or drying. Bitches may be seen straining due to the prolapsed tissue, and compression of surrounding structures may cause stranguria or tenesmus. Though a vaginal oedema mass may be very large, digital examination usually reveals the tissue as originating from a small area.

Treatment

For vaginal oedema, if the condition is acute and the protruding tissue viable, conservative treatment by lubrication and application of an Elizabethan collar to prevent self-trauma is appropriate. It may be possible to reduce the mass via an episiotomy followed by placement of vulvar sutures to maintain its position; the oedema will resolve spontaneously once oestrogen levels reduce. Ovariohysterectomy is recommended before the next cycle to prevent recurrence. If the mass is a vaginal prolapse (Fig. 5.11), then manual reduction of the tissue followed by OHE is recommended. However, with either condition, if the tissue is traumatised and non-viable, surgical excision is required. An episiotomy is performed to access the base of the mass, and the urethra is catheterised before resection. Haemorrhage is often significant during oestrus and therefore electrosurgery may be used for tissue transection. For vaginal oedema, the incision is made in the mucosa around the base of the mass on the ventral vaginal floor. This should be done in stages, and the resulting mucosal defect is closed with monofilament absorbable suture in a continuous or interrupted appositional pattern.

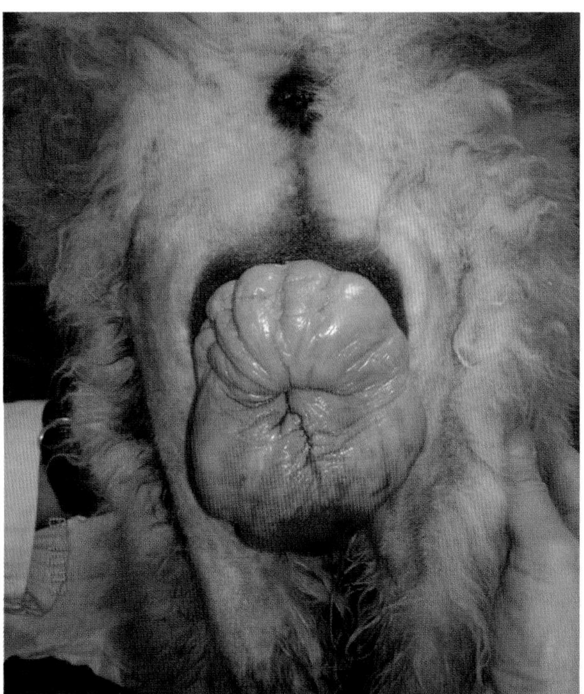

Fig. 5.11 Vaginal prolapse.

Vaginal, vestibular and vulvar neoplasia

The majority of vaginal, vestibular and vulval neoplasms are benign, with leiomyoma being the most common. Around one quarter of tumours are malignant, with leiomyosarcoma the most frequently diagnosed. Other reported malignancies include transmissible venereal tumour (TVT), transitional cell tumours and neuroendocrine tumours. The average age at diagnosis is around 11 years (Thacher and Bradley, 1983), and there are no reported breed predispositions. Malignant neoplasia can metastasise to the local lymph nodes, spleen, lungs or cervical spinal cord. Clinical signs include bulging of perineum, vaginal prolapse, tenesmus, dysuria, urinary incontinence, difficulty copulating and sanguinous or purulent discharge. Diagnosis is made by vaginoscopy, digital vaginal exam and rectal palpation in small dogs. Cytology should be performed, and thoracic radiography and abdominal radiography and ultrasound are recommended for full staging. Treatment of aggressive (i.e. malignant) tumours consists of surgical excision (vaginectomy) via an episiotomy or a combined (abdominal and perineal) approach. With the appropriate surgical expertise, splitting of the pelvis is not always needed, though this is a technically challenging surgery and referral to a specialist centre is recommended. TVT is best treated with vincristine, though radiotherapy is reported to be successful. Surgical excision carries a high rate of recurrence and therefore is considered a poor alternative. Treatment of benign tumours is performed by marginal excision via an episiotomy. Prognosis is good for both TVT and a completely excised leiomyoma, and guarded for malignant tumours. Adjunctive treatment is probably necessary after resection of malignant tumours.

Step by step: episiotomy

Episiotomy is an incision of the skin between the vulvar labia and the anus that allows exposure of the vestibule, vagina and urethral papilla (Fig. 5.12). The procedure is performed to allow reduction or resection of vaginal oedema and vaginal prolapse, excision of vestibulovaginal masses, vaginectomy and correction of congenital conditions such as vestibulovaginal stenosis.

Handy hints

The patient is positioned in ventral recumbency with the pelvic limbs placed over a padded end of the operating table to avoid inadvertent nerve or muscle injury, and the tail is wrapped and held dorsocranially using tape. The perineal skin is clipped, the vestibule flushed with dilute povidone-iodine and the skin aseptically prepared.

- A purse-string suture is placed in the anal orifice.
- An incision is made starting at the dorsal aspect of the vulval commissure and extending dorsally to the level of the most dorsal aspect of the vestibule, which is determined by placing a finger or blunt instrument into the vestibule.
- The incision is progressively deepened through subcutaneous tissue, vestibular constrictor muscle and vestibular mucosa, thus exposing the vestibule, clitoral fossa, urethral tubercle, vestibulovaginal junction and vagina.
- A stay suture placed at the distal aspect of each side of the incision and retracted laterally aids in visualisation of the structure(s) of interest.
- For incision closure, the mucosa and muscular layers are sutured separately using a rapidly absorbable suture material in a continuous or interrupted appositional pattern, followed by routine skin closure.

5.1.4 Mammary glands

Key points

- Around 40–50% of canine mammary tumours are malignant, whereas 80–90% are malignant in the cat.
- Mammary tumours are suggested as losing their hormonal dependency if they transform from benign to malignant.
- Disease-free interval is reported to be significantly shorter in the cat with mammary tumours when less aggressive surgery is performed.

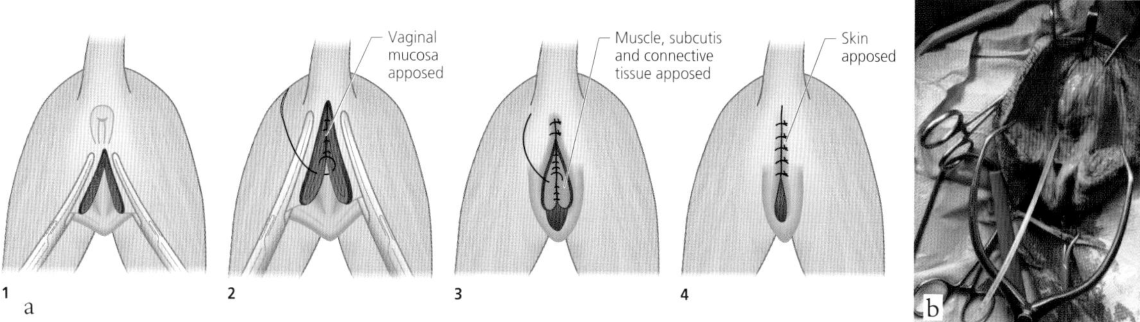

Fig. 5.12a,b Episiotomy. 1–4. The incision is made at the level of the dorsal vulvar commissure (between non-crushing forceps) and suturing of the incision is performed in three layers (mucosa, muscle and connective tissues, skin). b. Episiotomy performed to access a vaginal leiomyoma. A urinary catheter is placed. *Illustrator: Elaine Leggett*

- Chemotherapy is usually recommended for highly invasive cancers and high-grade carcinoma.

Neoplasia

Mammary tumours are the most common type of neoplasia in the dog, accounting for 42% of all tumours. In the cat, they account for 17% of all tumours. Males are rarely affected. Around 40–50% of canine tumours are malignant, whereas 80–90% are malignant in the cat. Metastatic spread is via the lymphatics and blood vessels to the regional lymph nodes and lungs. Less common sites of metastasis include the adrenal glands, kidneys, heart, liver and bone.

Mammary tumours are hormone dependent, and time of spaying significantly affects the risk of developing the disease; compared to an intact dog, the risk of a dog developing the disease when neutered before the first oestrus, second oestrus and after the second oestrus but before two years of age is 0.5, 8 and 26%, respectively (Schneider et al., 1969). Feline mammary tumours are similarly hormone dependent; compared to the intact cat, those spayed before 6 months and 1 year have a 91 and 86% reduction in risk for mammary carcinoma, respectively (Overley et al., 2005). However, tumours are suggested as losing their hormonal dependency if they transform from benign to malignant. This is demonstrated by the negative correlation between oestrogen/progesterone receptor expression and cell proliferation in malignant tumours. These receptors are found in normal mammary tissue and in 90% of benign tumours, but in only half of malignant tumours (and not in inflammatory carcinoma, the most aggressive mammary malignancy).

In the dog, the most common benign tumours are adenoma, fibroadenoma and mixed tumours. The most frequently diagnosed malignant tumours are carcinomas. These are sub-classified into complex carcinoma and simple carcinoma, the latter of which includes papillary, tubular, solid and anaplastic carcinomas. Less than 5% of malignant tumours are sarcomas. Inflammatory carcinoma is a highly aggressive tumour, usually of tubular, papillary, solid or anaplastic carcinoma classification. Initially it can appear like mastitis, but rapidly progresses and is highly metastatic.

Benign tumours in the cat include simple or complex adenomas and fibroadenomas. The majority (~90%) of feline mammary tumours are adenocarcinomas. The most common sub-types are tubular, solid, papillary and cribriform, which all metastasise rapidly to the lymph nodes and lungs. These are often not well differentiated, feel firm and appear ulcerated. Fibroadenomatous hyperplasia causes massive enlargement of the mammary glands and is caused by endogenous or exogenous progestins. Subsequent trauma or ischaemia of the glands can lead to ulceration which may appear like carcinoma, and therefore it is important to differentiate the two.

Diagnosis

Masses are usually detected on routine examination, though some animals may present with mammary discharge. In cases where pulmonary or bone metastasis has already occurred, the animal may be brought in with dyspnoea or lameness, respectively. On physical examination, mammary masses of varying size may be identified, most often affecting the caudal glands. Multiple masses occur in more than 60% of canine cases and 50% of feline cases, and these may be in one or both mammary chains. In dogs, masses are usually moveable and may be solid or cystic, sessile or pedunculated. When there is diffuse oedema (which may affect the limbs), and the mammary glands appear erythematous and ulcerated, inflammatory carcinoma should be suspected. Feline mammary masses are often ulcerated and adherent to the skin or abdominal wall.

Laboratory tests should include a complete blood count, biochemistry and urinalysis, in order to rule out concurrent disease and identify any paraneoplastic syndromes. Tumours in the dog are staged according to a modified WHO cutaneous tumour–node–metastasis

Table 5.1 Tumour–node–metastasis (TNM) stage classification of canine mammary tumours.

Stage	Description
T	**Primary tumour**
T_1	Tumour <3 cm maximum diameter
T_2	Tumour 3–5 cm maximum diameter
T_3	Tumour >5 cm maximum diameter
T_4	Inflammatory carcinoma
N	**Regional lymph nodes**
N_0	No evidence of regional lymph node involvement
N_1	Metastasis in ipsilateral nodes
N_2	Metastasis in contralateral or bilateral nodes
M	**Distant metastasis**
M_0	No evidence of distant metastasis
M_1	Distant metastasis detected
Stage	
I	$T_1N_0M_0$
II	$T_2N_0M_0$
III	$T_3N_0M_0$
IV	$T_xN_1M_0$
V	$T_xN_xM_1$

Note: x = any

Table 5.2 Modified World Health Organization clinical staging system for feline mammary tumours.

Stage	Description		
T	**Primary tumour**		
T_1	<2 cm maximum diameter		
T_2	2–3 cm maximum diameter		
T_3	>3 cm maximum diameter		
N	**Regional lymph nodes**		
N_0	No histological or cytological evidence of metastasis		
N_1	Histological or cytological evidence of metastasis		
M	**Distant metastasis**		
M_0	No evidence of distant metastasis		
M_1	Evidence of distant metastasis		
Stage			
I	T_1	N_0	M_0
II	T_2	N_0	M_0
III	T_1 or T_2	N_1	M_0
	T_3	N_0 or N_1	M_0
IV	Any T	Any N	M_1

(TNM) system (Owen, 1980; Table 5.1). In the cat, a different TNM classification system is used (Lana et al., 2007; Table 5.2).

Diagnostic imaging should include three-view thoracic radiographs or CT, and abdominal ultrasonography or CT. Regional lymph nodes should be aspirated using ultrasound guidance if there is lymphadenopathy. Since masses can transform from benign to malignant, sampling by fine needle aspiration or tissue biopsy is usually not necessary because treatments for benign and malignant lesions both involve surgical excision.

Treatment

Surgical excision should be performed if there is no evidence of metastasis and there are no contraindications to anaesthesia. The exception to this is in cases of inflammatory carcinoma, since prognosis is so poor and surgery is unlikely to affect the outcome. In the dog, the surgical technique chosen depends on the size of the mass and which gland is affected. However, it is presence of clean margins rather than the technique used which affects prognosis. In the cat, chain mastectomy of the affected side should always be performed regardless of the number or size of mammary masses, due to the high risk of early metastasis. As in any oncological surgery, it is critical to obtain clean margins (at least 1 cm of tissue with absence of microscopic disease). There are several methods of excision: lumpectomy, simple mastectomy, regional mastectomy and unilateral or bilateral (chain) mastectomy, as detailed below. The depth of excision should be to the pectoral muscles/abdominal wall fascia, except for tumours that are non-mobile, in which case the fascial layer (rectus sheath) should also be removed. It is important to implement good haemostasis and minimise tension and dead space by using walking sutures.

- Lumpectomy. This is appropriate only for known benign masses <0.5 cm in diameter. The mass is removed with a marginal rim of normal tissue. The disadvantage of this procedure is that milk and/or lymph can leak from the incised mammary tissue, causing local inflammation and pain.
- Simple mastectomy. For larger masses a simple mastectomy may be performed, which involves removal of a single gland. If there is suspicion over fixation to either the underlying muscle fascia or the skin, the fascia and first muscle layer and skin should be included in the surgical margin.
- Regional mastectomy. Regional mastectomy is indicated when masses are between glands. However, because of the confluence of venous and lymphatic anatomy between the mammary glands, *en bloc* removal of glands 1–3 or 3–5 is often performed even when the mass affects only one gland. These communications mean that it is actually often easier to perform regional mastectomy than simple mastectomy, and the problem of postoperative milk/lymph leakage is avoided. When the caudal glands are removed, the inguinal lymph node should also be removed. The

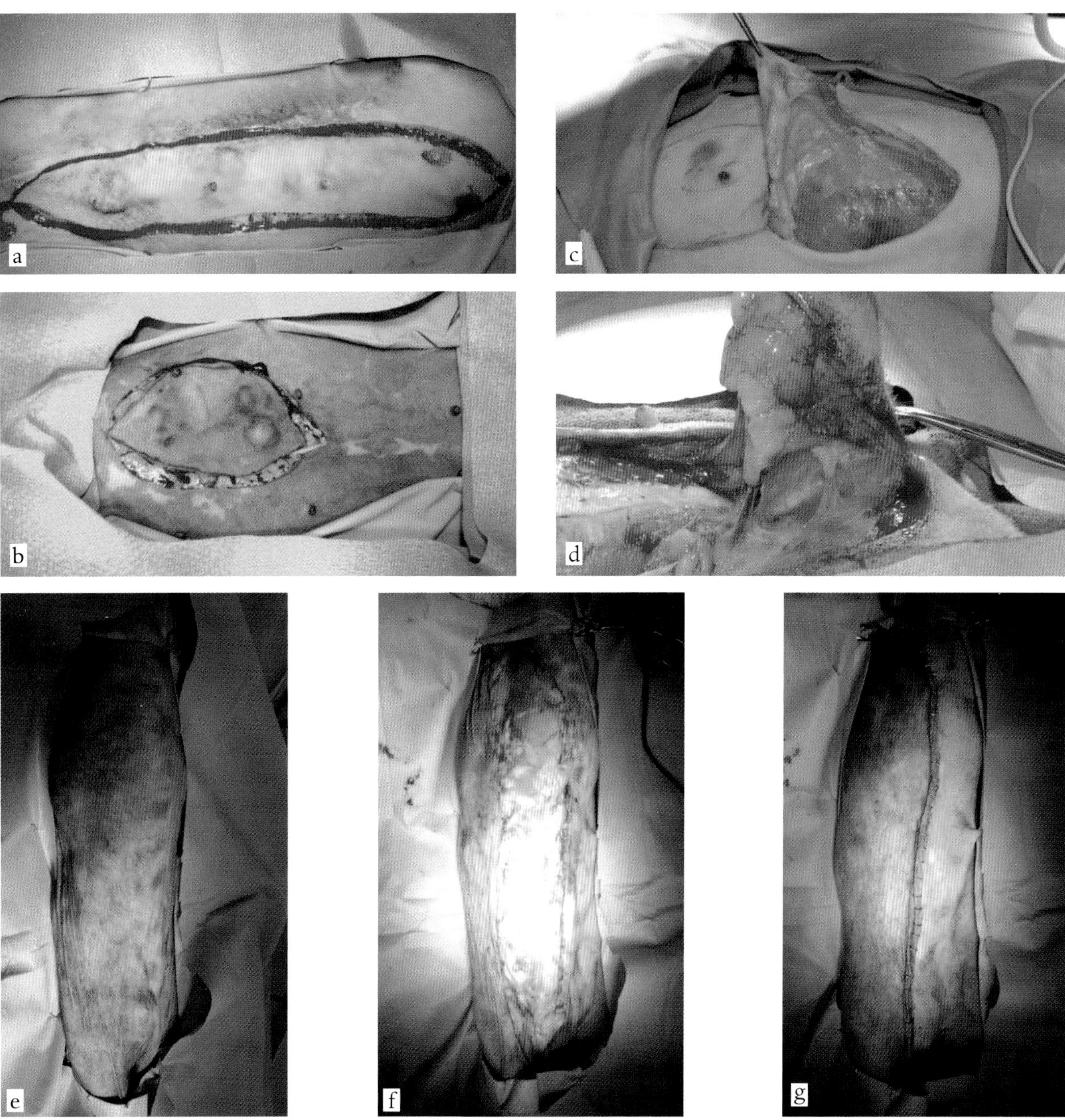

Fig. 5.13a–g a. Complete mammary chain resection. b. Regional mastectomy. In the dog, the type of resection needed (lumpectomy, simple mastectomy, regional mastectomy or unilateral mastectomy, bilateral mastectomy) is determined based on (1) the size and location of the mass and (2) the ability of the surgeon to create tumour-free margins. c. The dissection is performed at the level of rectus sheath (in the dog, there is no need to remove this unless the tumour is fixed). d. Haemostasis is performed by ligating the superficial epigastric artery (caudal and/or cranial) – the image shows the caudal superficial epigastric artery. e. Unilateral mammary tumour in a cat located at the level of the inguinal mammary gland (red arrow and red circle). In the cat, the treatment of choice is always a bilateral mammary chain resection irrespective of the size of the primary tumour. This operation is often staged. f. Unilateral mammary chain resection. g. Final closure. (Images a–d courtesy of Julius Liptak.)

axillary lymph node ideally should be removed when removing the cranial lymph nodes, though this is not always done unless it is enlarged or tumour cells have been identified on aspiration biopsy, because it is not usually in the surgical field.

- Chain mastectomy. Metastasis can be unpredictable due to lymphatic drainage of the third and sometimes fourth mammary glands to both the axillary and inguinal lymph nodes, and the possible existence of lymphatic communication between several other glands. For this reason, it may be preferable to remove all of the mammary glands by unilateral or staged bilateral chain mastectomy (Fig. 5.13a–g). However, studies have found no difference in the recurrence rate or survival time of simple mastectomy and radical mastectomy (Yamagami et al., 1996).

Evaluation of adjunctive therapy for mammary neoplasia is not widely published, and the use of radiotherapy has not been investigated. There are some reports of increased survival times when a combination of 5-fluorouracil and either cyclophosphamide or carboplatin is used alongside surgery (Karayannopoulou et al., 2001; Lavalle et al., 2012). Chemotherapy is usually recommended for highly invasive cancers and high-grade carcinoma.

Prognosis

In the dog, benign tumours carry a good prognosis with surgery. The prognosis for malignant mammary tumours depends on histological tumour type, tumour size, tumour stage, OHE status and extent of surgery. Approximately one-quarter of dogs with non-infiltrating carcinomas with well-differentiated nuclei will experience recurrence or metastasis 2 years postoperatively, in comparison to between 60 and 90% of those with infiltrating carcinoma with poorly differentiated nuclei. Solid carcinoma, anaplastic carcinoma, inflammatory carcinoma and sarcomas carry a worse prognosis than papillary or tubular carcinomas. Median survival time (MST) decreases as tumour size increases: dogs with tumours >3 cm and <3 cm had an MST of 14 and 22 months, respectively, in one study (Philibert et al., 2003). The presence of lymph node metastasis or distant metastasis further decreases survival time. Ovariohysterectomy at the time of surgery may improve survival time: one study found that OHE was more beneficial in dogs with complex carcinomas than in those with simple carcinomas (Chang et al., 2005).

In the cat, prognosis depends on histological type, tumour size, tumour grade and extent of surgery. Survival times for tumours >3 cm, 2–3 cm and <2 cm are reported to be 4–12 months, 15–24 months and >3 years, respectively (Viste et al., 2002). Another study found that the percentages of cats that died during the first postoperative year were 0, 42 and 100% for histological grades I, II and III, respectively (Seixas et al., 2009). Disease-free interval is reported to be significantly shorter when less aggressive surgery is performed (MacEwen et al., 1984).

5.2 Male reproductive tract

5.2.1 Surgical anatomy

The male reproductive tract is composed of the scrotum, testes, epididymides, spermatic cords, penis and prostate.

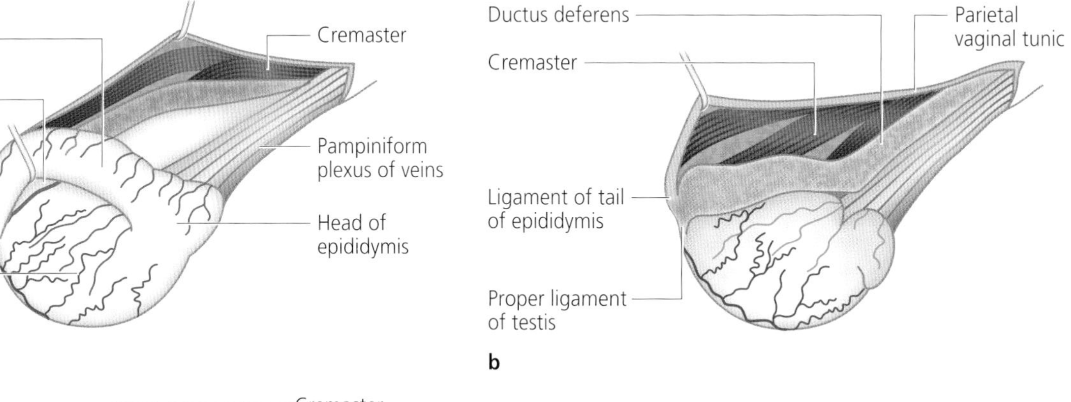

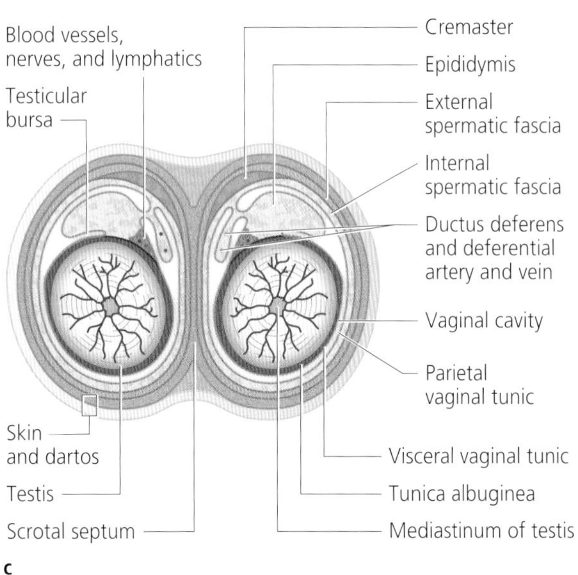

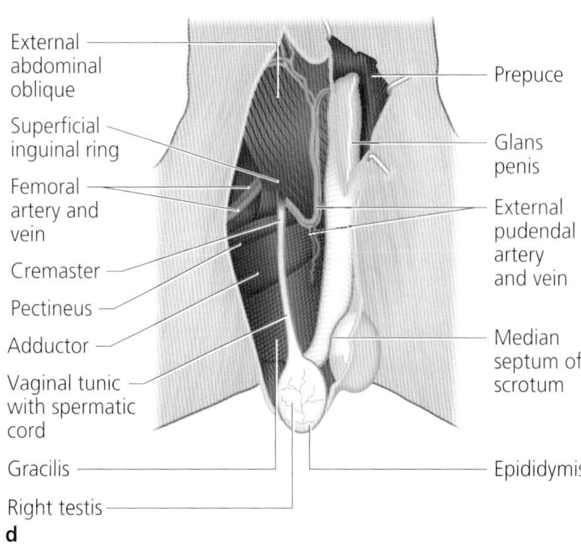

Fig. 5.14a–d Anatomy of the testis and inguinal ring. a. Right testes. b. Left testes, medial aspect. c. Cross section through scrotum and testes. d. Ventral aspect. *Illustrator: Elaine Leggett*

Scrotum, testes, epididymis and spermatic cord

The scrotum houses the testes, epididymides and distal spermatic cords, and is located between the inguinal region and the anus (Fig. 5.14). The epididymis is adherent to the dorsolateral aspect of the testis, and is a tube that connects the efferent ducts of the testes to the ductus deferens to allow exit of sperm and seminal fluid from the body. It has a head and a tail, the latter of which is attached to the testis via the proper ligament of the testis. The ligament of the tail of the epididymis attaches the testis and epididymis to the vaginal tunic and spermatic fascia. The epididymis continues as the ductus deferens and travels dorsocranially through the inguinal ring into the abdominal cavity before looping caudally, ventral to the ureter, and penetrating the dorsal aspect of the prostate where it terminates at the prostatic urethra. The spermatic cord, comprising external and internal spermatic fascia, spans the distance from the inguinal ring to the testis and contains the ductus deferens with its artery and vein, testicular artery, testicular vein, lymphatic vessels, nerves and cremaster muscle. The vascular supply to the testes is via the testicular artery and the artery of the ductus deferens, the latter being a branch of the prostatic artery. The testicular vein forms a network called the pampiniform plexus, which is responsible for testicular thermoregulation by counter-current heat exchange. The right testicular vein drains to the caudal vena cava, whereas the left drains to the left renal vein. The scrotal arteries (branches of the external pudendal artery) supply the scrotum, alongside satellite scrotal veins. Innervation to the testes is via the testicular plexus, part of the autonomic nervous system, and the scrotum is innervated by the superficial perineal nerve, a branch of the pudendal nerve. Testicular and epididymal lymphatics drain into the lumbar lymph nodes, and scrotal lymphatics drain to the superficial inguinal lymph nodes.

Penis and prepuce

The canine penis comprises the root, body and glans (Fig. 5.15). The root is attached by the left and right crura to the ischiatic tuberosity. The crura surround paired columns of cavernous tissue known as the corpus cavernosum, which extend distally from the root on the dorsal aspect of the penis, and are transformed into the os penis. The single corpus spongiosum surrounds the urethra for the length of the penis; proximally it forms the bilobed bulb, and distally it expands over the distal end of the corpus cavernosum and is confluent with the erectile tissue of the glans penis. The majority of erectile function of the glans penis is provided by the bulbus glandis, which is separated from the pars longa glandis by a fibrous septum. The os penis extends almost to the tip of the glans. The four extrinsic muscles of the penis are the ischiocavernosus, bulbospongiosus, retractor penis and ischiourethralis. The paired ischiocavernosus muscles originate from the ischial tuberosity and insert on the proximal corpus cavernosum. The bulbospongiosus covers the root and ventral surface of the penis and fuses with the retractor penis muscles at the proximal third of the penile body. The retractor penis is composed mainly of smooth muscle fibres that arise from the first two caudal vertebrae and run along the ventral surface of the penis, inserting on the penis at the level of the preputial fornix. The paired ischiourethralis muscles originate from the dorsal aspect of the ischial tuberosity and insert into a fibrous ring at the urethral bulb.

The vascular supply to the penis is via the artery of the penis, a branch of the internal pudendal artery. The artery splits into three anastomosing branches: the artery of the bulb, which supplies the corpus spongiosum, the deep artery of the penis, which supplies the corpus cavernosum, and the dorsal artery of the penis, which supplies the glans penis. Venous drainage is via the internal and external pudendal veins, and nerves from the pelvic and sacral plexuses innervate the penis. Lymphatic drainage is to the superficial inguinal lymph nodes.

The feline penis is much shorter than in the dog, and faces caudodorsally. Its structure is similar, though an os penis is evident only radiographically in approximately 40% of mature cats (Piola et al., 2010). The free part of the penis of a sexually mature cat is covered with caudally directed, cone-shaped keratinised papillae, called penile spines.

The prepuce is a tubular sheath that covers the non-erect penis to the level of the mid-bulbus glandis. Skin borders the prepuce laterally and ventrally, and dorsally it is attached to the ventral body wall. Parietal epithelium covers the inside of the prepuce to the level of the fornix, and this is continuous with the visceral epithelium which extends to the urethral orifice. Vascular supply to the parietal and visceral layers of the prepuce is by an anastomosis between the external pudendal artery and the artery of the penis. Venous drainage is via the superficial and deep veins of the glans, the dorsal vein of the penis and the external pudendal veins. The skin is supplied by the caudal superficial epigastric vessels, and preputial lymphatics drain to the superficial inguinal lymph nodes.

Prostate

The canine prostate is located at the neck of the bladder and completely surrounds the urethra (Fig. 5.16). In juvenile dogs, it lies in an intra-pelvic position and gradually migrates cranially into the abdomen; by 4 years of age half of the prostate occupies an intra-abdominal position. Adult size is variable dependent on breed, with the Scottish terrier generally having a larger

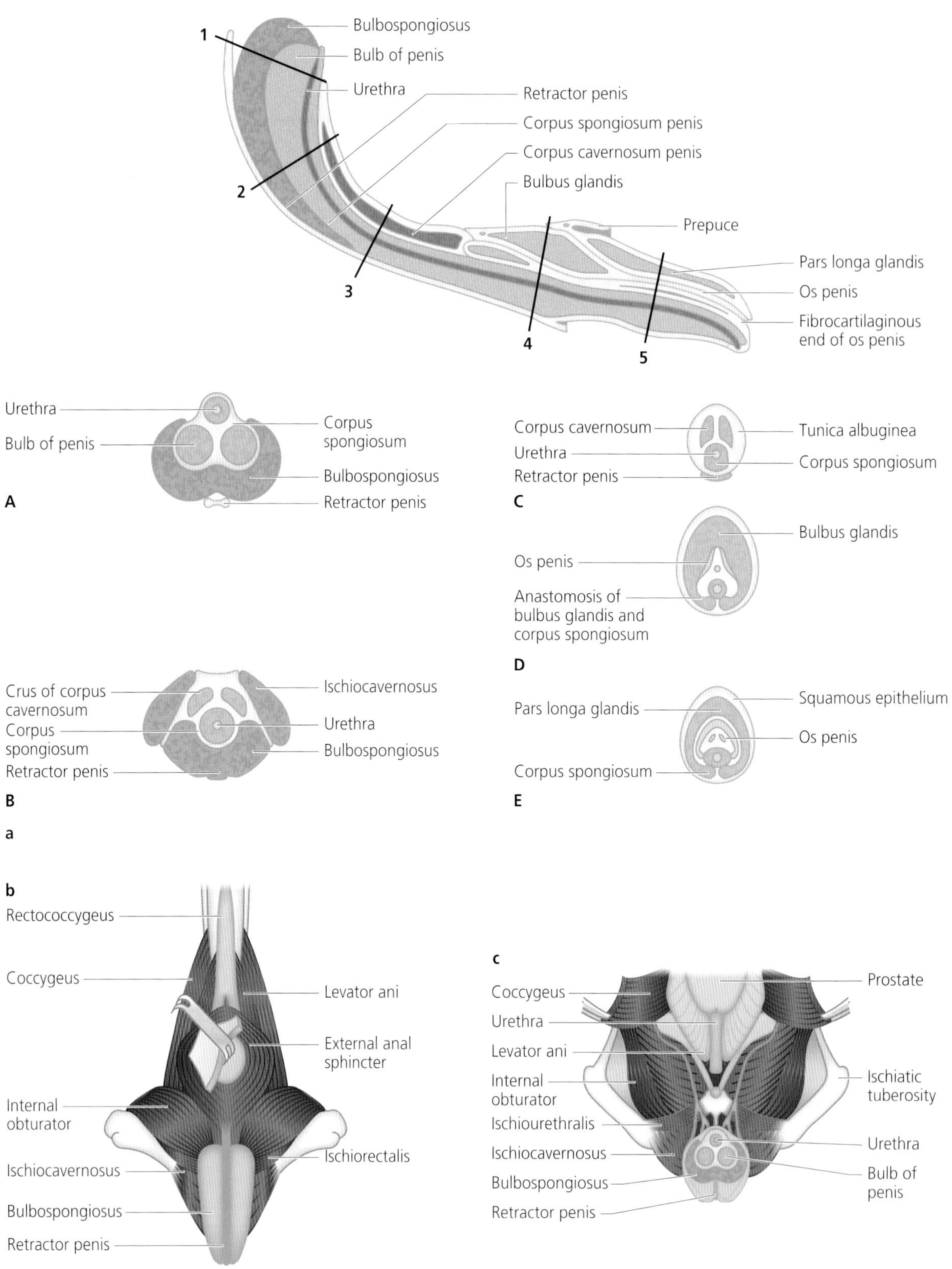

Fig. 5.15a–c a. Anatomy of the penis and male perineum: b. caudal aspect; c. dorsal aspect. *Illustrator: Elaine Leggett*

prostate than other breeds of a similar size. A fibromuscular capsule surrounds the prostate, and a mid-dorsal and ventral sulcus separates it into right and left lobes. The two ducti deferentes perforate the craniodorsal surface of the prostate before opening into the urethra via two slits at the colliculis seminalis. The parenchyma contains tubuloalveolar glands that secrete seminal fluid through ducts into the prostatic urethra. The prostate has an abundant vascular supply from the prostatic arteries, which branch from the internal pudendal arteries or umbilical arteries. Venous drainage from the gland is via the prostatic and urethral veins into the internal iliac veins, and lymphatic drainage is to the medial iliac and internal iliac lymph nodes. The autonomic nerve supply to the gland is via the hypogastric and pelvic nerves, which follow the vasculature and are responsible for micturition and continence.

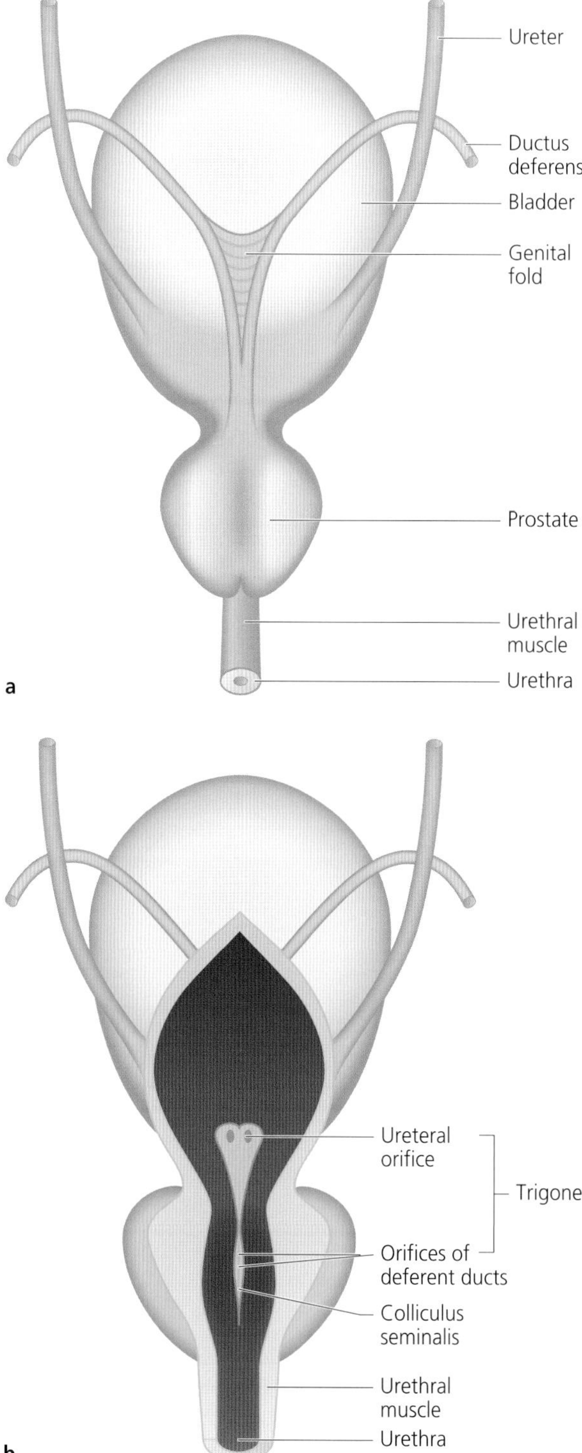

Fig. 5.16a,b Anatomy of the prostate. a. Dorsal aspect. b. Ventral aspect, partially opened at midline. *Illustrator: Elaine Leggett*

5.2.2 Testes and scrotum

Cryptorchidism

Failure of one or both testes to descend into the scrotum during development is termed cryptorchidism. Studies have shown that, normally, the testes have descended by 35 days (Kawakami et al., 1993), though diagnosis is often confirmed only once the animal reaches four to six months because anecdotally normal descent in some breeds is longer than this. The condition may be unilateral or bilateral, and may occur anywhere along the embryological path of testicular descent (termed abdominal, inguinal or pre-scrotal). Cryptorchidism is of significance as it can be a cause of ongoing 'intact male' symptoms in animals that are apparently neutered, though these animals are unlikely to be fertile due to thermal suppression of spermatogenesis. The condition is also associated with neoplastic transformation of the testicle or testicular torsion in the dog, and concurrent congenital anomalies in both the dog and cat. Cryptorchid dogs have been found to carry a risk of testicular neoplasia up to 13.6 times higher than normal dogs (Hayes and Pendergrass, 1976).

Diagnosis

Confirmation of cryptorchidism requires identification of the retained testicle. This can prove challenging, since a normal immature descended testicle can be retracted by the cremaster muscle in response to fear, stress or cold. The entire pre-scrotal and inguinal region should be palpated, and the descended testicle should be pushed dorsally and cranially to determine whether it is left or right. Abdominal testicles are not usually palpable unless they are neoplastic and enlarged, and therefore abdominal ultrasound or radiography is useful for identification. In adult animals when neoplasia or testicular torsion is suspected, complete blood count, serum biochemistry and urinalysis should be performed. Testosterone concentrations can be measured to confirm a bilateral cryptorchid patient versus an anorchid patient.

Treatment

Orchiectomy should be performed once the animal is of normal neutering age, and both testicles should be removed in the same procedure. An inguinal or prescrotal testicle is stabilised through the skin with the index finger and thumb, and the skin is incised directly over the testicle. A caudal midline laparotomy or laparoscopy is required for an abdominal testicle (Figs. 5.17, 5.18). To find the testicle, the abdomen can be explored from kidney to inguinal ring, or instead the prostate can be located and the ductus deferens followed until it is identified. If the vas deferens is found crossing the

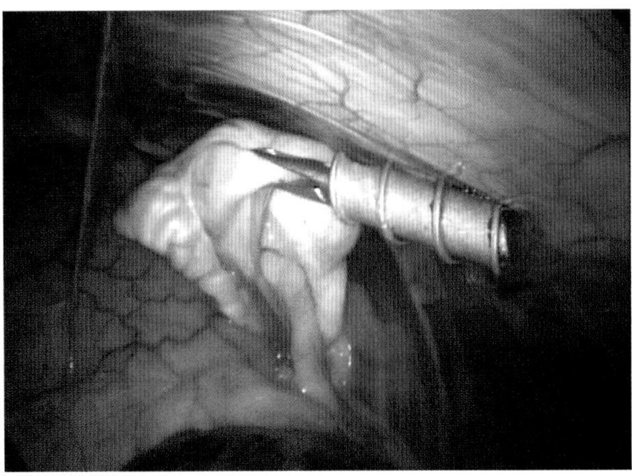

Fig. 5.17 Ectopic testicle found in the abdomen. Diagnosis and treatment can be performed via a laparoscopic approach.

inguinal ring internally, the testicle should be searched for in the inguinal region. Once found, the surgery is continued as for a routine castration.

Testicular torsion

Testicular torsion is a rare condition and is most often associated with abdominal testicles, though inguinal and scrotal testicular torsions have been reported (Pearson and Kelly, 1975; Fig. 5.19). Clinical signs are often non-specific (anorexia, vomiting, lethargy), though patients sometimes present with acute abdominal pain and shock. An abdominal mass may be palpable or, if scrotal, the torsed testicle may be enlarged and painful. Diagnostics should include complete blood count, acid–base analysis, serum biochemistry and abdominal imaging. Blood work may reflect dehydration, hypovolaemia and/or toxaemia. Abdominal radiography may reveal an ovoid soft tissue opacity. Ultrasonography is the most useful modality for confirmation of a torsed testicle; decreased testicular echogenicity is the most common finding and, with complete testicular torsion, blood flow within the spermatic cord is absent on colour Doppler. Treatment is by orchiectomy, following which there is generally a good prognosis.

Orchitis/epididymitis

Orchitis and epididymitis are both uncommon conditions and may be primary due to infection, or secondary to trauma or ascending infection from the urinary tract or prostate. Primary infection can be bacterial (e.g.

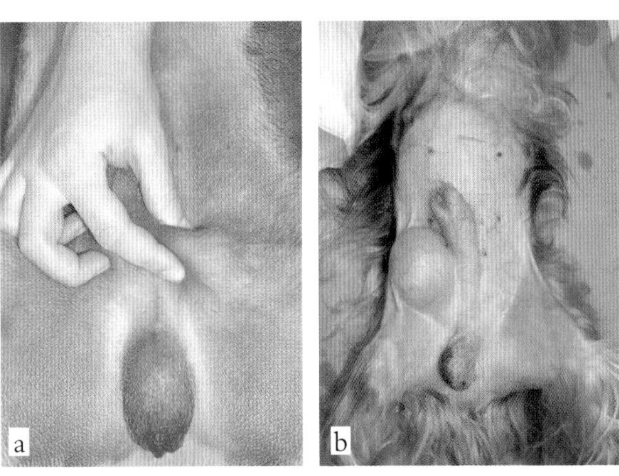

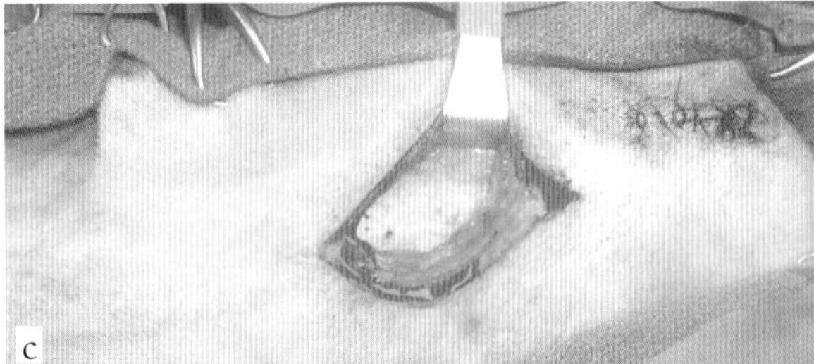

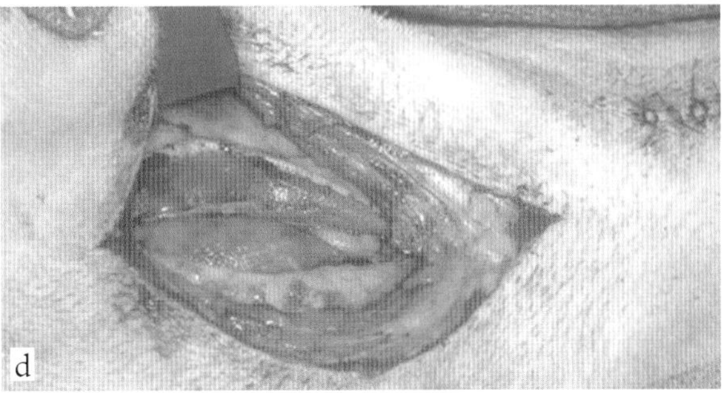

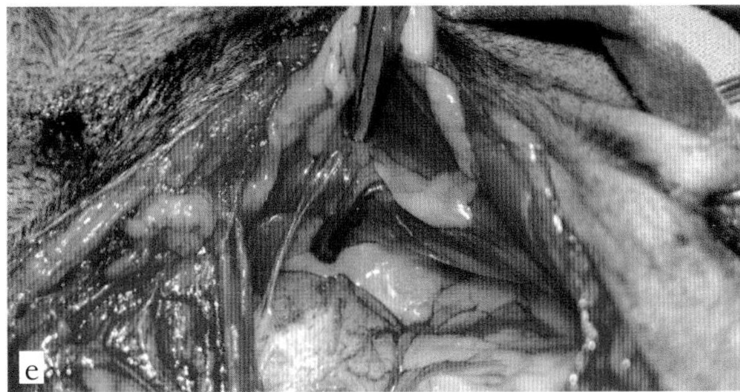

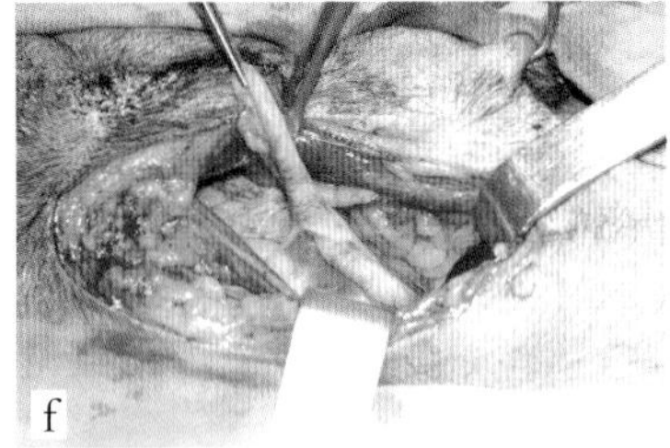

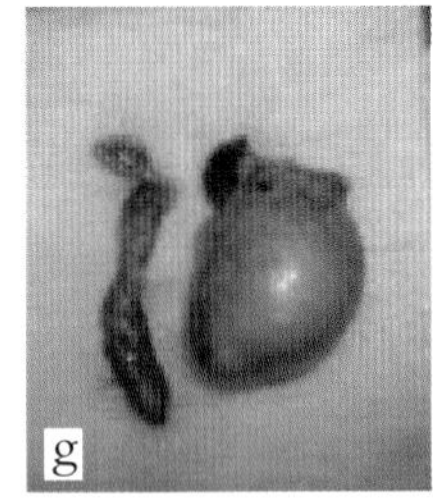

Fig. 5.18a–g Ectopic testicle. a. Palpation of the inguinal region (by the side of the prepuce) to identify the presence of an ectopic testicle (most common location). b. Inguinal ectopic testicle. The normal testicle is in the scrotum; the inguinal testicle is increased in size due to neoplastic changes. c. Para-preputial approach to identify ectopic testicle. The incision is made to the side of the prepuce. Normal orchiectomy has already been performed (suture line to the right of the picture). At this stage the inguinal region is carefully probed. d. If the ectopic testicle is not found, a caudal coeliotomy is performed. e. The internal inguinal ring is identified. The absence of ductus deferens passing through the ring confirms the intra-abdominal location of the ectopic testicle. f. The ectopic testicle is found and removed as per a normal orchiectomy. g. The shape of an ectopic testicle (left) can be very different from a normal testicle (right).

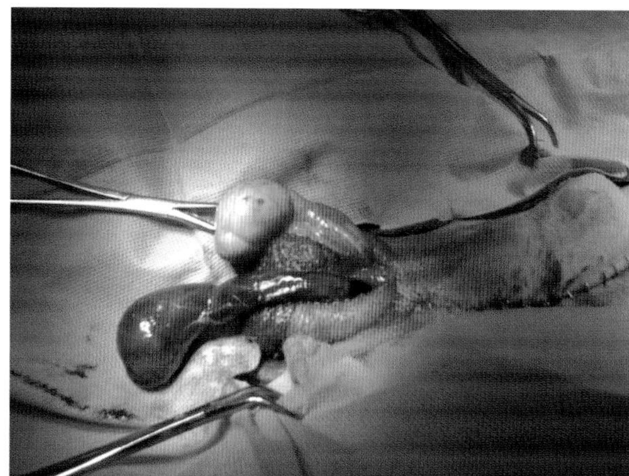

Fig. 5.19 Necrotic/thrombosed testicle following road traffic accident.

Brucella canis, *Klebsiella*), viral (canine distemper), fungal (*Rhodotorula glutinis*) or rickettsial (Rocky Mountain spotted fever). Clinical signs include pain, testicular swelling, inappetence, lethargy, pyrexia, vomiting and pelvic limb lameness. Testicular ultrasound and fine needle aspirate or biopsy can be used to rule out other causes such as neoplasia or torsion, and samples should be submitted for culture. Cure is achieved by orchiectomy, though in valuable breeding animals an attempt may be made to treat the underlying cause.

Testicular neoplasia

The three most common testicular neoplasms are interstitial cell (Leydig) tumour, Sertoli (sustentacular) cell tumour and seminoma, which are seen with near equal frequency. More than one type of tumour may be present (Dow, 1962), and Sertoli cell tumours and seminomas are more frequent in cryptorchid testicles. Sertoli cells are 'nurse cells' to the developing spermatozoa. Up to 40% of Sertoli cell tumours are functional (oestrogen-secreting) and cause signs of feminisation such as symmetrical alopecia, gynecomastia, galactorrhoea, pendulous prepuce and attractiveness to male dogs. Squamous metaplasia of the prostate may also occur, leading to prostatic cysts or abscessation, and bone marrow suppression may cause dullness, anaemia and thrombocytopenia. Seminomas are germ cell tumours and, as with Sertoli cell tumours, metastasise in up to 10% of cases. Leydig cell tumours rarely metastasise, but some are functional tumours (testosterone-secreting) and are associated with perineal hernia, perianal adenoma, perianal gland adenocarcinoma and prostatic disease. Diagnosis requires careful palpation of the testicles as bilateral involvement is common, and rectal examination to check for prostatic disease. Fine needle aspiration or testicular biopsy may be performed, though castration and submission of the testicles for histopathology is often preferred to obtain a definitive diagnosis. A complete blood count, serum biochemistry panel, urinalysis, three-view thoracic radiography or thoracic CT, two-view abdominal radiography or abdominal CT, and abdominal ultrasonography may be performed for complete staging of the tumour. Treatment of testicular neoplasia is by orchiectomy, and prognosis is excellent if there is no evidence of myelosuppression or metastasis.

Orchiectomy

Orchiectomy (castration) is routinely carried out to prevent breeding and undesirable behaviours and to reduce hereditary diseases, but may also be performed to control disease (e.g. *Brucella canis*, transmissible venereal tumour, feline virus) and to prevent and treat disease. Androgen-related conditions such as benign prostatic hyperplasia, prostatic disease, perineal adenoma and perineal hernia can be prevented by orchiectomy, and all testicular diseases can be prevented or treated. Other reasons for castration are inguinal-scrotal herniorrhaphy and control of endocrine abnormalities and epilepsy. Orchiectomy can be performed via either open or closed methods (see description below). The two methods have been compared in a prospective study showing that open castration was associated with higher scrotal complications including swelling, bruising and pain compared to closed castration (Hamilton et al., 2014). Orchiectomy with scrotal ablation may be performed in cases of scrotal neoplasia, trauma or abscess of the scrotum, and in scrotal urethrostomy. The disadvantages of castration include a slightly increased risk of developing prostatic carcinoma (Bryan et al., 2007; Sorenmo et al., 2003), delayed closure of growth plates and increased risk of hip dysplasia and cranial cruciate ligament disease, especially when castration is performed in dogs less than 6 months old (Hart et al., 2014). Castration may also increase the risk of developing urinary incontinence if performed late in life; where an enlarged prostate due to BPH had contributed to urethral pressure, prostatic shrinkage following castration may reduce pressure on the urethra and no longer maintain continence.

Step by step: canine orchiectomy

- The dog is positioned in dorsal recumbency and the pre-scrotal skin is clipped and aseptically prepared. The scrotum is not clipped (to prevent clipper irritation) and is draped out unless a scrotal ablation or scrotal incision is required; a pre-scrotal location is most commonly used, though in very young animals the testicle may slip down the inguinal canal when advanced cranially and in such cases a scrotal incision may be preferred.

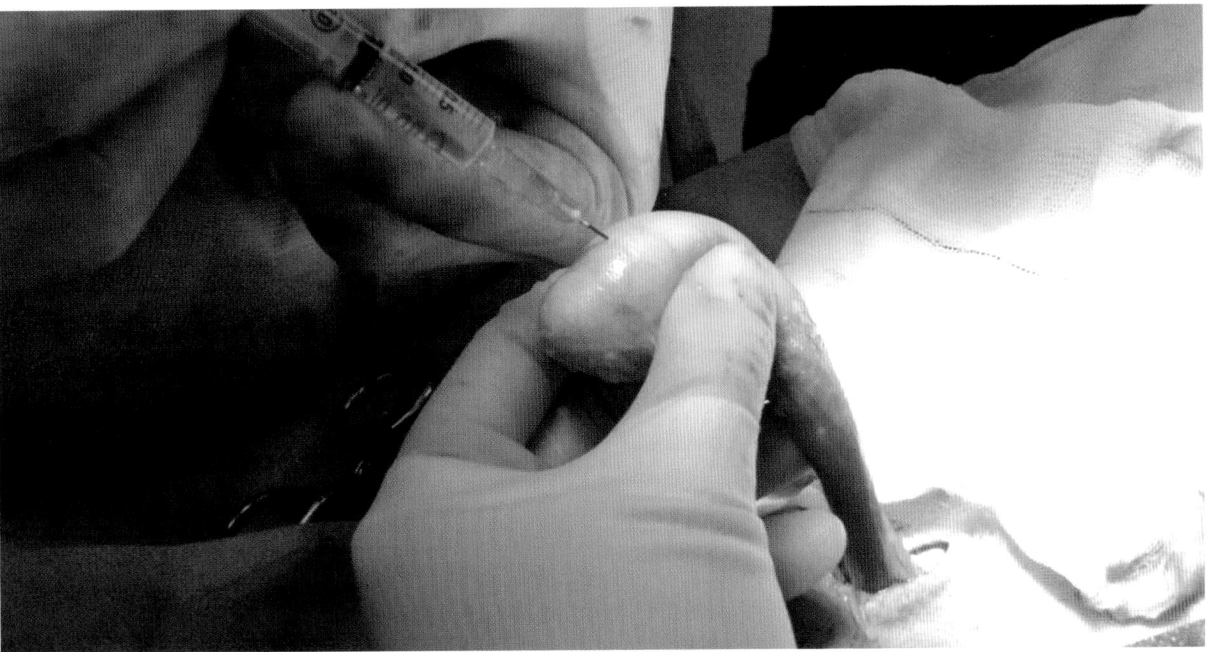

Fig. 5.20 Intra-testicular injection of bupivacaine during closed castration.

- Through the drape, pressure is applied to the scrotum and one testicle is pushed through to the pre-scrotal midline.
- The testicle is held between thumb and index finger, and the overlying skin and subcutaneous layer are incised on the midline. The skin is then squeezed to exteriorise the testicle.

Closed castration is performed as follows.

- A dry gauze swab is used to strip the parietal vaginal tunic of scrotal fat and fascia whilst gently pulling upwards on the testicle to maximise exposure of the spermatic cord.
- The cord is triple-clamped and ligated using two circumferential sutures, or one circumferential and one transfixation suture, with absorbable multifilament suture material of size 3-0 or 2-0 (2 or 3 metric).
- The first ligature is placed proximal to the most proximal clamp (i.e. closest to the body), and the second in the crush mark of this clamp once it has been removed.
- The cord can be severed with scissors between the two remaining clamps, or by twisting between them, which traumatises the vessel and causes spasm.

Open castration is performed as follows.

- The incision is continued below the spermatic fascia and through the vaginal tunic, so exposing the testicle. Care is taken not to incise the tunica albuginea, as this will result in testicular haemorrhage and may seed neoplastic cells in cases of testicular tumour.
- The tunica is torn free from the ligament of the tail of the epididymis using a gauze swab.
- A window is created in the fascia, separating the ductus deferens and its vessels from the spermatic vascular cord.
- The three-clamp technique is then performed on each group of structures.
- The incision is closed routinely – the vaginal tunic does not need to be closed.

Scrotal ablation is performed as follows (Fig. 5.21).

- An incision is made in the scrotal skin and a routine open or closed castration is performed.
- Allis tissue forceps are placed on the scrotum so that when lifted, the amount of skin for removal without causing undue tension can be established. Lifting also helps to avoid damage to the underlying urethra.
- An incision is made circumferentially around the scrotum and is continued through the dartos and fibrous connective tissue to fully excise it.
- The subcutaneous layer and skin edges are closed routinely.
- Alternatively, castration may be performed following a circumferential incision around the scrotum, and identification and dissection through the median raphe (Fig 5.21).

Step by step: feline orchiectomy

- The cat is positioned in lateral recumbency and the scrotal region is plucked free of hair and surgically prepped.

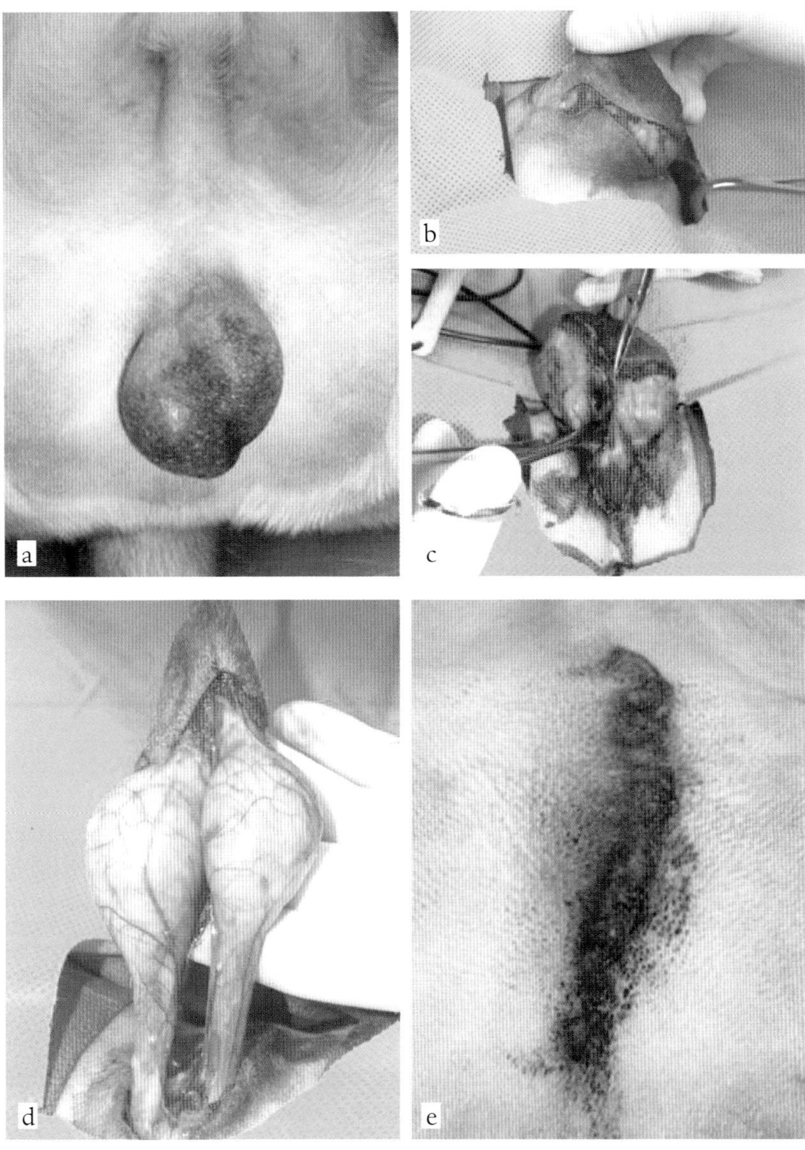

Fig. 5.21a–e Scrotal ablation. a. Preparation of the surgical site; the entre scrotum is clipped and prepped. b. A circumferential incision is made around the scrotal skin. c. The dissection is performed and the median raphe is identified (tip of the dissection scissors). d. Once the raphe is dissected, the orchiectomy is continued as per normal closed technique. e. Final result; there is no tension on the skin.

- The testicle is immobilised within the scrotum and an incision is made using a no. 15 scalpel blade.
- The incision is continued through the layers down to and including the tunica albuginea to create an open castration, and the ligament of the tail of the epididymis is broken off the testicle.
- Various methods of cord ligation are possible, but the authors prefer the square-knot open technique. This technique involves separating the vaginal tunic, cremaster muscle and ductus deferens and its associated vessels from the spermatic vascular cord (testicular artery, nerve and pampiniform plexus). The two structures are then tied together with two to three square knots (four to six throws) before distal transection.
- The knot is returned inside the scrotum by lifting the scrotal skin.
- Skin closure is not required – the wound is left to heal by secondary intention.

Complications following orchiectomy include infection, dehiscence, seroma and haemorrhage. Haemorrhage can be life-threatening if ligatures are ineffective; clotting disorders should be ruled out if an animal bleeds post-castration.

5.2.3 *Penis and prepuce*

Key points

- Hypospadias is a developmental abnormality of the external genitalia, most often seen in the Boston terrier.
- If the penile urethra has been damaged but not transected, catheterisation for 5–7 days will minimise the risk for stricture occurrence.

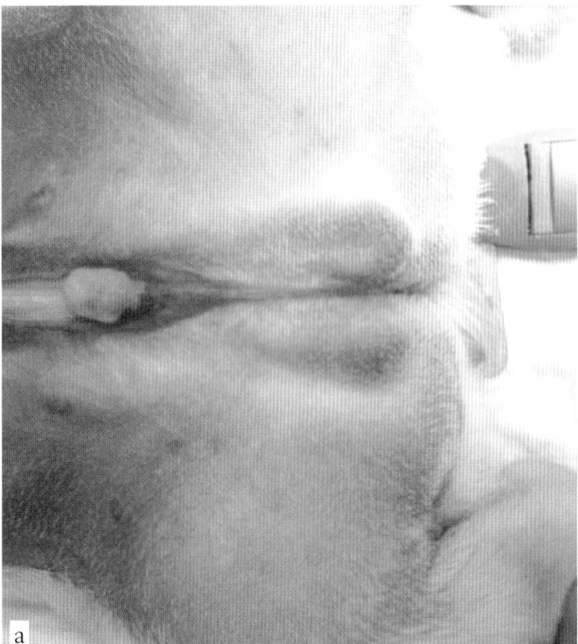

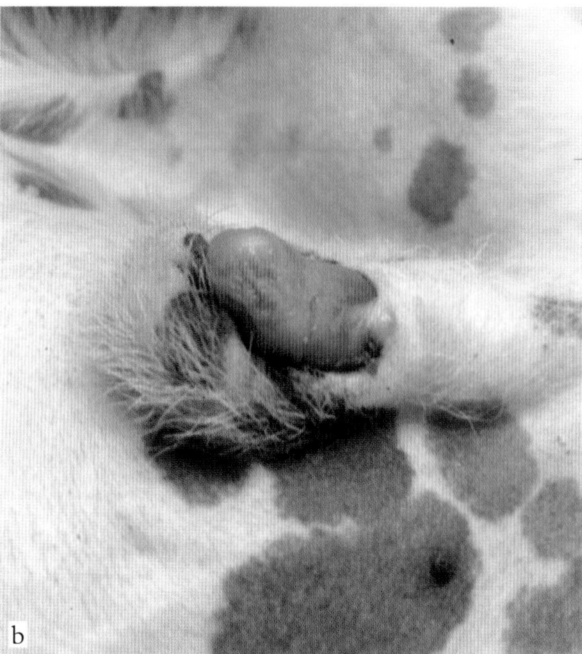

Fig. 5.22a,b Hypospadias. The urethral opening is located ventrally (at any location over the midline, from the tip of the penis to the perineal region) and the penis is usually atrophied and malformed. Ventral fusion of the prepuce is absent.

Hypospadias

Hypospadias is a developmental abnormality of the external genitalia where there is incomplete formation of the penile urethra due to a failure of fusion of the urogenital folds. The external urethral orifice is in an abnormal location, ventral and caudal to its normal position (Fig. 5.22). The classification of hypospadias is based on the location of the urethral opening (i.e. glandular, penile, scrotal, perineal or anal). The prepuce is usually ventrally incomplete, also from failure of fusion, and the penis often underdeveloped. The condition is rare, but is most often seen in the Boston terrier. Patients may be evaluated due to a chronically exposed penis, or there may be a history of urinary incontinence, skin irritation and infection. Clinical findings may include skin irritation or dermatitis, and penile/preputial inflammation or infection (balanoposthitis) from urine pooling. Diagnosis is made upon close examination of the penis and prepuce, and identification of an abnormally positioned external urethral orifice. Treatment may involve reconstruction of the penile defect, though this may not be possible as the urethra is usually deficient cranially. Enlargement of the urethral orifice or urethrostomy may be required, with excision of preputial and penile remnants.

Penile wounds

Trauma to the penis may occur following copulation, road traffic accident, fighting or jumping over fences (Fig. 5.23). Laceration or puncture of the cavernous tissue can cause profuse haemorrhage and lead to haematoma formation. Damage to the penile urethra causes subcutaneous swelling associated with urine extravasation. Sometimes trauma can cause fracture of the os penis. Whilst minor wounds may be treated with topical antimicrobial ointment and allowed to heal by secondary intention, more severe wounds often require surgery. If the urethra has been damaged but not transected, catheterisation for 5–7 days will minimise exposure of the healing urethra to urine and thus minimise risk for stricture occurrence. However, if there has been complete transection, urethral anastomosis should be performed and the urethra catheterised for up to 10 days. Tube cystostomy urinary diversion is an alternative to urethral catheterisation, and has been shown not to influence urethral function or healing (Cooley et al., 1999). Severe injuries may require partial penile amputation and scrotal urethrostomy. The prognosis for penile wounds is generally good unless the urethra has been transected, in which case urethral stricture may occur.

Penile and preputial tumours

Neoplasms of the penis and mucosal surface of the prepuce include transmissible venereal tumour (TVT), squamous cell carcinoma, haemangiosarcoma, papilloma and osteosarcoma of the os penis (Fig. 5.24). Any tumour affecting the skin can occur on the skin of the prepuce. Clinical signs are often licking, serosanguinous or purulent preputial discharge and unwillingness to copulate. Phimosis or paraphimosis may be present.

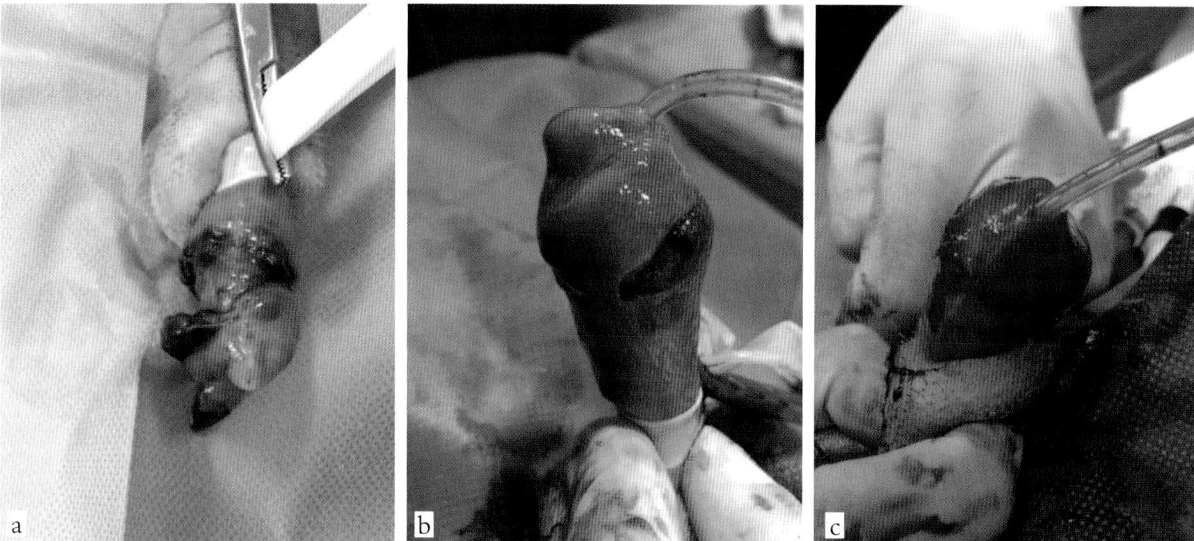

Fig. 5.23a–c Penile trauma due to laceration on a wired fence. a. The lacerations of the pars longa glandis and bulbus glandis are superficial and the urethra is intact. b. The tissues are debrided. c. Primary closure is performed using absorbable monofilament sutures.

Diagnosis may be obtained by cytological evaluation of fine needle aspirates or impression smears (especially with TVT), but biopsy may be required. Full staging should be performed i.e. three-view thoracic radiography or CT, two-view abdominal radiography or CT and/or ultrasound. Treatment depends on the type and extent of the neoplasm. TVTs generally respond best to chemotherapy (vincristine) or radiotherapy, whereas other types may require partial penile amputation or, sometimes, complete penile amputation and scrotal or perineal urethrostomy.

Phimosis

Phimosis is the inability to extrude the penis from the prepuce. It may be developmental, where the preputal opening is too small or absent, or it may be the result of preputial trauma and subsequent stenosis, or of neoplasia. Clinical signs may include pollakiuria and stranguria, and urine pooling may lead to balanoposthitis with associated licking and preputial swelling. Diagnosis is made based on the finding of being unable to exteriorise the penis. Further investigations are warranted if a preputial or penile mass is identified. Treatment of phimosis involves widening of the preputial opening. A V-shaped incision is made in the dorsal aspect of the preputial opening (or the ventral aspect in the cat), and a wedge of skin, subcutaneous tissue and preputial mucosa is excised. Enough should be removed so that the penis can be easily extruded but still be completely covered by prepuce. The ipsilateral skin and mucosa are then sutured together using a monofilament absorbable or non-absorbable suture in a simple interrupted pattern.

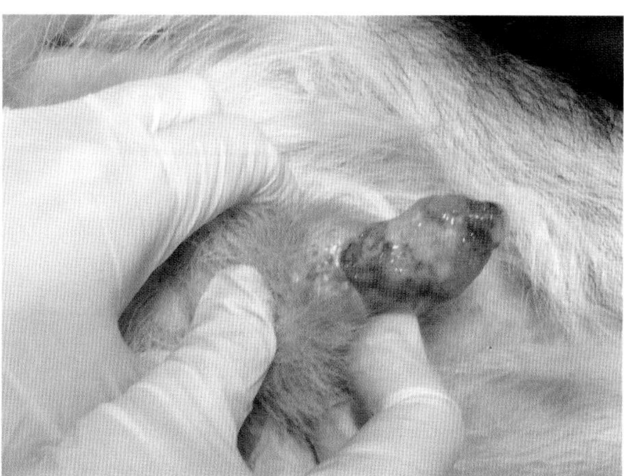

Fig. 5.24 Penile tumour in a dog.

Paraphimosis

Paraphimosis is the protrusion of the penis and inability to retract it into the prepuce (Fig. 5.25). This may be due to a congenitally narrowed or shortened prepuce, or be acquired due to trauma, constriction by preputial hairs, neoplasia or priapism. The condition is often seen following coitus or masturbation. Clinical signs initially are a penis that is unable to retract into the prepuce, pain and licking. The edges of the preputial orifice may be rolled inwards, and may appear too small for the penis which becomes swollen or engorged. Circulation to the penis becomes impaired due to the constriction, and it is easily traumatised. Fissures, lacerations and haemorrhage may be evident. With time the penis, becomes oedematous and the circulation is further compromised. Tissue necrosis ensues and the penis may appear purple or black. Diagnosis is made based on the physical examination, and further investigations are warranted if a preputial or penile mass is identified.

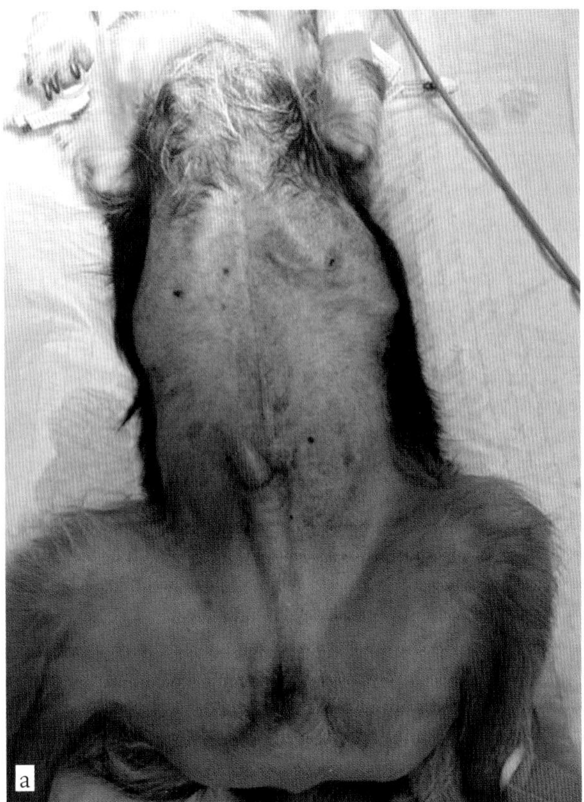

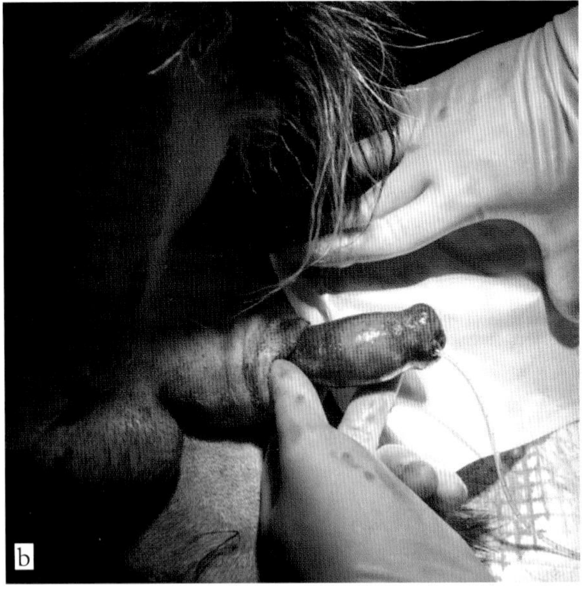

Fig. 5.25a,b a. Paraphimosis in a dog. b. Penile necrosis following placement of purse-string suture on a recurrent paraphimosis. Purse-string sutures must be carefully monitored.

Treatment is dependent on the cause and severity. Acute paraphimosis may be treated conservatively using lubrication, hyperosmolar agents such as sugar or local application of heat or cold to aid in replacement of the penis. Occasionally a loose purse-string suture can be placed. In that case, it is advised to place an indwelling urinary catheter and recheck the penile colour and shape twice a day. This suture is typically not left in place for more than 36–48 hours. If this is unsuccessful, a preputiotomy can be performed to allow retraction of the penis, and preputial reconstruction, phallopexy or penile amputation may be required. Preputial reconstruction may involve widening or narrowing of the preputial opening if it is too narrow or wide, respectively, or preputial lengthening if the prepuce is too short. Castration should be performed in cases where paraphimosis is a result of sexual activity.

Step by step: phallopexy

Phallopexy is indicated in cases of paraphimosis, once the penis has been replaced into the prepuce. It may be performed following preputial advancement (Fig. 5.26).

- The dog is positioned in dorsal recumbency and the ventral abdomen, including the prepuce, is clipped and aseptically prepared.
- A full-thickness incision measuring approximately one-third of the preputial length is made on the dorsolateral aspect, and a small strip of skin is removed.
- A strip of the same size is removed from the underlying penile mucosa. This is most readily achieved by marking the strip length with a scalpel and then extruding the penis to remove the strip.
- The penile and preputial mucosae are then sutured to one another using two lines of simple continuous or simple interrupted sutures, using 3-0 or 4-0 absorbable monofilament suture material.
- The preputiotomy is closed in two layers.

Step by step: preputial advancement

Preputial lengthening is performed when there is a deficiency in the length of the prepuce (Fig. 5.27).

- The dog is positioned in dorsal recumbency and the ventral abdomen, including the prepuce, is clipped and aseptically prepared.
- A semi-circular incision just cranial to and following the preputial opening is made, and the surrounding skin is freed from its attachments to the body wall.
- The prepuce is pulled forwards until the penis is covered, and a surgical marker pen is then used to mark the position.
- Another semi-circular incision is then made joining up with the first, and the segment of ventral abdominal skin is removed.
- The preputial muscles can be transected, shortened and re-apposed, or plicated and secured with a suture.
- The subcutaneous tissues and skin are closed routinely.

Step by step: partial penile amputation (dog)

This procedure may be necessary in cases of distal and benign neoplastic lesions, congenital abnormalities,

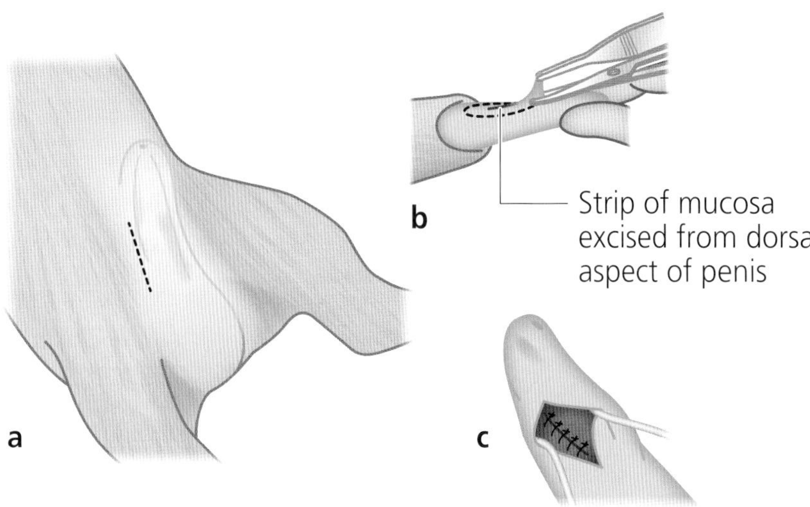

Fig. 5.26a–c Phallopexy. a. An incision is made in the prepuce 2–3 cm proximal to the preputial opening, at the junction between the prepuce and the skin of the body wall. b. A strip of mucosa is excised from both the dorsal aspect of the penis and the prepuce at the same level (just proximal to glans penis). c. The preputial and penile incisions are apposed using 3-0 or 4-0 monofilament absorbable sutures. *Illustrator: Elaine Leggett*

severe penile trauma or irreparable urethral damage (Fig. 5.28).

- The dog is positioned in dorsal recumbency and the ventral abdomen, including the prepuce and ventral pelvic region, is clipped and aseptically prepared. A urinary catheter is placed.
- The penis is extruded and a tourniquet is placed caudal to the proposed site of amputation – this also serves to keep the penis out of the prepuce.

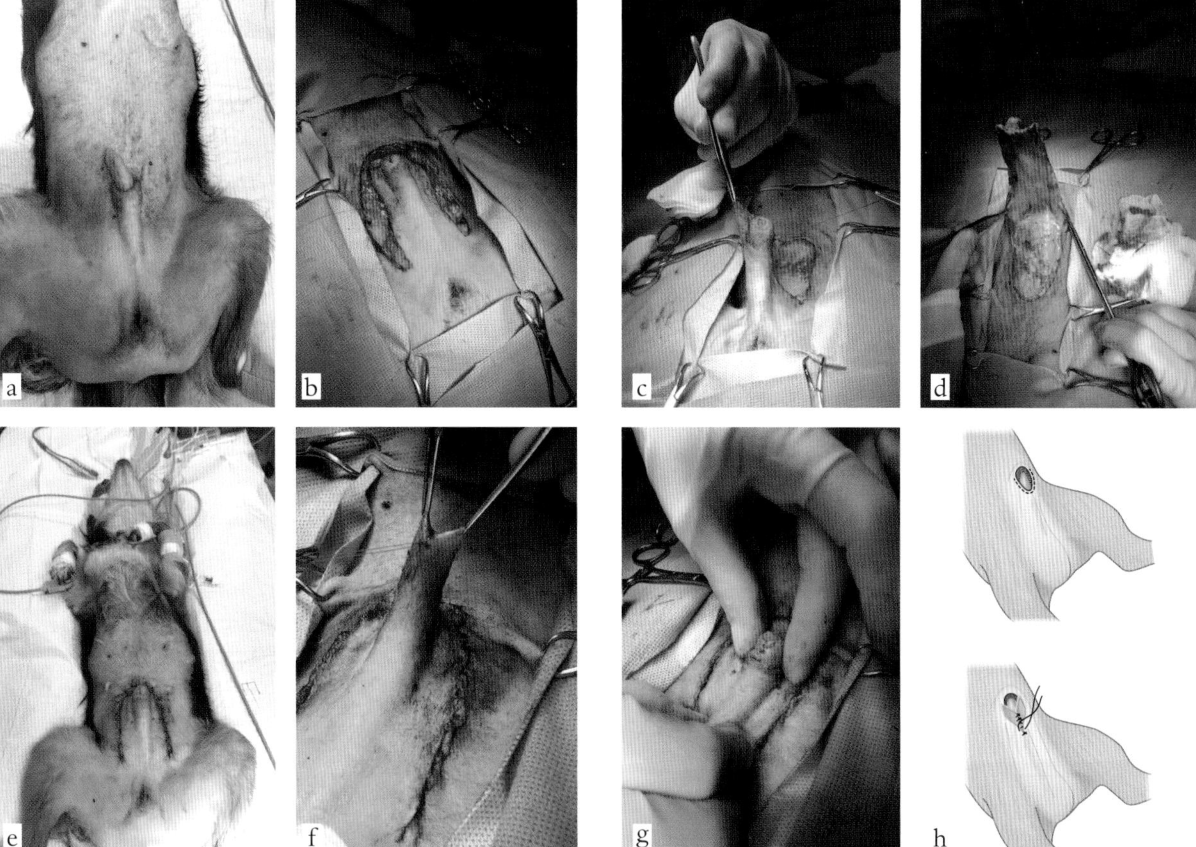

Fig. 5.27a–h Preputial advancement. a. Paraphimosis. b. Crescent-shaped incision made around the prepuce. The preputial flap is dissected from the body wall attachment. c. Dissection is performed until the prepuce is entirely free to allow advancement. Another semi-circular skin incision is then made at the cranial aspect of the flap. This should be pre-marked with a surgical pen and is the amount required to provide coverage of the penis once excised and the new skin edge advanced forward. This segment of ventral abdominal skin is then removed. d. The caudal superficial epigastric arteries and preputial vessels are visible on both sides and should be preserved. e. Complete closure. The preputial flap is attached to the body wall rostrally. f,g–h. In addition to preputial advancement (or in some cases as a sole procedure), it is also possible to perform a preputioplasty and narrow the preputial office by apposing two incisions made on the ventral part of the preputial opening (the opposite procedure can be done in the case of phimosis). *Illustrator: Elaine Leggett*

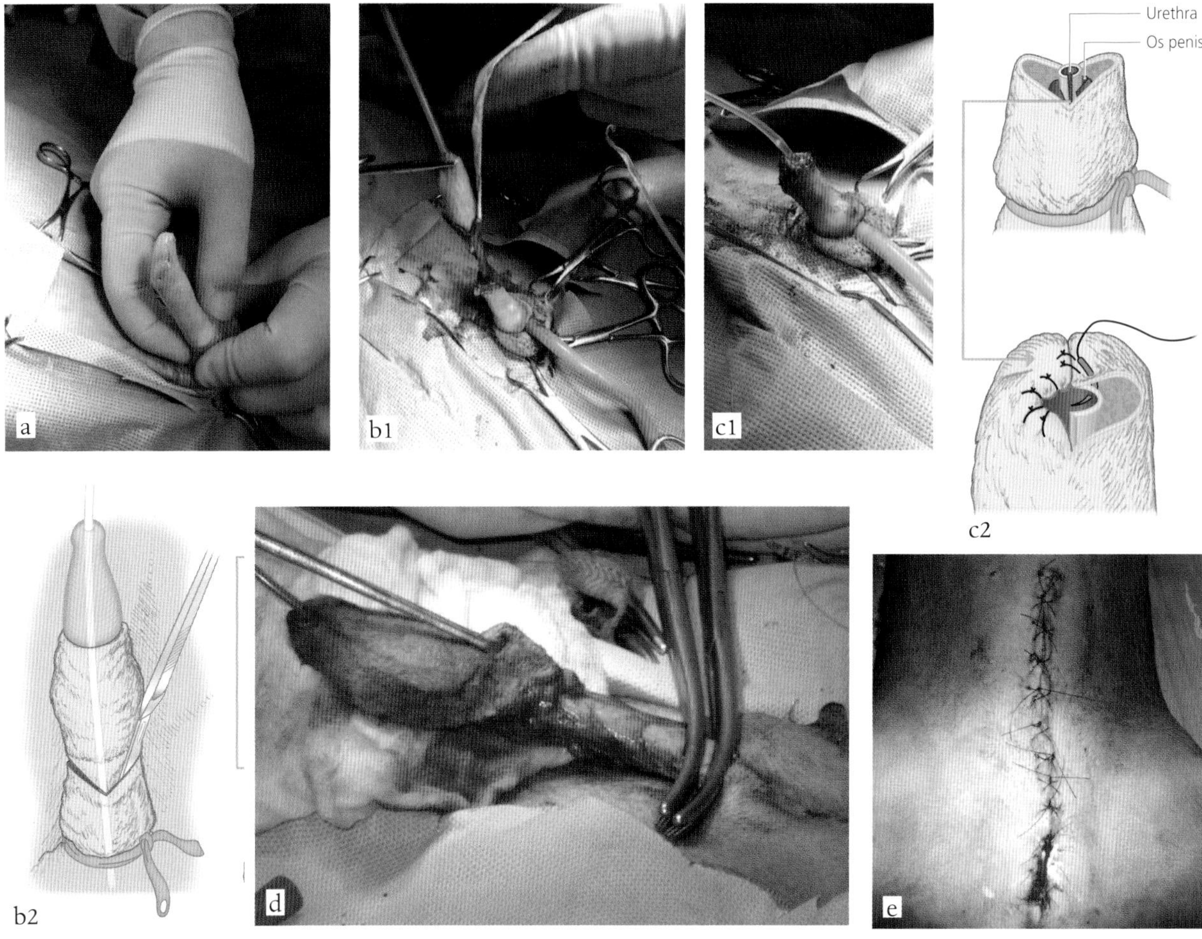

Fig. 5.28a–e Penile amputation: partial (a,b,c), complete (d,e) a. The penis is extruded and the urethra catheterised. b. A tourniquet is placed at the base of the penis and two incisions are made in a V shape. The urethra is isolated and transected distal to the proposed osteotomy of the os penis. c. The cavernous tissue and the tunica albuginea are closed and the urethra is anastomosed to the penile mucosa using simple interrupted absorbable sutures. d. When performing complete resection, the penis is isolated between two clamps with the distal one located immediately proximal to the os penis. Haemostasis is performed by suturing the cavernous tissues to the tunica albuginea. e. Final postoperative view: the penis is entirely resected and the peri-preputial skin is closed using cruciate sutures. A scrotal urethrostomy is performed. *Illustrator: Elaine Leggett*

- A V-shaped incision is made in the tunica albuginea and cavernous tissue, the urethra is dissected from the groove in the os penis and the latter is amputated using bone rongeurs as far caudally as possible.
- The urinary catheter is then removed and the urethra is transected and spatulated just distal to the amputation site.
- The tourniquet is loosened to allow identification and ligation of bleeding vessels in the erectile tissue, and then sutures are placed between the erectile tissue and the tunica albuginea to close the dead space.
- The spatulated urethral mucosa is sutured to the penile mucosa, and the remainder of the defect in the penile mucosa is closed.
- The prepuce must then be shortened by removing a full-thickness hexagonal segment of the ventral wall of the prepuce.
- The prepuce is closed in three layers – the preputial mucosa, subcutaneous tissue and skin.

5.2.4 Prostate

Key points

- The presence of prostatic enlargement is not necessarily indicative of disease, since this occurs with age in the majority of dogs.
- Surgical treatment by castration is preferred in patients with benign prostatic hyperplasia.
- Prostatitis and prostatic abscesses usually occur in middle-aged and old uncastrated male dogs, suggesting that their formation is associated with benign prostatic hyperplasia.
- Drainage of large abscesses during diagnostic aspiration is recommended, to relieve tension on the abscess capsule.

Benign prostatic hyperplasia

Benign prostatic hyperplasia (BPH) causes prostatic hypertrophy due to androgenic hormone stimulation (primarily dihydrotestosterone), which may be glandular, cystic or stromal. However, the presence of prostatic enlargement is not necessarily indicative of disease since it occurs with age in the majority of dogs. Many dogs do not show any clinical signs, but some may have dyschezia, ribbon-like faeces, haematuria and/or urethral bleeding. Dysuria is not usually seen because urethral intrusion or compression is rare.

Diagnosis

Diagnosis is made on the basis of physical examination and diagnostic tests to rule out other diseases. On rectal examination a large, non-painful and symmetrical mass cranial to the pelvic brim is identified. Abnormalities on haematological and biochemical analysis are not usually present. Similarly, urinalysis is often normal, though if there are cystic prostatic changes then sometimes red blood cells or squamous epithelial cells are present.

Abdominal radiography shows symmetric prostatomegaly and sometimes colorectal compression; enlargement is defined as being greater than 70% of the distance between the pubis and sacral promontory on lateral radiographs.

Ultrasonography may detect small cysts, and the parenchyma will be homogenous or mildly hyperechoic. Multiple fine needle aspirates should be taken during the ultrasound exam to rule out other disease; cytology of BPH shows sheets of uniform, mature, well-differentiated prostatic epithelial cells arranged in a honeycomb pattern.

Treatment

Surgical treatment by castration is preferred, as this results in involution of the hypertrophic glandular tissue within a few weeks. When this is not an option (i.e. in valuable breeding animals), medical management may be successful, though relapses are likely to occur once medication is stopped. Delmadinone acetate (Tardak, Pfizer; licensed in Europe) is a progestogen that reduces testosterone production by suppressing interstitial cell function. Finasteride (Proscar, Merck Sharp & Dohme) is a 5α-reductase inhibitor that reduces the rate of conversion of testosterone to dihydrotestosterone.

Prostatitis and abscessation

Prostatitis and prostatic abscess usually occur in middle-aged and old uncastrated male dogs, suggesting that their formation is associated with BPH. The cystic changes often found with BPH may be indicative of poor prostatic drainage, and may provide an environment compatible with bacterial growth. Infection is thought to be ascending from the urethra, with *E. coli* being the most common bacterial species, but *Pseudomonas* spp., *Streptococcus* spp., *Staphylococcus* spp. and *Proteus* spp. are also seen with some frequency. Mycotic infections, such as *Candida albicans* and *Cryptococcus neoformans*, are also possible but are much less common, and may be ascending or systemic in nature. Initially, multiple sites of infection are present and then micro-abscesses form. Larger abscesses develop when these coalesce into one area, and these may burst out into the peritoneal cavity (causing septic peritonitis) or retroperitoneal space. When communication exists between the abscess and urethra, a purulent urethral discharge is seen.

Diagnosis

Clinical findings can include tenesmus, pain on defecation and urination and sometimes purulent penile discharge, pyrexia and pelvic limb stiffness/lameness. Depending on the degree of abscessation and whether they have ruptured, there may be signs relating to sepsis such as vomiting, diarrhoea and collapse. Physical examination may reveal abdominal pain and the prostate may feel enlarged, asymmetric and soft in texture on rectal examination. Laboratory findings usually reveal neutrophilic leucocytosis with a left shift, and elevated alkaline phosphatase. Other findings may relate to sepsis, with dehydration or hypovolaemia such as azotaemia, hypoglycaemia, electrolyte disturbances and metabolic acidosis. Microorganisms and red blood cells are usually detected on urinalysis. Abdominal radiography and ultrasound will demonstrate prostatomegaly and free fluid if the abscess has ruptured into the peritoneal cavity. Retrograde contrast urethrography may indicate communication between the urethra and prostatic parenchyma. The characteristic finding on ultrasound is a multi-loculated appearance, with flocculent material bordered by capsular tissue. An ultrasound-guided fine needle aspirate should be performed to demonstrate septic neutrophilic inflammation and confirm the diagnosis.

Medical treatment

Shock therapy should be instituted as soon as possible in the dog with acute bacterial prostatitis and abscessation, and broad-spectrum antibiosis should be administered until culture and sensitivity results of aspirated material are obtained. Suitable choices are those with high lipid-solubility such as fluoroquinolones and trimethoprim-sulfonamides. Drainage of large abscesses during diagnostic aspiration is recommended to relieve tension on the abscess capsule. Ultrasound-guided percutaneous aspiration as a sole treatment, with or without infiltration of the abscess cavities with alcohol, has been described (Bussadori et al., 2000).

Surgical treatment

Various surgical techniques have been described for the drainage and resolution of prostatic abscess, such as omentalisation, active prostatic drainage, passive drainage with Penrose drains, stoma drainage (marsupialisation) and partial prostatectomy. Orchiectomy must also be performed, to trigger involution of the hypertrophic glandular tissue.

Ventral drainage, marsupialisation and partial prostatectomy are associated with complications such as urethrocutaneous fistula, premature drain loss, prolonged drainage, haemorrhage, urinary incontinence and recurrence. Postoperative complications following omentalisation are reported to be low (White and Williams, 1995), and the procedure is of only modest technical difficulty. Reported complications include inguinal oedema and recurrence. Omentalisation has the additional advantage of enabling shortened postoperative hospitalisation.

Step by step: approach to the prostate

- The dog is positioned in dorsal recumbency and the ventral abdomen is clipped and aseptically prepared.
- Placement of a urinary catheter can help identification of the prostatic urethra.
- A caudal midline coeliotomy is made from umbilicus to the pubic brim, and abdominal retractors are placed.
- The prostate is exposed by removal of peri-prostatic fat, and a small pair of Gelpis are placed around the gland to retract any surrounding fat.
- The prostate is then packed off from the abdomen using moist laparotomy swabs.
- The dorsal aspect of the gland should be avoided if possible, to prevent damage to the vascular supply and hypogastric and pelvic nerves.

Step by step: omentalisation (Fig. 5.29)

- An approach to the prostate is made as detailed previously.
- Stab incisions are made into the lateral aspects of the gland, and suction is used to drain purulent material.
- The incisions are then widened and the abscess cavity explored. Loculations are broken down digitally, and abscess chambers are connected.
- When abscessation is circumferential or involves the

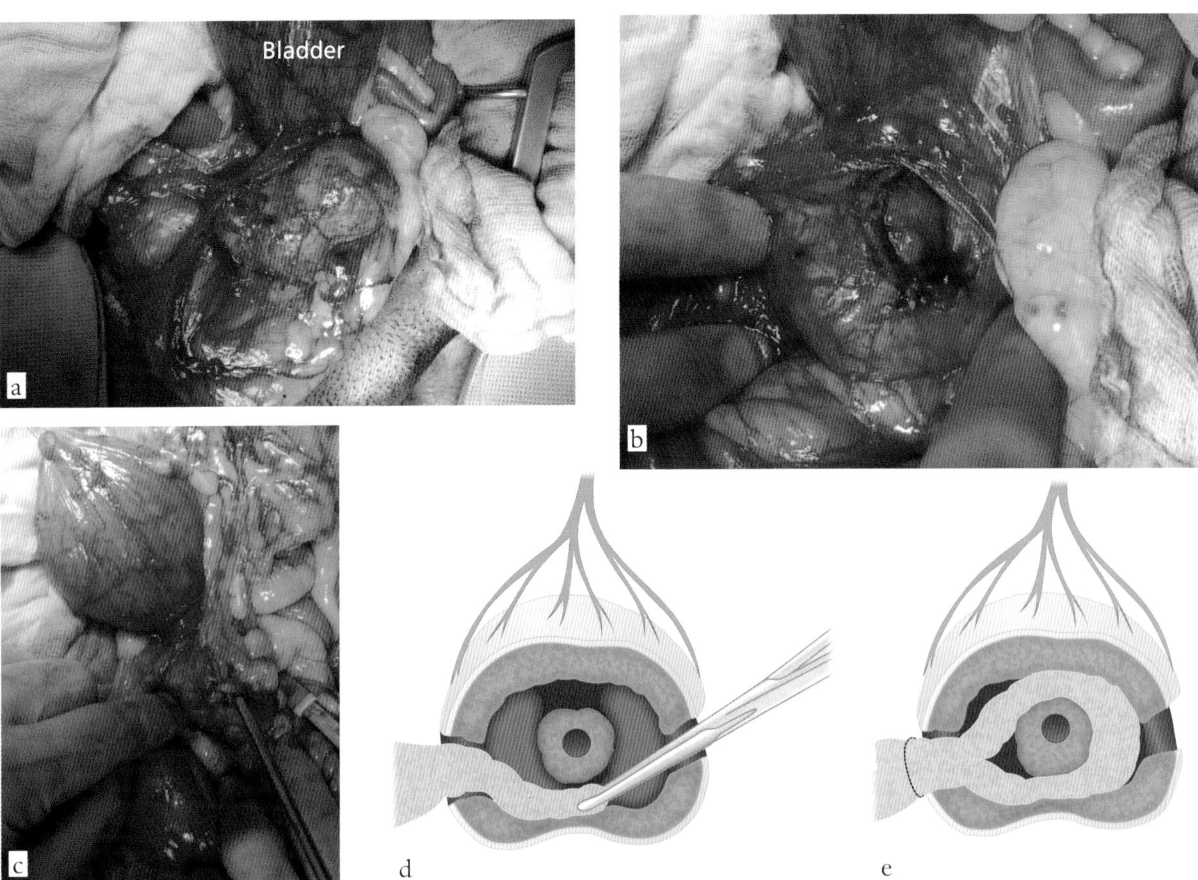

Fig. 5.29a–e Prostatic drainage via omentalisation. a. Prostate with prostatic abscesses (white arrows); the bladder is at the top of the image. b. The lateral position of the capsule and prostatic tissue of each lobe are incised and debrided. Tunnels are created dorsal and ventral to the urethra (catheterised). c. If omental lengthening is required to reach the abscess, the omental flap is divided (dorsal and ventral leaves of the omentum are separated) and brought caudally (omental flap (black arrow)). d. The omental flap is passed around the urethra dorsally and ventrally, and finally sutured on itself with mattress sutures. e. Omentalisation of the prostate completed; the omental flap is also attached to the remaining prostatic capsule. *Illustrator: Elaine Leggett*

dorsal prostate, the urethra should be identified by palpating the urinary catheter before carefully inserting a pair of haemostats around the urethra to connect the cavities.
- Warm saline is used to irrigate the common abscess cavity.
- The omentum is packed into the abscess cavity and secured with mattress sutures. It usually extends to the region without lengthening, though this may be necessary if the abscess is located very caudally. In the case of a circumferential abscess, haemostats are used to guide the omentum through both dorsal and ventral cavities, entering and exiting the same location. Urethral compression is avoided by not pulling the omentum tight.

Discrete prostatic cysts

Cystic changes within or on the surface of the prostate are a common finding in dogs with BPH, but development of solitary large cysts is rare. These cysts have been classified as 'prostatic', developing within the parenchyma, and 'para-prostatic', developing external to the prostate. Both types have a thick capsule of compressed epithelium and dense collagen, which are sometimes mineralised, and para-prostatic cysts are sometimes attached to the prostate by a stalk extending cranial to the bladder. The fluid origin of both types of cyst is likely to be prostatic secretions, which accumulate due to blocked ducts as a result of BPH or squamous metaplasia. The colour ranges from yellow to brown in colour, and they contain cellular debris.

Diagnosis

Discrete prostatic cysts may be an incidental finding, as clinical signs usually do not usually occur until there is rectal, urethral or bladder compression. Dysuria, urinary incontinence, haematuria, urethral haemorrhage and signs relating to azotaemia may be seen when the lower urinary tract is compressed, and rectal compression may cause dyschezia. Physical examination often reveals abdominal distension, and a palpable abdominal mass may be felt. Sometimes perineal rupture is evident due to chronic pressure on the pelvic diaphragm. Rectal exam may not be useful as the prostate is often displaced cranial to the pelvic brim, and cysts that are pelvic may make identification of landmarks difficult. Abdominal radiography will reveal a soft tissue opacity in the caudal abdomen or pelvis, sometimes with mineralised regions. Contrast studies may be required to distinguish between bladder and cyst. Ultrasound will confirm a fluid-filled mass and enable aspiration for sampling. Cytology of the fluid often shows only occasional inflammatory and epithelial cells, though culture should be performed to rule out infection. Sometimes fluid is found to be urine when fluid:serum creatinine ratio is performed. Laboratory findings are leucocytosis, elevated alkaline phosphatase and azotaemia if urinary obstruction is present.

Treatment

Discrete prostatic cysts should be treated by complete resection, or partial resection with omentalisation. Castration should also be performed to ensure prostatic involution.

Step by step: treatment of prostatic cysts

- The dog is positioned in dorsal recumbency and the whole ventral abdomen is clipped and aseptically prepared.
- A canine urinary catheter is inserted into the bladder.
- A caudal ventral coeliotomy is made, which can be extended cranially if the cyst is particularly large.
- The prostate should be examined for evidence of neoplasia that may account for the cyst, and a needle aspiration or biopsy taken.
- The cyst is then packed off from the abdomen with moist gauze laparotomy swabs, and a stab incision is made into it.
- Suction is used to drain the fluid and, if there are minimal attachments (i.e. to the prostatic capsule or other structures), the cyst is excised.
- Complete excision is best avoided when extensive intimal attachments to vital structures exist. Instead, the prostatic urethra and bladder neck are identified and avoided and the cyst capsule is partially excised, leaving the base of the attachment to the prostate intact. Omentum is then drawn into the cyst remnant and secured using a mattress suture.

Prostatic neoplasia

Prostatic neoplasia is seen in medium- to large-breed older dogs with a mean age of 10 years. The majority of prostatic tumours (98%) are carcinomas such as adenocarcinoma, transitional cell carcinoma, squamous cell carcinoma and undifferentiated carcinoma, with adenocarcinoma being the most frequently diagnosed. Mesenchymal tumours such as osteosarcoma, haemangiosarcoma, fibrosarcoma and leiomyosarcoma make up the other 2%. Carcinomas are classified according to their differentiation (i.e. glandular, urothelial, squamoid or sarcomatoid), and intra-tumoural heterogeneity is common; 50% show a mixed glandular and urothelial pattern. Hormonal influence is not a characteristic of prostatic tumours, and there is evidence that the disease occurs more frequently in castrated males (Bryan et al., 2007). The disease is aggressive in nature,

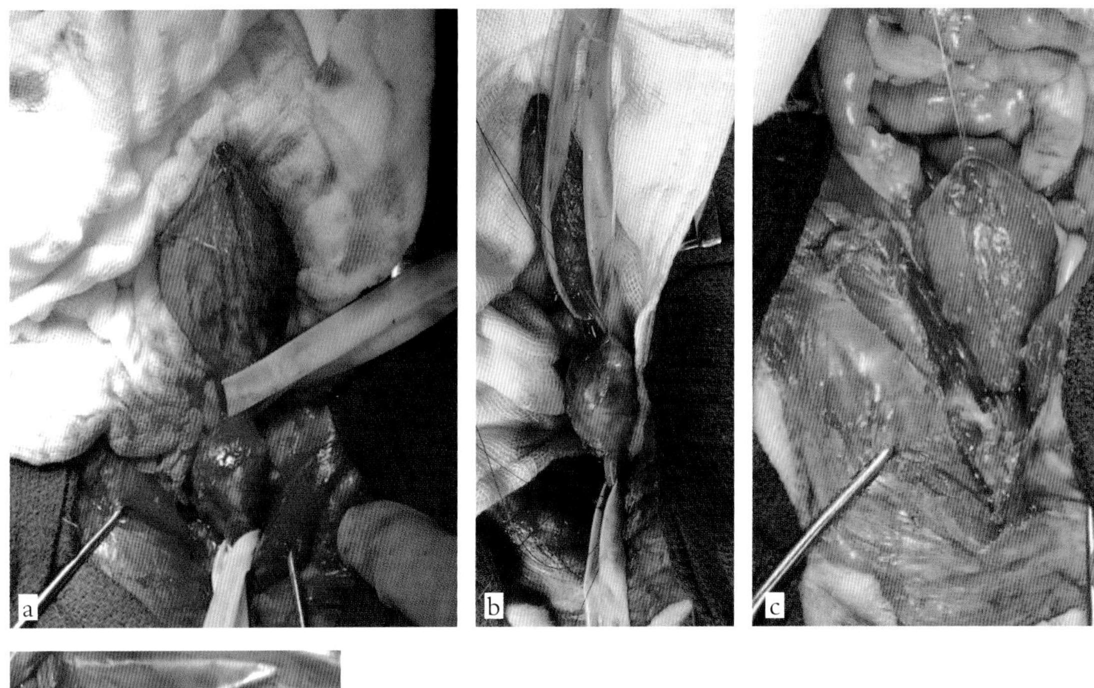

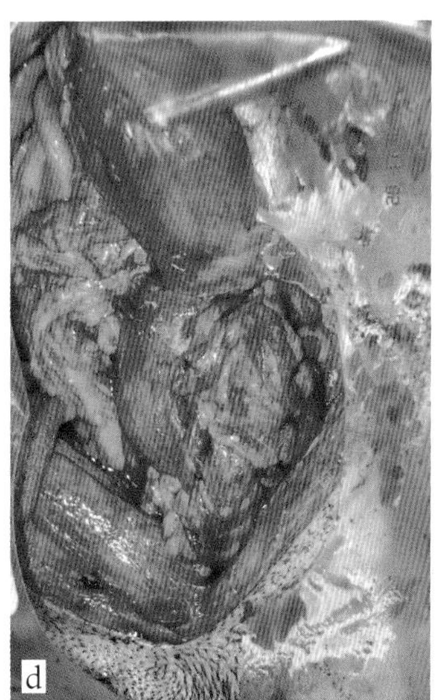

Fig. 5.30a–d Prostatectomy. a. The prostate is isolated, and Penrose drains are placed proximally and distally. The urethra is catheterised and a stay suture is placed at the apex of the bladder. b. The prostate is removed by incising the urethra proximal and distal to it. The urethral catheter is used as a guide. c. Final anastomosis (simple interrupted sutures placed circumferentially). d. The anastomosis is omentalised.

with metastases to lymph nodes, lungs and/or skeletal sites in 70–80% of cases at diagnosis.

Diagnosis

Clinical signs are similar to other prostatic diseases such as dyschezia and dysuria, though signs relating to metastasis may be present – for example, dyspnoea with pulmonary metastasis (Lévy et al., 2014). Progressive lethargy, vomiting and collapse may occur if there is urinary obstruction, and weight loss is common. Physical examination may reveal an abdominal or pelvic mass, enlarged sublumbar lymph nodes, significant pain on abdominal and rectal palpation, or pelvic limb lameness or neurological deficits due to tumour invasion to surrounding skeletal and neurologic structures. Abdominal and pelvic radiography or CT should be performed, and three-view thoracic radiography or CT is essential for staging. Abnormalities include prostatomegaly, prostatic mineralisation, lymph node enlargement and osteolytic or proliferative bony lesions (vertebra/pelvis). Retrograde urethrocystography often shows urethral invasion, and abdominal ultrasonography determines whether the prostatic mass is solid or cystic and facilitates ultrasound-guided prostatic aspiration. Blood tests and urinalysis findings are often non-specific. Definitive diagnosis is made on cytology or histopathology from prostatic aspirates or transurethral biopsy, though exfoliation of cells is less reliable with the latter technique.

Treatment

Prostatic neoplasms can be aggressive, and many dogs already have metastasis at the time of diagnosis. As such, treatments rarely extend the dog's life by more than a few months, and greater than 50% are euthanised at the time of diagnosis. Chemotherapy and radiation therapy have been attempted but are seldom effective, and complete surgical resection by prostatectomy is often not possible due to the size and extent of the tumour. In addition, prostatectomy is associated with high rates of urinary incontinence due to resection or damage to the trigonal innervation (Fig. 5.30). In cases when neoplasia is diagnosed early, or in the case of a transitional cell carcinoma that involves the prostate gland but not the trigone, prostatectomy may be possible. However, the procedure carries significant risk of haemorrhage and postoperative urinary incontinence, and so referral to a specialist centre should be considered. Total prostatectomy has been attempted, nonetheless, with some positive results (Bennett et al., 2018). The persistent incontinence rate in that study was 34%, and the median survival time was 231 days. Palliative treatments include partial prostatectomy via a neodymium:yttrium-aluminium-garnet (Nd:YAG) laser-filleting technique, urethral stenting, tube cystostomy and administration of prazosin to improve dysuria. There is some evidence that the use of COX-inhibitors (piroxicam or carprofen) may improve median survival times (Sorenmo et al., 2004). Survival time in dogs with prostatic malignancies varies widely, from 17 to 654 days depending on the stage of diagnosis and treatment pursued.

References

Bennett, T.C., Matz, B.M., Henderson, R.A., Straw, R.C., Liptak, J.M., Selmic, L.E., Collivignarelli, F., and Buracco, P. (2018) Total prostatectomy as a treatment for prostatic carcinoma in 25 dogs. *Veterinary Surgery* 47, 367–377.

Bergström, A., Fransson, B. and Olsson, K. (2006a) Primary uterine inertia in 27 bitches: aetiology and treatment. *Journal of Small Animal Practice* 47, 456–460.

Bergström, A., Nødtvedt, A., Lagerstedt, A.S. and Egenvall, A. (2006b) Incidence and breed predilection for dystocia and risk factors for cesarean section in a Swedish population of insured dogs. *Veterinary Surgery* 35, 786–791.

Børresen, B. and Skrede, S. (1980) Pyometra in the dog – a pathophysiological investigation. V. The presence of intrahepatic cholestasis and an "acute phase reaction." *Nordisk Veterinaermedicin* 32, 378–386.

Bryan, J.N., Keeler, M.R., Henry, C.J., Bryan, M.E., Hahn, A.W. and Caldwell, C.W. (2007) A population study of neutering status as a risk factor for canine prostate cancer. *The Prostate* 67, 1174–1181.

Bussadori, C., Bigliardi, E., D'Agnolo, G., Borgarelli, M. and Santilli, R.A. (2000) The percutaneous drainage of prostatic abscesses in the dog. *La Radiologia Medica* 98, 391–394.

Chang, S.C., Chang, C.C., Chang, T.J. and Wong, M.L. (2005) Prognostic factors associated with survival two years after surgery in dogs with malignant mammary tumours: 79 cases (1998–2002). *Journal of the American Veterinary Medical Association* 227, 1625–1629.

Cooley, A.J., Waldron, D.R., Smith, M.M., Saunders, G.K., Troy, G.C. and Barber, D.L. (1999) The effects of indwelling transurethral catheterization and tube cystostomy on urethral anastomoses in dogs. *Journal of the American Animal Hospital Association* 35, 341–347.

Darvelid, A.W. and Linde-Forsberg, C. (1994) Dystocia in the bitch: a retrospective study of 182 cases. *Journal of Small Animal Practice* 35, 402.

Davidson, E.B., Moll, H.D. and Payton, M.E. (2003) Comparison of laparoscopic ovariohysterectomy and ovariohysterectomy in dogs. *Veterinary Surgery* 33, 62–69.

Devitt, C.M., Cox, R.E. and Hailey, J.J. (2005) Duration, complications, stress, and pain of open ovariohysterectomy versus a simple method of laparoscopic-assisted ovariohysterectomy in dogs. *Journal of the American Veterinary Medical Association* 227, 921–927.

Dow, C. (1962) Testicular tumours in the dog. *Journal of Comparative Pathology* 72, 247–265.

Egenvall, A., Hagman, R., Bonnett, B.N., Hedhammar, A., Olson, P. and Lagerstedt, A.S. (2002) Breed risk of pyometra in insured dogs in Sweden. *Journal of Veterinary Internal Medicine* 15, 530–538.

Evans, K.M. and Adams, V.J. (2010) Proportion of litters of purebred dogs born by caesarean section. *Journal of Small Animal Practice* 51, 113–118.

Feldman, E.C. and Nelson, R.W. (2004) *Canine and Feline Endocrinology and Reproduction*. Elsevier Saunders, St. Louis, Missouri.

Fieni, F., Topie, E. and Gogny, A. (2014) Medical treatment for pyometra in dogs. *Reproduction in Domestic Animals* 49, 28–32.

Forster, K., Anderson, D., Yool, D.A., Wright, C. and Burrow, R. (2011) Retained surgical swabs in 13 dogs. *Veterinary Record* 169, 337.

Gibson, A., Dean, R., Yates, D. and Stavisky, J. (2013) A retrospective study of pyometra at five RSPCA hospitals in the UK: 1728 cases from 2006 to 2011. *Veterinary Record* 173, 396.

Gunn-Moore, D.A. and Thrusfield, M.V. (1995) Feline dystocia: prevalence, and association with cranial conformation and breed. *Veterinary Record* 136, 350–353.

Hagman, R. (2018) Pyometra in small animals. *The Veterinary Clinics of North America: Small Animal Practice* 48, 639–661.

Hamilton, K.H., Henderson, E.R., Toscano, M. and Chanoit G.P. (2014) Comparison of postoperative complications in healthy dogs undergoing open and closed orchidectomy. *Journal of Small Animal Practice* 55, 521–526.

Hammel, S.P. and Bjorling, D.E. (2002) Results of vulvoplasty for treatment of recessed vulva in dogs. *Journal of the American Animal Hospital Association* 38, 79–83.

Hart, B.L., Hart, L.A., Thigpen, A.P. and Willits, N.H. (2014) Long-term health effects of neutering dogs: comparison of Labrador Retrievers with Golden Retrievers. *PLoS ONE* 9, e102241.

Hayes, H.M. and Pendergrass, T.W. (1976) Canine testicular tumours: epidemiologic features of 410 dogs. *International Journal of Cancer* 18, 482.

Jitpean, S., Ambrosen, A., Emanuelson U. and Hagman R. (2017)

Closed cervix is associated with more severe illness in dogs with pyometra. *BMC Veterinary Research* 13, 11.

Karayannopoulou, E., Kaldrymidou, E., Constantinidis, T.C. and Dessiris, A. (2001) Adjuvant post-operative chemotherapy in bitches with mammary cancer. *Journal of Veterinary Medicine. A, Physiology, Pathology, Clinical Medicine* 48, 85–96.

Kawakami, M., Yamada, Y., Tsutsui, T., Ogasa, A. and Yamauchi, M. (1993) Changes in plasma androgen levels and testicular histology with descent of the testis in the dog. *The Journal of Veterinary Medical Science* 55, 931–935.

Lana, S.E., Rutteman, G.R. and Withrow, S.J. (2007) Tumours of the mammary gland. In: Withrow, S.J. and Vail, D.M. (eds) *Withrow & MacEwen's Small Animal Clinical Oncology*, 4th edn., Elsevier Saunders, St. Louis, Missouri.

Lavalle, G.E., De Campos, C.B., Bertagnolli, A.C. and Cassali, G.D. (2012) Canine malignant mammary gland neoplasms with advanced clinical staging treated with carboplatin and cyclooxygenase inhibitors. *In Vivo* 26, 375–379.

Lévy, X., Niżański, W., von Heimendahl, A. and Mimouni, P. (2014) Diagnosis of common prostatic conditions in dogs: an update. *Reproduction in Domestic Animals* 49, 50–57.

MacEwen, E.G., Hayes, A.A., Harvey, H.J., Patnaik, A.K., Mooney, S. and Passe, S. (1984) Prognostic factors for feline mammary tumours. *Journal of the American Veterinary Medical Association* 185, 201–204.

Moon, P.F., Erb, H.N., Ludders, J.W., Gleed, R.D. and Pascoe, P.J. (1998) Perioperative management and mortality rates of dogs undergoing cesarean section in the United States and Canada. *Journal of the American Veterinary Medical Association* 213, 365–369.

Okkens, A.C., vd Gaag, L., Biewenga, W.J., Rothuizen, J. and Voorhout, G. (1981) Urological complications following ovariohysterectomy in dogs (author's transl.). *Tijdschrift Voor Diergeneeskunde* 106, 1189–1198.

Overley, B., Shofer, F.S., Goldschmidt, M.H., Sherer, D. and Sorenmo, K.U. (2005) Association between ovariohysterectomy and feline mammary carcinoma. *Journal of Veterinary Internal Medicine* 19, 560–563.

Owen, L.N. (1980) TNM classification of tumours in domestic animals. World Health Organization, Geneva, Switzerland.

Pearson, H. and Kelly, D.F. (1975) Testicular torsion in the dog: a review of 13 cases. *Veterinary Record* 97, 200.

Pereira, C.T., Rahal, S.C., de Carvalho Balieiro, J.C. and Ribeiro, A.A. (2003) Lymphatic drainage on healthy and neoplasic mammary glands in female dogs: can it really be altered? *Anatomia, Histologia, Embryologia* 32, 282–290.

Philibert, J.C., Snyder, P.W., Glickman, N., Glickman, L.T., Knapp, D.W. and Waters, D.J. (2003) Influence of host factors on survival in dogs with malignant mammary gland tumours. *Journal of Veterinary Internal Medicine* 17, 102–106.

Piola, V., Posch, B., Aghte, P., Caine, A. and Herrtage, M.E. (2010) Radiographic characterization of the os penis in the cat. *Veterinary Radiology & Ultrasound* 52, 270–272.

Sandholm, M., Vasenius, H. and Kivistö, A.K. (1975) Pathogenesis of canine pyometra. *Journal of the American Veterinary Medical Association* 167, 1006–1010.

Schneider, R., Dorn, C.R. and Taylor, D.O. (1969) Factors influencing canine mammary cancer development and postsurgical survival. *Journal of the National Cancer Institute* 43, 1249–1261.

Seixas, F., Palmeira, C., Pires, M.A., Bento, M.J. and Lopes, C. (2009) Grade is an independent prognostic factor for feline mammary carcinomas: a clinicopathological and survival analysis. *Veterinary Journal* 187, 65–71.

Sorenmo, K.U., Goldschmidt, M., Shofer, F., Goldkamp, C. and Ferracone, J. (2003) Immunohistochemical characterization of canine prostatic carcinoma and correlation with castration status and castration time. *Veterinary and Comparative Oncology* 1, 48–56.

Sorenmo, K.U., Goldschmidt, M.H., Shofer, F.S., Goldkamp, C. and Ferracone, J. (2004) Evaluation of cyclooxygenase-1 and cyclooxygenase-2 expression and the effect of cyclooxygenase inhibitors in canine prostatic carcinoma. *Veterinary and Comparative Oncology* 2, 13–23.

Thacher, C. and Bradley, R.L. (1983) Vulvar and vaginal tumours in the dog: a retrospective study. *Journal of the American Veterinary Medical Association* 183, 690–692.

Viste, J.R., Myers, S.L., Singh, B. and Simko, E. (2002) Feline mammary adenocarcinoma: tumour size as a prognostic indicator. *The Canadian Veterinary Journal* 43, 33–37.

White, R.A. and Williams, J.M. (1995) Intracapsular prostatic omentalization: a new technique for management of prostatic abscesses in dogs. *Veterinary Surgery* 24, 390–395.

Yamagami, T., Kobayashi, T. and Takahashi, K. (1996) Influence of ovariectomy at the time of mastectomy on the prognosis for canine malignant mammary tumours. *Journal of Small Animal Practice* 37, 462.

Case 5.1

A 7-year-old female entire Border collie presents with a slightly distended, pendulous abdomen and lethargy.

- What further clinical history is important in reaching a diagnosis?
- What further clinical examination do you wish to perform?

On further discussion with the owner, you discover that the dog is a farm collie and lives outside. The owner doesn't know when her last season was. Two weeks previously the dog had a more rounded appearance to the abdomen. She has been inappetent and polyuric/polydipsic for the past few days.

On examination the dog has a heart rate of 140 beats/minute, respiratory rate of 36 breaths/minute, mucous membranes pale pink and tacky, capillary refill time of 2.5 seconds, moderate quality peripheral pulses, and normal rectal temperature. The abdomen is painful on palpation and has a slightly 'doughy' feel.

- What are your differentials at this stage?
- What diagnostic procedures would you like to perform?
- Would you do anything first?

Top differential diagnoses in this case include septic peritonitis (e.g. due perforation of viscus (intestinal/uterine), abscess or other cause), or pyometra.

Haematology revealed a leukocytosis (21.6 x 10^9/l; ref. interval 5.2–13.9 x 10^9/l) and neutrophilia (17.28 x 10^9/l; ref. interval 3.00–11.50 x 10^9/l) with band neutrophils present, consistent with inflammation. Serum biochemistry revealed a hypoalbuminaemia (21.0 g/l; ref. interval 32.0–38.0 g/l) and hyperglobulinaemia (52.1 g/l; ref. interval 20.0–35.0 g/l) consistent with an acute phase inflammatory response. A metabolic acidosis with elevated lactate was present.

A FAST scan identified free abdominal fluid. Cytology of the abdominal fluid revealed septic neutrophilic inflammation.

Following fluid resuscitation, abdominal radiographs were performed.

- What are the findings on the radiographs?
- Is any other diagnostic imaging required?
- What is the most likely diagnosis?

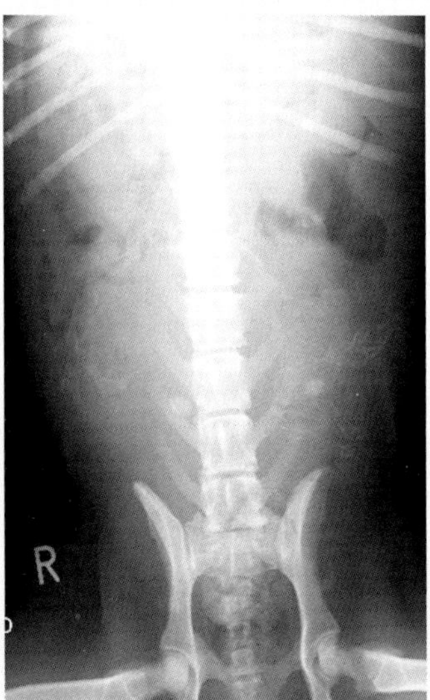

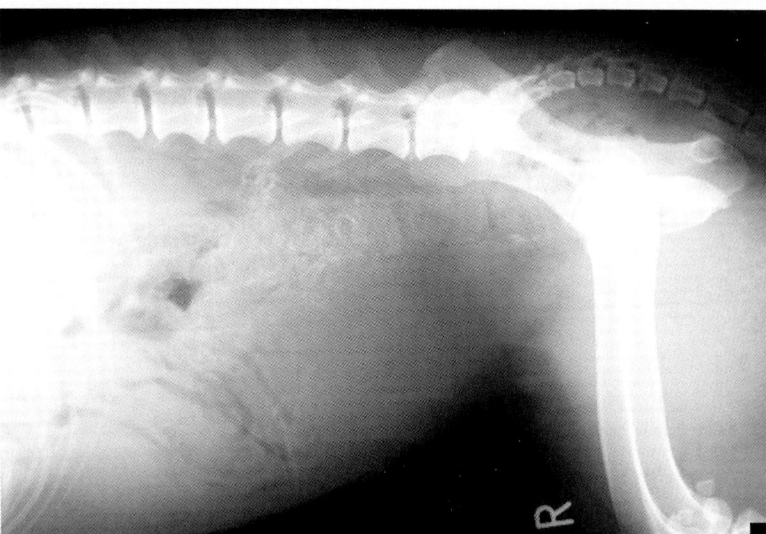

Fig 5.31a,b Laney Pike, case number 10014174

The radiographs (Figs 5.31a,b) show loss of serosal detail consistent with free abdominal fluid. Within both uterine horns, and within the body of the uterus just cranial to the pubic brim, there are remnants of partially mineralised foetal bones. There are also multiple small gas foci within the horns adjacent to the bones.

Abdominal ultrasound would be an alternative/additional imaging modality.

A diagnosis of an emphysematous ruptured uterus with macerated foetuses was made.

- What treatment options are available to the owner?
- What complications may be encountered?

Following initial stabilisation (to correct hypovolaemia, hydration and acidaemia), and initiation of broad spectrum antibiosis, treatment is ovariohysterectomy or, for valuable breeding animals, removal of foetuses and unilateral removal of the ruptured horn. When generalised peritonitis is present the abdomen should be copiously lavaged with warm saline. Complications of include development of SIRS, haemorrhage, incomplete removal of the ovaries, wound swelling, wound infection, and fistulous tracts. Surgical repair of the uterus may predispose to re-rupture in future pregnancies or to infertility.

Case 5.2

A 7-year-old male entire Weimaraner presents with stranguria and dyschezia.

- What further clinical history is important in reaching a diagnosis?
- What further clinical examination do you wish to perform?

On further discussion with the owner, you discover that a month previously the dog had developed penile bleeding and was diagnosed with benign prostatic hyperplasia at a different veterinary practice. He was treated with chemical castration, antibiotics and NSAIDs following which there was an improvement. However one week prior to presentation he developed stranguria and dyschezia.

On examination the dog's cardiovascular parameters are within normal limits, and the rectal temperature is normal. On rectal examination the prostate is bilaterally enlarged, and there is pain on caudal abdominal palpation.

- What are your differentials at this stage?
- What diagnostic procedures would you like to perform?

Prostatic cysts or abscessation are top differentials in this case. Prostatic neoplasia or other intrapelvic neoplasia causing compression of the colon and urinary tract should also be considered.

Haematology revealed a mild neutrophilia (11.68 x 10^9/l; ref. interval 3.00–11.50 x10^9/l) consistent with inflammation. Serum biochemistry revealed a mild hypoalbuminaemia (24.8g/l; ref. interval 32.0–38.0g/l) and hyperglobulinaemia (40.2g/l; ref. interval 20.0–35.0g/l) consistent with an acute phase inflammatory response. Urinalysis revealed dilute urine concentration (USG 1.014) but was otherwise unremarkable.

An abdominal CT scan with contrast was performed (Figs. 5.32, 5.33).

- What are the findings on the CT images?
- Is any other diagnostic imaging required?
- What is the most likely diagnosis?

On the right side of the prostate there is a well-defined fluid opacity structure consistent with a prostatic or paraprostatic cyst. Due to the presence of this mass lesion the colon and bladder (bladder seen on the first image) are displaced towards the left side and the urethra appears compressed. A retrograde urethrogram with fluoroscopy is unremarkable (Fig. 5.34).

- What treatment options are available to the owner?
- What complications may be encountered?

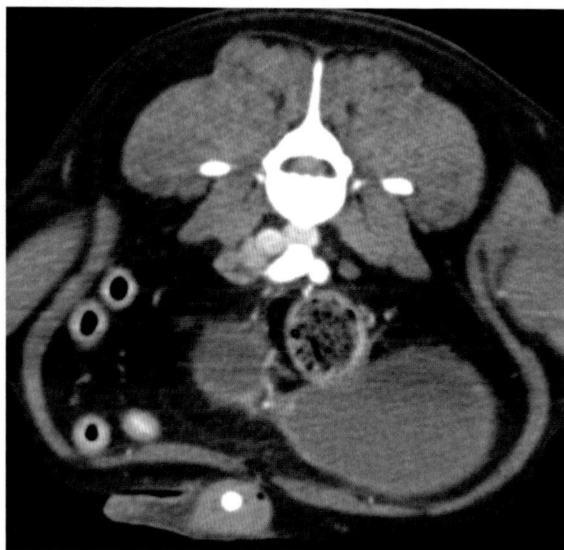

Fig 5.32 Transverse CT at the level of L6 vertebra, arterial phase.

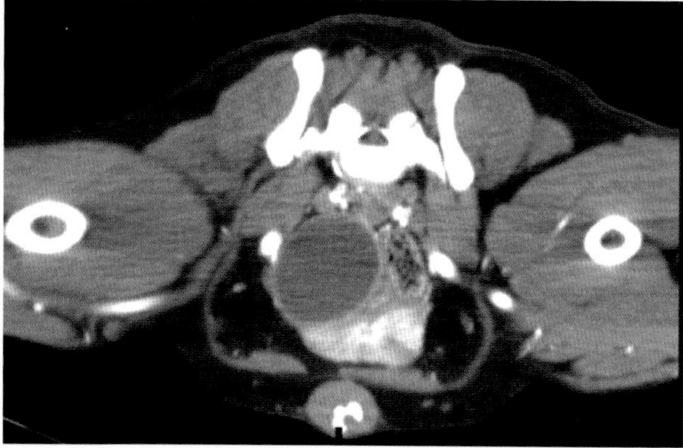

Fig 5.33 Transverse CT at the level of the sacroilial joint, arterial phase.

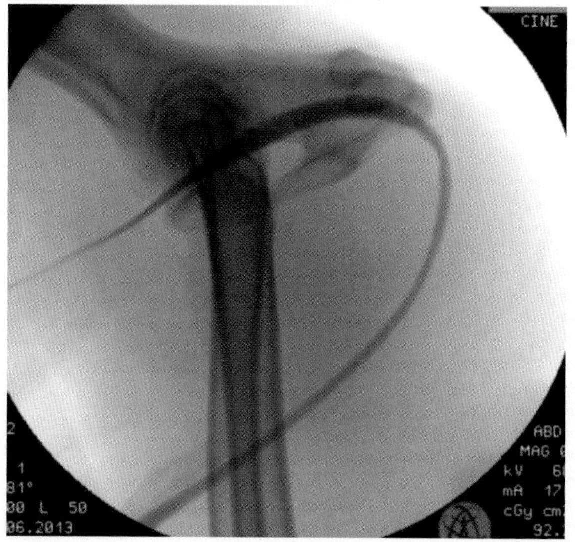

Fig 5.33 Retrograde urethrogram.

Discrete prostatic cysts should be treated by complete resection, or partial resection with omentalisation. If urinary obstruction is present due to urethral compression, ultrasound-guided cyst drainage may be performed prior to surgery whilst azotaemia resolves. Castration should always be performed to ensure prostatic involution.

Intra-operative complications include damage to neurovascular structures around the prostate and bladder neck, or damage to the urethra if it is not identified by use of a urinary catheter. Postoperative urinary incontinence may occur due to pressure changes around the urethra, as during growth of the cyst the urethra's structure may have changed to compensate for the compression. Inadequate cyst resection may lead to recurrence.

Oral and pharyngeal surgery

6

Donald Sheahan

Chapter summary

6.1 Preoperative preparation and surgical considerations

The oral cavity contains large numbers of bacteria, and oral surgery is classified as contaminated. The use of prophylactic antibiotics is debatable owing to the rich blood supply to the oral cavity and the antibacterial properties of saliva.

Surgical access to the oral cavity can be limited. Dental gags are useful to improve exposure, and placement of temporary tracheostomy tubes may be necessary to facilitate performance of the procedure.

Cuffed endotracheal tubes should be used to prevent aspiration of surgical fluids, and the oral cavity should be suctioned prior to recovery from general anaesthesia. Oesophagostomy or gastrostomy tubes may be placed in animals that are unable to eat after surgery.

The oral cavity may be disinfected with dilute povidone-iodine solution or 0.2% chlorhexidine solution prior to surgery.

Healing of the oral cavity is rapid owing to its rich blood supply. The use of 4-0 polyglactin 910 or poliglecaprone-25 is adequate for closure of most oral cavity wounds. Polydioxanone can be used if prolonged healing times are anticipated.

The tissues of the oral cavity are delicate, and hence fine instruments should be used. Stay sutures or skin hooks should be used when manipulating tissues, and care must be taken not to crush tissue or to allow it to desiccate.

6.2 Lips and cheek

Key points

- Typical presentations for animals with oral cavity disease include ptyalism, mouth pain, oral haemorrhage and difficulty in eating.
- Definitive treatment for excessive folding of the lower lip requires excision of the infected tissue.
- Tight lip syndrome in Shar-Peis is treated by incising the lip mucosa at the gingival margin to allow the lower lip to retract.
- Anti-drool cheiloplasty technique involves lifting a mucocutaneous flap in the lower lip.

6.2.1 Functional anatomy and physiology

The lips and cheeks are the lateral boundaries of the oral vestibule. They function to retain saliva in the oral vestibule and are composed of three layers: an outer skin, a middle fibro-elastic and muscle layer, and inner mucosa. Sensory innervation is from the trigeminal nerve (cranial nerve V) and motor innervation is by the facial nerve (cranial nerve VII). The blood supply to the upper lip and cheek is from the infraorbital artery and to the lower lip and cheek is from the facial artery (Evans, 2012).

6.2.2 Investigation

Typical presentations for animals with oral cavity disease include ptyalism, mouth pain, oral haemorrhage and difficulty in eating. A complete physical examination should be performed on all animals prior to focusing on the oral cavity, particularly in cases that are anticipated to be painful. Diagnostic tests commonly performed in patients with oral cavity disease include haematology, biochemistry, radiography and CT imaging. A clotting profile should be performed if significant haemorrhage is anticipated.

6.2.3 Disorders of the lips and cheek

Primary cleft palate

This is a largely cosmetic defect. Surgical repair requires re-establishing the normal separation between the nasal and oral cavities. This surgery will be discussed in more detail in the section on palate surgery.

Abnormal lip fold conformation

Excessive folding of the lower lip leads to trapping of saliva and a secondary dermatitis. Discolouring of the

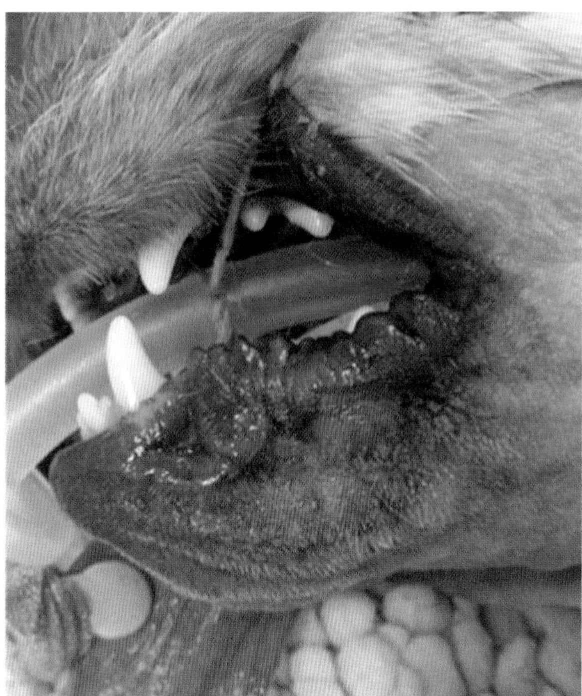

Fig. 6.1 Dermatitis secondary to abnormal lip fold conformation.

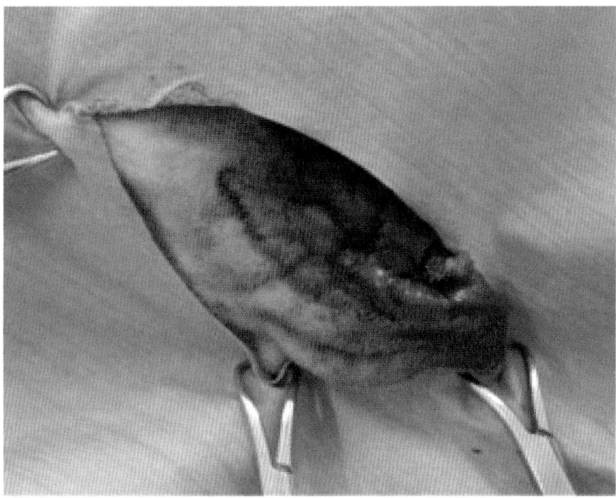

Fig. 6.2 Preoperative surgical planning to remove abnormal lip fold.

skin and halitosis are the common presenting signs (Fig. 6.1). Definitive treatment requires excision of the infected tissue (Fig. 6.2). An elliptical incision is made in the skin around the infected skin, usually starting just below the mucocutaneous junction. The underlying orbicularis oris muscle is preserved (Fig. 6.3). Meticulous haemostasis with bipolar cautery is beneficial. The skin is closed with fine intradermal sutures (Winkel, 2006; Fig. 6.4).

Tight lip syndrome in the Shar-Pei

The rostral edge of the lower lip is pulled over the lower incisors and is traumatised during mastication. Treatment involves incising the lip mucosa at the gingival margin to allow the lower lip to retract. Healing occurs by second intention. During this time, the lip can be digitally retracted to prevent the lip healing in its original position. Previously described alternatives to this technique include excision of a portion of skin on the ventral chin and deepening of the oral vestibule (Eisner, 2008).

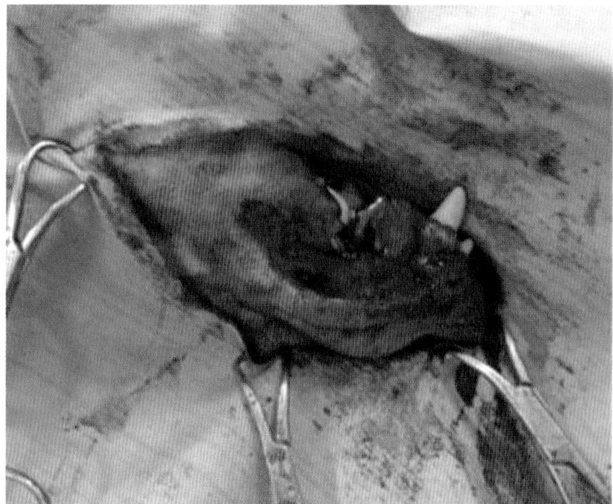

Fig. 6.3 Abnormal lip fold removed with elliptical incision. Note preservation of orbicularis oris muscle.

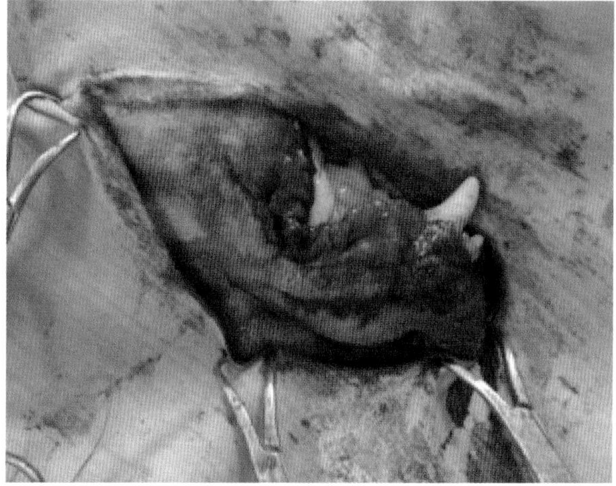

Fig. 6.4 Two-layer closure of surgical incision using fine intradermal sutures.

Redundancy and eversion of the lower lip

This condition is common in large- and giant-breed dogs. Surgery is performed to limit the amount of saliva leaking from the oral vestibule. The anti-drool cheiloplasty technique has been described in six dogs with favourable results. The procedure involves lifting a mucocutaneous flap in the lower lip, which is then pulled through a full-thickness incision made in the caudodorsal vestibule and out through the cheek (Smeak, 1989). Alternatively, the redundant fold of tissue near the commissure can be resected with a full-thickness wedge resection. Resection involves any region of hyperplasia, ulceration or dermatitis. Once the affected

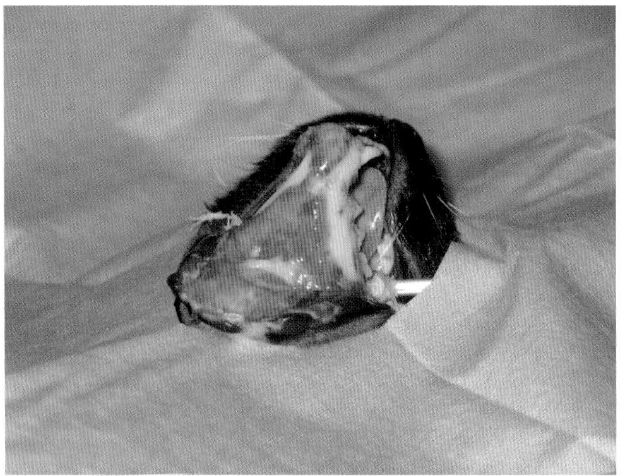

Fig. 6.5 Avulsion injury of lower lip.

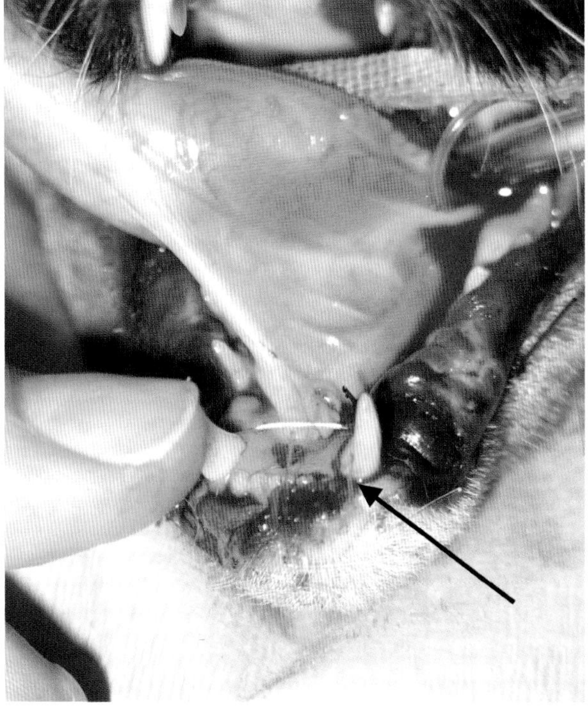

Fig. 6.6 Suture placed around canine tooth to repair avulsion injury.

tissue is excised a stay suture is placed at the edge of the lip margin to allow accurate reconstruction. The wound is closed in three layers in a simple continuous pattern using 1.5 or 2.0 metric rapidly absorbable monofilament suture in the mucosa, muscular layer and skin.

Trauma

Avulsion of the lower lip is usually seen following a road traffic accident. Avulsion usually occurs along the gingival margin (Fig. 6.5). Owing to the poor holding power of gingival mucosa, sutures can be placed around the canine or incisor teeth or through small drill holes in the mandible using monofilament sutures

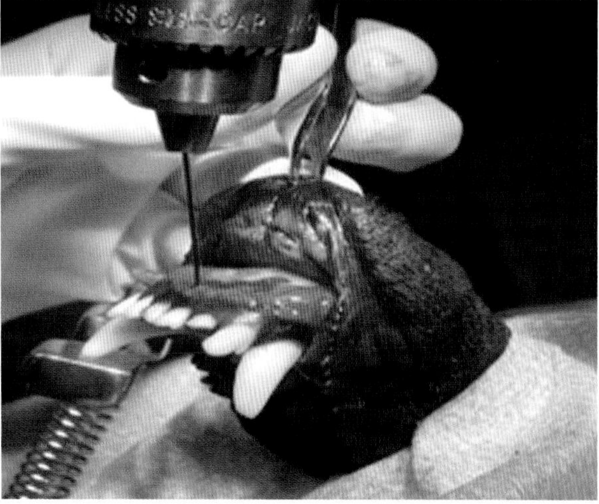

Fig. 6.7 Drill holes placed into mandible using 1.0 mm K-wire.

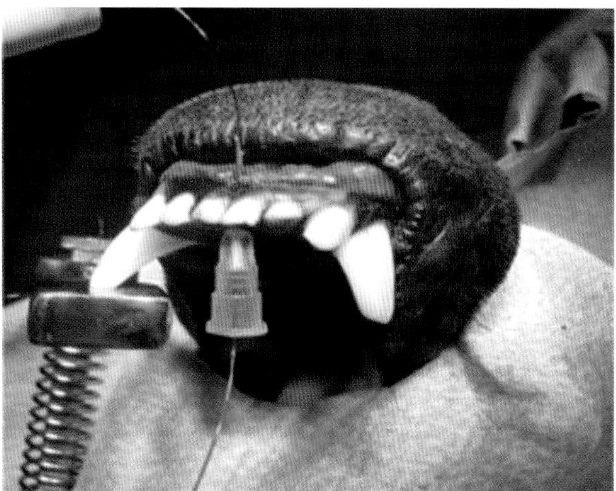

Fig. 6.8 Monofilament suture placed through mandible.

(Figs. 6.6, 6.7, 6.8). A Penrose drain can be placed if necessary (Farrow, 1973; Pavletic, 1990).

Neoplasia

The most common tumour affecting the lips is melanoma. Most tumours can be removed with a simple wedge resection. While the majority of defects can be closed primarily (Figs. 6.9, 6.10), larger defects require full-thickness labial advancement or rotation flaps (Dorn and Priester, 1976).

6.3 Tongue

Key points

- Partial glossectomy is an effective treatment for macroglossia.
- Frenuloplasty can be recommended in ankyloglossia.

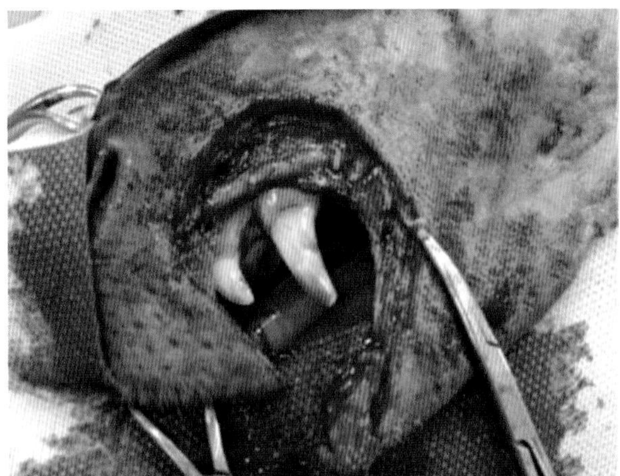
Fig. 6.9 Full-thickness labial excision.

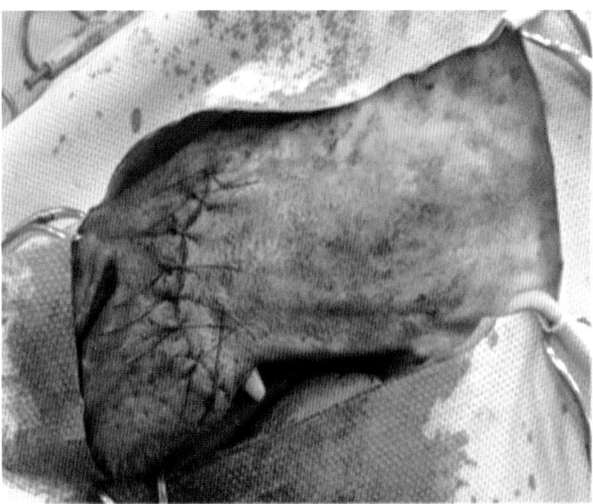
Fig. 6.10 Primary closure of full-thickness labial excision.

- Most injuries of the tongue will resolve without surgery.
- Malignant melanoma and squamous cell carcinoma (SCC) are the most common lingual tumours in the dog.

6.3.1 Functional anatomy

The functions of the tongue are prehension, thermoregulation, grooming and vocalisation. The root of the tongue is anchored to the oropharynx. The body extends rostrally and is attached to the floor of the oral cavity via the frenulum. The apex is the most rostral part of the tongue and is not attached to the frenulum. Sublingual folds run along each side of the frenulum and end at the sublingual caruncle. These folds contain the mandibular and sublingual salivary ducts which open at the caruncle.

The root of the tongue contains three pairs of extrinsic muscles, all of which are innervated by the hypoglossal nerve.

- Styloglossus. This muscle originates from the stylohyoid bones and inserts on the ventral aspect of the tongue. It functions to draw the tongue caudally and to depress it.
- Hyoglossus. This muscle originates from the basihyoid bone and inserts on the caudal two-thirds of the tongue. It retracts and depresses the tongue.
- Genioglossus. This muscle originates from the medial mandible and separates into three bundles. These depress and protrude the tongue.

The intrinsic muscles are concerned with protruding the tongue and with intricate movements. They are also innervated by the hypoglossal nerve.

The lyssa is a tube-like structure of muscle, fat and cartilage that lies on the median plane of the ventral aspect of the tongue. Its function is unknown. Gustatory papillae on the dorsal surface of the tongue contain taste buds. These include fungiform, vallate and foliate papillae. Non-gustatory papillae include filiform and conical papillae. These facilitate grooming, particularly in cats.

The blood supply to the tongue is through paired lingual arteries. These anastomose throughout the tongue. The lingual vein starts at the apex of the tongue and runs alongside the arteries before emptying into the facial vein (Evans, 2012).

6.3.2 Disorders of the tongue

Congenital

Macroglossia, microglossia and tongue deviations are rare. Care must be taken not to diagnose macroglossia in brachycephalic dogs. In true macroglossia the tongue hangs from the mouth and is often traumatised. Treatment by partial glossectomy is effective. Ankyloglossia is a congenital disorder in which the lingual frenulum is abnormally short and thickened, restricting movement. Affected animals have difficulty suckling, swallowing and vocalising resulting in stunted growth, ptyalism and difficulty eating. This condition has only been described in Anatolian shepherd dogs. Three dogs were successfully treated by frenuloplasty (Temizsoylu and Avki, 2003).

Trauma

Penetrating trauma to the oral cavity is occasionally seen in the dog and cat and can lead to lingual abscess formation, with the commonest site directly beneath the tongue. Positive culture results in the few reported cases include *Escherichia coli* and *Pasteurella multocida* (Kelmer et al., 2007; Von Doernberg et al., 2008). Lethargy, anorexia and ptyalism are typically seen, but

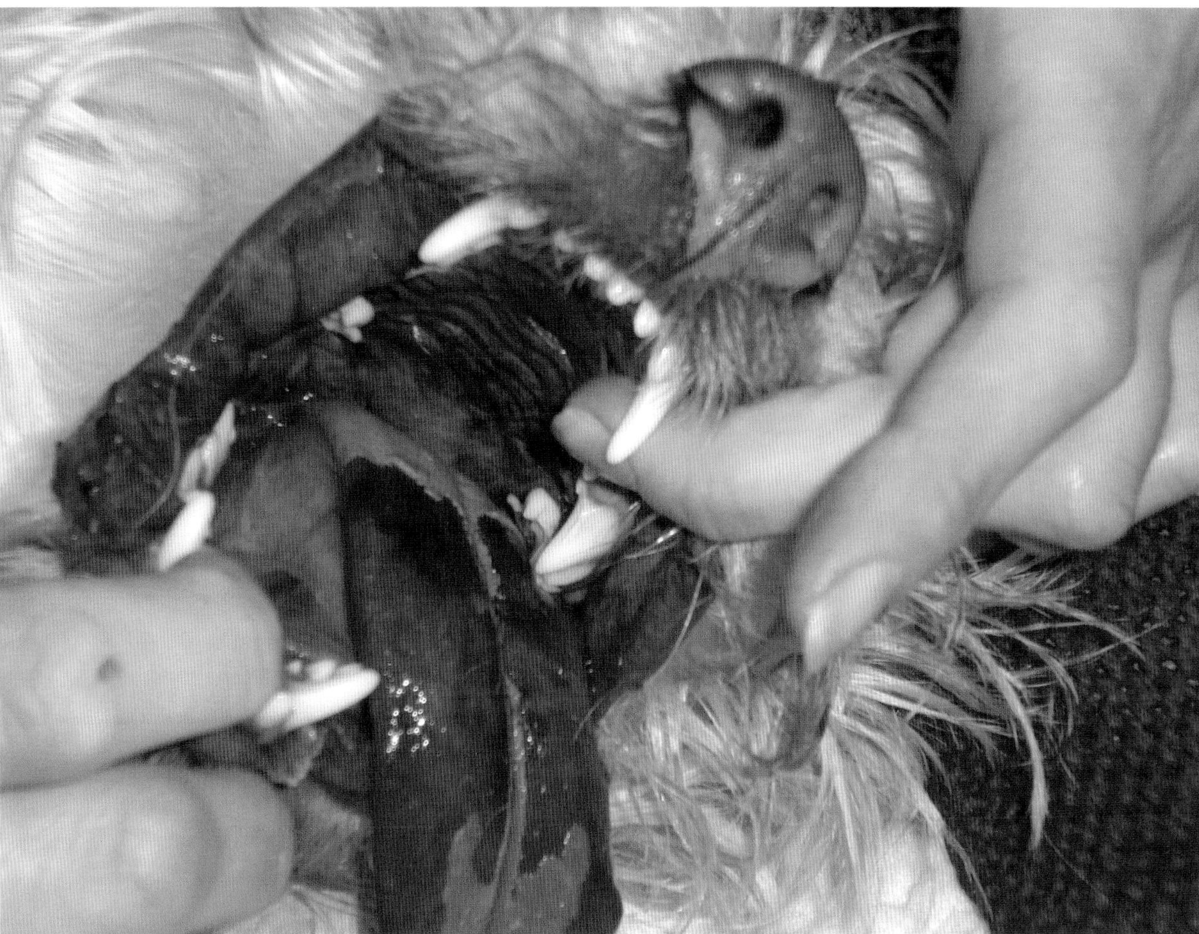

Fig. 6.11 Lingual burn injury.

occasionally animals will present in respiratory distress. Treatment involves either active or passive drainage. Other reported traumatic injuries include lacerations and burns (Fig. 6.11). Most injuries will resolve without the need for surgical intervention. It may occasionally be necessary to debride or repair an injury to the tongue in order to control haemorrhage or to remove foreign material. This should be kept to a minimum in order to preserve the function of the tongue, particularly in the cat. Normal tongue conformation is maintained by accurate apposition of deep muscular tissue and then epithelium with fine, rapidly absorbable, synthetic monofilament suture (1.5 or 2.0 metric). Dogs will usually eat immediately after surgery but cats are less predictable.

Miscellaneous conditions

Calcinosis circumscripta is an uncommon syndrome of ectopic deposition of hydroxyapatite crystals or amorphous calcium phosphate (Fig. 6.12) (Tafti et al., 2005). It is thought to occur as a result of tissue injury (dystrophic) or abnormal calcium or phosphate metabolism secondary to renal failure (metastatic) or is of unknown aetiology (idiopathic). The tongue is the second most common site (23% of all cases). Clinical signs vary but are typically due to the physical presence of the lesion and subsequent abnormal tongue function. Surgical management is warranted only in cases of dysphagia.

Oral papillomatosis results from a viral infection and affects dogs less than one year of age. White, translucent nodules on the tongue and gingiva can be numerous but will usually regress within 4 to 8 weeks. Adult dogs that present with this condition should be screened for immunosuppressive conditions. Surgical intervention is not typically indicated other than for diagnosis or palliative purposes.

Neoplasia

Primary neoplasia of the tongue is rare, comprising only 4% of all oropharyngeal tumours in the dog. Malignant melanoma and SCC are the most common lingual tumours in the dog. Chow chow and Chinese Shar-Pei breeds are at increased risk for lingual melanoma development (Dennis et al., 2006). Canine SCC can be located anywhere on the tongue and is over-represented in female dogs. Granular cell myoblastoma is the next most common canine lingual tumour. This tumour appears large and invasive, but is usually removed with

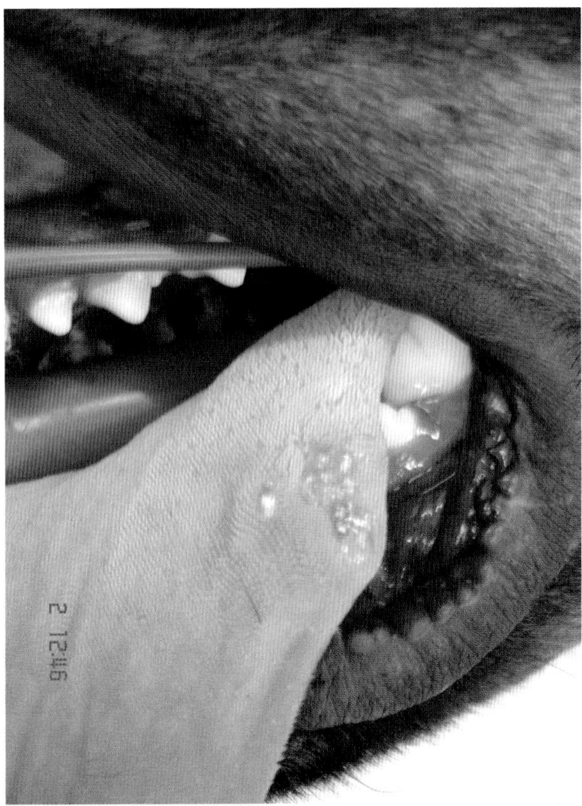

Fig. 6.12 Calcinosis circumscripta.

conservative, narrow margins. Permanent control is possible in 80% of cases. Late recurrence is possible, but serial resections can be successfully performed. These tumours rarely metastasise. Melanomas can be controlled by local excision or radiation therapy. The metastatic rate is less than 50%.

Lingual tumours comprise approximately 24% of all oropharyngeal tumours in the cat (Dorn and Priester, 1976). SCC accounts for 61% of feline lingual tumours, with most located on the ventral surface near the frenulum (Stebbins et al., 1989).

Diagnosis

The majority of dogs with lingual tumours are asymptomatic but, when clinical signs are present, these include dysphagia, halitosis, bleeding and stridor (Syrcle et al., 2008). Cats typically present with signs of poor oral health or general well-being. Wedge incisional biopsies should be taken to differentiate neoplastic lesions from non-neoplastic. Ultrasound can be used to delineate the margins of tongue tumours in order to aid in resection. Regional lymph nodes should be biopsied or aspirated, and thoracic radiographs or preferably CT images obtained to rule out lung metastasis.

Prognosis

The prognosis for lingual tumours depends on the site, type and grade of the tumour (Culp et al., 2013). Grade I SCC has significantly better median survival time than grades II and III (16 months vs 3–4 months). Rostral tumours have a better prognosis than caudal tumours, owing to earlier detection, rich lymphatic and vascular channels caudally and easier resection with wide margins; 37% of canine SCC metastasise, and this is more common in high-grade and caudally located tumours. The prognosis for feline SCC is grave, with 1-year survival rates of less than 25%.

Treatment

Partial glossectomy is the treatment of choice for lingual tumours (Culp et al., 2013). A wedge glossectomy is adequate for the removal of benign tumours or small malignant tumours (Figs. 6.13, 6.14, 6.15). Malignant tumours of medium or large size or those near the midline often require total glossectomy to achieve complete excision. Wedge glossectomy extending more than 50% of the width of the tongue may result in loss of blood supply and function to the rostral tongue. Transverse glossectomy is a better option in these cases. Tumours that are unilateral or confined to the free rostral portion of the tongue are more easily removed, and up to 50% of the tongue can be removed without adverse effects. Unfortunately, 54% of canine tumours are midline or bilateral, which may limit a complete resection. However, total glossectomy has been successfully performed in dogs with only mild impairment of eating and drinking.

Control of haemorrhage should be considered prior to surgery. Electrosurgery may facilitate haemostasis, but care must be exercised to prevent thermal injury and subsequent tissue necrosis. In the author's experience, acceptable haemostasis with minimal tissue damage can be achieved with monopolar electrocautery using a fine needle tip, a low coagulation setting and gentle traction on the tongue. Laser excision has also been shown to be acceptable. Alternatively,

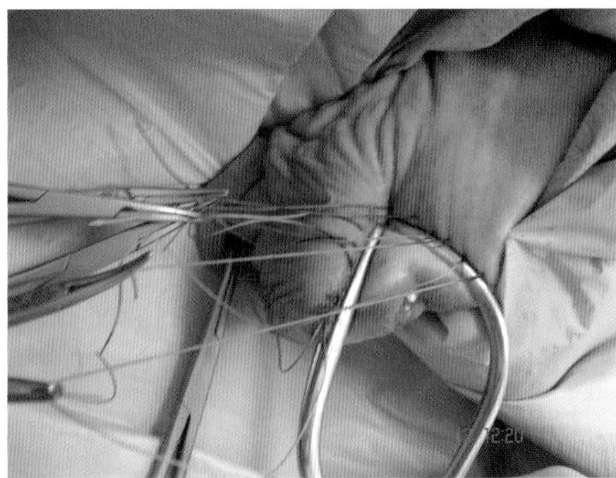

Fig. 6.13 Pre-placement of clamps and mattress sutures prior to wedge resection.

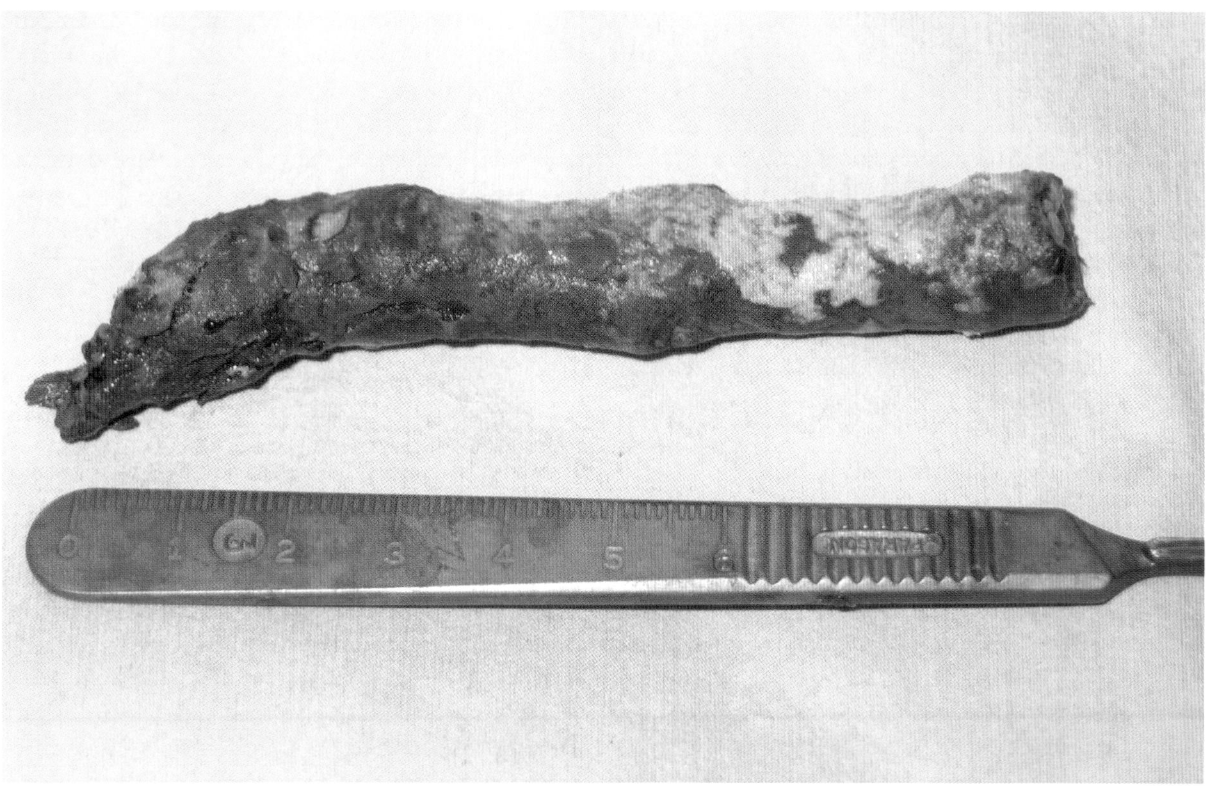

Fig. 6.20 Large stick seen in Fig 6.19 removed from cervical region.

- oesophageal (primary motility disorder)
- other oesophageal (stricture, vascular ring anomaly, mass)
- lower oesophageal sphincter/hiatus.

A functional cause should be suspected if a mass or congenital structural abnormality is not found on physical examination or advanced diagnostics. Functional dysphagia can be idiopathic, congenital or secondary to an acquired neurological condition such as polyneuropathy or myasthenia gravis, so a thorough neurological examination is warranted.

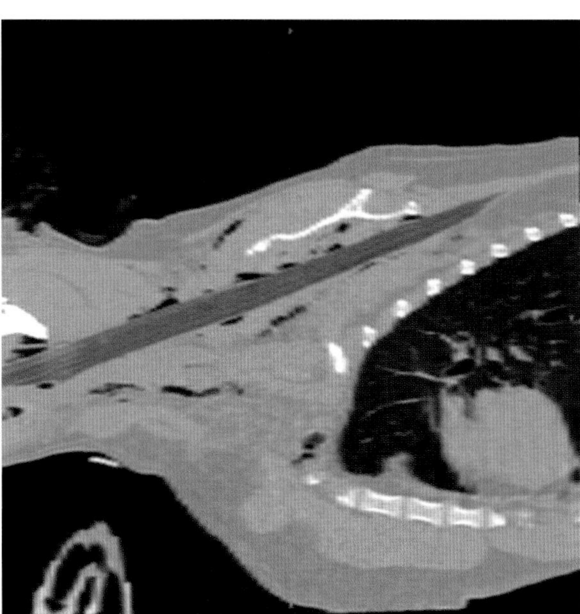

Fig. 6.21 CT image showing penetrating stick foreign body.

Oropharyngeal dysphagia may be congenital owing to a polyneuropathy of the glossopharyngeal, vagal or hypoglossal nerves, structural as a result of a foreign body, neoplasia or trauma, or functional (achalasia or chalasia).

Cricopharyngeal achalasia is a condition characterised by failure of the upper oesophageal sphincter to open at the end of the oropharyngeal phase of swallowing, which prevents the bolus of food from entering the oesophagus. Clinical signs of regurgitation immediately after attempted swallowing are usually seen at weaning. Secondary aspiration pneumonia may occur.

Advanced imaging using a fluoroscopic barium contrast-swallowing study is needed to diagnose this condition. Fluoroscopy demonstrates normal barium movement into the posterior pharynx. Powerful pharyngeal contraction causes marked dilation of the pharyngeal wall. There is inadequate relaxation of the cricopharyngeal sphincter and a thin stream of barium is seen in the oesophagus. Residual barium enters the trachea as the epiglottis relaxes and opens the larynx. There is a significant delay between swallowing (closure of the epiglottis) and opening of the upper oesophageal sphincter.

Cricopharyngeal myotomy is curative. It is essential to differentiate this condition from pharyngeal dysphagia prior to surgery, as that is worsened by cricopharyngeal myotomy. It is also important to rule out concurrent oesophageal dysfunction.

To perform a cricopharyngeal myotomy, a ventral midline approach is made to the larynx. The larynx is rotated 180° to expose the thyropharyngeus (cranial) and cricopharyngeus (caudal) muscles. The cricopharyngeus muscle is incised on its median raphe to the level of the pharyngeal mucosa and extended 1–2 cm caudally along the oesophagus (Fig. 6.22). The prognosis is excellent, assuming that the correct initial diagnosis has been made (Niles et al., 2001).

6.5 Tonsils

Key points

- Clinical signs of tonsillitis include coughing, retching, anorexia, pyrexia and lethargy.
- Squamous cell carcinoma is the most common tonsillar tumour in the dog.

6.5.1 Anatomy

The tonsillar fossa is located rostral to the dorsolateral aspect of each palatopharyngeal arch. Each palatine tonsil has a large fusiform portion which occupies the majority of the fossa and a smaller portion which lies in the rostrolateral wall of the fossa. The blood supply is via the tonsillar artery, which is a branch of the lingual artery. The tonsils are involved in the immune response to antigens that enter the oral cavity, and they do not have afferent lymphatics. Efferent lymphatics feed into the mandibular and medial retropharyngeal lymph nodes. In addition to the palatine tonsils, dogs and cats possess a lingual tonsil (tonsilla lingualis) located in the base of the tongue and a pharyngeal tonsil (tonsilla pharyngea) located in the roof of the nasopharynx (Evans, 2012).

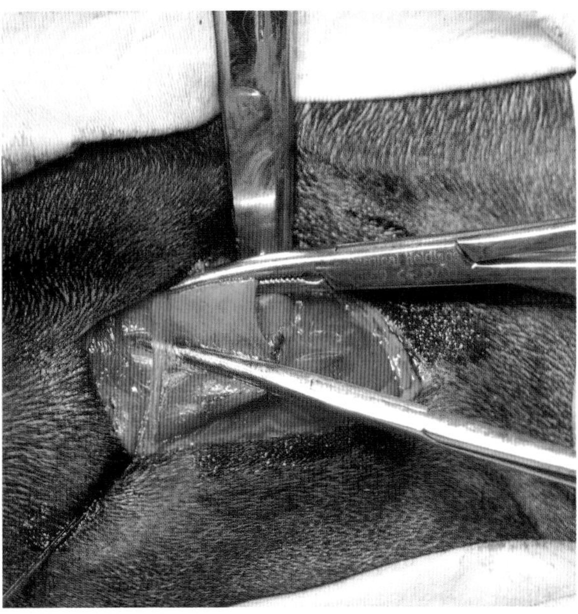

Fig. 6.22 Elevation of cricopharyngeal muscle prior to myectomy.

6.5.2 Disorders of the tonsils

Tonsillar inflammation

Tonsillitis is usually secondary to any upper respiratory tract infections. Primary tonsillitis occurs in young dogs. Clinical signs include coughing, retching, anorexia, pyrexia and lethargy. This condition is self-limiting, though antibiotics and analgesics are often used. Tonsillectomy is indicated in cases of recurrent primary tonsillitis.

Tonsillar neoplasia

Squamous cell carcinoma is the most common tonsillar tumour in the dog (Fig. 6.23). Clinical signs are similar to those of primary tonsillitis (Todoroff et al., 1979). This tumour metastasises early in the disease process, and the disease is considered systemic in 90% of cases. A recent study showed a 1- and 2-year survival rate of 40% and 20%, respectively. The same study also showed a significant difference in long-term survival in cases with no evidence of metastatic disease at the time of diagnosis (637.5 days) compared to those with local (134 days) or distant (75 days) metastasis present (Grant and North, 2016). Thoracic radiographs are positive in 10–20% of cases at the time of presentation. Tonsillectomy is recommended for biopsy and to palliate clinical signs, even if complete margins cannot be obtained (Fig. 6.24). Adjunctive chemotherapy or radiation therapy is indicated in these cases.

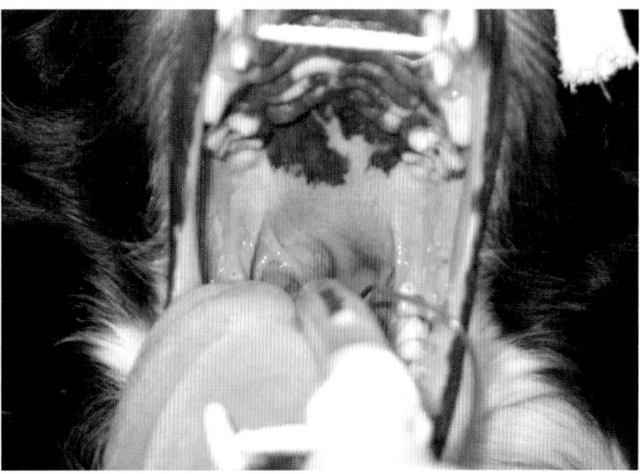

Fig. 6.23 Tonsillar carcinoma.

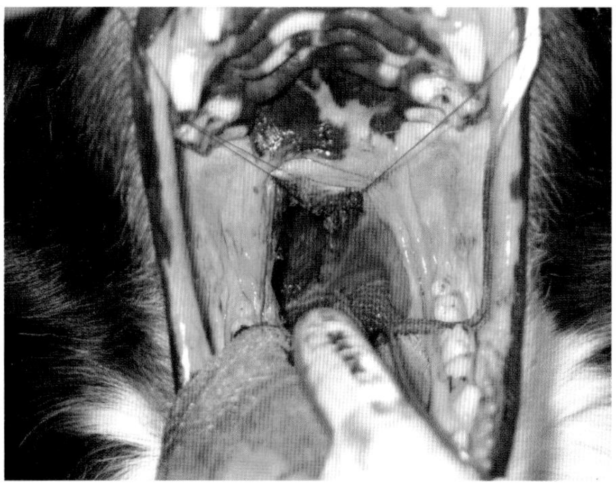

Fig. 6.24 Resection of tonsillar carcinoma seen in Fig 6.23.

6.5.3 Tonsillectomy

Tonsillectomy is indicated for the treatment of tonsillar neoplasia and recurrent primary tonsillitis and in brachycephalic syndrome. The tonsil is grasped and pulled out of the tonsillar crypt. The base is transected and ligated if necessary. Electrocautery or vessel-sealing systems facilitate this procedure (Belch et al., 2017). The crypt mucosa is closed with a continuous suture of 3-0 to 4-0 absorbable material.

6.6 Palate

Key points

- Clefts of the primary palate rarely cause clinical signs other than mild local rhinitis.
- Clinical signs of patients suffering from clefts of the secondary palate (hard and soft palates) may initially go unnoticed but are likely to progress to rhinitis, coughing, aspiration pneumonia and failure to thrive.
- The medially positioned flap technique is used for hard palate repair but has the disadvantage of locating the suture line directly over the defect.
- A nasal pharyngeal mucosal flap is used to close a lateral cleft.
- Overlapping flap technique for hard palate repair results in less tension on the suture line.
- The medially positioned flap technique for soft palate repair is suitable for midline clefts of the soft palate.
- Labial-based mucoperiosteal flaps are used to repair oronasal fistulas.
- The modified split palatal U-flap technique is used in situations where there is a large defect of the caudal hard palate.

6.6.1 Anatomy

The palate separates the nasal passages, choanae and nasopharynx from the oral cavity. Congenital failure of the palate to fuse, or trauma to the hard or soft palate, results in an abnormal communication between the oral cavity and nose and the oropharynx and nasopharynx. The hard palate comprises the palatine, maxillary and incisive bones, and the palatal mucoperiosteum. The oral surface is lined by stratified squamous epithelium and contains six to ten transverse ridges and depressions. The incisive papilla opens at, or just rostral to, the first transverse ridge. The major palatine foramina are located medial to the carnassials (4th premolars). The major palatine artery exits these foramina and runs rostrally to supply the hard palate. Numerous rami are present, one of which runs between the canine and third incisor to anastomose with the infraorbital artery. Sensory innervation to the oral surface of the hard palate is by the major palatine branch of the maxillary division of the trigeminal nerve. This nerve also exits the major palatine foramen.

The soft palate is continuous with the hard palate and extends just caudal to the last molar in non-brachycephalic breeds. The blood supply to the soft palate is via the minor palatine arteries. Venous drainage is via the palatine plexus lateral to the palatine muscles. Sensory innervation to the soft palate is by the minor palatine branch of the maxillary division of the trigeminal nerve. The glossopharyngeal and vagus nerves supply the pterygopharyngeal and palatopharyngeal muscles. The soft palate muscles include the palatinus and levator and tensor veli palatini. The palatinus muscle runs from the palatine process of the palatine bone to the caudal edge of the soft palate. It functions to shorten the soft palate. The tensor veli palatini muscle arises rostral to the tympanic bulla and inserts on the palatine aponeurosis. It functions to stretch the soft palate between the pterygoid bones. The levator veli palatini muscle has a similar origin and inserts on the caudal soft palate. It functions to elevate the soft palate during swallowing (Evans, 2012).

6.6.2 Palate defects

Congenital palate defects arise owing to incomplete fusion of the maxillofacial structures during fetal development. Acquired palate defects arise following infection, trauma, neoplasia, surgery and radiation therapy. Brachycephalic breeds are reported to be at greater risk due to differential growth of the palatine portions of the facial bones in relation to the growth of the head. Causes of acquired defects of the palate include chronic infection (severe periodontal disease,

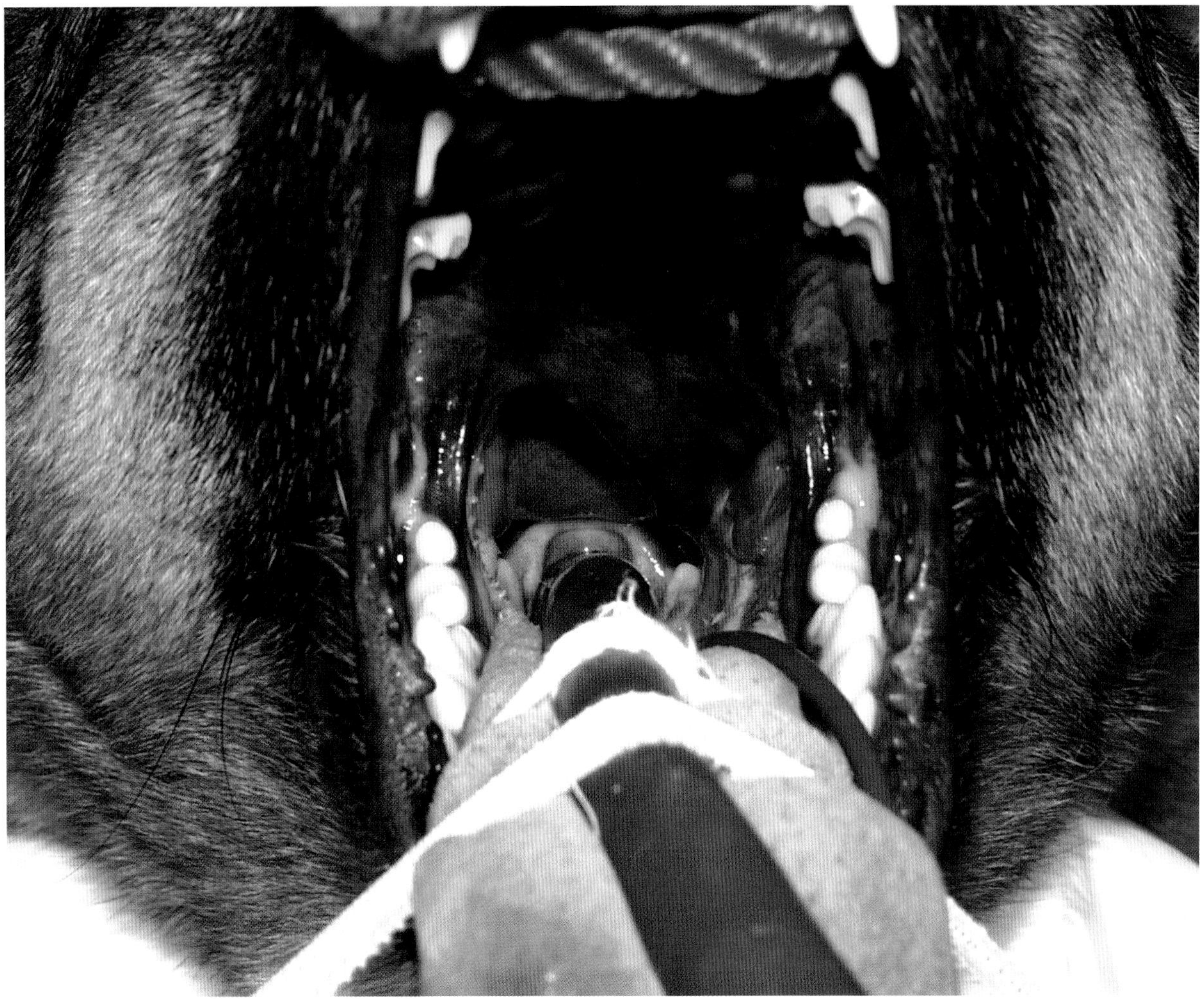

Fig. 6.25 Congenital defect of the soft palate.

osteomyelitis or osteonecrosis), trauma (high-rise syndrome, motor vehicle trauma, electric cord, gunshot trauma, foreign body penetration and chronic pressure wounds due to malocclusion), neoplasms and radiation therapy.

Clefts of the primary palate (lip and premaxilla) are more commonly left-sided. These rarely cause clinical signs other than mild local rhinitis. They can, however, be associated with clefts of the secondary palate. Successful surgical repair requires reconstruction of the lip, the philtrum, the floor of the nasal vestibule and rostral hard palate with flaps harvested from oral and nasal tissues.

Clefts of the secondary palate (hard and soft palates) may initially go unnoticed. Clinical signs are failure to create a negative pressure when suckling, drainage of milk from the nares during suckling, rhinitis, coughing, aspiration pneumonia and failure to thrive. Congenital hard palate defects are almost always midline and are usually associated with a midline soft palate defect. Soft palate clefts may be midline or unilateral (Fig. 6.25). Traumatic cleft palate in the cat is usually associated with a visible misalignment along the midline of the maxillary dental arch. Puppies and kittens with cleft of the secondary palate can be tube-fed until at least 8 weeks of age. Surgery before this age is difficult as the soft tissues are soft and friable. Surgery is not delayed beyond 4–5 months as the cleft may widen as the animal grows (Harvey, 1987).

6.6.3 Treatment of palate defects

The aim of surgery is closure of the defect with a well-vascularised, tension-free graft harvested for the oral and nasal cavities. The best chance of success is usually with the first procedure. Oral tissues are delicate and should be handled with fine forceps and stay sutures. Tissues shouldn't be crushed or allowed to desiccate. Considerable haemorrhage can occur during surgery; however, electrocautery is to be avoided as this may delay wound healing. Digital pressure with gauze swabs will usually be sufficient to control any bleeding. Suture lines should not be under tension and, if possible, should not be located directly over the defect.

Patients should be fed soft food only for 10–14 days after the surgery, and access to chew toys should be restricted. Dehiscence remains a major complication, and owners should be warned that multiple procedures may be required (Fiani et al., 2016).

Repair of rostral defects

Repair of rostral defects is complicated by the lack of a connective tissue bed to provide support for simple sliding grafts. Repair of the floor of the nasal vestibule and rostral hard palate is achieved with a combination of advancement, rotation, transposition or overlapping flaps followed by reconstruction of the overlying cutaneous structures. The presence of teeth in the incisive bone and maxilla may impede flap elevation. Removal of one or more incisors and the canine tooth several weeks prior to definitive repair can facilitate flap elevation (Howard et al., 1976).

Step by step: overlapping flap technique for hard palate repair

This technique is used for repair of midline cleft of the hard palate (Howard et al., 1974). It results in less tension on the suture line, which is not located directly over the defect. It provides a larger area of opposing connective tissue which, in turn, provides a stronger scar.

- A mucoperiosteal incision is made along the dental arch 1–2 mm from the teeth and to the rostral and caudal margins of the defect. This will form the overlapped flap.
- A second mucoperiosteal incision is made on the other side of the palate along the medial margin of the defect. This will form the envelope flap.
- Both flaps are undermined with a periosteal elevator. It is essential that the major palatine artery, which exits the major palatine foramen, is preserved on each side.
- The overlapped flap is inverted at its base so that the periosteal surface is exposed. This flap is secured under the envelope flap with horizontal mattress sutures (Fig. 6.26).
- Granulation and epithelialisation of the exposed bone are complete within 3–4 weeks.

Step by step: medially positioned flap technique for hard palate repair

This technique has the disadvantage of locating the suture line directly over the defect. There is a smaller area of opposing connective tissue over the defect. This technique is best suited for repair of traumatic midline clefts in cats (Reiter and Smith, 2018).

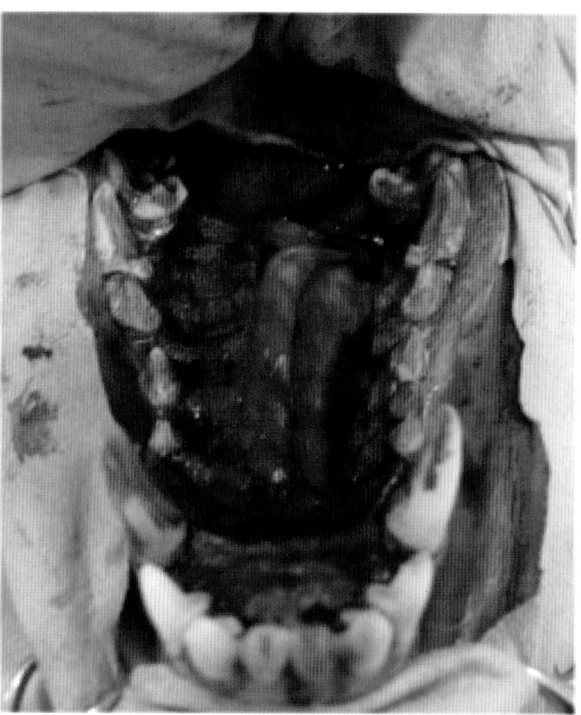

Fig. 6.26 Overlapping flap elevated and sutured in place to close cleft of the hard palate.

- Paired mucoperiosteal incisions are made along the dental arcade 1–2 mm from the teeth and along the margins of the defect.
- Both flaps are undermined with a periosteal elevator. It is essential to preserve the major palatine arteries.
- The two flaps are moved medially and sutured to each other. The exposed bone will granulate and epithelialise within a few weeks (Fig. 6.27).

Step by step: medially positioned flap technique for soft palate repair

This technique is suitable for midline cleft of the soft palate (Reiter and Smith, 2018). The tensor and levator veli palatini muscles exert lateral tension on the suture line. This can be nullified by lateral relaxing incisions transecting the tensor veli palatini muscle. The palatine muscles place a shearing force on the sutures, particularly near the free edge of the soft palate. A three-layer closure is desirable. However, the nasal mucosa is often friable and this layer is frequently closed with the muscle layer.

- Paired incisions are made along the medial margins of the defect to the level of the caudal palatine tonsils. The palatal tissues are bluntly dissected and separated into a dorsal (nasopharyngeal) and ventral (oropharyngeal) flap on each side.
- The palatal tissues are repaired separately with simple interrupted sutures.

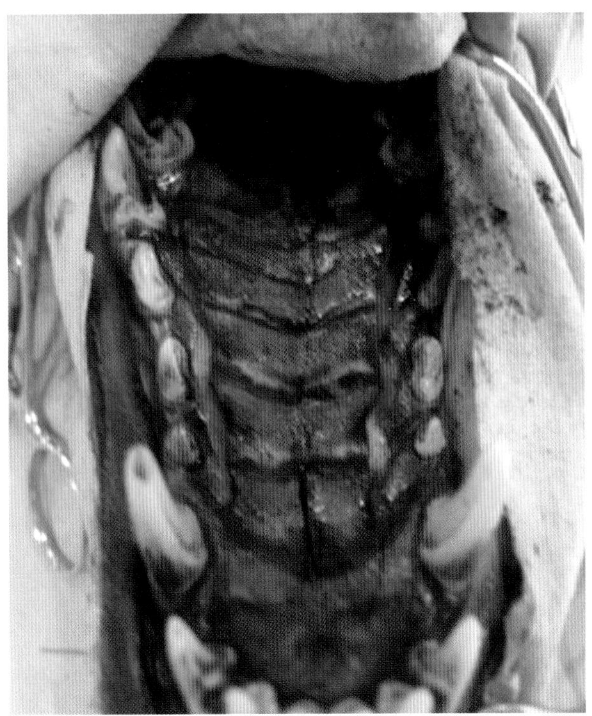

Fig. 6.27 Medially positioned flaps elevated and sutured in place to close defect of hard palate.

- Paired incisions through the levator veli palatini muscles are made lateral to the suture line, to minimise tension across the repair.

Step by step: labial-based mucoperiosteal flap for repair of oronasal fistula

Oronasal fistula typically develops in the canine tooth region. Repair involves the creation of a labial-based mucoperiosteal flap over the defect (Bojrab et al., 1986).

- The fistula is debrided by removing any granulation tissue and the epithelial lining on the oral aspect of the fistula.
- Incisions are made rostral and caudal to the fistula. The alveolar and labial mucosae are undermined with a periosteal elevator.
- The periosteal attachment is incised at its base with a scalpel blade to mobilise the flap completely.
- The flap is sutured to both the alveolar and labial mucosa in a simple interrupted pattern. Ensure there is no tension across the repair.

Step by step: modified split palatal U-flap technique

This technique is used in situations where there is a large defect of the caudal hard palate. The flaps are based on the major palatine arteries (Reiter and Smith, 2018).

- Paired incisions are made in the mucoperiosteum of the hard palate. The longer incision extends to the first or second maxillary premolar; the shorter incision is to the second or third maxillary premolar.
- A third incision is made on the midline, splitting the flaps in two.
- The shorter flap is rotated and sutured to the caudal aspect of the debrided defect.
- The longer flap is similarly rotated. The medial aspect of the longer flap is sutured to the rostral aspect of the shorter flap.
- The donor site is allowed to heal by granulation and epithelialisation.

Step by step: repair of lateral clefts of the soft palate

These clefts occur lateral to the palatine muscles. The tensor and levator veli palatini muscles or the palatopharyngeal muscles pull the free edge of the cleft laterally. Bilateral cleft can also be seen. A nasal pharyngeal mucosal flap is used to close a lateral cleft.

- The flap is based just dorsal to the palatine tonsil and includes the vestige of the lateral portion of the palate.
- The free edge originates from the dorsolateral wall of the nasopharynx.
- The width of the flap is 2 mm wider than the width of the defect.
- The medial edge of the cleft is incised to form two layers of tissue, and is deepened by 1–2 mm to receive the free edge of the pharyngeal mucosa.
- The defect is closed in one or two layers with simple interrupted sutures.
- The nasal surface is left to granulate and epithelialise.

Prostheses

The use of prostheses made from metal alloy, non-aqueous elastomeric impression material or synthetic resin has been described (Reiter and Smith, 2018). Fabrication and placement of an obturator usually requires two anaesthetic episodes. First, an impression of the defect is taken which allows the construction of a cast. From the cast the prosthesis is created, trial-fitted, adjusted and secured in place. Halitosis is a common complication with palatal obturators. Dogs and cats fitted with obturators should be examined every 6–12 months under general anaesthesia to clean the edges of the defect and to scale and polish the obturator.

6.6.4 Postoperative care

Regional nerve blocks of the maxillary, infraorbital and major palatine nerves can be performed using long-acting 0.5% bupivacaine hydrochloride. The total dose should not exceed 2 mg/kg in both dogs and cats. Postoperative pain can also be controlled with injectable, transdermal and oral opioids. Non-steroidal anti-inflammatory medication should be used to control postoperative swelling. Food should be withheld for the first 8–12 hours after surgery, except in paediatric patients. The diet should be a soft gruel consistency for the first two weeks after surgery. Chlorhexidine mouthwashes can be used, but postoperative antibiotics are typically not needed due to the rapid healing of oral tissues. Feeding tubes are also not typically needed after surgery but may be considered in cases of poly-trauma.

The commonest complication after surgery of the soft and hard palate is dehiscence of the flap due to excessive tension or compromised vascular supply. An Elizabethan collar should be used for two weeks to prevent self-trauma. Sedation or anaesthesia may be required to assess the degree of repair. Any revision surgery should not be attempted before healing of all tissues involved.

6.6.5 Management of elongated soft palate

This topic is covered in this volume, Chapter 7.3, Brachycephalic obstructive airway syndrome.

6.7 Mandible and maxilla

Key points

- Malignant melanomas are locally invasive and have a very high metastatic rate.
- Squamous cell carcinoma (non-tonsillar) is locally invasive but has a low metastatic rate.
- Fibrosarcoma appears benign on histology, but aggressively invades bone and requires wide excision.
- Osteosarcoma frequently metastasises to the lungs.
- Fibromatous and ossifying epulis are locally invasive but do not metastasise. Acanthomatous ameloblastoma is non-metastatic but locally invasive.
- Dehiscence over the bone ends following rostral mandibulectomy, and at the labial mucosa–palate suture line following maxillectomy, are of greater concern.
- Cats are often unwilling to eat after mandibulectomy, and feeding tubes should be placed at the time of surgery.

6.7.1 Anatomy

Anatomy of the mandible

The mandible consists of left and right halves divided into a horizontal body and a vertical ramus. These halves are joined rostrally at the mandibular symphysis, which is a strong fibrous joint.

The major muscles of mastication insert on the mandible.

- The masseter muscle extends from the zygomatic arch to the lateral surfaces of the caudal body and vertical ramus.
- The temporalis muscle extends from the temporal region of the skull to the dorsal portion of the ramus.
- The pterygoid muscle extends from the pterygoid, palatine and sphenoid bones to the angular process of the ramus.
- The digastricus muscle extends from the occipital region of the skull to the ventral border of the body of the mandible.

The majority of the blood supply to the mandible comes from the mandibular alveolar artery, which is a branch of the maxillary artery and enters the mandible via the mandibular foramen on the medial surface of the bone at the angle of the mandible. It exits laterally via the mental foramen immediately caudal to the canine.

Sensory innervation to the mandible is through the mandibular alveolar nerve, which is a branch of the trigeminal nerve. It enters the mandible via the mandibular foramen and exits via the mental foramina as mental nerves, which innervate the lower teeth and surrounding tissues.

The mandibular and sublingual salivary ducts run medially to the body of the mandible below the gingiva. They exit at the sublingual papilla caudal to the symphysis (Evans, 2012).

Anatomy of the maxilla

The muzzle comprises three bones. The maxilla is the largest bone and contains the canines, premolars and molars. The incisive bone or premaxilla contains the incisor teeth. The nasal bone runs along the dorsal midline of the muzzle.

The blood supply to the maxillary region is via two major branches of the maxillary artery:

- The major palatine artery runs through the caudal nasal cavity and exits the hard palate via the caudal palatine foramen. This artery can be safely ligated during maxillectomy.
- The infraorbital artery runs through the caudal nasal cavity, maxillary foramen and infraorbital canal of the maxilla and exits via the infraorbital foramen at the level of the rostral margin of the carnassial tooth. The infraorbital artery branches into dorsal and lateral nasal arteries.

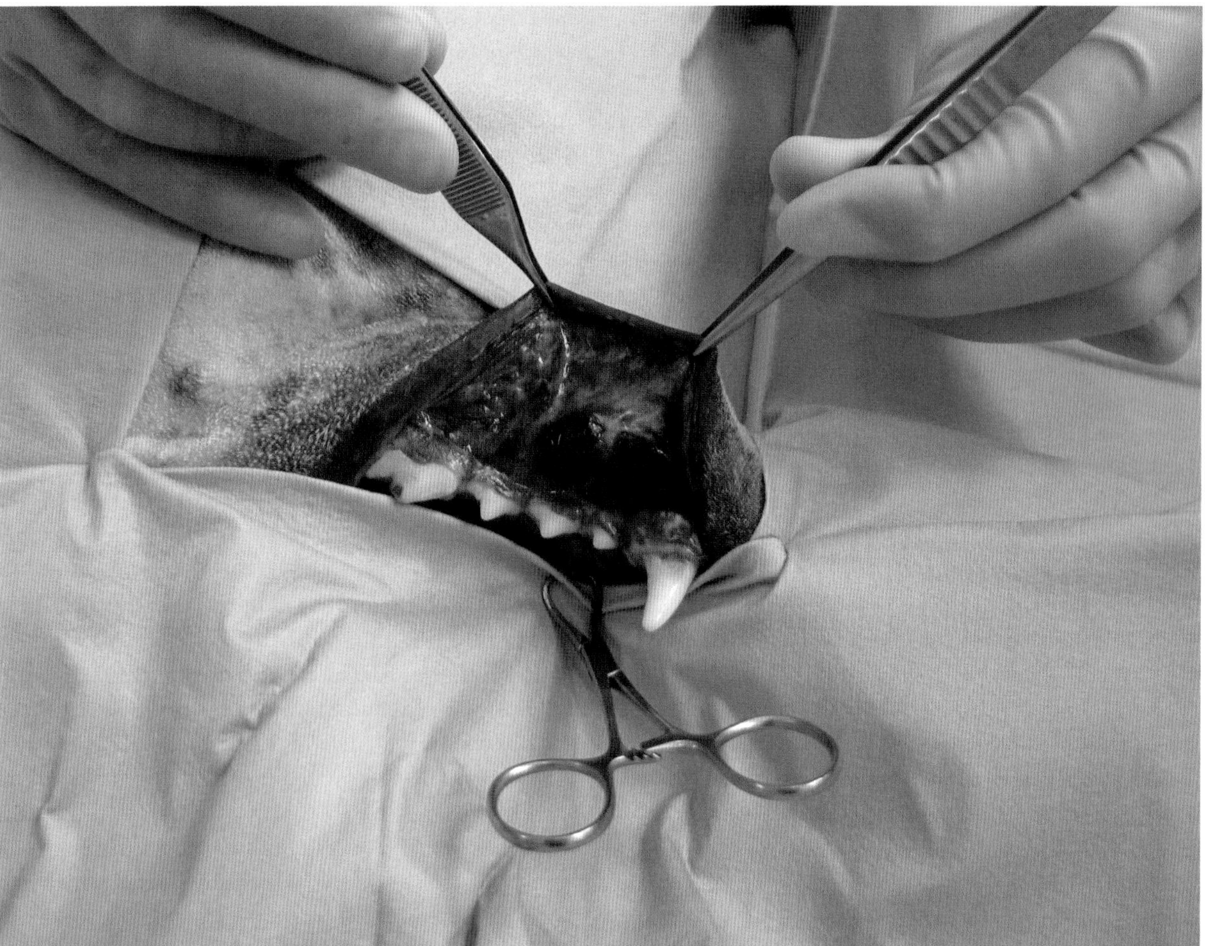

Fig. 6.28 Malignant melanoma.

The infraorbital nerve, which is a branch of the maxillary nerve, runs through the infraorbital canal. This nerve provides sensory innervation to the upper teeth.

The parotid salivary duct terminates lateral to the carnassial, and the zygomatic salivary gland lies just medial to the rostral portion of the zygomatic arch. These ducts can be transected during maxillectomy without adverse effects (Evans, 2012).

6.7.2 Canine oral tumours

A number of specific tumours can affect the oral cavity of dogs. They all carry the potential for aggressive invasion of the surrounding tissues, including bone. Their metastatic potential can vary significantly.

Malignant melanoma

This is the commonest oral tumour found in the dog. They tend to occur in older, small-breed dogs, but can also affect larger breeds such as chow chows and golden retrievers. They are usually darkly pigmented but also can be amelanotic (Fig. 6.28). These tumours are locally invasive and have a very high metastatic rate (81%) (Todoroff and Brodey, 1979).

Squamous cell carcinoma (non-tonsillar)

This tumour tends to occur in older, large-breed dogs. It is a typically flat, ulcerative tumour with minimal external mass. It is locally invasive but has a lower metastatic rate (20%) (Theon et al., 1997).

Fibrosarcoma

This tumour tends to occur in middle-aged to older large-breed dogs, particularly golden retrievers and Labradors. It has a proliferative appearance and usually arises from the gingiva close to the carnassial (Fig. 6.29). It is locally invasive and has a metastatic rate of around 35% (Todoroff and Brodey, 1979). A variation of this tumour is the histologically low-grade, biologically high-grade fibrosarcoma. This tumour appears benign on histology but aggressively invades bone and requires wide excision.

Osteosarcoma

This tumour arises from the bone of the mandible or maxilla. It frequently metastasises to the lungs. Survival times are superior to those for appendicular osteosarcoma following amputation (Farcas et al., 2014).

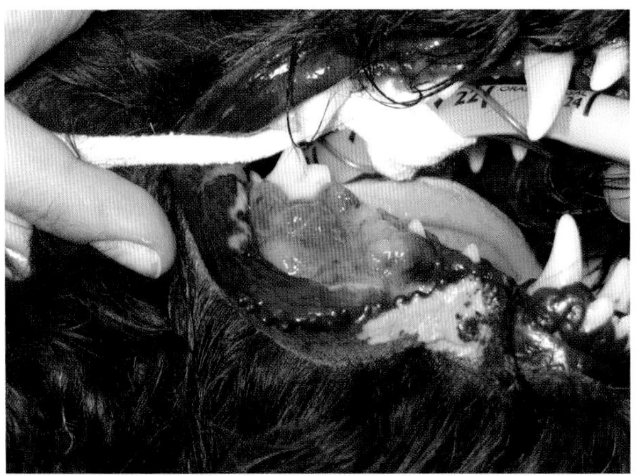

Fig. 6.29 Fibrosarcoma arising from mandible.

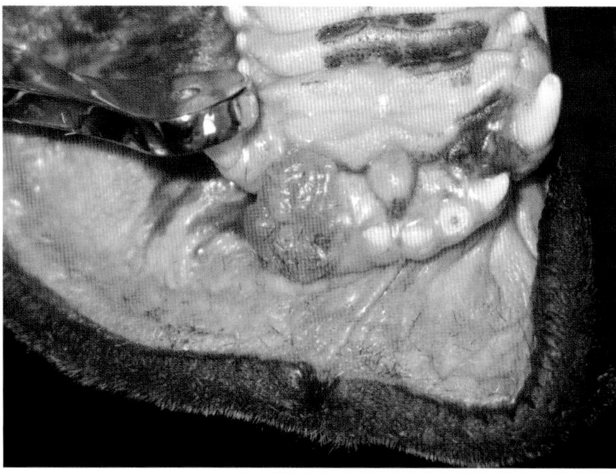

Fig. 6.30 Acanthomatous ameloblastoma causing disruption of incisor arcade.

Tumours arising from the periodontal ligament or odontogenic epithelium

These tumours were originally classified into fibromatous, ossifying and acanthomatous epulis based on their histological criteria. Fibromatous epulis truly arise from the periodontal ligament. The origin of ossifying epulis is unclear. Acanthomatous epulis arises from the odontogenic epithelium rather than the periodontal ligament, and the term acanthomatous ameloblastoma is now used.

Fibromatous and ossifying epulis are benign lesions, which are slow growing and often occur in the premaxillary region. These tumours are locally invasive but do not metastasise. Local excision without bone removal typically provides excellent long-term palliative care. Curative intent surgery for these tumours involves removal of the tooth and a small margin of alveolar bone.

Acanthomatous ameloblastoma is a non-metastatic but locally invasive tumour. It has a similar appearance to SCC and can cause spreading of the teeth (Fig. 6.30). It is best treated by mandibulectomy or maxillectomy (Goldschmidt et al., 2017).

6.7.3 Staging of oral tumours

Oral radiographs should be taken to assess the extent of the primary tumour. Around 60–80% of gingival tumours cause radiographically apparent bone lysis, but plain radiographs often underestimate the extent of bone destruction and give little information about the extent of involvement of local soft tissues; CT and MRI are superior. These modalities are particularly useful for assessing caudal tumours, tumours that cross the midline and those that invade the nasal cavity, pharynx or orbit.

Incisional biopsies are useful, as gingival tumours tend to have different metastatic rates. This can help make the decision on whether surgery is likely to be curative, and whether adjunctive radiation therapy is appropriate. A deep wedge of tissue must be taken as most gingival tumours are covered by inflamed, infected or necrotic tissue. The biopsy incision should be in the gingival mucosa so that the biopsy tract can be removed at the time of definitive surgery. The skin and labial mucosa should be preserved.

Regional lymph nodes should be assessed for metastasis. The oral cavity drains to the mandibular, parotid and medial retropharyngeal lymph nodes. Only the mandibular lymph node is palpable. The sensitivity and specificity of lymph node size for predicting the cytological and histological presence of metastasis was only 70 and 51%, respectively (Williams and Packer, 2003). Fine needle aspirates can be taken from the mandibular lymph node, but a better option is to excise all three drainage lymph nodes. This can be done through a single incision. A study of this procedure showed that 35.5% of dogs had histological evidence of metastasis to one or more of the three lymph nodes, but only 54.5% of these were to the mandibular lymph node (Smith, 1995).

Thoracic radiographs should be taken to identify pulmonary metastases, but thoracic CT is more sensitive and can be performed at the time of oral CT.

6.7.4 Preoperative preparation

It is essential to make clients aware of the cosmetic and functional results following mandibulectomy or maxillectomy. Post-surgical images are useful for this. Surgery of the oral cavity is considered to be a clean-contaminated procedure. Surgical infections are rare owing to the oral cavity's rich blood supply. Prophylactic broad-spectrum antibiotics can be used.

Handy hints

- Local nerve block with 0.5–1.0 ml of 0.5% bupivacaine should be considered.
- The rostral mandible and incisor region can be blocked by injecting at the level of the second premolar at the mental foramen.
- The mandibular nerve can be injected for more extensive mandibulectomy as it leaves the mandibular foramen at the medial angle of the jaw.
- The infraorbital nerve can be blocked at the level of the infraorbital foramen, which is located dorsal to the rostral aspect of the carnassial. This is used for rostral maxillectomy procedures.
- The entire maxillary area can be blocked by blocking the maxillary nerve rostral to the ramus and below the ventral border of the zygomatic arch just caudal to the lateral canthus of the eye.

Control of haemorrhage is essential. The mandibular alveolar artery and major palatine artery will need to be identified and ligated during mandibulectomy and maxillectomy procedures, respectively. The nasal cavity is often entered during extensive maxillectomy. In the majority of cases haemorrhage can be controlled by electrocautery, gelatine sponges or topical administration of epinephrine. If severe haemorrhage is encountered, then temporary or permanent carotid artery occlusion can be used to control it within the nasal cavity.

Positioning of the patient is dependent on the area of bone to be removed. A mouth speculum should be placed and the oropharynx should be packed with swabs.

- Dorsal recumbency is best for bilateral rostral mandibulectomies and rostral maxillectomies.
- Lateral recumbency is best for segmental removal of the mandible or any part of the ramus.
- Oblique lateral recumbency is best for central and caudal maxillectomy.

6.7.5 Technique for mandibulectomy

The area and amount of bone to be removed are determined by the site of the tumour and by the radiographic or CT appearance. At least 1 cm of bone either side of the tumour should be removed. Bone should be transected between tooth roots. It is safer to consider removal of the entire hemi-mandible if the tumour is extensively invading the medullary cavity.

Step by step: rostral and central mandibulectomy

- The patient is positioned in dorsal recumbency for rostral mandibulectomy (Fig. 6.31), or in lateral recumbency for segmental hemi-mandibulectomy.
- The gingiva is incised 0.5 cm beyond the level at which the bone is to be transected, and is elevated from the bone.
- Oral mucosa, labial mucosa and muscular attachments are transected to give at least 1 cm margins. It is usually possible to obtain wider margins owing to the redundant skin and mucosa adjacent to the mandible. Haemorrhage can be controlled by use of electrocautery.
- The mandibular body is transected with an oscillating saw. The area is irrigated during cutting to prevent heat necrosis (Fig. 6.32). Care must be taken if an osteotome is being used not to split the bone longitudinally. The mandibular alveolar artery is ligated or cauterised.
- The mandibular symphysis is separated with an oscillating saw or osteotome. For small tumours confined to the incisors, it may be possible to preserve the symphysis by transecting the bone across the canine tooth then extracting the roots. This preserves stability and reduces postoperative pain.
- Closure is achieved by suturing labial mucosa to gingival mucosa and sublingual mucosa using a synthetic monofilament. The skin can be sutured directly to the sublingual mucosa following rostral mandibulectomy.

Step by step: caudal mandibulectomy and hemi-mandibulectomy

- The patient is positioned in lateral recumbency. A full-thickness incision can be made in the cheek from

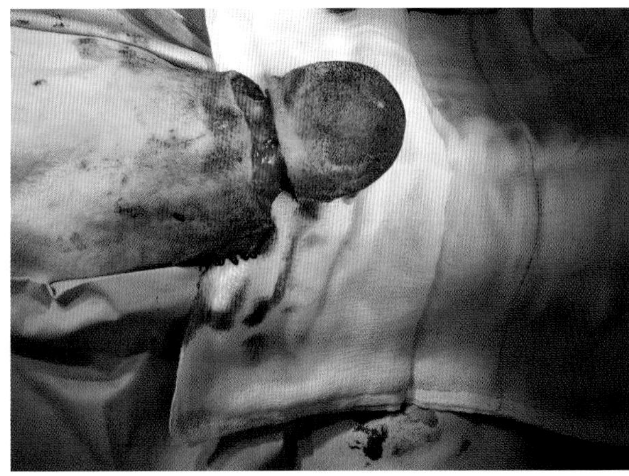

Fig. 6.31 Patient positioned in dorsal recumbancy for bilateral rostral mandibulectomy.

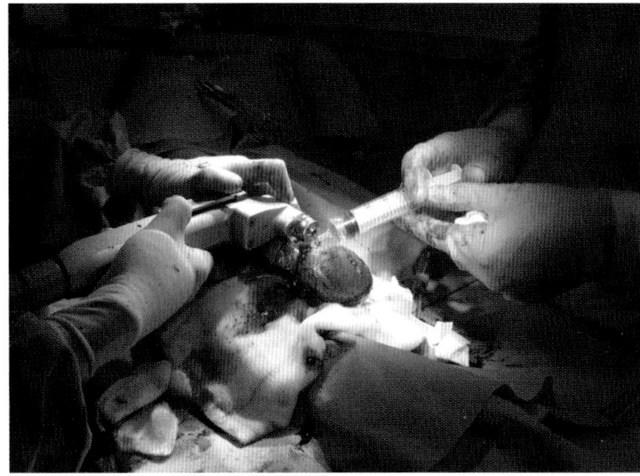

Fig. 6.32 Rostral mandibulectomy being performed using oscillating saw.

the commissure to the level of the caudal border of the ramus, to improve exposure. Removal of the zygomatic arch improves exposure of the dorsal ramus and temporomandibular joint. This can be replaced using orthopaedic wire; there are no functional and only minor cosmetic problems if the zygomatic arch is not replaced.

- For hemi-mandibulectomy, the soft tissues including the masseter, digastricus, temporalis and pterygoid muscles are transected. This allows lateral retraction of the mandibular body and exposure of the medial ramus.
- The mandibular alveolar nerve is ligated and divided at the level of the mandibular foramen.
- The remaining muscles of mastication are transected and the temporomandibular joint is disarticulated. It is easier to transect the mandible through its angle or the cranioventral ramus if the tumour is confined to the caudal body. The residual ramus can be left in place.
- The labial mucosa is sutured to the gingival and sublingual mucosa. Advancement of the commissure rostrally to the level of the first or second premolar prevents the tongue hanging out of the mouth.

Mandibular rim excision

Mandibular rim excision using a bi-radial saw has been described (Arzi and Verstraete, 2010). Its only indication is for tumours located between the canine and ramus that have not invaded the underlying bone. It was suggested that 10 mm of bone is left to prevent postoperative fracture, though it is not clear how important this is. It may be an acceptable treatment for acanthomatous ameloblastoma.

6.7.6 Technique for maxillectomy

Step by step: rostral and central maxillectomy

- The patient is positioned in oblique lateral recumbency. Incise the labial mucosa, gingiva and palate at the proposed sites of bone transection. Electrocautery assists in controlling haemorrhage.
- It may be necessary to ligate and divide the major palatine and infraorbital arteries during central maxillectomy. These vessels are not encountered during rostral maxillectomy.
- The thin bone of the maxilla and hard palate can be transected with an osteotome.
- It is difficult to control haemorrhage from the nasal turbinates and, in some cases, to ligate the major arteries until after the segment of bone has been removed. It is best to perform the caudal osteotomy last of all as this is the area where the major vessels will be encountered.
- After removal of the bone and control of haemorrhage, remove any remaining mucosal and turbinate attachments (Fig. 6.33). Bleeding from the nasal cavity is controlled with electrocautery, direct pressure and diluted adrenaline solution.
- Suture the labial mucosa to the gingival and palatine mucosa (Fig. 6.34). This may require a dorsally based labial advancement flap. Pre-placed drill holes in the hard palate may help to prevent dehiscence. The dorsal nasal cartilage can be sutured to drill holes in the nasal bone to prevent ventral drooping of the nose.

Step by step: caudal maxillectomy

- The patient is positioned in oblique lateral recumbency. Exposure can be increased by incising the cheek from the commissure to the caudal margin of the ramus.
- A dorsolateral skin incision can be made over the maxilla to further improve exposure of the dorsal osteotomy site, ventral orbit and zygomatic arch. This incision is continued through the labial mucosa to create a bi-pedicled flap of skin and labial mucosa.
- Labial, gingival and palatine incisions are made as for rostral and central maxillectomies.
- As the caudal osteotomy is beyond the carnassial, the major palatine artery must be ligated in the nasal cavity. It is best to perform this osteotomy last, to delay transection of this artery as long as possible. The tumour is then removed by transecting attached turbinates before the vessel is ligated.

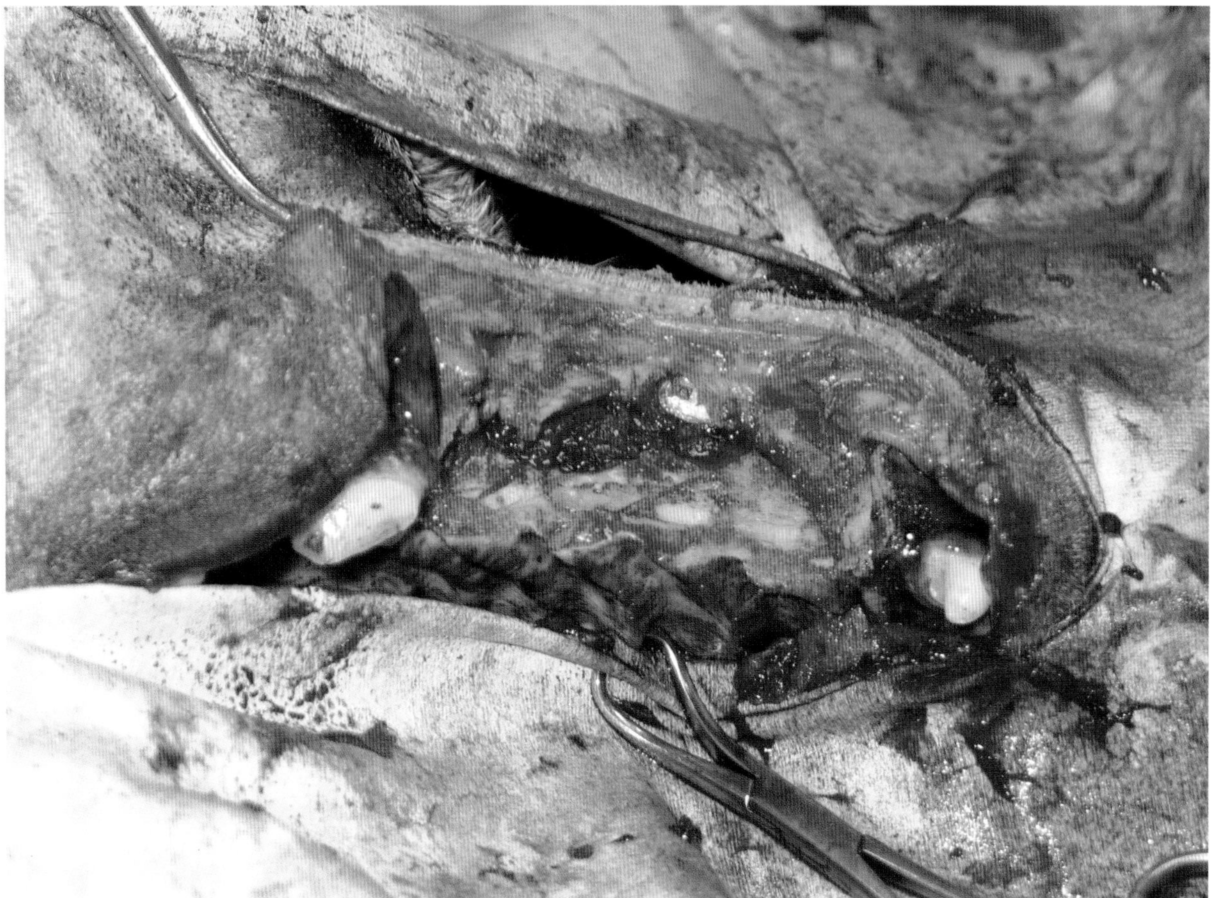

Fig. 6.33 Central maxillectomy performed to remove malignant melanoma seen in Fig 6.28.

- The rostral portion of the zygomatic arch and part of the ventral orbit can be removed if necessary.
- The labial mucosa is sutured to the gingival and palatine mucosa. It is often necessary to create a labial mucosal advancement flap.

6.7.7 Postoperative care

The pharynx should be suctioned prior to recovery from general anaesthesia, to remove blood and saline. Opioid analgesia should be continued for the first 48 hours after surgery or longer if required. Food and water can be reintroduced the day after surgery. Patients should be restricted to soft food for 10–14 days and there should be no access to chew toys. Feeding tubes are rarely necessary following either mandibulectomy or maxillectomy. Facial and sublingual swellings are common, particularly after hemi-mandibulectomy and caudal mandibulectomy. These usually resolve with conservative management. The skin over maxillectomy sites may rise and fall with respiration, but this resolves within a few weeks. If subcutaneous emphysema occurs it is self-limiting. Postoperative antibiotics are not necessary.

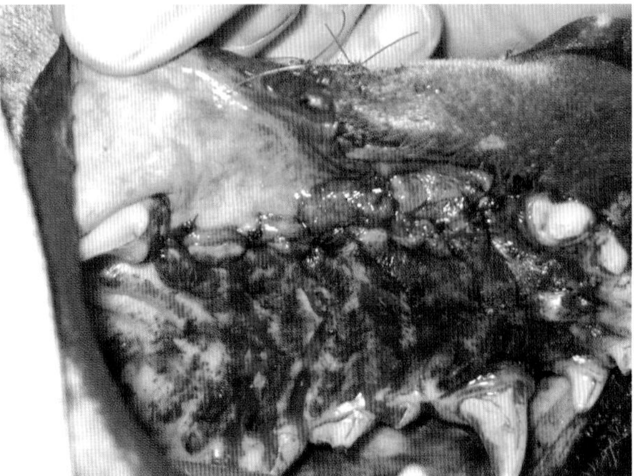

Fig. 6.34 Closure of maxillectomy site by suturing labial mucosa to palatine mucosa.

6.7.8 Complications

Minor intra-oral dehiscence is relatively common. The majority of these cases will heal by second intention and further surgical intervention is not warranted. Dehiscence over the bone ends following rostral mandibulectomy and at the labial mucosa–palate suture line following maxillectomy is of greater concern. Dehiscence of the mandibular site requires debridement, removal of additional bone and re-suturing.

Breakdown of the labial mucosa–palate suture line can lead to oronasal fistula development, which can be monitored. If clinical signs of food impaction, nasal discharge and halitosis develop then debridement, further elevation of the labial mucosa and tension-free closure should be performed. Damage to residual tooth roots may necessitate future dental extractions.

The tongue may fall from the mouth and drooling may be excessive following hemi-mandibulectomy. This can be prevented by rostral advancement of the commissure. Mandibular drift rarely causes clinical problems. If the lower canine is causing an ulcer on the palate, it can be extracted.

Dogs that undergo removal of at least half the length of both bodies may have difficulty prehending food initially. Dogs undergoing almost complete removal of both bodies will require lifelong hand-feeding.

6.7.9 Prognosis

Close monitoring of the incision site should be performed every 3–4 months. This should be performed by the surgeon, as most owners are not capable of inspecting the oral cavity adequately. Sedation may be required to inspect incision sites in the caudal aspect of the oral cavity.

The literature currently supports a number of broad conclusions:

- Aggressive surgical management improves the survival rate for dogs with aggressive oral neoplasia (Sarowitz et al., 2017) – 1-year survival rates of 70–90% have been reported following mandibulectomy and maxillectomy (White, 1991). Most reported local recurrence rates are less than 50%.
- The tumour type significantly influences survival time. Tumours with a high metastatic potential are usually associated with shorter survival times (Sarowitz et al., 2017).
- Tumour location influences local recurrence rates. Tumours on the caudal aspect of the oral cavity are associated with a poorer prognosis. These tumours are more difficult to resect and may not be noticed by owners until they are more advanced.
- The adequacy of excision is the biggest determinant of local recurrence. Local recurrence rates of only 15% have been reported for completely excised tumours, compared with 62–65% for incompletely excised tumours (Sarowitz et al., 2017).
- The best outcomes are achieved with SCC and acanthomatous ameloblastoma. Fibrosarcomas are associated with a high incidence of local recurrence owing to their frequently caudal location. Although being metastatic, malignant melanomas have a median survival time of almost one year. The prognosis for mandibular osteosarcoma is better than that for appendicular osteosarcoma (Sarowitz et al., 2017).

6.7.10 Adjunctive therapy

Current knowledge regarding the response rate of oral malignancies to radiation therapy is derived from retrospective studies of either dogs that did not have surgery or those had residual gross disease following incomplete excision. The median survival times for dogs with SCC, fibrosarcoma and melanoma treated with megavoltage radiation were 36, 26 and 7.9 months, respectively (Theon et al., 1997) – indicated for incompletely excised tumours, large tumours and caudally located tumours. Radiation is best given after surgery, as it is most effective against microscopic volumes of tumour rather than against large tumours.

Platinum-based drugs have been used to treat malignant melanoma, and have been associated with a reduction in tumour bulk. They may lead to increased survival times if used postoperatively, but there are few data to substantiate this.

6.7.11 Feline oral tumours

The most common feline oral tumour is SCC. This usually arises in the sublingual or gingival mucosa and is highly invasive, making it difficult to treat surgically (Cotter, 1981). Mandibular tumours often have extensive intramedullary invasion. Maxillary tumours often invade the periocular region. Fibrosarcoma and osteosarcoma are locally invasive but have low metastatic rates.

Feline oral tumours should be staged in a similar manner to their canine equivalent. CT or MRI is advisable owing to the invasive nature of feline oral tumours.

Cats are often unwilling to eat after mandibulectomy, and feeding tubes should be placed at the time of surgery. Long-term inappetance is more of a problem in cats undergoing removal of over 50% of the mandible. Small maxillectomy is well tolerated; however, most maxillary tumours have extensive nasal and periocular involvement and cannot be excised.

In one study of feline mandibulectomy, 48% had incomplete excision and the local recurrence rate was 43%; the 1- and 2-year survival rates were 56 and 49%, respectively (Northrup et al., 2006). Squamous cell carcinoma was associated with shorter survival times than fibrosarcoma and osteosarcoma. There are few data available on adjunctive radiation therapy or chemotherapy.

6.8 External ear

Key points

- Treatment options for aural SCC include partial and total pinnectomy; in more extensive cases, vertical canal ablation may be needed in addition.
- Aural haemangiosarcomas are rapidly growing and invasive and metastasise to the lungs and parenchymal organs.
- Mast cell tumour of the pinna accounts for 59% of all cutaneous mast cell tumours of the head in the cat, with the Siamese breed over-represented.
- CT is the most useful imaging modality to investigate external and middle ear disease.
- The most common cause of para-aural abscess is incomplete debridement of the epithelial lining of the tympanic bulla during total ear canal ablation.
- The prognosis following lateral wall resection is variable. Failure rates of 42.3–55% have been reported.
- Vertical ear canal ablation is indicated for irreversible hyperplastic otitis, severe trauma and neoplasia limited to the vertical canal.
- Total ear canal ablation is indicated for the management of chronic proliferative otitis externa/media, external ear canal neoplasia, severe trauma involving the external ear canal, atresia of the external auditory canal and failed lateral wall resection.

6.8.1 Pinna

Anatomy

- The pinna functions to direct sound towards the middle ear.
- The auricular cartilage, or scapha, is covered by haired skin on its convex surface and by relatively hairless skin on its concave surface. The skin is fixed to the perichondrium on the concave surface but is more mobile on the convex surface. Tiny channels in the perichondrium allow blood flow between the two surfaces.
- The antihelix is a cartilaginous protuberance on the medial surface which separates the scapha from the opening to the external ear canal. The tragus is opposite this and marks the lateral opening to the external ear canal. The antitragus marks the caudal opening to the external ear canal and is separated from the tragus by the intertragic incisure. The helix marks the cranial opening to the external ear canal. This is separated from the tragus by the pretragic incisure.
- The caudal auricular artery forms lateral, intermediate and medial vascular rami at the base of the ear on its convex surface. These pass through scapha foramina to supply the concave surface (Evans, 2012).

6.8.2 Conditions affecting the pinna

Aural haematoma

Aural haematoma is thought to arise from trauma to the pinna. This is often due to head shaking or scratching secondary to otitis externa, though a number of cases have no evidence of this. It is thought that repeated trauma damages the auricular cartilage and causes shearing of the vessels passing from the convex surface to the concave surface. The location of the haematoma has been proposed to be subcutaneous, subperichondrial and intrachondral. These shear forces create a dead space which fills with blood.

Affected animals present with an acutely hot, distended pinna. If this condition is not treated, fibrosis will occur and the cartilage will ossify, leading to distortion of the pinna and chronic irritation. This may obstruct the opening to the external canal in the cat and exacerbate any pre-existing otitis externa.

In acute haematoma, surgery is indicated to remove the blood clot and prevent its recurrence, and to retain a normal appearance to the pinna. This can be done most simply by needle drainage. However, not all animals are amenable to this and repeated treatments are necessary. Placement of a Penrose drain through proximal and distal stab incisions overcomes these problems. Penrose drains are well tolerated and should be left in place for 2 weeks.

Chronic haematoma is treated by incisional drainage. An S-shaped incision is made on the concave surface and the haematoma is drained. Full-thickness monofilament nylon mattress sutures are placed parallel to the vessels on the convex surface. The knots are tied on the convex surface and the sutures are left in place for 2 weeks. Bandaging the ear prevents further damage to the pinna and compresses the skin to the underlying cartilage.

Pinna trauma and lacerations

Lacerations commonly occur following bites and other head trauma. These may involve skin, skin and cartilage or be full thickness. Lacerations involving one skin surface may be sutured or left to heal by second intention. Two- or three-sided skin flaps should be sutured along the margins and through the centre of the flap.

Full-thickness lacerations are best sutured to prevent distortion to the pinna as a result of second-intention healing. Vertical mattress sutures are placed on one side with the deeper bite aligning the cartilage and the superficial bite aligning the skin. Suturing should start from the margin in order to prevent a step forming. The other skin surface can be repaired with simple interrupted sutures: 4-0 or 3-0 monofilament nylon should be used. Only the cutaneous surfaces need to be sutured in cats. Large defects are most easily and effectively treated by partial pinnectomy.

Neoplasia

Actinic keratosis

Actinic keratosis is caused by exposure of poorly pigmented skin to ultraviolet-B radiation. The lesions are erythematous and hyperkeratotic, and become crusting with chronicity. These lesions are considered pre-neoplastic. They progress to dysplasia, carcinoma *in situ* and invasive neoplasia, typically SCC, within 3–4 years. Lesions are usually bilateral. White cats are at 13.4 times greater risk of developing SCC than are coloured cats (Dorn et al., 1971). Treatment is by partial pinnectomy, total pinnectomy or laser surgery.

Squamous cell carcinoma

SCC is raised or erosive and invades the auricular cartilage. Cats often present with bleeding, cracked, non-healing wounds of the margins of the pinna. The diagnosis is confirmed by cytology or an incisional biopsy. Regional lymph nodes should be assessed and thoracic radiographs taken; however, the metastatic rate of pinnal SCC is low. Treatment options include partial and total pinnectomy and, in more extensive cases, vertical canal ablation may be needed in addition.

Haemangioma and haemangiosarcoma

Haemangioma and haemangiosarcoma are caused by exposure to ultraviolet-B radiation and are common in light-coloured cats. They are rare in the dog. Haemangiomas are small, benign dermal or subcutaneous lumps which are raised, alopecic and blue-tinged. Haemangiosarcomas are rapidly growing and invasive and metastasise to the lungs and parenchymal organs. The prognosis for these is poor.

Basal cell tumour

Presents as a well-demarcated, raised nodule. It is often pigmented and can be mistaken for melanoma. Siamese, Himalayan and Persian cats are thought to be predisposed. Narrow excision is usually curative.

Mast cell tumour

MCT of the pinna accounts for 59% of all cutaneous mast cell tumours of the head in the cat, with the Siamese over-represented (Miller et al., 1992). These are usually benign and narrow excision is usually curative. Incomplete excision is not associated with higher recurrence rates. Mast cell tumours of the pinna in dogs may be dermal or subcutaneous and are of variable appearance and location. One study found a 42% incidence of lymph node metastasis, suggestive of a more aggressive biological behaviour compared to MCT in other regions of the body. Excision with 1–2 cm margins and a deep margin of auricular cartilage is recommended.

Histiocytoma

Histiocytomas are usually seen in young dogs, with a male to female ratio of 2.5:1. These can be differentiated from other round cell tumours on cytology. Surgery can often be avoided as these tumours usually spontaneously regress. Some will become ulcerated and cause irritation, in which case surgery can be considered.

Sebaceous adenoma

Sebaceous adenomas are common in older dogs and can be diagnosed on cytology. Narrow excision is usually curative.

Infectious and inflammatory conditions

Infectious conditions affecting the pinna include canine leproid granuloma syndrome, dermatophytosis (*Microsporum* and *Trichophyton* spp.) *Malassezia* dermatitis, feline cowpox, sarcoptic mange and demodecosis. Contact dermatitis, food hypersensitivity, vasculitis and immune-mediated discoid and systemic lupus erythematosus are common inflammatory conditions. These are medical conditions but should be considered as part of the diagnostic work-up for pinna lesions.

6.8.3 External ear canal

Anatomy

- The scutiform cartilage is a small, boot-shaped cartilage medial to the ear and is considered part of the external ear canal. The vertical ear canal begins at the external acoustic opening. It travels ventrally and rostrally for 2–3 cm before turning medially into the horizontal canal. It tends to taper ventrally in the cat.
- The annular cartilage is a tube which connects the base of the auricular cartilage to the osseus external auditory meatus. It is attached to the auricular cartilage

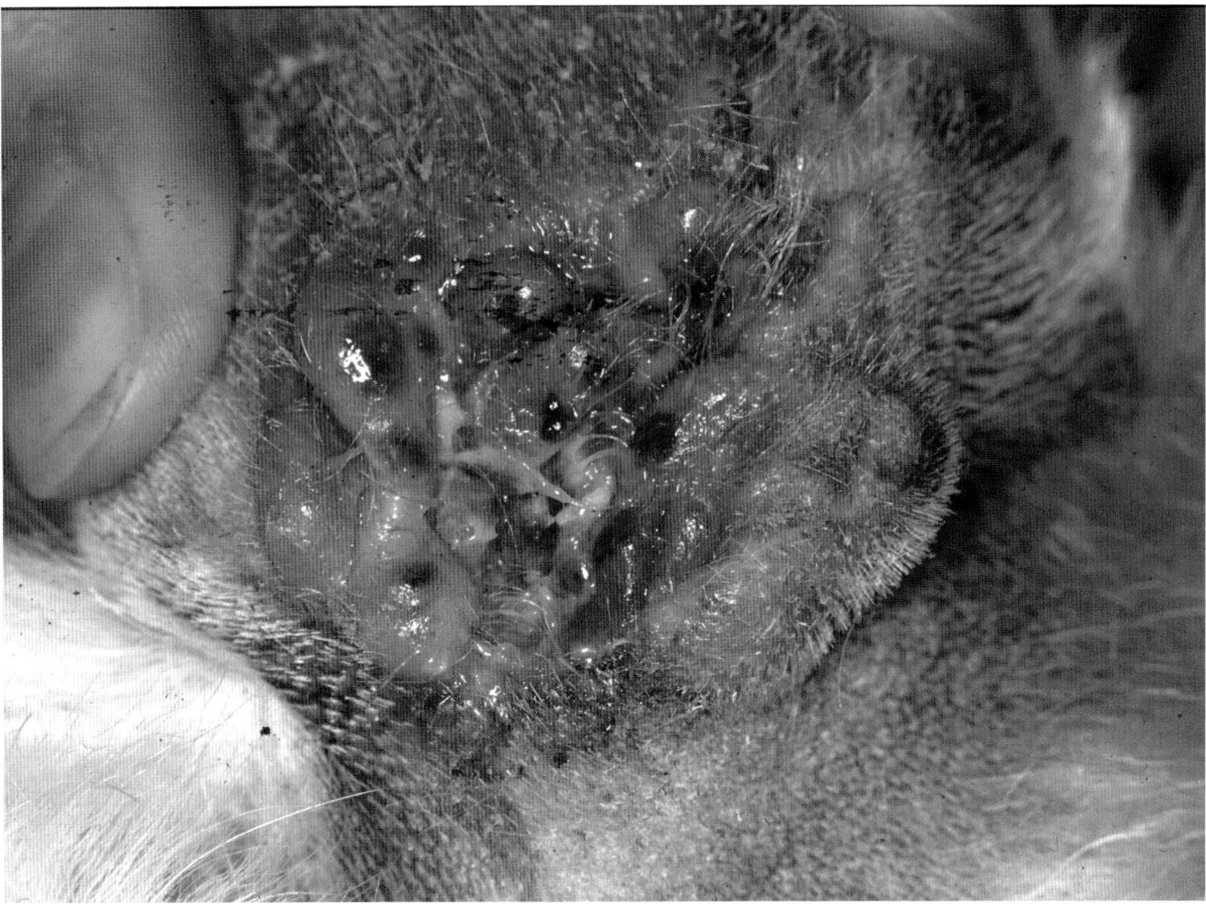

Fig. 6.35 Irreversible otitis externa.

and temporal bone by fibrous connective tissue, and is about 2 cm long.

- The osseous auditory meatus is a 5–10 mm extension of the temporal bone. It has a more pronounced flare in the cat.
- The ear canal is lined by stratified squamous epithelium which contains hair follicles and adnexal structures. It also contains superficial sebaceous glands and deeper tubular ceruminous glands (modified apocrine). These are more numerous in the vertical canal than in the horizontal canal. Cerumen is a product of these glands, combined with desquamated epithelium.
- The facial nerve exits the cranial vault through the internal acoustic meatus with the vestibulocochlear nerve. It runs through the facial canal of the petrous temporal bone, through the middle ear and exits via the stylomastoid foramen caudodorsally to the external osseous ear canal. It crosses the ventral aspect of the horizontal canal and sends off motor branches to the caudal auricular muscles. It then runs over the masseter and gives off cervical, buccal and auriculopalpebral branches. Auricular branches of the vagus nerve supply sensory innervation to the external ear canal.
- The great auricular artery provides the blood supply to the external ear canal. This arises medial to the dorsal apex of the parotid salivary gland. The external carotid artery and maxillary vein are ventral to the bulla. The retro-articular vein is immediately rostral to the osseous ear canal and can be damaged during total ear canal ablation. The internal carotid artery is medial to the bulla (Evans, 2012).

6.8.4 Conditions affecting the external ear canal

Otitis externa/media

Otitis externa is very common in the dog (Fig. 6.35). Clinical signs include head shaking, ear scratching and aural discharge. Chronic cases are characterised by hyperkeratinisation, hyperplasia of the sebaceous and ceruminal glands and infiltration by inflammatory cells. This can lead to stenosis, fibrosis, mineralisation and occlusion of the external ear canal. Infection can spread through an intact or ruptured tympanic membrane to cause otitis media and otitis interna.

The causes of otitis have historically been classified into primary, predisposing and perpetuating factors:

- Primary factors
  - Parasites: *Otodectes cynotis* accounts for 50% of otitis externa cases in the cat and 5–10% in the dog.
  - Foreign bodies: these include grass awns, dead insects and dried secretions.
  - Hypersensitivity: this includes atopic dermatitis and food allergies. In 5% of cases of atopy and 25% of cases of food allergy, the animal presents solely with signs of otitis externa (Griffin and DeBoer, 2001).
  - Endocrine disease: this includes hypothyroidism, hyperadrenocorticism and sex hormone imbalances. They result in altered keratinisation, increased cerumen gland production and consequently a seborrhoeic otitis externa.
  - Autoimmune disease: pemphigoid diseases, discoid lupus erythematosus and vasculitis can affect the pinna and external ear canal but are rare.
- Predisposing factors
  - Abnormal ear conformation. Common examples are pendulous ears in spaniels and narrow ears in the Shar-Pei.
  - Excessive hair in the external canal in the poodle.
  - Excessive cerumen production in the cocker spaniel.
  - Chronic ear moisture.
  - Inappropriate antibiotic use.
  - Obstruction of drainage owing to tumour.
- Perpetuating factors
  - Secondary bacterial infection.
  - Secondary yeast infection.
  - Otitis media.

Patients with otitis should be examined for generalised skin disease. Those with middle ear disease may show signs of facial nerve paralysis, vestibular disease and a head tilt. Osteomyelitis of the tympanic bulla may extend to the temporomandibular joint and cause pain on opening of the mouth. Otoscopic examination should be performed in all cases of recurrent or chronic otitis. This is typically painful and general anaesthesia may be required. Normal ear canals are light pink and have minimal exudate. The tympanic membrane is translucent and the ossicles can be seen. The tympanic membrane is intact in 71% of cases of otitis media, so myringotomy should be performed in suspected cases of otitis media. Cytology can be performed to identify and characterise the presence of secondary bacterial and yeast infections.

Bacteriology is useful to determine whether secondary bacterial overgrowth is likely to be susceptible to antibiotic treatment. *Staphylococcus intermedius* is the most commonly isolated pathogen. Most animals are affected with multiple bacteria. A study found a single microorganism in 18% of samples, two in 62% of samples and three or more in 20% of samples. There was a significant difference between the bacteria isolated from left and right ears in 68% of cases (Oliveira et al., 2008).

CT is the most useful imaging modality for investigation of external and middle ear disease. It provides excellent images of the tympanic bullae and gives fewer false negative results for otitis media than radiography (Fig. 6.36). It can help with evaluating the external ear canal for mineralisation, neoplasia and para-aural abscessation. Contrast CT can be performed if necessary. Abscesses have a central hypo-attenuating region with ring enhancement; tumours don't have ring enhancement and only large tumours have a hypo-attenuating central zone of necrosis.

Medical treatment of chronic otitis includes topical and systemic antibiotics, ear cleaners, corticosteroids and management of any underlying systemic disorders. Lateral wall resection is a useful adjunctive treatment for chronic otitis externa. Total ear canal ablation is reserved for the management of end-stage otitis externa / media.

Middle ear polyps

These are easily identified as red, spherical, proliferative lesions. They can be successfully treated by ventral bulla osteotomy or total ear canal ablation and lateral osteotomy (Fig. 6.37).

Neoplasia

Most aural tumours are epithelial in origin and are malignant (London et al., 1996). Aural tumours occur

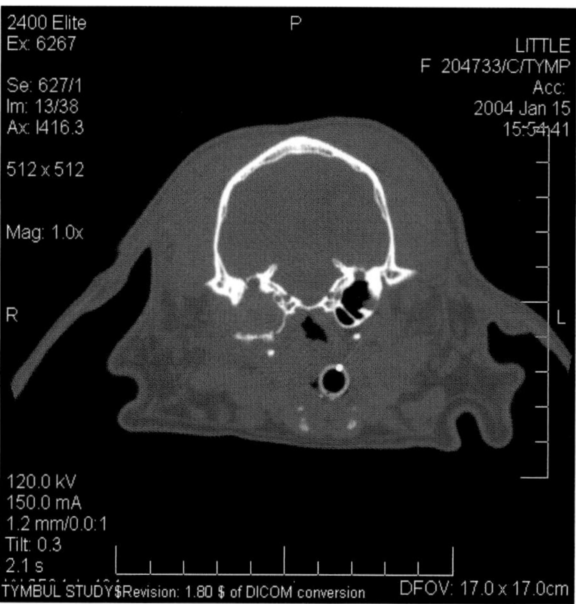

Fig. 6.36 CT image showing destruction of tympanic bulla secondary to otitis media.

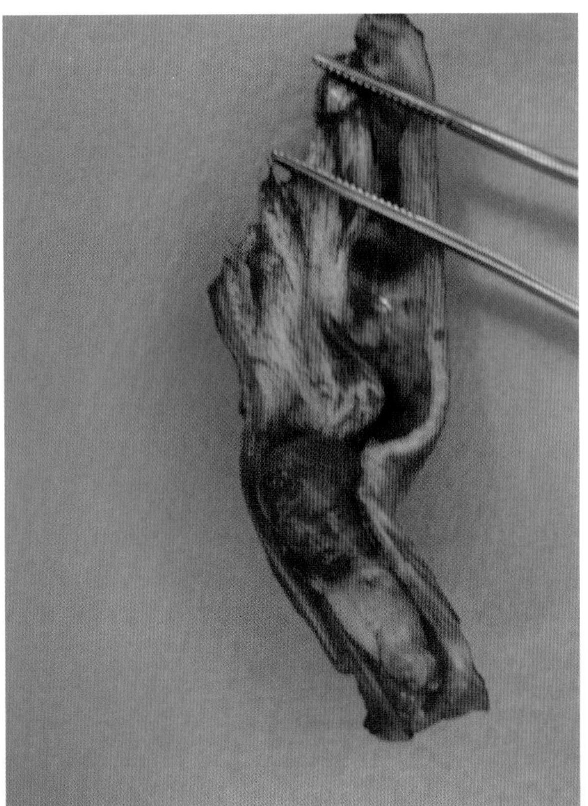

Fig. 6.37 Polyp located in external ear canal.

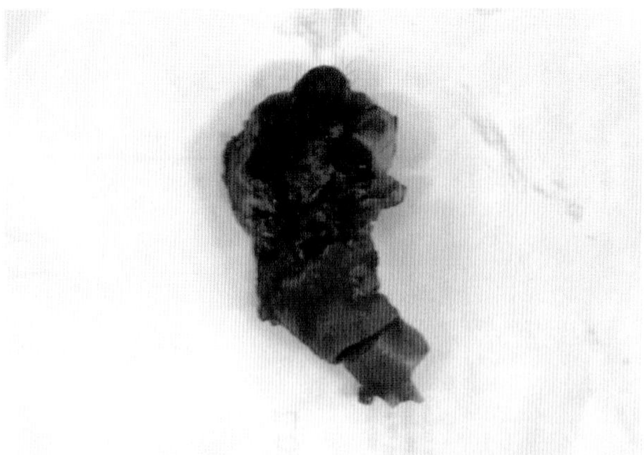

Fig. 6.38 Ceruminous gland tumour removed via total ear canal ablation.

in older cats and dogs, and cocker spaniels are over-represented. Clinical signs include the presence of a mass at the external auditory meatus, aural discharge, odour, pruritus and pain. Neurological signs are present in 10% of dogs and 25% of cats with malignant tumours. Benign tumours are raised, pedunculated and rarely ulcerated. Malignant tumours are ulcerated, haemorrhagic and have a broad base of attachment. Most benign tumours can be managed by conservative surgical resection.

Otoscopic examination under general anaesthesia and skull CT are an essential part of the diagnostic work-up. Around 25% of malignant tumours have bulla involvement.

Ceruminous gland adenocarcinoma is the most common malignant tumour in dogs (Fig. 6.38). In cats, this tumour and SCC appear to be equally common. These tumours are locally invasive, with invasion of the auricular cartilage in 50% of dogs and 60% of cats (London et al., 1996). Invasion into the peri-aural tissues and deeper auditory structures is less common, and local control of disease can usually be obtained by total ear canal ablation.

The median survival time in dogs after total ear canal ablation is 2 years. Approximately 10% of dogs have evidence of metastasis at the time of diagnosis. Bulla involvement and conservative surgery are negative prognostic indicators. The median survival time in cats is 1 year, with 5–15% showing evidence of metastasis. The presence of neurological signs, SCC or anaplastic carcinoma, lymphatic or vascular invasion and conservative surgery are negative prognostic indicators.

Trauma and avulsion

Traumatic rupture between the auricular and auditory canals can lead to obstruction of the proximal vertical canal by a pseudo-tympanic membrane. Accumulation of ceruminous and infectious debris in the horizontal canal can lead to pain, head tilt, facial swelling and aural discharge (Connery et al., 2001). The remnant of the horizontal canal can be identified, debrided and sutured to the skin.

Traumatic separation of the junction between auricular and annular cartilages has been described. This can be managed by either total ear canal ablation (TECA) or primary repair through a caudal approach to the ear (Tivers and Brockman, 2009).

Congenital external auditory canal atresia

This has been associated with haired skin covering the external auditory meatus, blind termination of the vertical canal midway along its length, or atresia between the auricular and annular cartilages. Accumulation of ceruminous material can lead to facial pain and discomfort (Caine et al., 2008; House, 2001). The horizontal canal can be sutured to the overlying skin if atresia is limited to the vertical canal; otherwise total ear canal ablation is required.

Para-aural abscess

This can occur due to extension of infection from the external ear, bites, trauma or neoplasia (Fig. 6.39). However, the most common cause is incomplete debridement of the epithelial lining of the tympanic bulla during TECA (Mason et al., 1988). Surgical exploration, debridement and drainage are indicated.

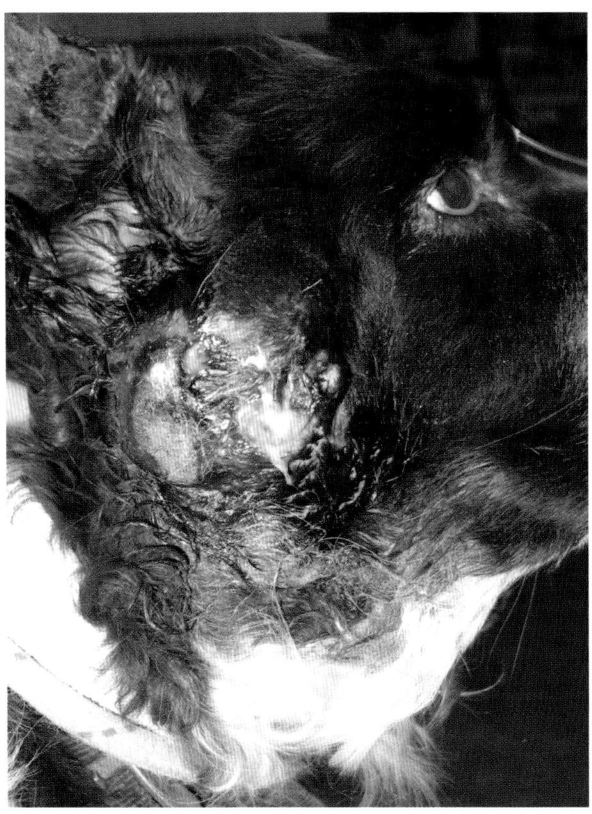

Fig. 6.39 Para-aural abscess secondary to aural carcinoma.

6.8.5 Surgery of the external ear

Handy hints

Lateral wall resection is indicated as an adjunct in the management of recurrent or chronic otitis externa. It increases the ventilation and drainage of the horizontal canal, and facilitates the application of topical treatments. It is essential to make clients aware that this is not a curative procedure, and that long-term management of the otitis and any underlying skin disease will still be required. This procedure is best performed early in the disease process.

Step by step: lateral wall resection

- The patient is positioned in lateral recumbency. A sandbag can be placed under the neck to elevate the head slightly. The surgical clip should be circumferential from the lateral canthus to the mid-cervical region and should include the pinna.
- Artery forceps can be placed in the external auditory meatus to delineate the vertical canal. Paired skin incisions are made cranial and caudal to the vertical canal, starting from either side of the tragus and extending ventral to the junction between the vertical and horizontal canals. The incisions are joined ventrally, and the resulting thin skin flap is elevated from the vertical canal all the way to its attachment on the tragus.
- The vertical canal is sharply dissected from the surrounding loose peri-auricular tissues. Bipolar cautery is useful to control haemorrhage from the numerous small vessels in this area. The parotid salivary gland overlies the ventral aspect of the vertical canal. This can be retracted or incised without adverse effects. Dissection should continue until the rostral and caudal edges of the vertical canal and the junction between the auricular and annular cartilages are visible.
- The rostral and caudal edges of the vertical canal are transected to release the lateral wall of the vertical canal. Rotating the scissors so that the handles are parallel with the skin creates a cartilage incision parallel to the skin which helps with accurate apposition of the ear canal epithelium and skin. The incisions are continued to the junction of the auricular and annular cartilages. This allows the lateral wall to be reflected ventrally without tension.
- The proximal end of the cartilage flap and attached skin flap are removed to leave a drainage board. This is reflected ventrally and the proximal end is sutured to the distal skin incision with simple interrupted sutures of 4-0 or 3-0 monofilament nylon. The sutures at the junction between the auricular and annular cartilage are then placed. The remaining sutures are then placed between the skin and epithelium.

Opioids should be continued for the first 24 hours, after which NSAIDs are adequate. An Elizabethan collar is required to prevent self-trauma to the surgical wounds. Some patients tolerate this surgery poorly, and additional analgesics and sedatives may be required. A second general anaesthetic is necessary 10–14 days after surgery to allow suture removal and cleaning of the surgical wounds.

Wound dehiscence is a common complication and is usually the result of poor patient selection, poor surgical technique or self-trauma. It is essential to achieve good apposition between the skin and ear canal epithelium. A common mistake is to suture the skin to the cartilage rather than to the epithelium, which results in excessive granulation. Failure to adequately dissect out the vertical canal can lead to incorrectly positioned incisions in the lateral wall, excessive tension at the surgical site and distortion of the stoma.

The prognosis following lateral wall resection is variable. Failure rates of 42.3–55% have been reported. One study found a poor outcome in 86.5% of cocker spaniels. Case selection is important. Shar-Peis, animals with excessive hair in the external canal and patients with fewer chronic changes are likely to have better outcomes (Sylvestre, 1998). Poor surgical technique is another cause of poor outcome. Finally, clients should have realistic expectations prior to surgery and should be aware that long-term management of the otitis will still be necessary following surgery.

Step by step: vertical ear canal ablation

This procedure is indicated for irreversible hyperplastic otitis, severe trauma and neoplasia limited to the vertical canal. It is unusual for only the vertical canal to be affected, so this procedure is rarely performed (Lanz and Wood, 2004).

- The patient is positioned and the surgical site prepared as for lateral wall resection.
- A skin incision is made over the vertical canal extending from the tragus to just ventral to the junction between the auricular and annular cartilages. The incision is extended circumferentially around the external auditory meatus.
- The vertical canal is sharply dissected from the surrounding peri-auricular soft tissues. Bipolar cautery is useful to control haemorrhage. Dissection is continued to the level of the horizontal canal.
- The vertical canal is amputated and the medial and lateral walls of the horizontal canal are spatulated and sutured to the skin to act as drainage boards. The dorsal skin wound is closed in a T-shape. Simple interrupted sutures of 4-0 or 3-0 monofilament nylon are used.

Step by step: TECA

This procedure is indicated for the management of chronic proliferative otitis externa/media, external ear canal neoplasia, severe trauma involving the external ear canal, atresia of the external auditory canal and failed lateral wall resection; 59–85% of dogs undergoing total ear canal ablation had chronic proliferative otitis, with cocker spaniels being the most common breed undergoing this procedure (43–60%; Angus et al., 2002). One study in the cat found that 50% had chronic inflammatory disease and 41% had neoplastic disease (Bacon et al., 2003).

- The patient is positioned and the surgical site prepared as for lateral wall resection.
- A T-shaped incision is made over the vertical canal from the tragus to just ventral to the junction between the auricular and annular cartilages. The dorsal skin incision is continued around the opening of the external ear canal. The medial incision should not extend too far up the pinna in order to prevent ischaemic necrosis.
- The ear canal is sharply dissected from the surrounding soft tissues. It is best to stay close to the perichondrium to avoid damage to the surrounding neurovascular structures. It is advisable to work circumferentially and to use Gelpi retractors to improve exposure (Fig. 6.40).
- The facial nerve exits the stylomastoid foramen and runs caudoventrally to the terminal horizontal canal (Fig. 6.41). It is better to deliberately avoid this nerve rather than to dissect it out and retract it.
- The horizontal canal is transected as close as possible to the osseous external auditory meatus. The remaining hyperplastic epithelium is then removed from the meatus with a combination of scissors and rongeurs. The external osseous meatus can be removed with rongeurs to facilitate this (Fig. 6.42). Care must be taken to avoid damage to the retro-articular vein rostrally.

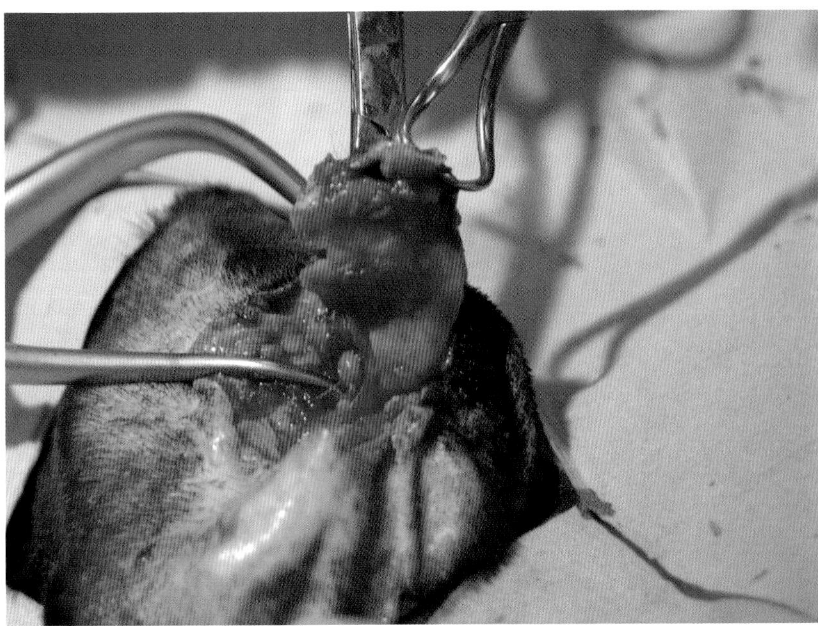

Fig. 6.40 Dissection of external ear canal during TECA.

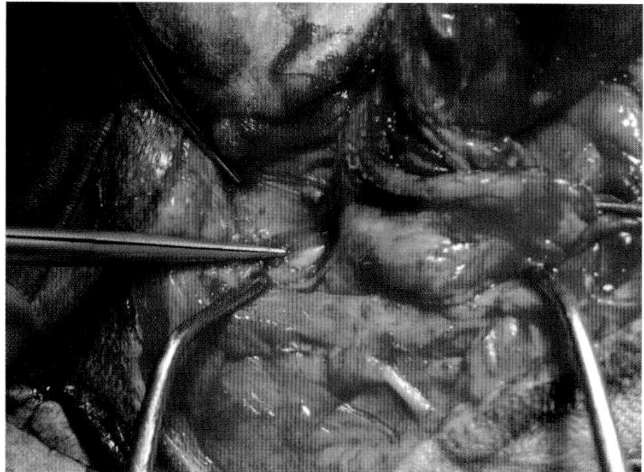

Fig. 6.41 Identification of facial nerve during TECA.

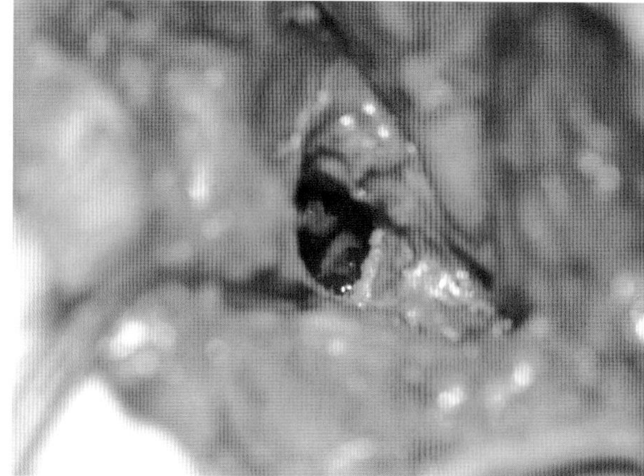

Fig. 6.42 View of tympanic cavity following lateral bulla osteotomy (LBO).

- Residual epithelium must then be removed from the mesotympanum. This is done with a combination of saline irrigation and curettage. If the ossicles are still present in the epitympanum, they can be preserved. Aggressive dorsal curettage is avoided. The hypotympanum can be visualised through its communication with the mesotympanum. This is also carefully debrided. Lateral bulla osteotomy can be performed to facilitate debridement of the tympanic bulla, but it is rarely necessary to do so.
- The subcutaneous tissues and skin are closed routinely. A Penrose drain can be placed but it is not necessary to do so. Excision of small triangles of skin on the rostral and caudal pinna can help to retain ear carriage in erect-eared dogs. In the cat, the caudal part of the pinna can be folded forwards and sutured to the rostral part. The use of a single pedicle advancement flap has also been described.

Opioids are continued for 24 hours postoperatively, after which NSAIDs are usually adequate. Postoperative antibiotics can be given, but they have not been shown to decrease the incidence of post-surgical wound infections. Bandages can be used to improve patient comfort and to reduce post-surgical swelling and dead space.

Facial nerve damage is a commonly reported complication following total ear canal ablation (Fig. 6.43). This causes drooping of the ipsilateral lip and ear and loss of the ipsilateral blink reflex. This has been reported in 13–40% of dogs after surgery, and can be permanent in 4–13% (Coleman and Smeak, 2016). The incidence is higher in the cat, with rates of 12–56% reported and up to 28% being permanent (Bacon et al., 2003).

Horner's syndrome can result from damage to the postganglionic sympathetic fibres running through the middle ear. This causes enophthalmos, third eyelid protrusion, miosis and ptosis. Horner's syndrome usually occurs following excessive debridement of the tympanic bulla. The incidence is higher in the cat owing to the fragility of the sympathetic plexus, with rates of 27–42% reported (Fig. 6.44). It is permanent in 14–27% of cases (Bacon et al., 2003).

Intra-operative haemorrhage from the retro-articular vein occurs in 3% of cases (White and Pomeroy, 1990). This can be prevented by avoiding debridement rostral to the bulla. The vein tends to retract into the retro-articular foramen when damaged, which prevents ligation. The foramen can be packed with bone wax in a dorsomedial direction.

Fistulae can occur following total ear canal ablation as a result of inadequate removal of hyperplastic epithelium and accumulated debris; the incidence is between 6 and 10%. Antibiotic treatment is ineffective, and

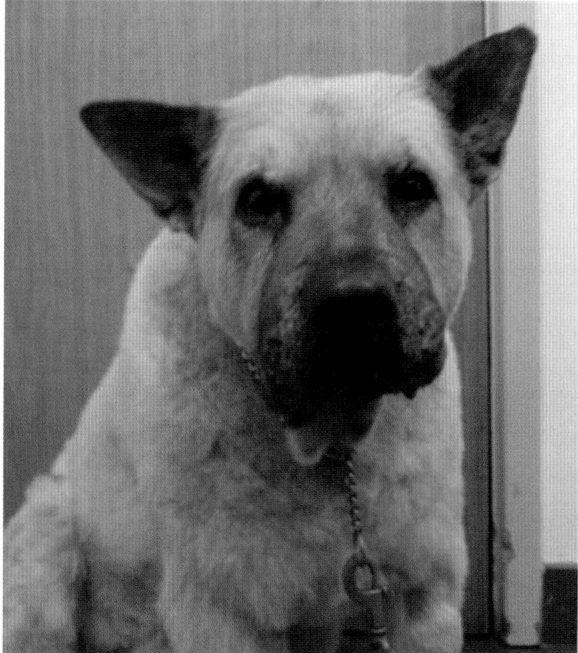

Fig. 6.43 Facial nerve paralysis following a TECA–LBO procedure.

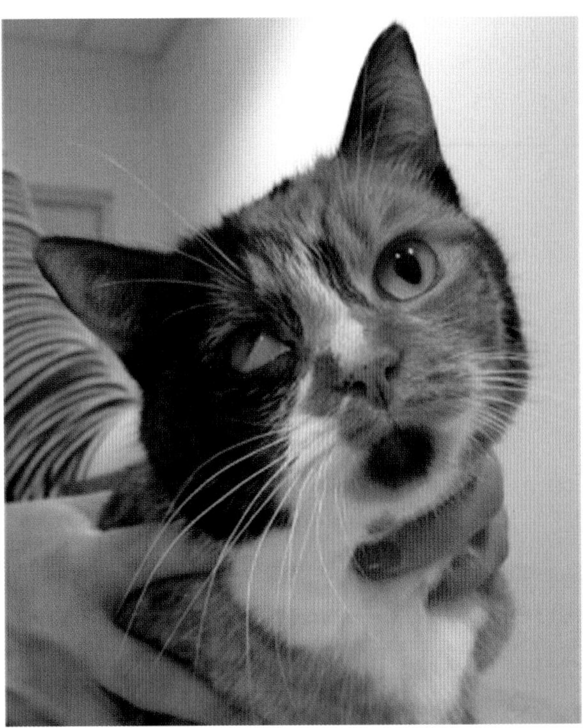

Fig. 6.44 Horner's syndrome following TECA–LBO.

exploratory surgery of the bulla is required to remove residual epithelium. This can be done via a lateral or ventral approach (Smeak, 2016).

Deafness is a common concern after this surgery. Most patients have reduced or absent hearing prior to surgery owing to the severity of their end-stage otitis. There is probably sound conduction through bone, and most owners report that their pets retain some hearing following surgery.

The prognosis following total ear canal ablation is excellent, and significant improvement is seen in up to 92% of patients.

6.9 Middle ear

Key points

- The most common cause of otitis media in the dog is spread of infection from the external ear across the tympanic membrane.
- Removal of polyps by traction followed by oral prednisolone resulted in recurrence of clinical signs in 10% of cats with nasopharyngeal polyps and 50% of cats with external ear polyps.
- The prognosis for cholesteatoma is guarded, and advanced lesions can recur.
- Lateral bulla osteotomy allows the removal of the chronically diseased tissue of the external meatus and exposure of the tympanic bulla.
- Ventral bulla osteotomy is most commonly performed for the removal of feline inflammatory polyps.

6.9.1 Canine anatomy

The tympanic cavity is located in the tympanic bulla of the temporal bone caudomedial to the zygomatic arch and temporomandibular joint. It is lined with respiratory epithelium and is continuous with the nasopharynx. It is divided into three chambers:

1. The *epitympanum* or epitympanic recess is the smallest chamber and is located dorsally. It contains the incus and part of the malleus. It is lined by cuboidal or squamous epithelium with few cilia.
2. The *mesotympanum* or true tympanic chamber has four sides and is lined with cuboidal or columnar epithelium with variable numbers of cilia. The tympanic membrane is lateral and the smaller cochlear membrane is posterior. The bone promontory that accommodates the cochlear structure is medial.
3. The *hypotympanum* is the largest component of the tympanic cavity and communicates with the mesotympanum through an anterolateral facing opening on its dorsal aspect. It is lined with cuboidal or squamous cells.

Two membranes are present in the mesotympanum: the tympanic membrane separates the external acoustic meatus from the mesotympanum.

- The pars flaccida occupies the dorsal portion of the membrane.
- The pars tensa comprises the majority of the membrane.

The malleus is embedded in its dorsal surface. It is made up of three layers, being derived from the pharyngeal pouch and ectoderm of the outer ear. A constant centrifugal movement of cells clears debris from the surface of the membrane and allows its repair. The cochlear (or round) membrane separates the mesotympanum from the inner ear. The opening to the auditory tube (eustachian tube or pharyngotympanic tube) is found in the rostral mesotympanum. It is supported by cartilage in the nasopharyngeal region, by the petrous temporal bone and laterally by the tensor veli palatini muscle.

The ossicles of the middle ear concentrate sound waves striking the tympanic membrane and focus them on the smaller vestibular (or oval) window. They are connected by a series of ligaments and muscles.

- The malleus is embedded in the tympanic membrane; its head articulates with the incus.
- The incus lies entirely within the epitympanum and articulates with the stapes.
- The stapes is attached to a cartilaginous ring around the vestibular window. This separates the tympanic cavity from the perilymphatic space of the inner ear.

A number of nerves supply or pass through the tympanic cavity.

- The facial nerve enters the internal auditory meatus with the vestibulocochlear nerve. It enters the facial canal and exits the bulla at the stylomastoid foramen. It is exposed in the dorsal tympanic cavity near the vestibular window. In the facial canal, it gives branches into the stapedius nerve and the chorda tympani (tympanic nerve). The chorda tympani mixes with preganglionic parasympathetic vagal branches and exits the petrotympanic fissure to join the lingual nerve.
- The tympanic plexus is formed from the tympanic branches of the glossopharyngeal nerve and the caroticotympanic nerve. It spreads across the bone promontory and enters the lesser petrosal nerve. It gives rise to preganglionic parasympathetic fibres to the parotid and zygomatic salivary glands, postganglionic fibres to the parotid gland and sensory fibres to the middle ear cavity.
- Postganglionic sympathetic fibres arise from the cranial cervical ganglion deep to the bulla. These supply the smooth muscle of the dilator pupillae and the nictitating membrane. They run with the internal carotid artery and join the tympanic branch of the trochlear nerve.

The blood supply to the middle ear is the tympanic artery, which is derived from the maxillary artery, along with meningeal and pharyngeal arteries (Evans, 2012).

6.9.2 Feline anatomy

The feline tympanic cavity is divided into a larger ventral cavity which corresponds to the hypotympanum, and a smaller rostrolateral component which corresponds to the epitympanum and mesotympanum.

The two compartments are separated by a bony septum. They communicate on their medial aspect through a small, slit-like opening that widens into a distinct foramen caudally. This gives the double-shell profile on anteroposterior radiographs.

The tympanic plexus distributes widely across the bone promontory. It is more exposed, or more sensitive, to iatrogenic trauma (Evans, 2012).

6.9.3 Physiology

The primary function of the middle ear is the conduction of sound from the external auditory meatus, across the air-filled tympanic cavity, to the fluid-filled inner ear and receptor cells of the cochlea. The ossicles focus sound striking the tympanic membrane to the vestibular window. This compensates for the change of impedance caused by the fluid–air interface.

Cellular debris and mucous secretions are expelled to the pharynx by mucociliary clearance and muscular contractions of the auditory tube. The auditory tube is periodically opened during swallowing by the tensor veli palatini muscles to allow equilibration of atmospheric pressure with that of the tympanic cavity.

6.9.4 Septic otitis media

The most common cause of otitis media in the dog is spread of infection from the external ear across the tympanic membrane. The mechanism by which this occurs is unknown, but may be as a result of rupture or trans-membrane migration. Another proposed mechanism is by bacterial invasion of the integument that lines the osseous external auditory prominence. Spread of infection from the nasopharynx via the auditory tube and haematogenous spread are less commonly seen in dogs. The most common organisms isolated in canine middle ear infections are *Staphylococcus intermedius*, *Pseudomonas* and *Malassezia* (Cole et al., 1998). Middle ear infections in the cat usually arise as a result of ascending infection via the auditory tube associated with episodes of viral nasopharyngeal infection. These infections are implicated in the development of middle ear polyps.

Clinical signs include otorrhoea, otalgia and head shaking. A purulent discharge may be present at the external meatus. The head may be carried lower on the affected side. Extension of inflammation to the temporomandibular joint causes pain on opening the mouth. These signs are similar to those seen with otitis externa. As most cases of otitis media occur following chronic otitis externa, otitis media can be overlooked. Facial nerve palsy may be present in 10% of cases. Damage to the parasympathetic fibres of the chorda tympani may lead to decreased tear production. Horner's syndrome is less commonly seen. Otitis media may spread to the inner ear. Signs of otitis interna include loss of hearing and vestibular signs.

Otoscopic examination should be performed in all cases. This usually requires general anaesthesia. The normal tympanic membrane is shiny, pink and translucent. The malleus and vascular structures should be visible, as should the concavity of the membrane. Bulging, loss of translucency, change in colour or perforation is suggestive of middle ear disease. If the tympanic membrane is intact but abnormal, myringotomy can be performed. Samples can be collected for cytology, histopathology and bacteriology. CT gives excellent images of the tympanic bulla and adjacent bony structures (Belmudes et al., 2018). However, it may lack sensitivity in early disease. MRI is the most sensitive modality for detecting middle and inner ear disease. It can identify early disease in the middle ear and fluid in the inner ear.

Medical management of otitis media is only likely to be effective if the underlying disease in the external ear canal can be controlled. In many cases this is not possible and surgical management is preferred. The middle ear should be lavaged with warm saline to remove debris. Topical and systemic antibiotics are administered for 4–6 weeks, preferably based on bacteriology results. Medical management is unlikely to be successful in cases with established infection in the tympanic bone or with stenotic changes in the external ear. Total ear canal ablation with or without lateral bulla osteotomy will be more successful in these cases.

6.9.5 Middle ear polyps

Inflammatory polyps originate from the epithelium of the tympanic cavity or auditory tube. They may remain in the middle ear, extend into the nasopharynx or disrupt the tympanic membrane and extend into the external ear canal. This is often preceded by upper respiratory viral infection in cats. Obstruction of drainage of the auditory tube may also be a factor (Tos et al., 1984).

Clinical signs are related to the location of the polyp and include vestibular signs, Horner's syndrome, difficulty swallowing, nasal discharge, respiratory stertor and purulent aural discharge.

Diagnosis is made by otoscopic examination and examination of the nasopharynx by retraction of the soft palate under general anaesthesia. CT is useful to determine the number and location of inflammatory polyps.

Removal of polyps by traction followed by oral prednisolone resulted in recurrence of clinical signs in 10% of cats with nasopharyngeal polyps and 50% of cats with external ear polyps (Anderson et al., 2000). Patients with neurological signs and those with external ear polyps are best managed surgically. Ventral bulla osteotomy gives good visualisation of the tympanic cavity and allows complete removal of the polyp.

6.9.6 Cholesteatoma

This is characterised by destructive and expanding keratinising squamous epithelium. Congenital forms have not been reported in the dog, and most seem to arise secondary to otitis media. They have been likened to a human condition called cholesteatoma because of their cystic structure and the presence of cholesterol clefts. Treatment is by total ear canal ablation and lateral bulla osteotomy or by ventral bulla osteotomy. The prognosis is guarded and advanced lesions can recur. The presence of neurological signs significantly correlated with recurrence after surgery (Hardie et al., 2008).

6.9.7 Disorders of middle ear drainage

Secretory otitis media results in the accumulation of mucinous material in the tympanic cavity. This condition is increasingly recognised, particularly in the Cavalier King Charles spaniel. The cause may be a congenital dysfunction of drainage via the auditory tube. Dogs with congenital hypoplasia or malformations of the soft palate are reported to be at risk of middle ear disease and impaired hearing (Stern-Bertholtz et al., 2003).

Primary ciliary dyskinesia is a rare congenital condition. This leads to failure of middle ear drainage and a sterile otitis media (Edwards et al., 1992).

Myringotomy provides only a temporary resolution of the clinical signs. Placement of tympanostomy tubes or grommets in the pars tensa is reported to produce long-term resolution. Insertion is complex and requires microscopy. Total ear canal ablation is an alternative to this.

6.9.8 Surgery of the middle ear

Lateral bulla osteotomy

Lateral bulla osteotomy is most commonly performed along with total ear canal ablation. This allows the removal of the chronically diseased tissue of the external meatus and exposure of the tympanic bulla. It is possible in most cases to adequately lavage and debride the tympanic cavity without performing a bulla osteotomy. Lateral bulla osteotomy is occasionally performed in the cat for the management of tumours of the external ear. Access to the bulla is easier, but the incidence of neurological complications is higher.

Case 6.2

A 5-year-old mixed-breed dog was involved in a dog fight, resulting in significant trauma to the soft tissues and fractures of the maxilla and premaxilla. The initial soft tissue repair had failed due to necrosis of the involved palatal tissues. No attempt had been made to stabilise the maxillary fractures (Fig 6.49).

- In your opinion, what is the likely reason(s) for the wound dehiscence?
  - vascular compromise
  - instability and movement across the suture lines due to the underlying maxillary fractures
  - infection.

- What techniques would be suitable for stabilising the maxillary/palatal fractures?
  - inter-fragmentary wires
  - inter-fragmentary locking titanium plates
  - inter-fragmentary wires and wire/composite resin splint.

Inter-fragmentary wires on their own would be unlikely to provide adequate stability. The use of locking titanium plates has been described in the veterinary literature, but it was decided to use a combination of inter-fragmentary wires and a wire/resin composite splint as this would result in less soft tissue trauma during placement (Figs. 6.50, 6.51).

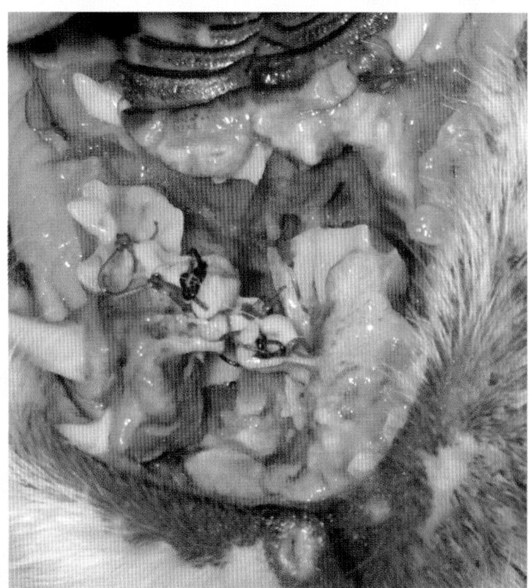

Fig 6.49 Preoperative intra-oral image showing significant breakdown of the soft tissues of the palate with multiple fractures of the palatal bones visible. (Image courtesy of David Crossley.)

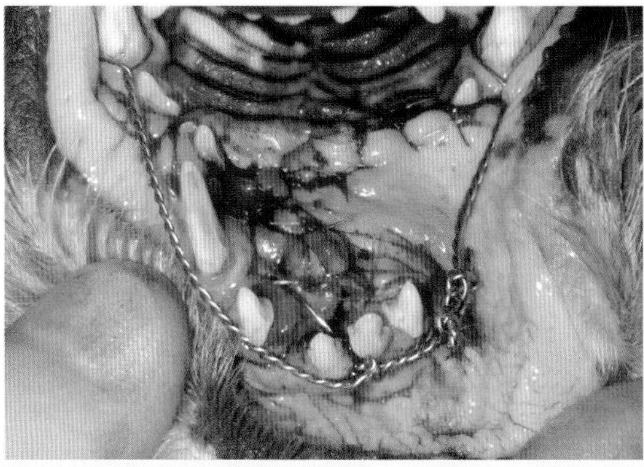

Fig 6.50 Postoperative intra-oral image showing inter-fragmentary wires, wire splint and labial mucosal flap sutured in place prior to resin application. (Image courtesy of David Crossley.)

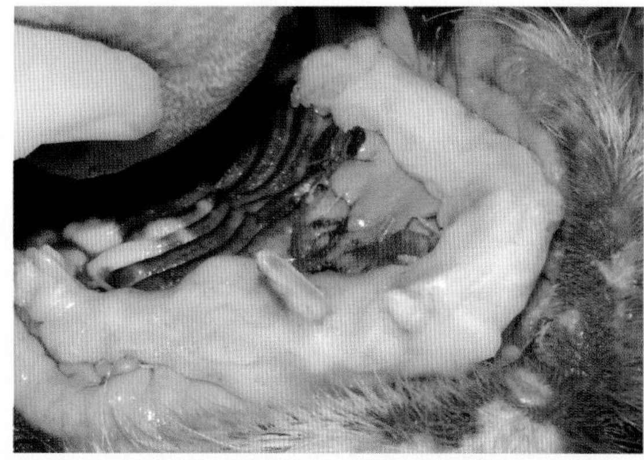

Fig 6.51 Postoperative intra-oral image showing the wire/resin composite splint. (Image courtesy of David Crossley.)

- What further procedures should be considered at the time of surgery to help manage this case during the postoperative period?

Placement of an oesophageal feeding tube, as some animals, particularly cats, can be anorexic due to pain and loss of the sense of smell.

- What potential postoperative complications can occur with this injury and repair?
  - wound dehiscence
  - bone sequestrum
  - implant failure
  - stomatitis
  - vascular damage to the teeth, leading to discoloration in the future.

Surgery of the upper airway

7

Kate Forster

Chapter summary

7.1 Nasal surgery

Key points

- The key to successful nasal surgery is the preoperative planning. CT or MRI is required to evaluate the extent of the tumour and therefore guide the clinician to appropriate margins.
- Significant haemorrhage may well be seen with nasal surgery. Monitoring of pre-, peri- and postoperative PCV may be required and blood products administered accordingly.
- The challenges of nasal surgery should not be underestimated, and referral to an experienced specialist surgeon may be appropriate in certain cases.

7.1.1 Investigation of nasal disease

History

Typical presentation for nasal or nasopharyngeal disease includes nasal discharge, sneezing, reverse sneezing, stertorous respiration and epistaxis. In the cat, stertorous respiration and phonation changes are more commonly associated with nasopharyngeal disease, but cats with nasal disease alone exhibit sneezing and nasal discharge. The nasal discharge will vary in consistency, colour and localisation (unilateral/bilateral). Studies have investigated the correlation between types of nasal discharge (mucopurulent/haemorrhagic) and aetiology. The characteristics of nasal discharge and associated clinical signs are not considered pathognomonic, and a combination of both clinical history and diagnostic imaging is therefore required to achieve an accurate diagnosis (Plickert et al., 2014; Tasker et al., 1999).

Physical findings

A complete physical examination should be performed in all animals before focusing on specific attention to the skull, oral cavity and upper respiratory tract. Although there are few systemic manifestations of nasal disease, attention should be made to the general body condition and mental status of the animal.

Palpation and visual evaluation of the skull should be performed to identify the presence of any facial swelling, pain or distortion. Facial distortion is more commonly associated with neoplasia, and soft fluctuant masses may be palpable if a tumour has eroded through the nasal or frontal bones. Retrobulbar extension of a nasal tumour may cause exophthalmos. The nostrils should also be assessed for symmetry, obstruction and distortion and neoplastic erosion. Airflow through both nostrils can be assessed by placing a few strands of cotton wool in front of each nostril and assessing symmetry of movement.

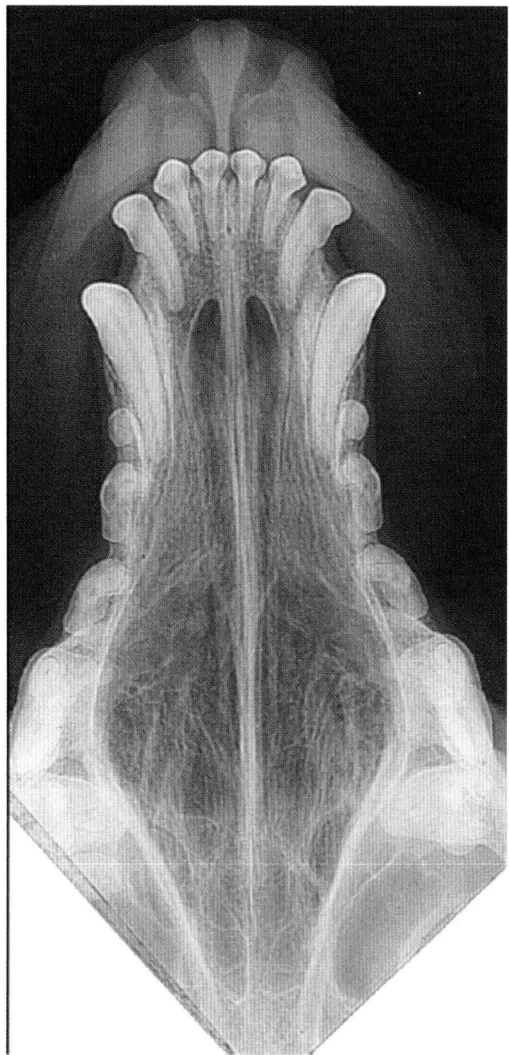

Fig. 7.1 Dorsoventral intra-oral radiograph showing a normal nasal cavity. Note the symmetry between the left and right turbinates.

Diagnostic evaluation

For investigation of epistaxis, a complete haematological, biochemical and clotting profile should be performed. APTT (intrinsic and common coagulation pathway) and PT (extrinsic and common coagulation pathway) are used to assess the intrinsic, extrinsic and common coagulation pathways. A buccal mucosal bleeding time (BMBT) may be appropriate to exclude a primary clotting problem (i.e. formation of a clot). Haematology is important in detection of platelet numbers and assessment of anaemia. In the cat, serological testing for FeLV and FIV should be performed. Serological testing for aspergillosis can be performed; however, test sensitivity varies and both false-positives and negatives can occur. As such, a definitive diagnosis would still require further diagnostic imaging and culture of fungal plaques (Garcia et al., 2001).

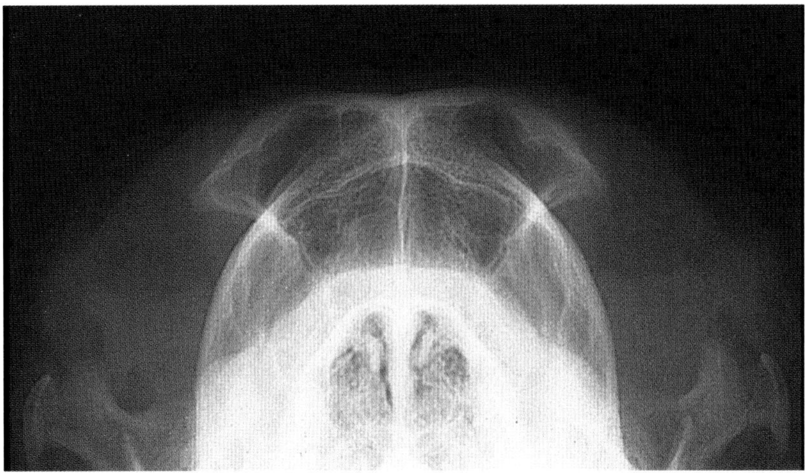

Fig. 7.2 Rostro-caudal horizontal radiograph showing a normal frontal sinus. Note the symmetry between the left and right frontal sinuses.

Radiography

Ideally, three views are recommended for assessment of nasal disease: lateral, dorsoventral intra-oral (Fig. 7.1) and rostro-caudal horizontal (Fig. 7.2) for evaluation of the frontal sinuses. The intra-oral view is best for evaluating the nasal cavity. Destructive changes of the turbinates and nasal septum are more typically associated with either aspergillosis or neoplasia. Although neoplasia is more likely to cause erosion of the nasal or facial bones, aspergillosis may also cause an osteomyelitis and periosteal reaction of the facial bones. An increase in soft tissue density within the nasal chambers may be associated with neoplasia, a polypoid growth or accumulation of discharge. Aspergillosis typically causes a reduction in density and, in severe cases, the nasal chamber can appear almost empty.

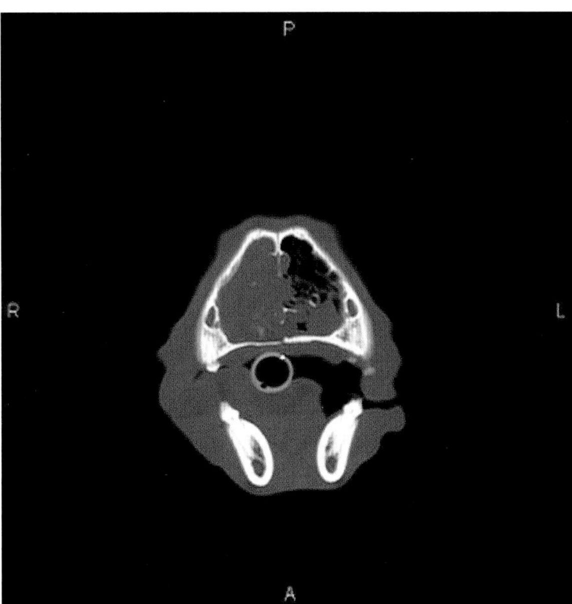

Fig. 7.3 Transverse CT of the nasal cavity showing a right-sided nasal mass and erosion through the nasal septum. An accurate assessment of the extent and invasiveness of the tumour can be gained with 3D imaging techniques such as CT.

Turbinate detail, frontal sinus involvement and the degree of extra-nasal extension of the tumour can be accurately assessed with CT/MRI (Fig. 7.3). CT/MRI has revolutionised the assessment of nasal disease, not only in aiding a definitive diagnosis but also in assisting in the exclusion of other differential diagnoses.

Rhinoscopy

Both anterior and posterior (retrograde) rhinoscopy should be completed. Examination with a rigid 2.7 or 3.0 mm arthroscope permits a thorough inspection of all structures within each nasal fossa. The scope should be navigated along the dorsal, middle and ventral meatuses to examine completely all regions of the nose. Retrograde rhinoscopy (using a flexed bronchoscope) allows examination of the nasopharynx and choanal region.

Culture

Secondary bacterial infection will develop with nasal disease, regardless of the underlying aetiology. A routine nasal swab is therefore of limited diagnostic value and should be reserved only for culture of fungal plaques identified via rhinoscopy.

Nasal flush

Cytological examination of the fluid or soft tissue collected during vigorous flushing of the nasal cavity with saline may occasionally identify the underlying aetiology. A large swab should be packed at the back of the throat and saline forced in through the nostrils. The vigorous flushing may result in dislodgement of tissue into the swab placed at the back of the throat, although the diagnostic yield of this technique is often low.

Nasal biopsy

This can be achieved by blind nasal grab biopsies or under direct visualisation using rigid rhinoscopy (Fig. 7.4). However, with blind nasal grab biopsy techniques,

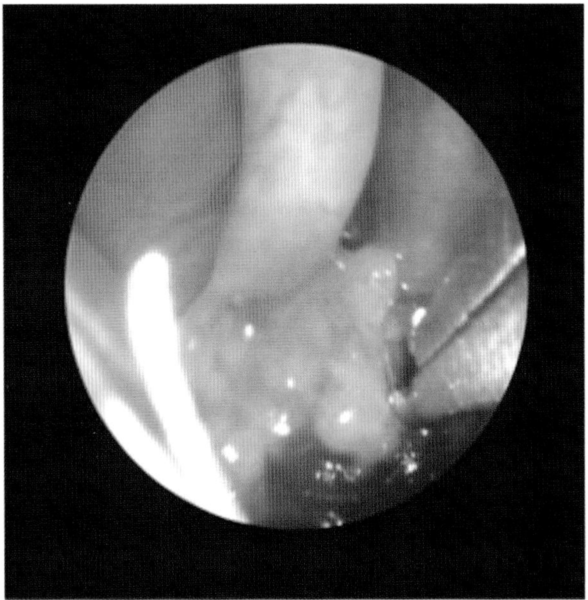

Fig. 7.4 Biopsy of focal nasal mass under direct visualisation.

non-diagnostic samples can be frustrating. It is very common for nasal haemorrhage to be noted following this procedure, which explains the requirement for preoperative clotting profiles to be performed. In dogs with a high index of suspicion of neoplasia, blind nasal grab biopsies have been shown to be as diagnostic as rhinoscopically guided biopsy techniques, and repeated biopsies are frequently required for definitive diagnosis (Harris et al., 2014).

Exploratory rhinotomy

Very few diseases are considered to benefit from complete turbinectomy, and the indications for rhinotomy are now limited. Rhinotomy is invasive and can be associated with considerable haemorrhage. Complications are minimised by swiftness and by packing off areas of

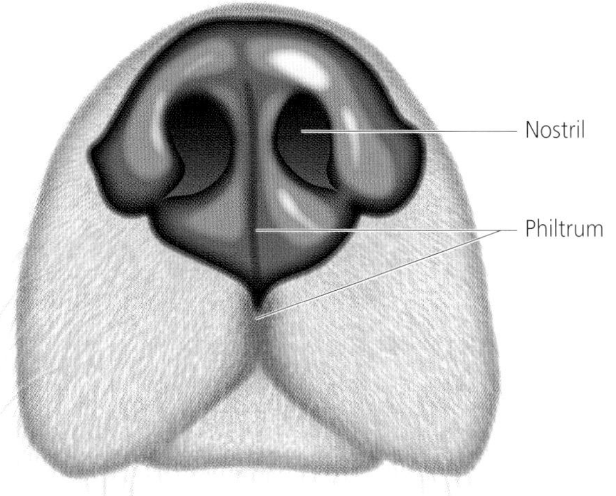

Fig. 7.5 Anatomy of the nostril and nasal philtrum. *Illustrator: Elaine Leggett*

the nose during exploration to control blood loss. The nose can be packed prior to closure, with packing material removed via the nostril after surgery.

7.1.2 Anatomy of the nostrils and nasal cavity

The nasal cavity begins at the nostril (Fig. 7.5) and ends at the choanae. The cavities are separated by the cartilaginous nasal septum. Nasal conchae fill the nasal fossae; the ventral concha is the most prominent in the dog and the middle concha the most prominent in the cat. The conchae define the air passages which are named the dorsal, middle, ventral and common nasal meatuses (Fig. 7.6). The roof of the nostrils is supported by the dorsolateral (alar) cartilage (Fig. 7.7). The alar fold occupies the nasal vestibule and limits air flow into the nose. It is supported and suspended by

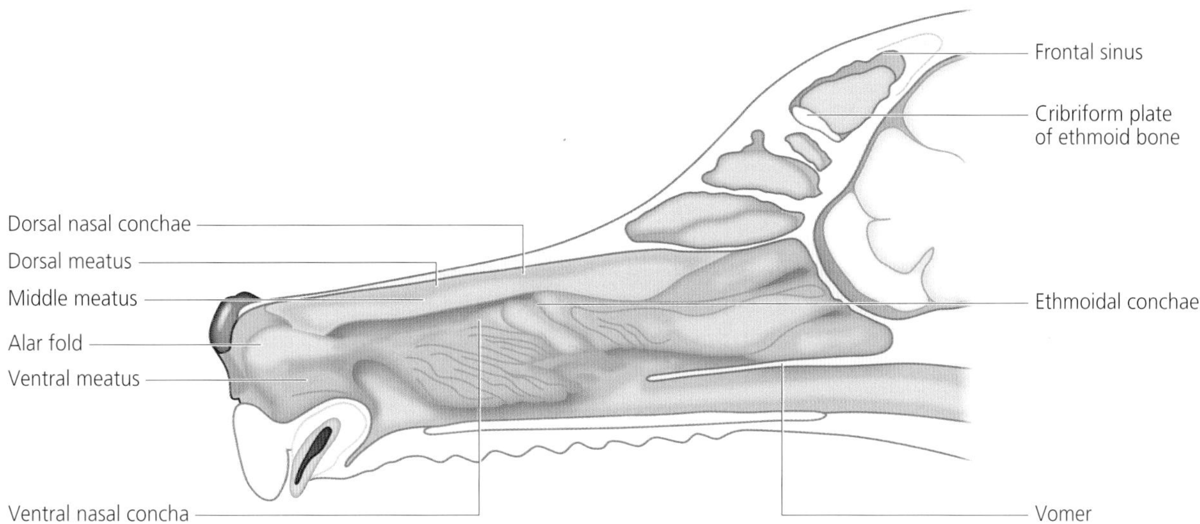

Fig. 7.6 Anatomy of the dorsal, middle and ventral nasal meatuses. A methodical approach to rhinoscopy should be performed, assessing each meatus in turn. *Illustrator: Elaine Leggett*

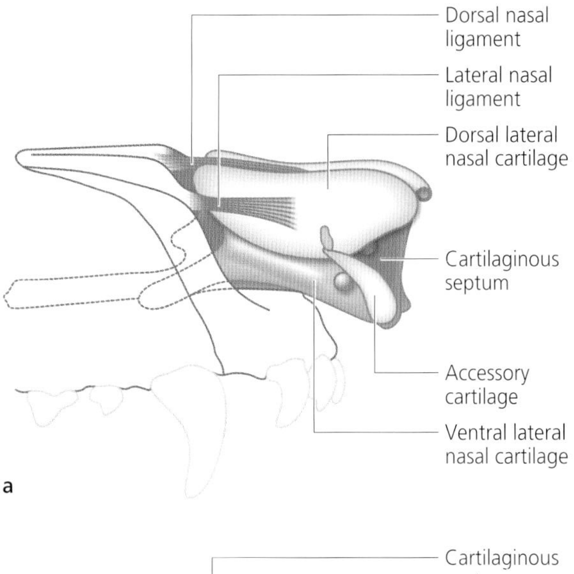

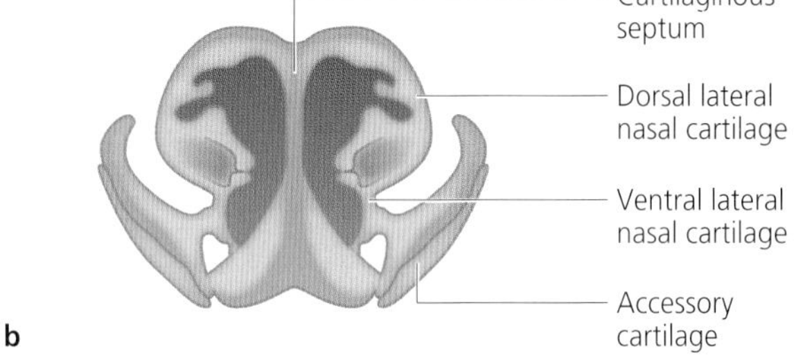

Fig. 7.7 Anatomy of the nasal cartilages. *Illustrator: Elaine Leggett*

the alar cartilage. The infraorbital vessels supply the nostrils.

7.1.3 Nasal planum neoplasia

Neoplasia of the nasal planum is more common in the cat than in the dog, and squamous cell carcinoma is the most common nasal planum tumour in both the cat and dog.

Other tumours reported include lymphoma, fibrosarcoma, melanoma, fibroma, haemangioma, haemangiosarcoma and eosinophilic granuloma (Withrow, 2013).

Squamous cell carcinoma of the nasal planum of the cat and dog

Squamous cell carcinoma is more common in older cats and dogs, and often reflects chronic exposure to UV radiation. The pinnae, nasal planum and eyelids of white cats are most affected (Macy and Reynolds, 1981). In dogs, squamous cell carcinoma usually originates in the mucous membranes of the nostril or external planum. The tumour originates as a pre-malignant form with superficial crusting and ulceration. The disease progresses into carcinoma *in situ*, followed by superficial and then invasive squamous cell carcinoma. Squamous cell carcinoma is a locally invasive malignancy that invades adjoining soft tissue and bone. Exposure to sunlight plays an important role in the malignant transformation of normal squamous epithelial cells in both dogs and cats.

Diagnosis and staging

A deep wedge biopsy assists diagnosis, the degree of invasiveness and the histological type of the disease. Although the risk of metastasis is considered low, evaluation of regional lymph nodes (mandibular) and inflated thoracic radiographs for staging should always be performed. CT or MRI is of particular use in assessing the extent of the tumour, and therefore surgical planning.

Treatment

In the cat, superficial squamous cell carcinoma can be managed by a number of techniques including photodynamic therapy, radiotherapy, intra-lesional carboplatin, cryosurgery and strontium plesiotherapy. Surgery may also be recommended for superficial lesions, and is considered the treatment of choice for more extensive squamous cell carcinomas in both cats and dogs.

Surgery

Wide local excision is the treatment of choice for all dogs and many cats with extensive disease. The surgery usually involves resection of the entire nasal planum together with the nasal cartilage. The surrounding skin is sutured to the cut edge of the nasal mucosa. Stenosis of the surgical site and wound dehiscence can be a complication of the procedure. In a study comparing surgery, radiation and cryotherapy in cats with squamous cell carcinoma of the nasal planum, surgery alone resulted in the longest median disease-free interval of 549 days (Lana et al., 1997). In dogs, a comparison of surgery alone, megavoltage radiotherapy alone and a combination of the two treatments showed that surgery gave a more favourable outcome (Lascelles et al., 2000). Surgery alone for nasal planum squamous cell carcinoma has a 67–100% cure rate and recurrence is associated with incomplete margins (Lascelles et al., 2000; Rogers et al., 1995).

Handy hints

Cautious use of monopolar electrocautery can be used to facilitate resection of the nasal planum and reduce haemorrhage. However, overuse of electrocautery may result in excessive tissue heating causing wound breakdown and dehiscence. A scalpel blade alone can be used to resect the nasal planum but the visibility may be limited from excessive bleeding. Often, once the nasal planum is resected and removed, adequate haemostasis can be achieved.

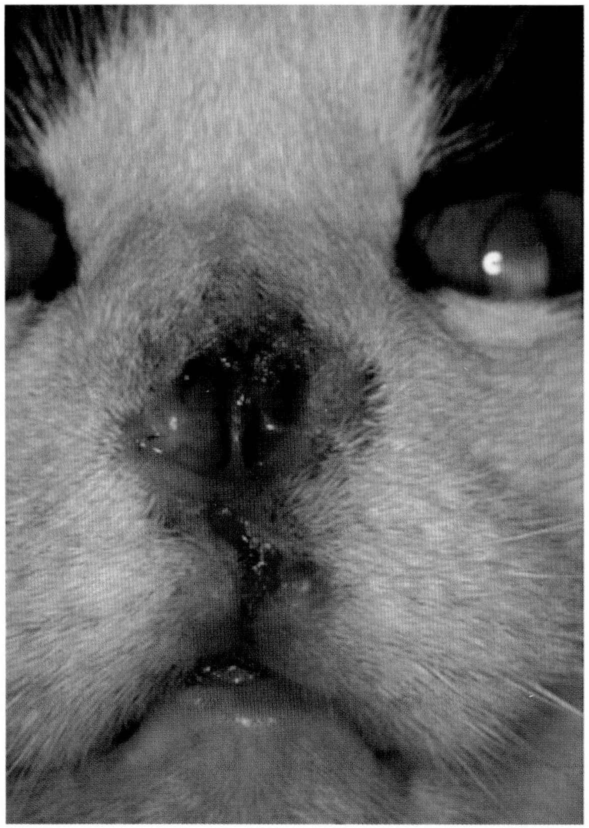

Fig. 7.8 Surgical resection of the nasal planum of the cat, showing good wound healing of the skin to the edge of the resected nasal mucosa. The nasal septum is evident here, covered with pink nasal mucosa. (Image courtesy of Professor R.A.S. White.)

Step by step: feline nosectomy

- A circumferential incision is made (using a scalpel or monopolar electrocautery) around the nasal planum, allowing for appropriate margins according to the extent of the tumour. The level of this resection will vary on an individual case-by-case basis depending on the degree of tumour invasiveness.
- Bipolar electrocautery is used to assist in haemostasis of the skin. Care is taken to avoid excessive use of electrocautery on the nasal mucosa.
- The skin edges are apposed directly to the nasal mucosa using non-absorbable monofilament suture material in a simple interrupted pattern.

Initially, following surgery, the nasal planum is visible and yellow/white in appearance. However, once the healing process progresses, the nasal septum is covered in healthy nasal mucosa. The nasal septum and nasal mucosa will be directly exposed and visible to the owner (Fig. 7.8).

Step by step: canine nosectomy

Canine squamous cell carcinoma typically presents as an erosion of the nasal planum/septum, although a visible mass can also be seen (Fig. 7.9).

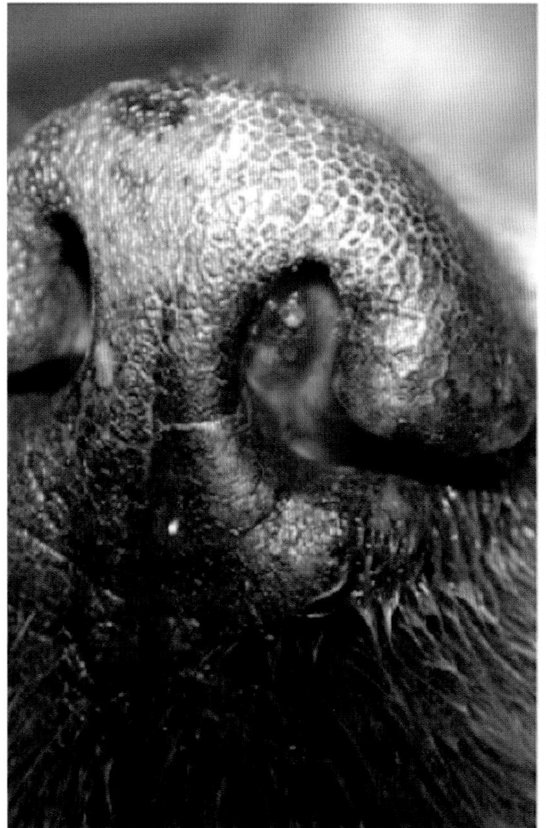

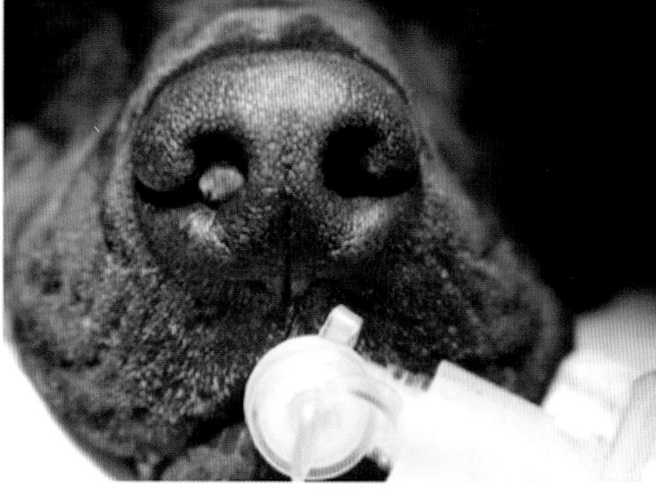

Fig. 7.9 Typical appearance of nasal squamous cell carcinoma in the dog, causing ulceration of the nasal planum (left) and a visible mass (right).

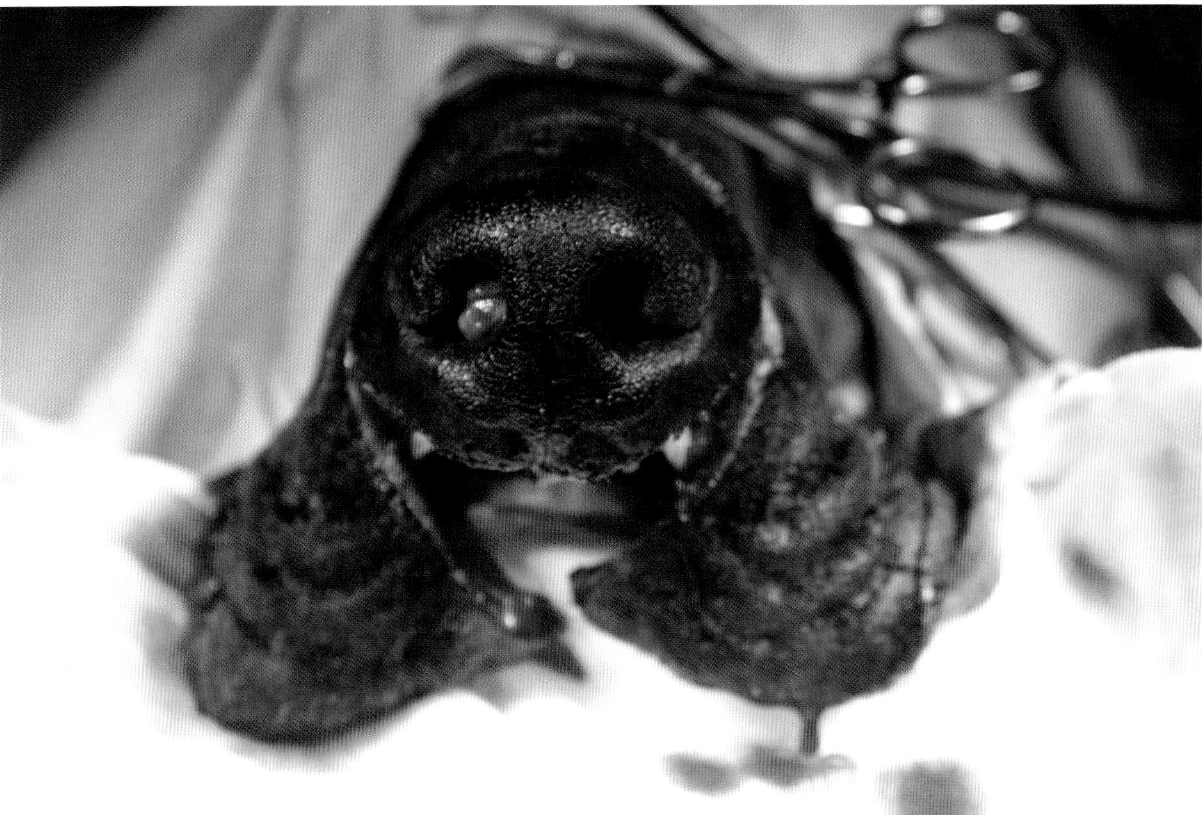

Fig. 7.10 A circumferential skin incision is performed, allowing for appropriate planned margins based on preoperative imaging.

Handy hints

The extent of surgery, determined by the caudal margin, will vary on a case-by-case basis. Resection of the nasal planum, incisive bone and rostral aspects of the nasal bone and maxilla may be required to achieve clean surgical margins. These surgeries can be lengthy and challenging. They can often involve blood loss, which should not be overlooked as some cases may require blood products perioperatively. Preoperative imaging, such as MRI or CT, is invaluable in determining the extent of surgical margins.

- A circumferential skin incision allowing for appropriate caudal margins (Fig. 7.10) is performed using a scalpel blade or monopolar electrocautery. Appropriate bone resection with an oscillating saw, osteotome or mallet may also be required depending on the invasiveness of the tumour (Figs. 7.11, 7.12).
- Reconstruction is achieved through direct apposition of the skin to the cut surface of the nasal mucosa (Fig. 7.13) using a non-absorbable monofilament suture.

Whilst simple apposition of skin to nasal mucosa achieves a successful result in most, if not all, cases, a more cosmetic technique for reconstruction of the nose following resection of the nasal planum in conjunction with a premaxillectomy has been reported (Gallegos et al., 2007). This technique is based on reconstruction using the non-haired pigmented margins of bilateral labial mucocutaneous rotational advancement flaps. The technique can be used successfully in breeds with pendulous lips, such as the dogue de Bordeaux. A technique for removal of very rostral nasal septum squamous cell carcinomas has also been reported (Ter Haar and Hampel, 2015), offering less radical surgery and a cosmetic outcome that is potentially more acceptable to owners. However, case selection using this technique is crucial.

Photodynamic therapy

Photodynamic therapy involves three components: a photosensitising agent, light of a specific activating wavelength and the presence of oxygen in the tissues. 5-aminolaevulinic acid (5-ALA) cream is applied to the tumour and preferentially binds to tumour cells. The agent is 'activated' by illumination with a light source of a specific wavelength which, in the presence of oxygen, results in the production of oxygen radicals and superoxide anions. These free-radical molecules cause localised cytotoxicity and tumour cell necrosis within 24–48 hours. The biggest advantage is the non-invasive nature of the treatment compared with surgery. This is performed under general anaesthesia for approximately 30 minutes. The therapy is reserved for

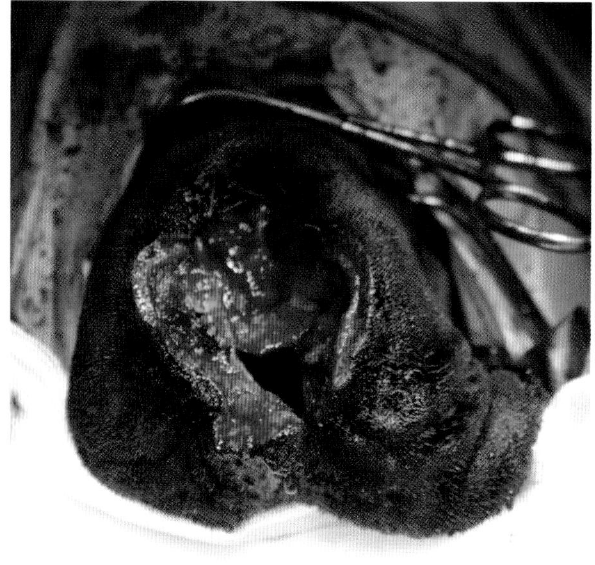

Fig. 7.11 Surgical site following resection of nasal planum, incisive and nasal bone.

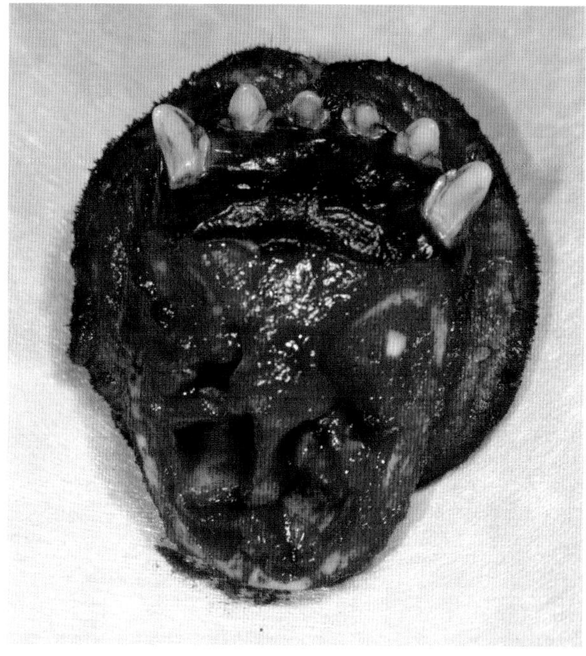

Fig. 7.12 Resected nasal planum, incisive and nasal bones.

superficial lesions only. In a study of 55 cats treated with photodynamic therapy, 96% responded to therapy with a complete response in 85%, while 11% showed a partial response. Of those cats that had a complete response to a single treatment, 51% recurred, with a median time to recurrence of 157 days (Bexfield et al., 2008).

Radiotherapy

Radiotherapy in feline patients is an effective method of treatment for superficial squamous cell carcinomas and is well tolerated by patients, although the equipment is costly and not readily available. A study assessing the response of 15 cats treated with proton beam radiation showed a complete response in 60%, a partial response in 33% and no response in 6.6%. Tumour control rate at one year was 64% and no cat showed evidence of tumour recurrence after one year. The median survival time was 946 days (Fidel et al., 2001).

Strontium-90 plesiotherapy

Strontium plesiotherapy is suitable for superficial lesions only. The radioactive source emits beta-particles which penetrate over a short distance (approx. 2–3 mm).

Sedation or general anaesthesia is required for each application, and often five fractions (50 Gy total) are delivered over a 10-day period. In a retrospective study of strontium-90 plesiotherapy used in the treatment of 15 cases of feline squamous cell carcinoma of the nasal planum, 85% achieved a complete response. Of these, there was no recurrence of disease during a follow-up period of 134–2043 days (median 652). In addition to prolonged disease-free survival, strontium-90 therapy produced excellent cosmetic results from the owners' perspective (Goodfellow et al., 2006). In a second study assessing 49 cases of feline squamous cell carcinoma treated with strontium-90 plesiotherapy, 98% had a response to treatment and 88% showed a complete response. Median progression-free and overall

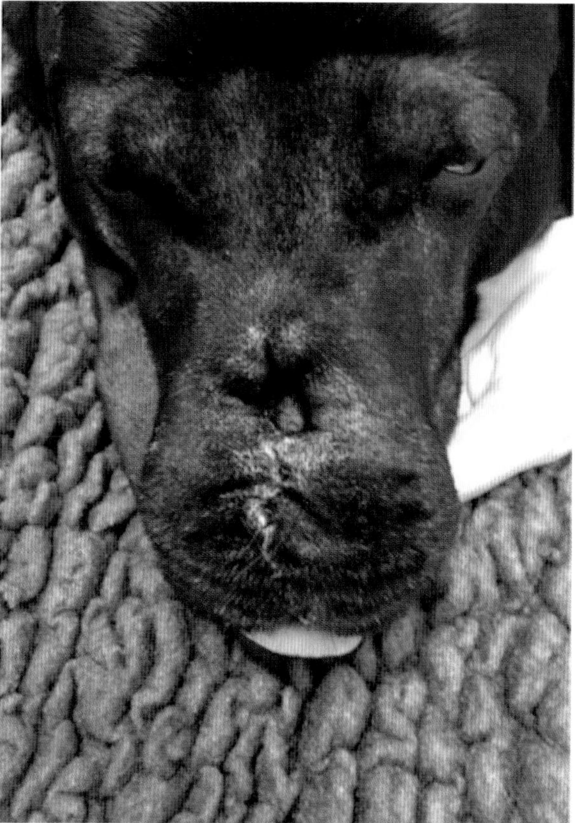

Fig. 7.13 Reconstruction via apposition of the skin to the nasal mucosa with non-absorbable sutures.

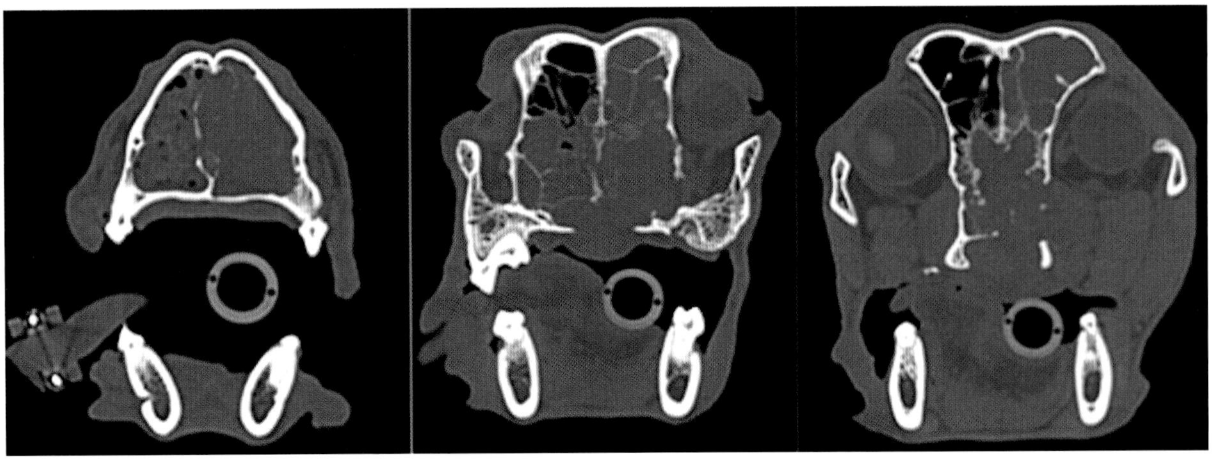

Fig. 7.14 Transverse CT image of a destructive nasal tumour at the rostral (left), mid- (middle) and caudal (right) nasal cavity showing the advantage of CT imaging to highlight the extent of both tumour and nasal bone destruction.

survival times were 1710 and 3076 days, respectively (Hammond et al., 2007).

Chemotherapy

Chemotherapy has not been widely used or reported for the treatment of squamous cell carcinoma. Intra-lesional carboplatin has been reported to have some efficacy in conjunction with concurrent radiotherapy. Results from the treatment of advanced stage squamous cell carcinoma of the nasal planum in the cat, using a combination of intra-lesional carboplatin and superficial radiotherapy, showed a complete response in 100%. The median follow-up for all cats was 268 days, and the median time-to-recurrence, time-to-progression and overall survival were not reached at the time of writing (de Vos et al., 2004).

Cryosurgery

Cryosurgery has been reported as a method of treatment for squamous cell carcinoma in cats (Lana et al., 1997). The technique involves damage to tissues through intracellular and extracellular ice formation. Necrosis occurs, with the defect healing by granulation and epithelialisation. The inability to assess the exact margins of treatment is a significant problem with the use of cryosurgery.

7.1.4 Nasosinal tumours

Canine nasosinal tumours

The average age of dogs with nasosinal tumours is 10 years, and medium- to large-breed dogs are more commonly affected (Patnaik et al., 1984). The metastatic rate is usually low at time of diagnosis (although 40–50% of cases have usually metastasised at time of death; Patnaik et al., 1984). The regional lymph nodes and lungs are the most common sites of metastasis (Henry et al., 1998; Patnaik et al., 1984). Carcinomas (adenocarcinoma, squamous cell carcinoma, undifferentiated carcinoma) comprise nearly two-thirds of all tumours; sarcomas (fibrosarcoma, chondrosarcoma, osteosarcoma, neurofibroma, undifferentiated sarcoma) make up the remainder (Madewell et al., 1976; Patnaik et al., 1984). In the dog, round cell tumours, including lymphoma, mast cell tumours and transmissible venereal tumour, are considered rare tumours of the nasosinal region.

Clinical signs associated with canine nasosinal tumours involve epistaxis, mucopurulent nasal discharge, facial deformity, oral pain on opening the mouth, sneezing, dyspnoea, stertorous breathing, exophthalmos and ocular discharge (Patnaik et al., 1984; Madewell et al., 1976).

Whilst conventional radiographs can assist in the diagnosis of nasosinal tumours, the use of cross-sectional imaging, including CT and MRI, is far superior in terms of accurate assessment of the extent of the tumour and degree of invasiveness into surrounding structures (Fig. 7.14). CT imaging also assists in accurate localisation of the tumour with respect to biopsy and radiation treatment planning. Full staging should be performed with all nasosinal tumours, including biopsy of the primary tumour, aspirates of local lymph nodes and thoracic imaging. Figures 7.15 and 7.16 show combined CT and rhinoscopy used to assist accurate localisation and subsequent biopsy of a small and focal nasal tumour, confirmed histologically as a squamous cell carcinoma.

Untreated nasal carcinomas have a reported survival time of 95 days (Rassnick et al., 2006). A median survival of <6 months is described with exenteration (Laing and Binnington, 1988), suggesting that surgical management alone has yet to prove beneficial in terms of long-term survival. Survival times ranging from 8 to 19.7 months have been documented with mega-voltage

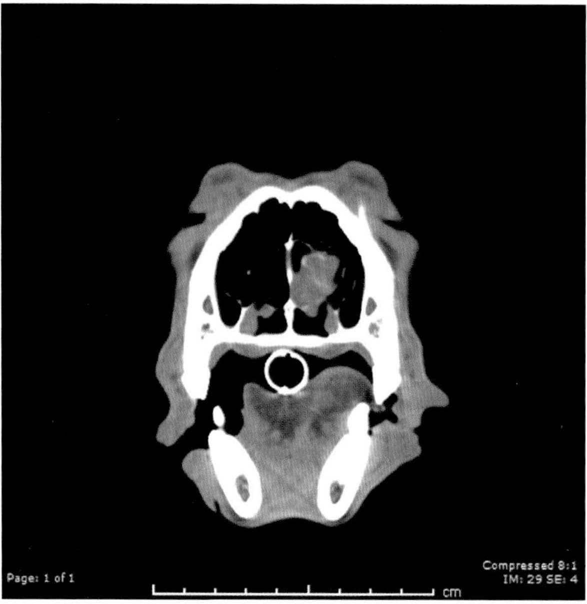

Fig. 7.15 Transverse CT image of the nose showing focal, contrast-enhancing, nasal mass in the right nasal cavity.

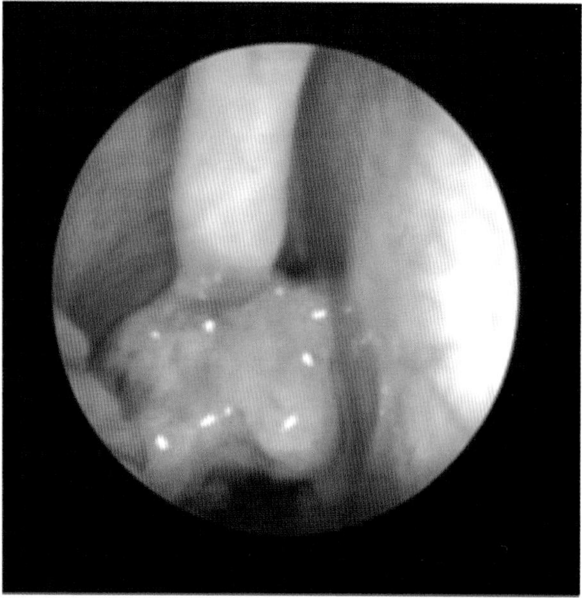

Fig. 7.16 Rhinoscopy used to identify and subsequently biopsy the focal nasal mass noted in the transverse CT image in Fig. 7.15.

radiotherapy alone (Adams et al., 1998, 2005; Theon et al., 1993). A combination of accelerated radiotherapy in conjunction with exenteration of the nasal cavity performed ≥6 weeks following radiation therapy has a reported 47.7 months' survival (Adams et al., 2005). Whilst severe rhinitis with subsequent progression to chronic osteomyelitis and bone necrosis was identified in a number of these patients, this treatment protocol may still prove appropriate for a select subset of patients with small, well-defined nasal tumours.

Feline nasosinal tumours

The average age of cats with nasosinal tumours is 9–10 years (Henderson et al., 2004; Mukaratirwa et al., 2001). Lymphoma is the most commonly diagnosed feline nasal tumour, with others such as carcinoma, adenocarcinoma, squamous cell carcinoma, fibrosarcoma, osteosarcoma, chondrosarcoma, mast cell tumour, melanoma and plasmacytoma being less commonly reported (Rogers et al., 1995). Diagnosis again relies on CT imaging of the nose (Fig. 7.17) and thorax. Biopsy of the mass and cytology of regional lymph nodes is also required, despite a low metastatic rate. Radiotherapy is the treatment of choice for feline nasosinal tumours. For non-lymphoproliferative tumours, reported survival with definitive radiotherapy is approximately 12 months (Theon et al., 1994). The role of chemotherapy in the management of feline nasal lymphoma is yet to be elucidated.

7.1.5 Autoimmune diseases associated with the nasal planum

The external nose can be a primary site for the clinical manifestations of autoimmune diseases such as pemphigoid lesions and discoid lupus. Clinical signs include severe ulceration and erosion (Fig. 7.18), crusting and hyperkeratotic changes. Confirmation of these relies on immunofluorescent staining of deep biopsies, and it is important to differentiate these lesions from neoplasia. Treatment usually involves long-term immunosuppressive agents.

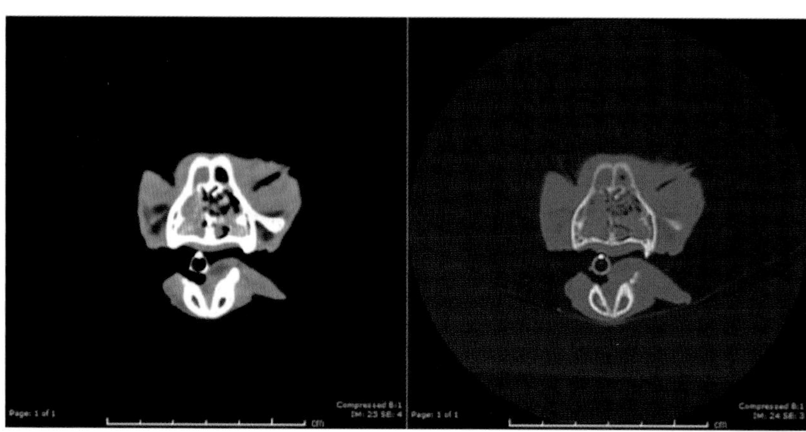

Fig. 7.17 Transverse CT images showing feline nasal lymphoma. Left: soft tissue window; right: bone window.

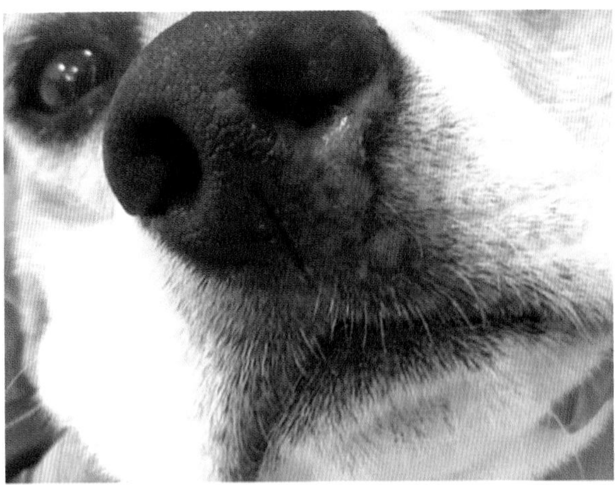

Fig. 7.18 Erosion noted with autoimmune diseases associated with the nasal planum. A biopsy is clearly needed to exclude neoplasia.

7.2 Nasal sinuses and mycotic nasal disease

Key points

- *Aspergillus fumigatus* commonly causes mycotic nasal disease in mesocephalic and dolichocephalic dogs. Sneezing, epistaxis, mucopurulent nasal discharge and nasal depigmentation may be noted.
- Trephination of the nasal sinuses with a clotrimazole cream deposition and a 1-hour clotrimazole liquid soak of the nasal cavity are the most common treatment methods.
- Multiple treatments are often necessary to achieve a successful outcome.
- Diagnostic imaging including CT or MRI are very useful in determining the severity of the disease and the integrity of the cribriform plate prior to treatment.

7.2.1 Nasal sinuses

In the dog, the frontal sinus is divided by a median septum and each side is further divided into lateral, medial and rostral compartments. These compartments communicate via the nasofrontal ostium which opens into the nasal cavity (Figs. 7.6, 7.19). The patency of this nasofrontal ostium must be confirmed if successful treatment via the frontal sinus is to be achieved. A saline flush through the frontal sinus, exiting at the nostril, verifies a patent nasofrontal ostium.

7.2.2 Mycotic nasal disease

Both *Aspergillus* and *Penicillium* species cause mycotic nasal disease in dogs.

The majority of clinical cases are associated with *A.*

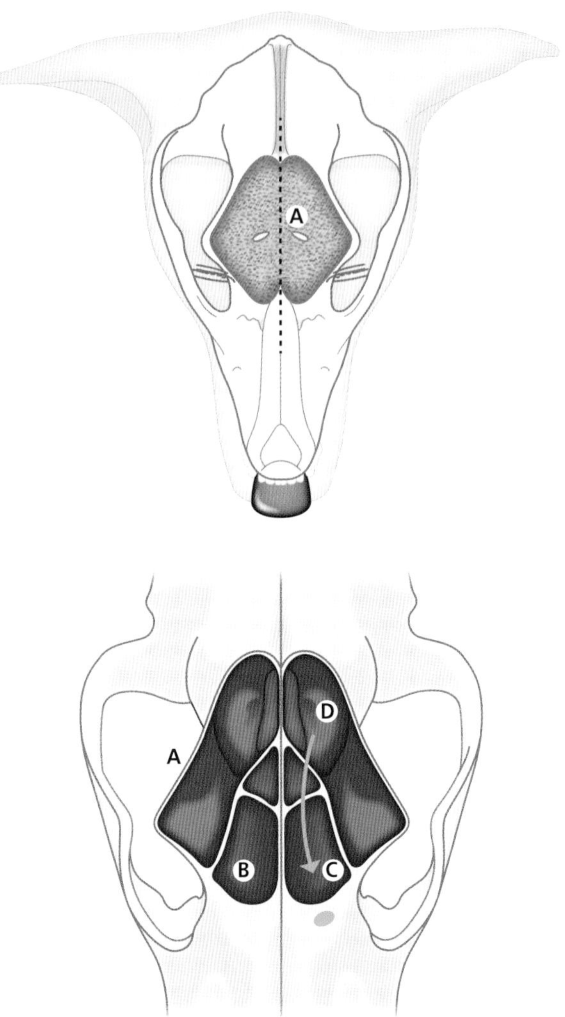

Fig. 7.19 Anatomy of the frontal sinus, approximate location of nasofrontal osteum (green). *Illustrator: Elaine Leggett*

fumigatus infection, although *A. niger* and *A. nidulans* are also reported (Peeters and Clercx, 2007). *A. fumigatus* is ubiquitous in the environment. The fungus releases spores containing conidia, which are inhaled through the nostril and are small enough to reach the alveoli of the lung. The mucociliary escalator and the innate immune system are usually adequate to clear the fungus. However, the virulence of the fungus and the immunocompetence of the host determine the ability to prevent infection.

In the dog, aspergillosis is usually limited to the nasal and paranasal sinuses, although disseminated or systemic forms have been reported (Day et al., 1986). Marked nasal turbinate destruction is noted, with extension into the nasal sinus and destruction of the cribriform plate in severe cases. Interestingly, fungal hyphae have not been shown to invade the nasal mucosa; instead, bony destruction results from the necrolytic toxins that are produced from the fungus (Peeters et al., 2005).

Aspergillosis is typically identified in mesocephalic and dolichocephalic dogs. Dogs are usually young to

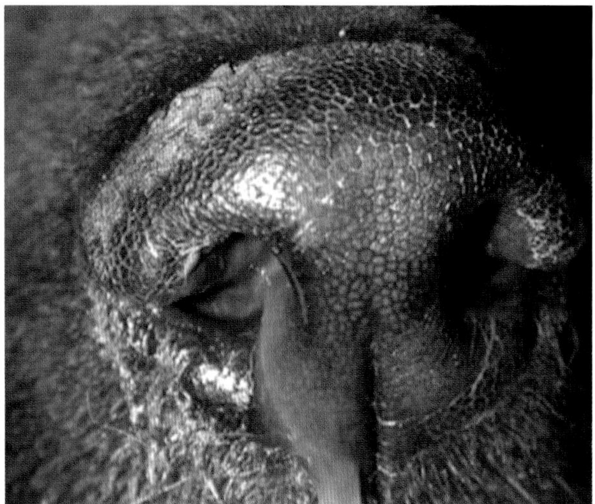

Fig. 7.20 Typical presentation of mucopurulent nasal discharge seen with nasal aspergillosis.

middle age, and although not consistent, a male predisposition has been reported (Sharp et al., 1991). Clinical signs include sneezing, epistaxis, mucopurulent nasal discharge, facial pain and ulceration/depigmentation of the nasal planum (Figs. 7.20, 7.21).

Diagnosis

Diagnosis of aspergillosis relies on a combination of techniques rather than on one single technique. Dorsoventral and lateral radiographs of the skull, intra-oral views of the nasal cavities and rostro-caudal views of the frontal sinus are suggested. Intra-oral radiographs typically show punctate lucencies or a generalised increase in radiolucency due to erosion of the nasal turbinates. Frontal sinus radiography often shows increased radiodensity within one or both nasal sinuses (Fig. 7.22). It is critical that frontal sinus radiography is performed in these cases; treatment of nasal disease alone will likely be unrewarding if concurrent sinus aspergillosis is present yet undiagnosed.

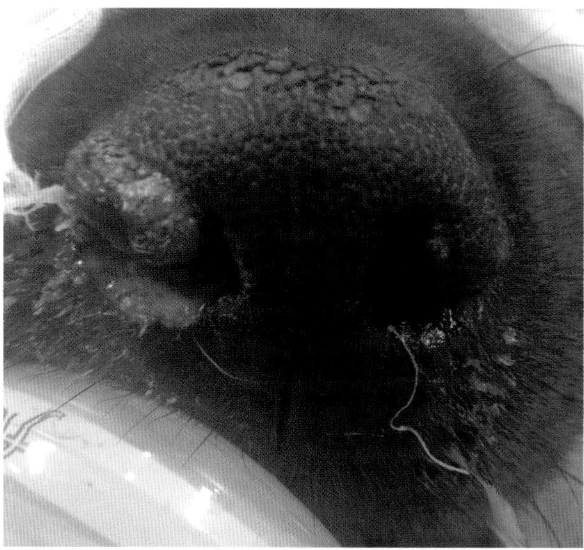

Fig. 7.21 Depigmentation of the nasal planum seen typically in nasal aspergillosis.

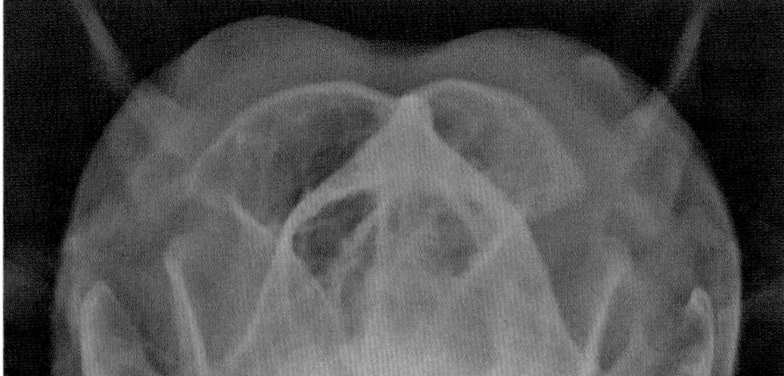

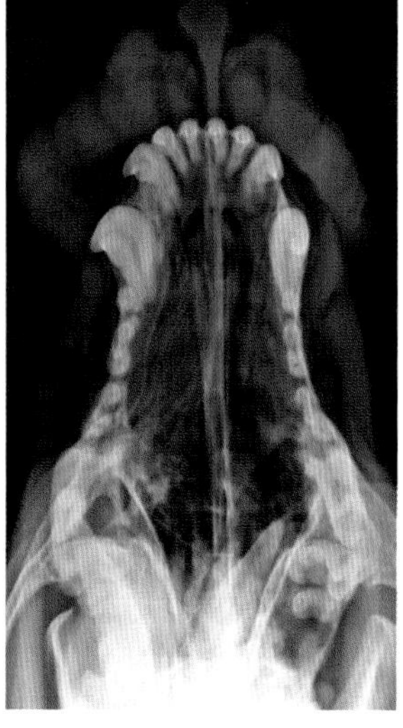

Fig. 7.22 Intra-oral (left) and horizontal frontal sinus (right) radiographic views showing nasal aspergillosis. The former shows right-sided radiolucency and loss of turbinate detail, while the latter shows increased opacity within the right frontal sinus.

Both CT (Figs. 7.23, 7.24) and MRI have been shown to significantly increase sensitivity in comparison with radiography (Saunders and van Bree, 2003). CT allows a three-dimensional assessment of the nasal cavity and nasal sinus and also, importantly, allows assessment of the cribriform plate (Fig. 7.25). Identification of erosion of the cribriform plate (Fig. 7.26) may exclude certain treatment options. Topical antifungal treatment in the presence of an eroded cribriform plate may result in life-threatening seizures. Rhinoscopy, direct visualisation of fungal plaques (Fig. 7.27), biopsy (identifying fungal hyphae) and culture is the gold standard for diagnosis of mycotic nasal disease. Serology can be unreliable due to variable sensitivities and specificities (Garcia et al., 2001) and should therefore be avoided in the diagnosis of nasal aspergillosis.

Treatment

The large variety of treatment protocols suggested for the management of nasosinal aspergillosis only highlights the difficulties in achieving effective control. Topical and systemic antifungal treatments have been reported. Systemic treatment involves oral antifungals, including itraconazole, ketoconazole and fluconazole, although cure rates of only 60–70% have been reported (Sharp and Sullivan, 1986; Sharp et al., 1991). Reported

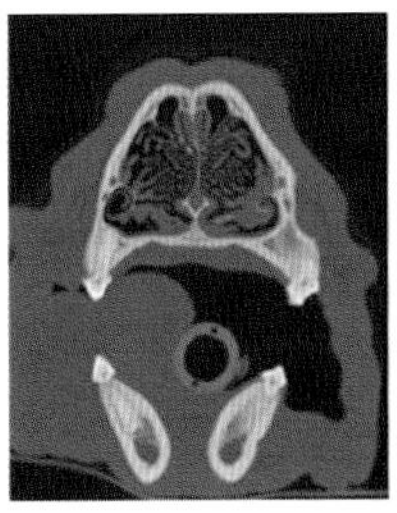
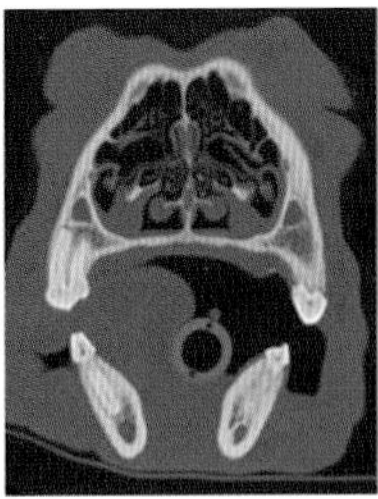
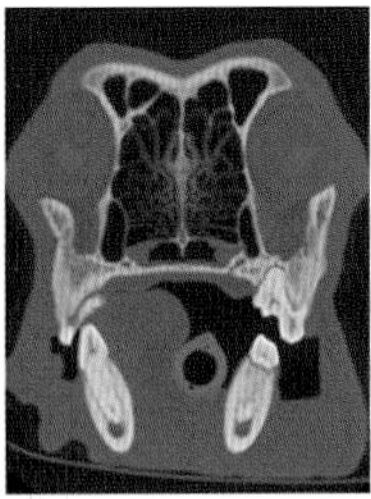

Fig. 7.23 Transverse CT images of a normal nose, showing bilaterally symmetrical nasal turbinates with no evidence of turbinate destruction.

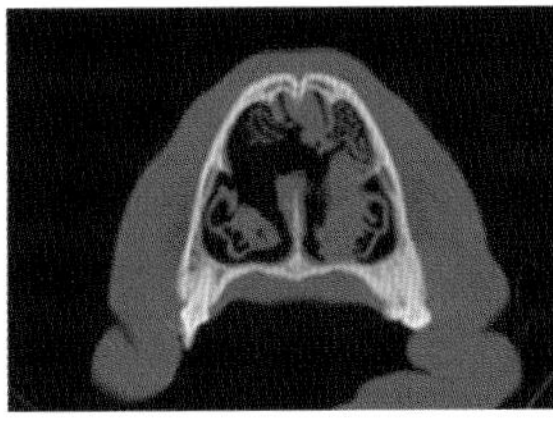
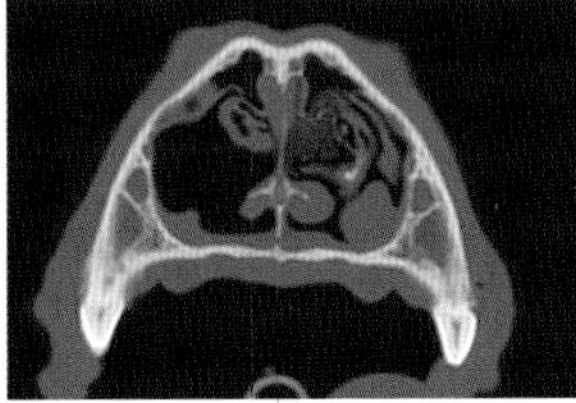

Fig. 7.24 Transverse CT images of a nose affected by nasal aspergillosis showing destruction of the nasal turbinates.

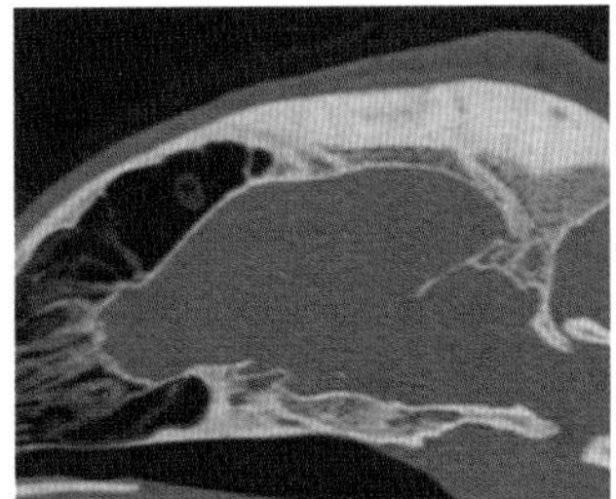
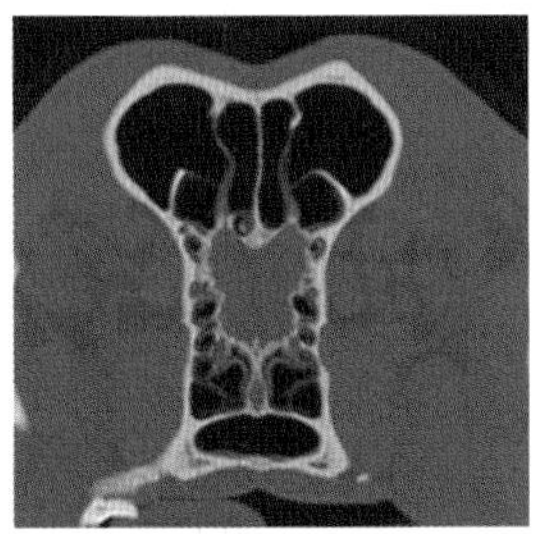

Fig. 7.25 Sagittal (left) and transverse (right) CT showing a normal intact cribriform plate.

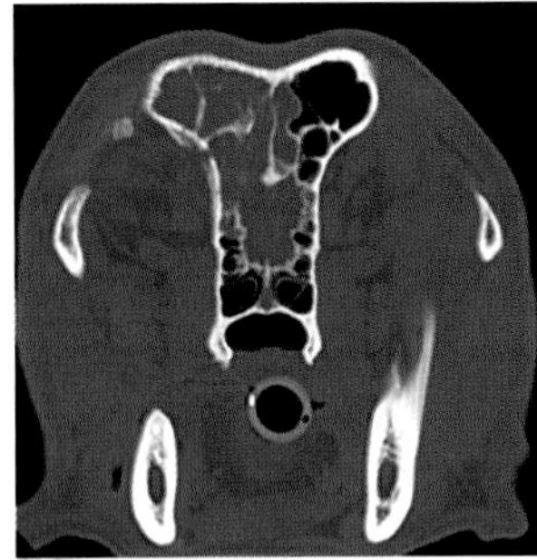
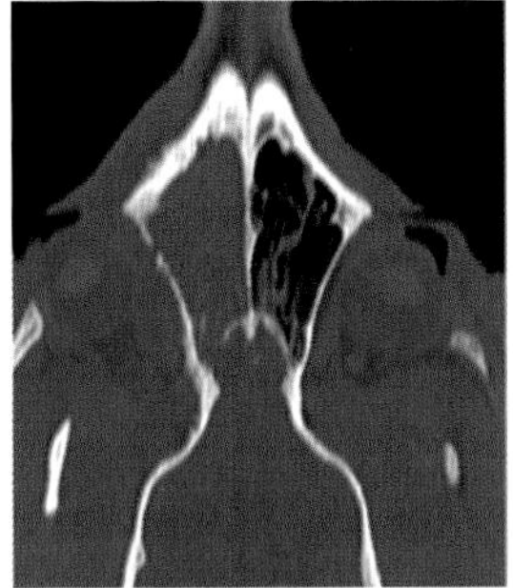

Fig. 7.26 Transverse (left) and dorsal (right) CT showing an eroded cribriform plate.

side effects with systemic antifungals include hepatotoxicity, hepatocutaneous syndrome and anaemia (Legendre et al., 1996).

Topical treatment involves surgical trephination into the frontal sinus (Davidson et al., 1992) or non-surgical placement of Foley catheters into the nostrils and dorsal to the soft palate, via retroflexion of the Foley catheter around the soft palate (Mathews et al., 1998). With either technique, infusion or deposition of enilconazole or clotrimazole has been reported. Enilconazole or clotrimazole infusion with non-surgical placement of

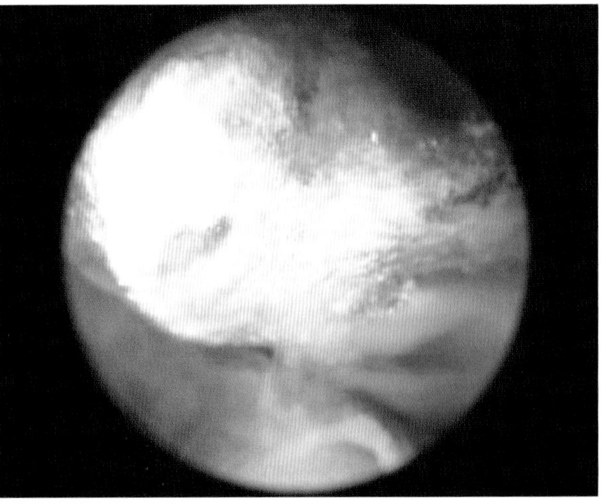

Fig. 7.27 Rhinoscopy showing typical yellow/white appearance of a fungal plaque. Rhinoscopic biopsy of the fungal plaque for histopathology and culture is required for definitive diagnosis.

Foley catheters has a reported success with first treatment of 46.6–69.5% (Mathews et al., 1998; Schuller and Clercx, 2007). The most successful reported treatment to date, however, involves trephination of the frontal sinus with deposition of 1% clotrimazole liquid followed by a deposition of 1% clotrimazole cream. A reported 86% response to first treatment was reported (Sissener et al., 2006).

Step by step: frontal sinus trephination

Handy hints

Using a drill bit to trephine the hole into the frontal sinus allows a gradual and controlled approach to the sinus. With this technique, the surgeon can appreciate engagement of the drill bit into the bone of the frontal sinus and, with continued gentle rotation, the drill bit is guided into the frontal sinus. Once a hole is made, rongeurs can be used to enlarge the hole, if necessary, should concurrent debridement of fungus within the frontal sinus be required.

- The dog is placed in sternal recumbency and the skin clipped in a rectangle at the level of the frontal sinus. The skin is surgically prepped.
- The trephination site is aimed at the centre of an imaginary triangle formed with its base along the middle of the skull, with the other landmarks being the frontal crest and the bony rim of the orbit (Sharp et al., 1991; Fig. 7.28).
- A 1 cm skin incision is made on the left / right side and blunt dissection using artery forceps used to identify the skull.
- A Jacobs hand chuck with an appropriately sized drill bit or Steinman pin is used to trephine into the sinus (Fig. 7.29). The diameter of the trephination hole can

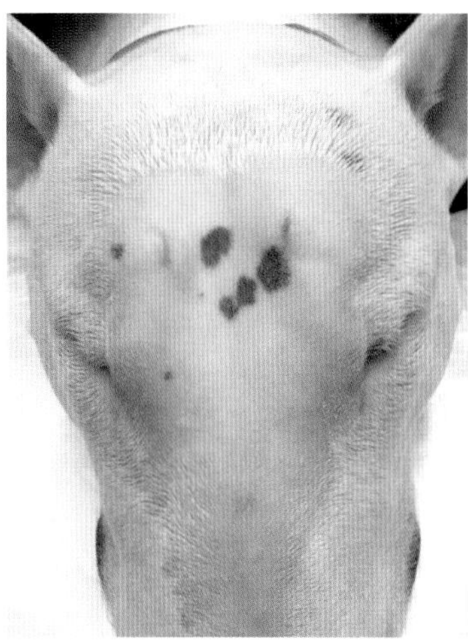
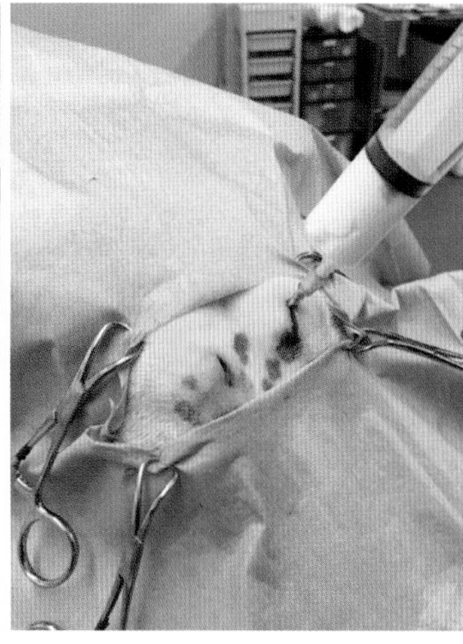

Fig. 7.28 Left: location of trephination sites; right: 1% clotrimazole cream deposition into the frontal sinus.

be enlarged, should rigid rhinoscopy or debridement/biopsy of the frontal sinus be required.

- A large 16 or 18G catheter with the stylet removed is placed in the trephination hole and clotrimazole cream/solution is deposited within the sinus (Fig. 7.28).
- The process is repeated on the contralateral side and the skin sutured with non-absorbable monofilament suture.
- Skin sutures are not always necessary. Some surgeons elect to leave the skin unsutured allowing excess cream to be removed.

Step by step: Foley catheter placement for a clotrimazole soak

Handy hints

Positioning of the dog in dorsal recumbency assists in the placement of the initial Foley catheter around the back of the soft palate. By doing this, the surgeon is not working against gravity when retroflexing the Foley catheter. Placement of the Foley catheter around the back of the soft palate can be challenging. Flexing the last 4–5 cm of the Foley catheter 180 degrees and grasping this with some long ratchet forceps can assist with the direction of the catheter around the soft palate.

- Inflation of the ET tube cuff is confirmed, preventing iatrogenic deposition of clotrimazole solution into the trachea and lungs.
- The nasal cavity is isolated by placing and inflating a Foley catheter up each nostril and a third Foley catheter around the back of the soft palate (Fig. 7.30).
- The caudal nasopharynx is packed with swabs to prevent iatrogenic deposition of clotrimazole solution into the trachea.
- A Backhaus towel clamp is placed across each alar fold to maintain a tight seal around the nasal catheters.
- A 1% clotrimazole solution is instilled into the nasal cavity via the nasal catheters until full – this can be identified via leakage from the vomeronasal organ.
- The clotrimazole is left for a 1-hour soak, and the head position is varied to ensure complete mucosal soaking. A 15-minute soak is recommended for every 90-degree head position.

Despite previously reported success rates with a single treatment for aspergillosis (Sissener et al., 2006), repeated treatments for severe cases of aspergillosis are often required. In the author's experience, three to four treatments performed every two weeks are usually required before resolution of clinical signs is achieved. The treatment process can often be lengthy and costly, and owners should be well informed of this prior to commencing treatment.

Feline aspergillosis

Fungal rhinitis is uncommon in the cat. Two forms of upper respiratory tract aspergillosis are identified: sino-nasal and sino-orbital. Both infections start in the nasal cavity, with sino-orbital aspergillosis being the more common form in 65% of cases (Barrs and Talbot, 2014). Brachycephalic breeds of cats, especially Persian

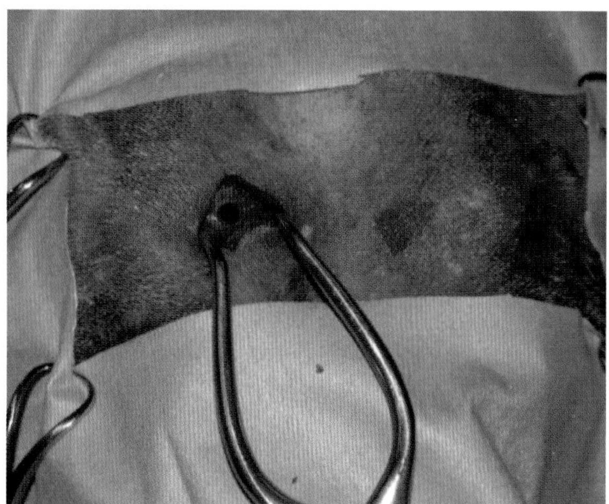

Fig. 7.29 Frontal sinus trephination.

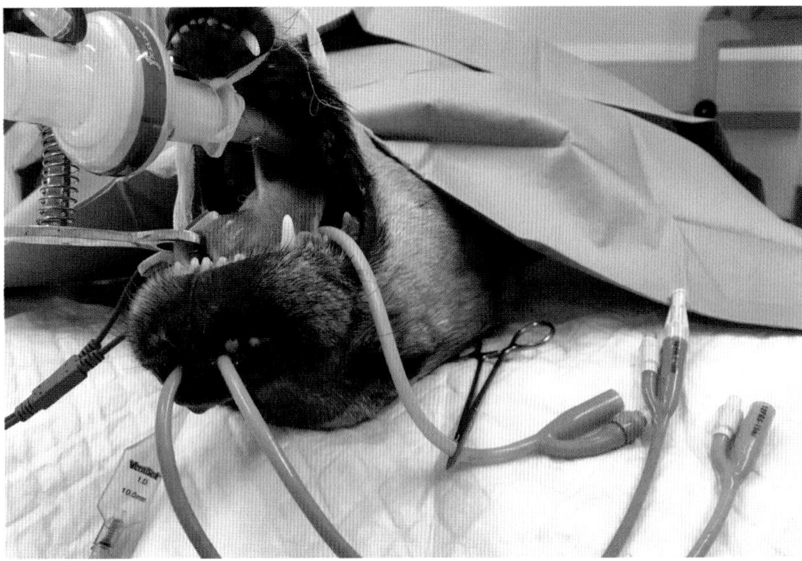

Fig. 7.30 Foley catheter placement into the nostrils and around soft palate for instillation of 1% clotrimazole solution.

and Himalayan, are predisposed. Unlike in dogs, where the fungus does not invade the nasal mucosa, invasive disease is seen in cats. Sino-nasal aspergillosis is most commonly caused by *A. fumigatus* and *A. niger*, whilst *A. felis* is documented with sino-orbital aspergillosis. Clinical signs often involve sneezing, stertor, serous to mucopurulent nasal discharge and mandibular lymphadenopathy. Less commonly, epistaxis, fever and a discharging sinus or soft tissue mass involving the nasal bone or frontal sinus are seen. The prognosis for feline aspergillosis is favourable with topical antifungal therapy alone (Tomsa et al., 2003), or combined with systemic antifungals such as oral itraconazole (Barrs and Talbot, 2014; Whitney et al., 2005).

7.3 Brachycephalic obstructive airway syndrome (BOAS)

Key points

- Both primary and secondary factors contribute to BOAS. Primary factors include stenotic nares, elongated soft palate and a hypoplastic trachea. Secondary factors include everted laryngeal saccules, everted tonsils and laryngeal collapse.
- Gastrointestinal signs, including regurgitation, vomiting and gastrointestinal reflux, are commonly reported in BOAS patients.
- H1 antagonists, such as omeprazole, are important in the medical management of BOAS patients.
- Surgeon experience and facilities available to perform pre-, peri- and postoperative care are critical in achieving a positive outcome.

The condition of BOAS is seen in brachycephalic breeds, including the English bulldog, French bulldog, Boston terrier, shih-tzu, Lhasa apso, Pekingese, pug and boxer. A rostro-caudal shortening of the skull (Fig. 7.31) results in compressed nasal passages and pharyngeal tissue. This compression of the nasal passages and distortion of the pharyngeal tissue results in increased airway resistance.

In brachycephalic breeds, resistance to airflow is increased by the narrowed airway, causing an increase in the intra-luminal pressure gradient during inspiration (Koch et al., 2003). When this pressure is excessively greater than the atmospheric pressure, the tissues become inflamed, tonsils and laryngeal saccules evert

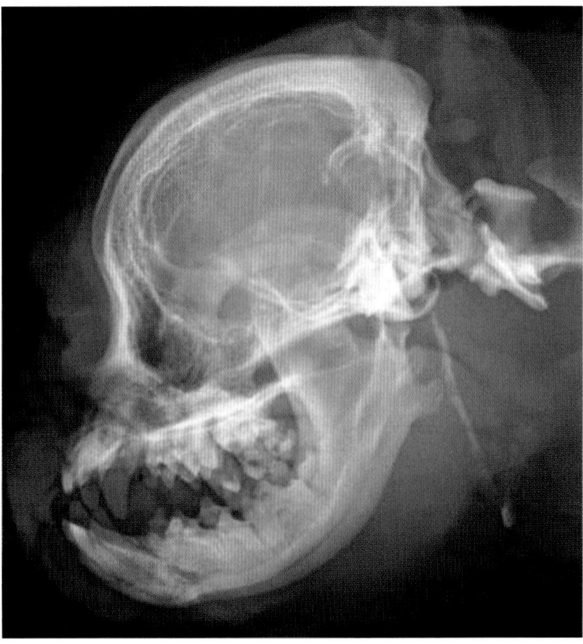

Fig. 7.31 Rostro-caudal shortening of the skull identified in brachycephalic breeds. The radiograph also highlights the thickened soft palate often noted in these breeds.

and the cartilaginous larynx becomes compromised and can collapse, decreasing the laryngeal lumen size and further increasing resistance to airflow (Koch et al., 2003). This increased resistance causes turbulent airflow, oedema and, thus, inspiratory noise. A vicious cycle can then self-perpetuate.

Both primary and secondary factors contribute to BOAS. Primary factors include stenotic nares, elongated soft palate and hypoplastic trachea. These primary factors create negative pressure in the airway, leading to the secondary components of BOAS. These secondary factors include everted laryngeal saccules, laryngeal collapse and everted tonsils.

In a study assessing 90 cases of dogs with BOAS (Fasanella et al., 2010), English bulldogs (61%), pugs (21%) and Boston terriers (9%) were the breeds most commonly affected. The most common components of BOAS were elongated soft palate (94%), stenotic nares (77%), everted laryngeal saccules (66%) and everted tonsils (56%). Dogs most commonly had three or four components of BOAS, with the most common combination being stenotic nares, elongated soft palate, everted laryngeal saccules and everted tonsils (Fasanella et al., 2010).

Abnormal inspiratory effort is also believed to result in low intrathoracic pressure, which may initiate or indeed worsen a hiatal hernia. Gastrointestinal disorders, including regurgitation, vomiting and gastro-oesophageal reflux, have been reported in brachycephalic dogs. In one study, 97.3% of brachycephalic dogs with upper respiratory signs had gastric, oesophageal or duodenal abnormalities confirmed histopathologically (Poncet et al., 2005) and a correlation between the severity of GI signs and respiratory signs was noted. Surgical management has been shown to result in an improvement of 88.3% in respiratory and of 91.4% in gastrointestinal disorders (Poncet et al., 2006). Gastro-oesophageal medical management (H1 antagonism) is also suggested to improve the outcome for surgically treated brachycephalic dogs (Poncet et al., 2006). Breed has been shown to influence the severity of gastrointestinal signs, with French bulldogs reported to present with more severe gastrointestinal signs than pugs (Haimel and Dupre, 2015).

7.3.1 Clinical signs and diagnosis

Clinical signs associated with BOAS include noisy, stertorous breathing, snoring, inspiratory dyspnoea, open-mouth breathing, cyanosis, exercise intolerance and collapse. Gastrointestinal signs including regurgitation and vomiting may also be present. Diagnosis is achieved primarily by a full clinical history and clinical examination, which, in conjunction with the appropriate signalment, may raise a high level of suspicion for the disease. Examination of the external nares will confirm the presence of stenotic nares, together with thoracic radiographs to assess the tracheal diameter and exclude aspiration pneumonia secondary to regurgitation. These radiographs can be performed conscious if the clinical examination reveals a high suspicion of pulmonary pathology. General anaesthesia is required for a full oral examination, including assessment of the soft palate, larynx and laryngeal saccules. Induction and recovery from anaesthesia in BOAS patients should not be treated lightly, and surgical correction should therefore be performed under the same anaesthetic. Should the surgical facilities, surgeon experience and availability of pre-, peri- and postoperative care be questioned, referral to a specialist centre would be highly recommended prior to induction of general anaesthesia.

7.3.2 Anaesthesia for BOAS surgery

It is possible that these patients present in respiratory distress. As such, oxygen therapy and sedation on admission may be required. These patients may also be hyperthermic and external cooling may be needed. As with all brachycephalic breeds, pre-oxygenation prior to anaesthesia is most important. Adequate preparation is vital and a previously prepared airway box would be recommended. This box includes a laryngoscope, multiple-sized ET tubes, a rigid urinary catheter for oxygen delivery, suction tubing and temporary tracheostomy tubes. Many brachycephalic intubations require suctioning prior to intubation; regurgitation is quite common under anaesthesia in these breeds. Administration of a proton pump inhibitor is advised either before surgery or at induction. Laryngeal and soft palate oedema may be noted following surgery, and corticosteroid administration may be required on completion of the surgery. The endotracheal tube should be maintained for as long as possible during recovery, and one-to-one monitoring is critical during the early postoperative period, observing for signs of obstruction, regurgitation and aspiration. Whilst placement of a temporary tracheostomy tube is not frequently required, patients with severe laryngeal collapse or laryngeal oedema may require emergency surgery. Arrangements should be made prior to all BOAS surgeries to prepare for this, and owners should be appropriately informed of the risks associated with this surgery.

7.3.3 Patient preparation for BOAS surgery

Correct positioning of the patient is critical for BOAS surgery, and the surgeon must select their preferred

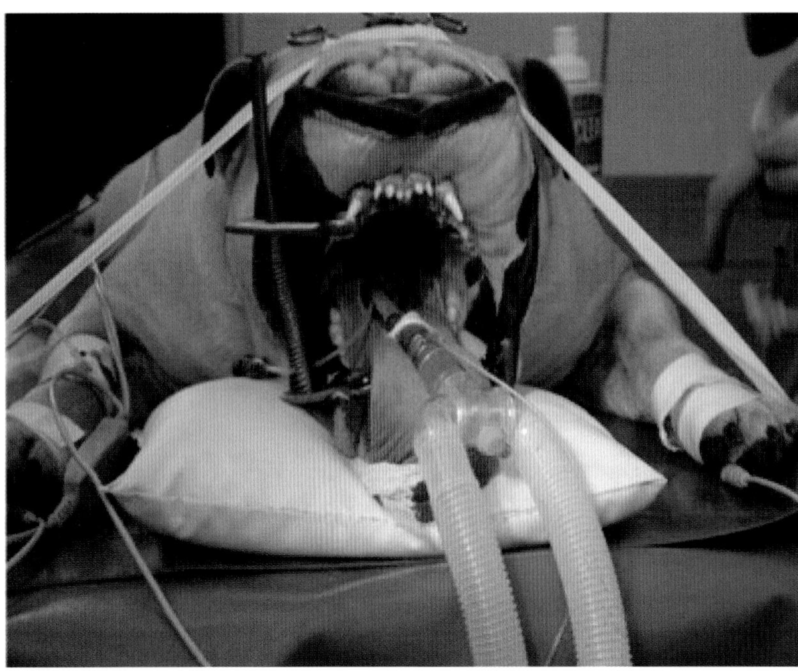

Fig. 7.32 The mouth is held open using a mouth gag. The lips are retracted using Allis tissue forceps, which are taped caudally. The eyes are protected with swabs preventing contact by the forceps.

positioning method to allow exposure of the soft palate and laryngeal saccules (Figs. 7.32, 7.33). Adequate time must be allowed for this surgical preparation, as failure to achieve stable surgical positioning with adequate exposure could result in significant intra-operative problems. Prior to surgery, the ET tube must be well cuffed and a swab placed at the back of the throat, preventing inhalation of blood during the procedure. Adequate lighting is vital for this procedure, and electrocautery is required if a folded-flap palatoplasty is to be performed.

7.3.4 Stenotic nares

As illustrated by Poiseuille's law, airway flow is proportional to the radius of the airway to the fourth power. Hence, a small increase in radius results in a large increase in airway flow. The aim of treatment therefore is to surgically increase the opening to the nostril.

Step by step: nasoplasty

Handy hints

When performing BOAS surgery, the staphylectomy/folded-flap palatoplasty is best performed first, with a swab placed in the throat prior to surgery. The swab should remain in place whilst the nasoplasty is performed, as this is often a haemorrhagic surgery and results in blood passing from the nose and pooling in the nasopharynx. Finally, the swab is removed and the laryngeal saccule resection is performed.

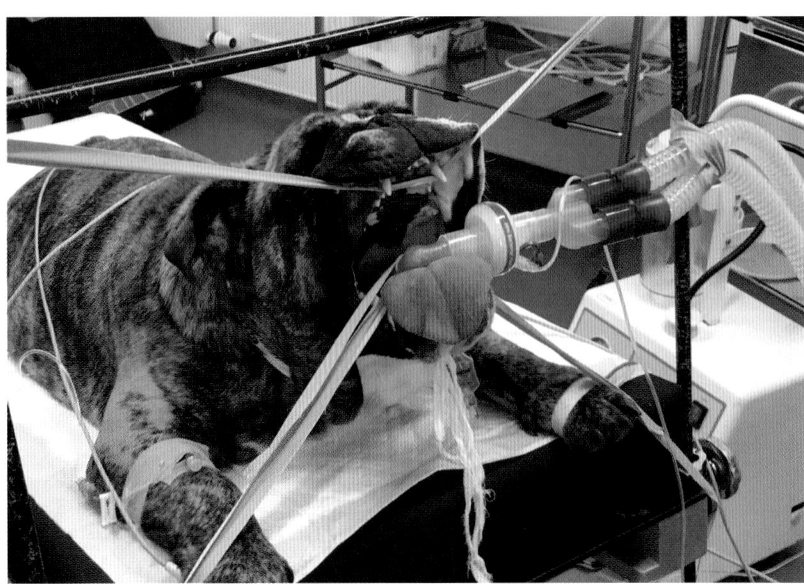

Fig. 7.33 The mouth is held open using bandage/Elastoplast attached to a frame.

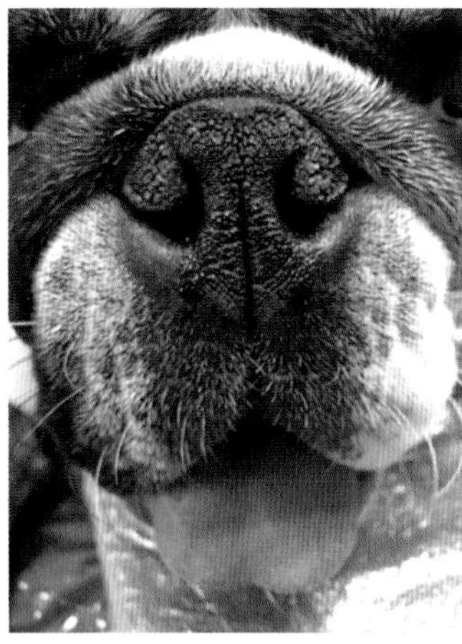

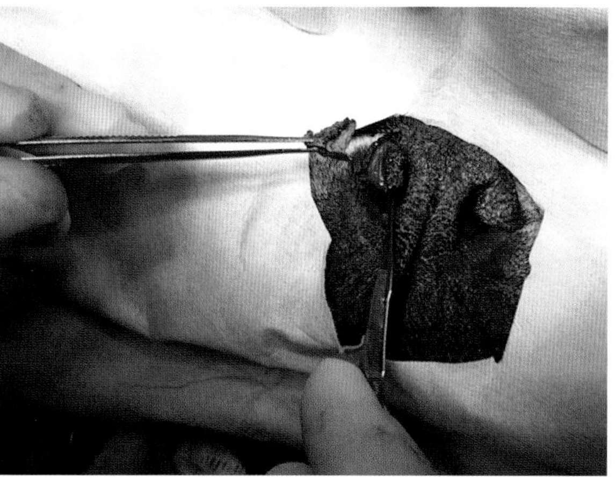

Fig. 7.34 Nasal stenosis resulting in increase in resistance to air flow (left) and nasoplasty (right) to remove a vertical wedge of tissue.

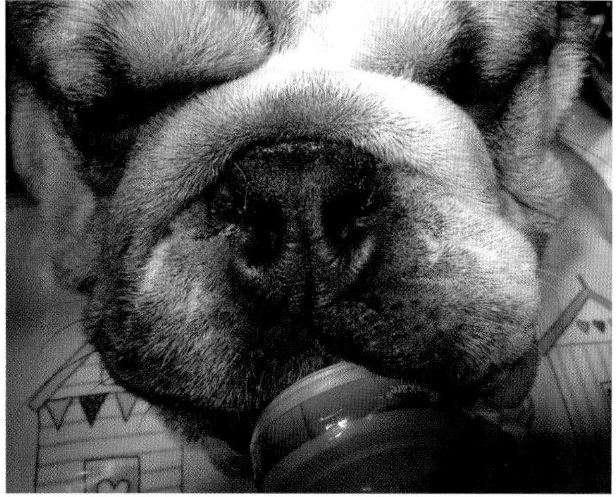

Fig. 7.35 Simple interrupted, absorbable sutures have been placed resulting in an increase in nostril size.

- A no. 11 scalpel blade is used to perform either a vertical or horizontal wedge resection.
- This resection should be deep into the wing of the narrowed nostril, including the alar fold (Fig. 7.34).
- Haemorrhage is profuse but usually subsides once the sutures are placed.
- Closure is performed using a rapidly absorbable suture in a simple interrupted pattern, resulting in a clearly visible increase in nostril size (Fig. 7.35).
- The procedure must be repeated in an identical manner on the opposite nostril to maintain nasal symmetry.

7.3.5 Elongated soft palate

Whilst no absolute guidelines have been set, a normal soft palate and epiglottis should overlap by approximately 1–3 mm. If the palate extends excessively beyond this level, it will obstruct the airway. Accurate assessment of soft palate length comes with experience. This assessment should always be performed under anaesthesia, prior to intubation. A probe is often useful to gently depress and elevate the epiglottis and manipulate the soft palate. Caution should be taken not to extend the tongue excessively during this assessment as a relatively neutral tongue position is more physiological.

Staphylectomy

During this procedure, the free edge of the soft palate is cut and sutured with a simple continuous suture placed through both the nasal and oral mucosae. Assessment of the length of the soft palate to be resected can be challenging. The soft palate should be trimmed to the level of the mid-caudal tonsillar crypt. If trimmed too short, the dog will continue to display clinical signs of upper airway obstruction. Over-trimming of the soft palate can lead to oronasal reflux. Care should also be taken to achieve a symmetrical incision. The surgeon should be aware that tying knots in the soft palate mucosa can be challenging due to the depth of the tissue and limited space available.

Step by step: staphylectomy

Handy hints

Two pairs of long DeBakey forceps are useful for manipulation of the soft palate.

- Using the 'cut–sew–cut–sew' technique, an absorbable suture is pre-placed and tied at the level of the initial cut, on the lateral edge of the palate.
- One end of the suture is cut and the needle end left long to continue the suture.
- The soft palate is then cut to the mid-point, and the pre-placed suture is used to suture the resected portion of the palate, taking care to suture both the nasal and oral mucosa.
- Once the first half of the palate is resected and sutured, the remaining section of palate is cut and sutured accordingly, using the same piece of suture.
- Alternatively, tonsillectomy forceps can be used to clamp the soft tissue to be resected. Once the palate is cut, the free edge of the soft palate can be sutured using a continuous pattern (Fig. 7.36).

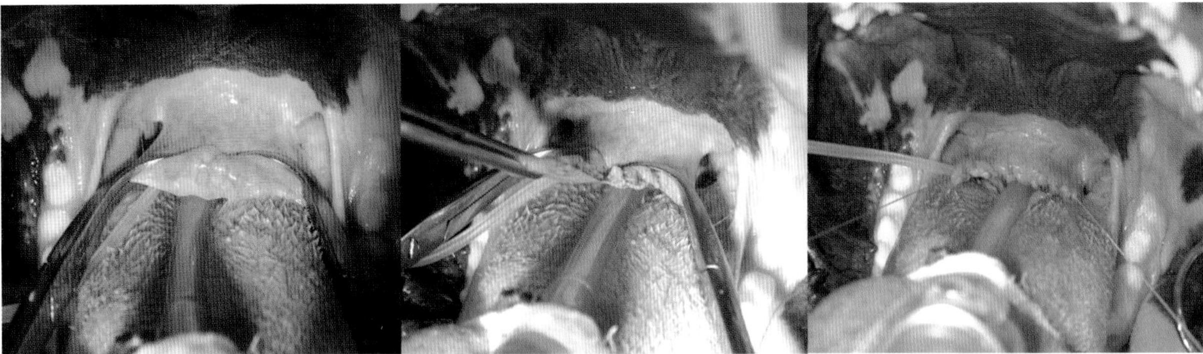

Fig 7.36 Tonsillectomy forceps clamping the free edge of the soft palate to be resected (left). Once the palate is resected, the oral and nasal mucosa can be sutured in a simple continuous pattern with absorbable suture (middle). Successful completion of a symmetrical staphylectomy (right).

Folded-flap palatoplasty

The conventional staphylectomy technique addresses the excessive length of the soft palate. However, elongated soft palates also commonly demonstrate excessive thickness (Findji and Dupre, 2009) resulting in nasopharyngeal and oropharyngeal obstructions. A folded-flap palatoplasty technique (Findji and Dupre, 2009) was introduced in order to address the excessive length and thickness of the palate. In a series of 55 dogs using this folded-flap palatoplasty technique, 97.5% of patients showed improvement of respiratory signs after surgery. A temporary tracheostomy was required postoperatively in 10.9% of cases (Findji and Dupre, 2009).

Step by step: folded-flap palatoplasty

Handy hints

Bipolar electrocautery is required with this technique.

- Long DeBakey forceps are used to grasp the caudal-most edge of the soft palate, which is retracted rostrally until the opening of the nasopharynx can be visualised (Fig. 7.37).
- The level at which the caudal edge of the soft palate makes contact with the ventral mucosa of the soft palate is marked with electrocautery (Fig. 7.38).
- Starting at the marked position (Fig. 7.39), the ventral aspect of the soft palate is then resected in a trapezoid shape, using electrocautery and blunt dissection.
- The palatinus muscle is resected. Some authors also resect the levator veli palatini muscles, whilst others keep this muscle *in situ* (Fig. 7.40) in order to preserve some muscular function of the palate during swallowing.
- Laterally, the sides of the trapezoid pass just medially to the tonsils.

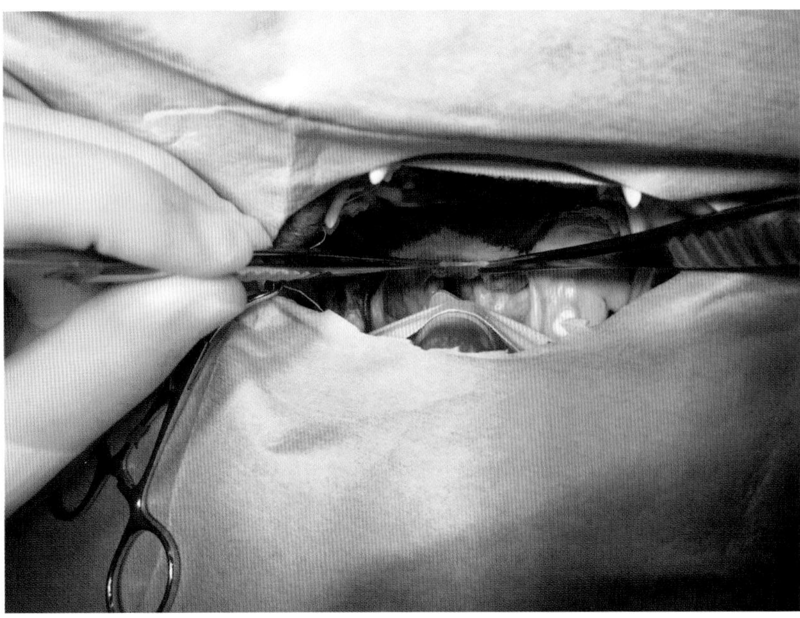

Fig. 7.37 Long DeBakey forceps used to grasp the caudal edge of the soft palate.

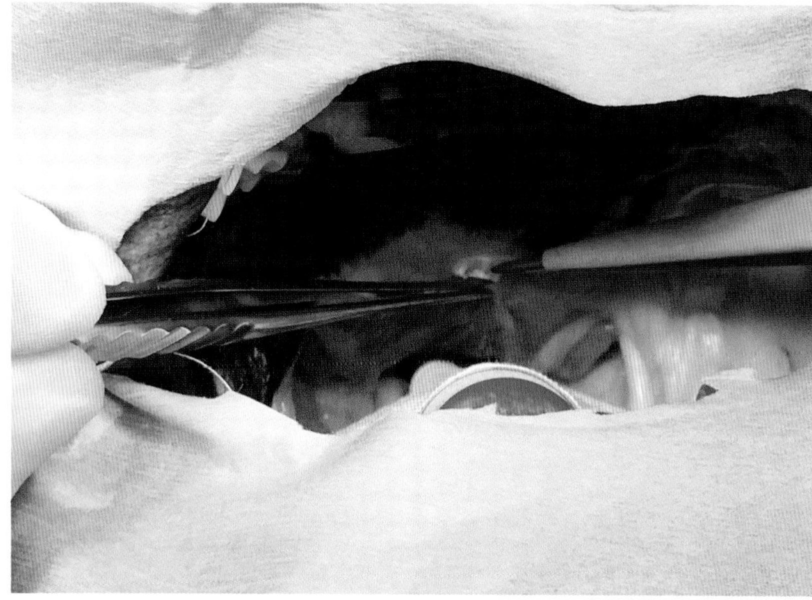

Fig. 7.38 The level at which the caudal edge of the soft palate meets the ventral mucosa of the soft palate is marked with electrocautery.

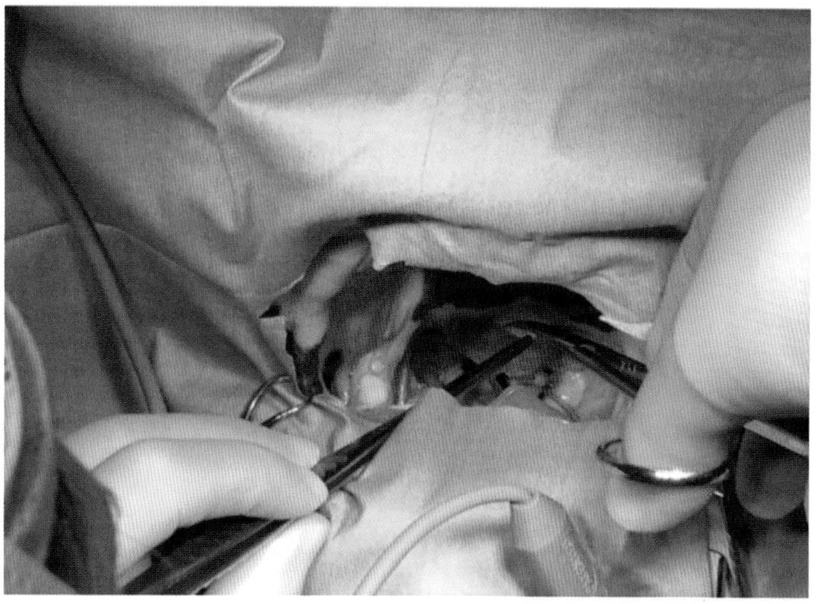

Fig. 7.39 The surgery is started at this marked position, and the ventral aspect of the soft palate is resected in a trapezoid shape.

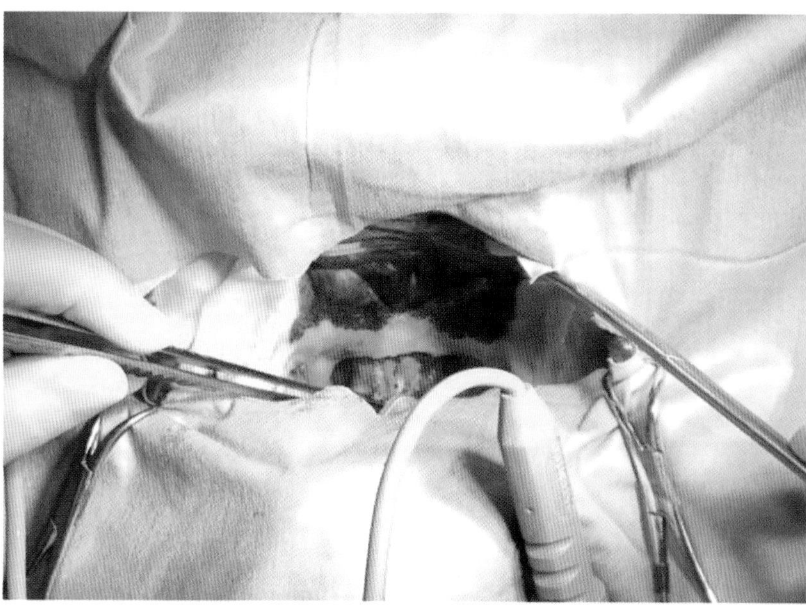

Fig. 7.40 The oral mucosa of the soft palate is resected. Here, the levator veli palatini muscles are left in situ and are easily visualised as two strap-like muscles.

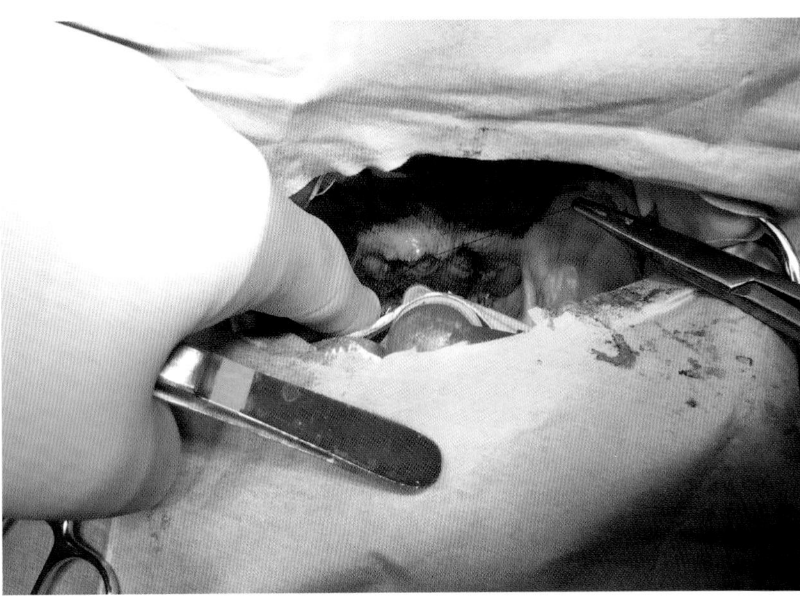

Fig. 7.41 The caudal edge of the soft palate mucosal incision is sutured to the rostral edge of the soft palate mucosal incision initially with submucosal simple interrupted sutures.

- The caudal edge of the soft palate is then retracted rostrally to the rostral edge of the trapezoidal incision and sutured with absorbable suture – initially with two submucosal simple interrupted sutures taking the initial tension (Fig. 7.41) and then with a continuous mucosal suture (Fig. 7.42).

7.3.6 Tonsillar hypertrophy

Some surgeons feel that tonsillar hypertrophy contributes to airway resistance, and tonsillectomy is therefore performed.

Step by step: tonsillectomy

- Tonsillectomy forceps are placed around the base of the tonsil, which will already be exteriorised from its tonsillar crypt due to hypertrophy.
- The tonsil is resected using a scalpel blade, and electrocautery is used to assist with haemostasis of the tonsillar artery if necessary. Absorbable suture is used in a continuous pattern to close the tonsillar mucosa (Fig. 7.43).

7.3.7 Laryngeal saccules

Everted saccules represent stage I laryngeal collapse, and can be present in up to 66% of brachycephalic breeds (Fasanella et al., 2010). The prolapsed saccules are frequently oedematous and result in ventral obstruction of the rima glottidis (Fig. 7.44). Most surgeons remove these laryngeal saccules after completion of soft palate and nares surgery. Reports describe an 88.3% improvement in respiratory signs from palatoplasty and rhinoplasty alone, without the need for sacculectomy (Poncet et al., 2006).

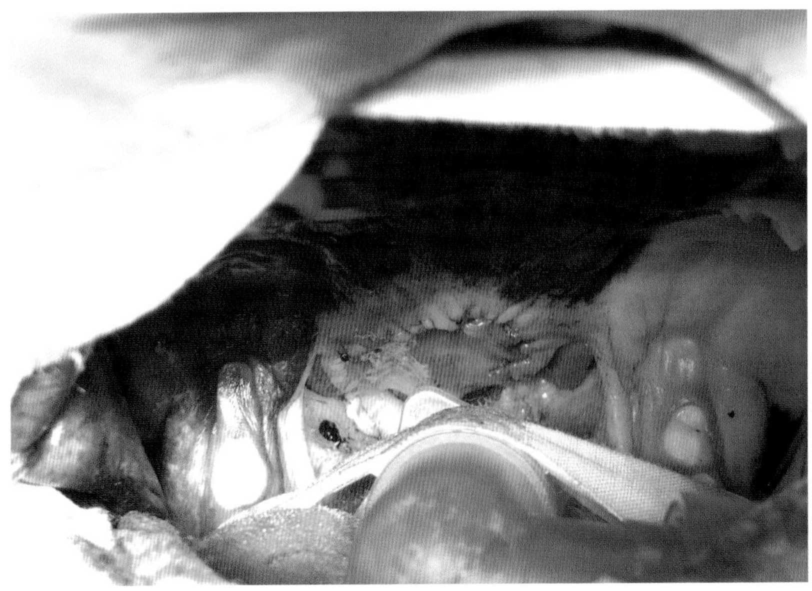

Fig. 7.42 A continuous suture pattern completes the mucosal apposition.

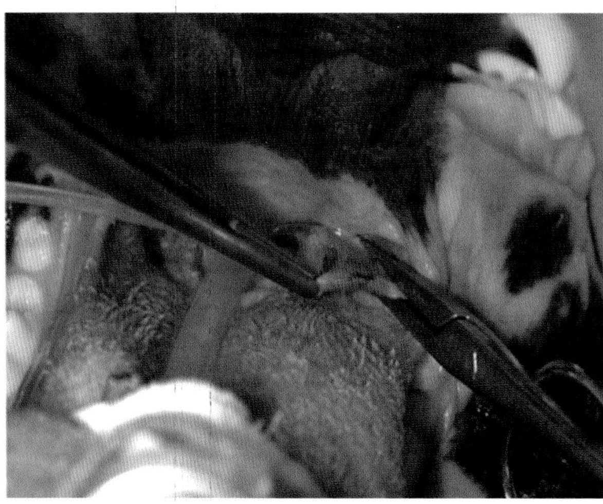

Fig. 7.43 Tonsillectomy forceps in position prior to resection of the tonsil with a scalpel blade.

Step by step: laryngeal sacculectomy

Handy hints

If the dog is to be extubated during the procedure, a clean ET tube will be required to re-intubate at the end of surgery. Grasping the saccule and visualising the base can be challenging and may take time. In this case, intravenous anaesthesia should be administered whilst providing flow-by oxygen.

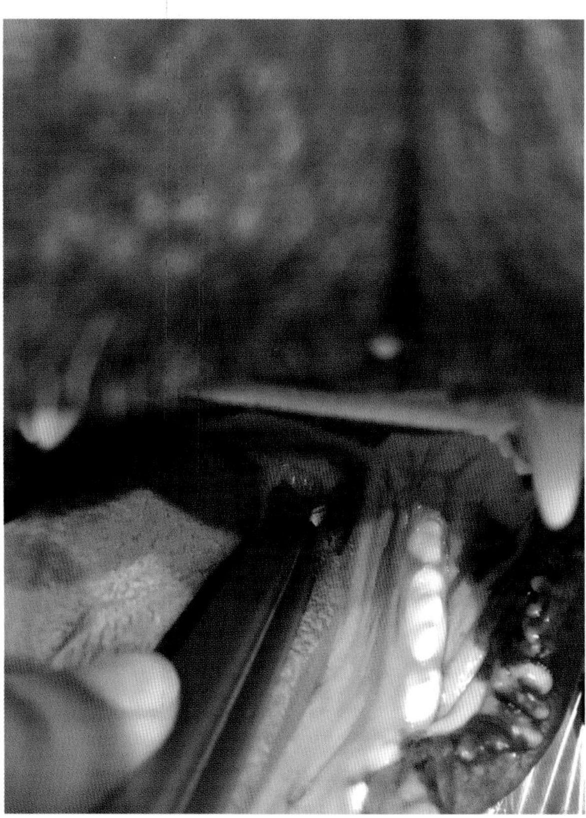

Fig. 7.44 Everted saccules: stage I laryngeal collapse.

- Extubation is often required for this procedure, although some surgeons manage to remove the everted saccules with the ET tube *in situ*.
- Removal is performed by grasping the saccules with long DeBakey forceps and amputating them at the base using Metzenbaum scissors. No suture is required.

7.3.8 Laryngeal collapse

Laryngeal collapse may be seen in animals affected by progressive, advanced secondary stage BOAS. The increased airway resistance and increased negative airway pressures result in displacement of the rostral laryngeal structures medially, with permanent cartilage deformation.

Three stages of laryngeal collapse are recognised in the dog. In stage I laryngeal collapse, eversion of the laryngeal saccules is seen. In stage II, there is loss of rigidity and medial displacement of the cuneiform processes of the arytenoid cartilage. Stage III collapse is defined as collapse of the corniculate processes of the arytenoid cartilages with loss of the dorsal arch of the rima glottidis (Leonard, 1960). All dogs with laryngeal saccule eversion therefore have stage I laryngeal collapse, with stage II and stage III describing the more severe medial deformation of the laryngeal cartilage.

We do not truly understand the relationship between the degree of laryngeal collapse, severity of clinical signs and prognosis. In dogs with stage I laryngeal collapse, sacculectomy, nasoplasty and soft palate resection has shown to significantly improve clinical signs (Torrez and Hunt, 2006). However, nasoplasty and soft palate resection alone is reported with good success (Poncet et al., 2006). It is possible that resection of the everted saccules may not significantly affect the clinical outcome in dogs with stage I laryngeal collapse. However, with an experienced surgeon, this simple and quick technique allows for immediate reduction in airway obstruction and reduction in airway resistance.

In one study comparing brachycephalic airway syndrome in French bulldogs and pugs, the grade of laryngeal collapse did not influence the grade of respiratory signs (Haimel and Dupre, 2015). Treatment based on clinical signs alone rather than the severity of laryngeal collapse is therefore required. Whilst laryngeal collapse is frequently diagnosed in brachycephalic breeds, surgical management including nasoplasty and rhinoplasty is often all that is required to reduce airway resistance and correct the negative inspiratory pressures.

In dogs displaying continuing respiratory signs as a result of stage II or III laryngeal collapse, where surgical correction of the elongated soft palate, stenotic nares and everted laryngeal saccules has not resulted in an improvement in clinical signs, further surgical intervention is required. In these severely affected cases, arytenoid lateralisation (White, 2012) or a permanent tracheostomy may be required. These are challenging cases to manage and successful outcomes are often best achieved in the referral setting.

7.3.9 Nasal conchae obstruction and laser-assisted turbinectomy (LATE)

A more recent development in the assessment of brachycephalic breeds has involved the use of CT to identify patients with excessive nasal conchae causing nasal obstruction (Schuenemann and Oechtering, 2014). The use of LATE has been described for these patients (Oechtering et al., 2016) in an attempt to reduce airway resistance. The long-term success of this surgery is yet to be truly identified, with regrowth of nasal turbinates being a potential complication (Oechtering et al., 2016).

7.3.10 Hiatal hernia

A type I hiatal hernia cannot be excluded in brachycephalic animals displaying severe or frequent episodes of regurgitation. In many cases, correction of the primary components of BOAS (nasoplasty, palatoplasty and sacculectomy) together with medical management (long-term proton pump inhibitor) results in a resolution of clinical signs. In cases where clinical signs persist, fluoroscopy may be required to confirm the diagnosis and appropriate surgery (plication of the phrenico-oesophageal ligament, oesophagopexy and gastropexy) performed. A full discussion into the diagnosis and management of hiatal hernias can be found in this volume, Chapter 3.

7.3.11 Postoperative complications and considerations

The importance of appropriate postoperative care and monitoring cannot be over-emphasised in dogs undergoing upper respiratory tract surgery. Patients may rapidly present in respiratory distress post-extubation due to laryngeal/pharyngeal swelling. Intravenous anaesthetic induction agents and endotracheal tubes should be placed next to the patient during and after recovery in case of emergency. The clinician should be well informed of the complications associated with airway surgery and should be prepared for re-intubation in the case of obstruction. An airway box should be immediately available, in the event of an emergency tracheostomy being required. The clinician should be adequately experienced to perform this emergency procedure.

Patients that have regurgitated during or even before the surgery are at higher risk of developing aspiration pneumonia. It is important to be aware of this possible complication, and antibiotic therapy ± thoracic radiographs may be warranted. Radiographic evidence of aspiration pneumonia occurs later than the clinical signs. Clinical signs of coughing and increased respiratory effort should be addressed immediately.

Whilst most brachycephalic surgeries are undertaken without complications, some patients rapidly deteriorate and require immediate surgical intervention. The surgeon's experience and facilities available to perform pre-, peri- and postoperative care are critical in achieving a positive outcome.

7.4 The larynx

Key points

- Acquired laryngeal paralysis has been shown to be part of a generalised peripheral neuropathy. Geriatric onset laryngeal paralysis polyneuropathy (GOLPP) is a more accurate term for dogs with idiopathic laryngeal paralysis.
- Inspiratory stridor, altered phonation, gagging after food/water and pelvic limb weakness are often noted in patients with laryngeal paralysis.
- Laryngoscopy is the gold standard for diagnosis.
- Surgical management of laryngeal paralysis should be performed under the same anaesthetic as laryngoscopy.
- Knowledge of the appropriate anatomy is critical in the success of this surgery, as is surgeon experience and the ability to provide perioperative care.

7.4.1 Anatomy

The larynx is attached cranially to the skull via the hyoid apparatus and caudally to the trachea by the cricoid cartilage. Figures 7.45, 7.46 and 7.47 show the anatomy of the larynx, which is structurally formed by four cartilages. The epiglottis is the most rostral cartilage. It is spade-shaped, with its apex pointing rostrally and resting on the soft palate when in normal position. Its function is to protect the airway from aspiration of food. The paired arytenoid cartilages consist of cuneiform, corniculate, vocal and muscular processes. The gap between them forms the dorsal part of the rima glottidis. The thyroid cartilage is a U-shaped cartilage forming a rigid base necessary for the movement of the other surrounding cartilages. Finally, the cricoid cartilage is a ring-shaped cartilage and is the most rigid of all, supporting the thyroid and arytenoids which articulate

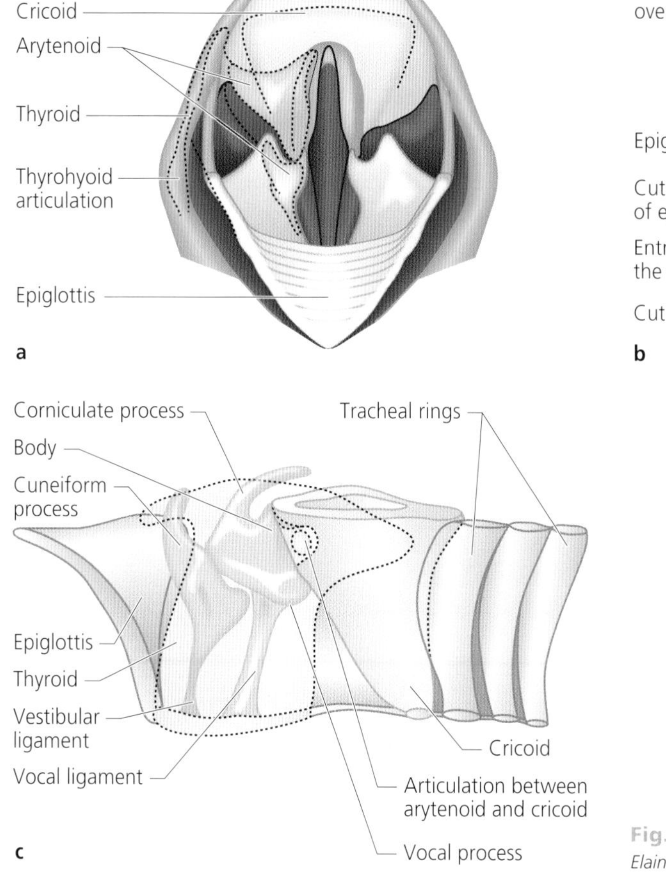

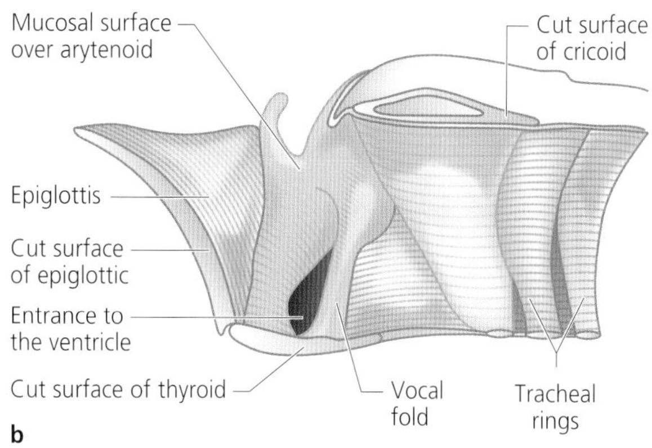

Fig. 7.45 The cartilaginous structure of the larynx. *Illustrator: Elaine Leggett*

with it. The main articulations of the larynx are the cricothyroid articulation, the cricoarytenoid articulation and the inter-arytenoid sesamoid band, which hinges the dorsal part of each arytenoid cartilage. The vocal ligaments originate from the ventral portion of the arytenoids and meet at the internal midline of the thyroid cartilage, forming the core of the vocal folds and the ventral part of the rima glottidis.

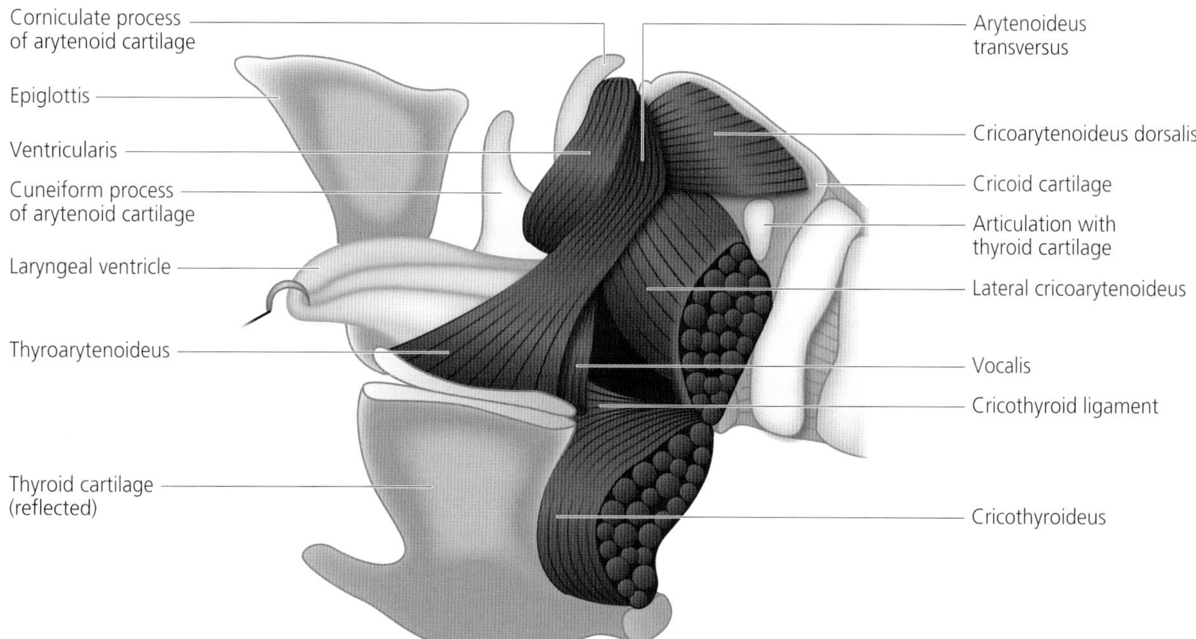

Fig. 7.46 The intrinsic muscles of the larynx. *Illustrator: Elaine Leggett*

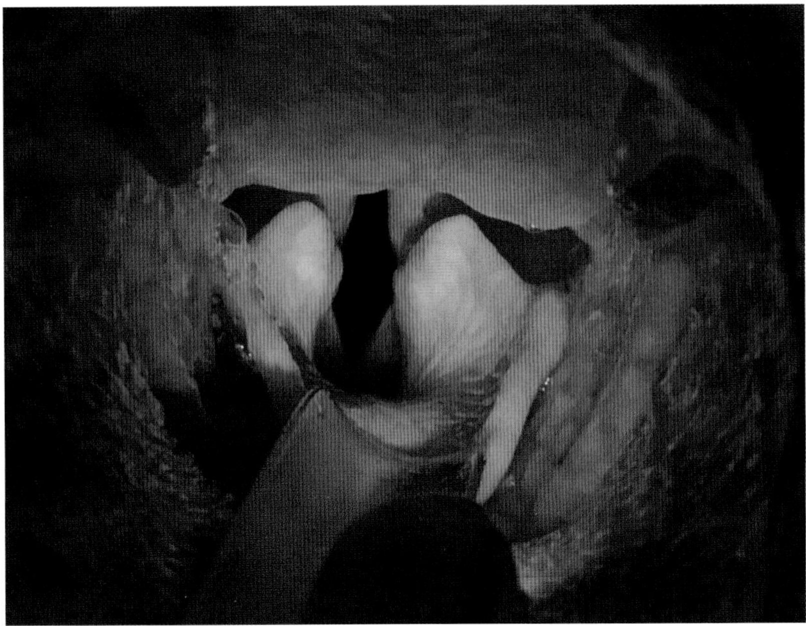

Fig. 7.47 Intra-oral view of the larynx showing the paired arytenoid cartilages. The laryngoscope here is depressing the epiglottis.

Both intrinsic and extrinsic muscles can be identified within the larynx. The intrinsic muscles are responsible for laryngeal function. The most important muscle is the dorsal cricoarytenoid muscle, which is responsible for abducting the arytenoid cartilage to open the glottis. This muscle arises from the dorsolateral surface of the cricoid cartilage and inserts on the muscular process of the arytenoid. Often, the dorsal cricoarytenoid muscle is atrophied in dogs with laryngeal paralysis. The caudal laryngeal nerve provides innervation to all the muscles of the larynx except the cricothyroid muscle.

7.4.2 Function of the larynx

The larynx has three functions. First, during swallowing, the larynx and hyoid apparatus are pulled cranially, bringing the rima glottidis under the epiglottis to block the laryngeal opening. Second, the larynx is responsible for controlling airway resistance; abduction of arytenoid cartilages during inspiration decreases airway resistance. Finally, the larynx is responsible for voice production by changing tension on the vocal cords. In cats, rapid narrowing and widening of the glottis by the laryngeal muscles and fast twitching of the diaphragm cause vibrations of the respiratory air that result in purring.

7.4.3 Laryngeal paralysis

There are two forms of laryngeal paralysis; congenital and acquired. Congenital laryngeal paralysis is the less common form and has been reported in a number of large pure breeds including Dalmatians, bull terriers, Rottweilers, Siberian huskies and Bouvier des Flandres. In the Siberian huskies, laryngeal paralysis starts as a progressive degeneration of neurons within the nucleus ambiguous in the medulla of the brain, with subsequent Wallerian degeneration of the laryngeal nerves. The onset of clinical signs in dogs with congenital laryngeal paralysis is usually before one year of age.

Acquired laryngeal paralysis is the most common form and mainly affects large- and giant-breed dogs, particularly Labrador retrievers, golden retrievers, St Bernards and Irish setters. The average age at the time of presentation is approximately 10 years. Acquired laryngeal paralysis may result from trauma or iatrogenic injury to the recurrent laryngeal nerve (e.g. during thyroidectomy) or compression of the recurrent laryngeal nerve by a cranial mediastinal or cervical mass. It has also been inconsistently associated with hypothyroidism and myasthenia gravis. More commonly, however, acquired laryngeal paralysis is classified as idiopathic and has been shown to be part of a generalised peripheral neuropathy (Jeffery et al., 2006). In a study assessing 11 dogs with laryngeal paralysis, biopsies performed on the cranial tibial muscle showed neurogenic atrophy with concurrent axonal degeneration of the peroneal nerve suggesting evidence of a more generalised neurological disease (Thieman et al., 2010).

The abbreviation GOLPP has been proposed as a more accurate term for dogs with idiopathic laryngeal paralysis (Stanley et al., 2010). Fluoroscopic assessment of oesophageal function in dogs with laryngeal paralysis showed that all individuals with laryngeal paralysis had some degree of oesophageal dysfunction (Stanley et al., 2010). On concurrent neurological examination of these dogs, 31% showed evidence of generalised neurological disease at the time of examination whilst 100% went on to develop generalised neurological

is often determined by the frequency of build-up of mucous/fluid. Some clinicians will suction the tube regularly every 4 hours, whilst others chose only to do so if a noticeable change in noise is noted during inspiration as a result of a mucus/fluid build-up. Changing of the tube once daily is often performed; pulling the proximal and distal sutures assists in opening the tracheostomy hole.

Removal of the tube is performed when there is resolution of the inciting event. It is best to occlude the tube first for 10–15 minutes whilst observing the patient's breathing. If no change in the breathing pattern or effort is noted during occlusion of the tube, removal can be performed. The tube is removed simply by gentle traction and the tracheostomy wounds are left to heal by second intention, usually achieved by 7–10 days.

A high complication rate of 86% has been reported with the use of temporary tracheostomy tubes (Nicholson and Baines, 2012). Reported complications include pneumomediastinum, obstruction of the tube or airway, dislodgement of the tube and aspiration pneumonia, with bulldogs being more likely to dislodge the tube. Despite a high complication rate being reported, a good outcome was achieved in most dogs. In summary, the placement of these tubes is relatively straightforward, although the requirement for their careful management following placement should not be overlooked.

7.5.4 Permanent tracheostomy

Indications for a permanent tracheostomy include permanent laryngeal obstruction, including a laryngeal mass or laryngeal collapse.

Step by step: permanent tracheostomy

Handy hints

A fine instrument set, if available, can be useful when dissecting the tracheal cartilages from the tracheal mucosa.

- A ventral cervical midline approach through the skin and subcutaneous tissues is made, and the sternohyoid muscles are separated at their midline to expose the ventral trachea.
- The sternohyoid muscle is apposed dorsally to the trachea, using mattress sutures to help elevate the trachea closer to the skin. This is achieved via placement of a suture through the sternohyoid muscle. The suture is then passed dorsally around the trachea (this can be a little tricky depending on the curvature of the needle) and finally the suture is passed through the contralateral sternohyoid muscle. The needle is reversed and the process repeated, creating a mattress suture. On tying the suture, the sternohyoid muscle is elevated dorsally and the trachea nicely exposed (Fig. 7.56).
- The ventral half of the cartilage of three or four rings is removed using a no. 11 blade. Ideally, the mucosa of the trachea is left intact whilst removing this cartilage.

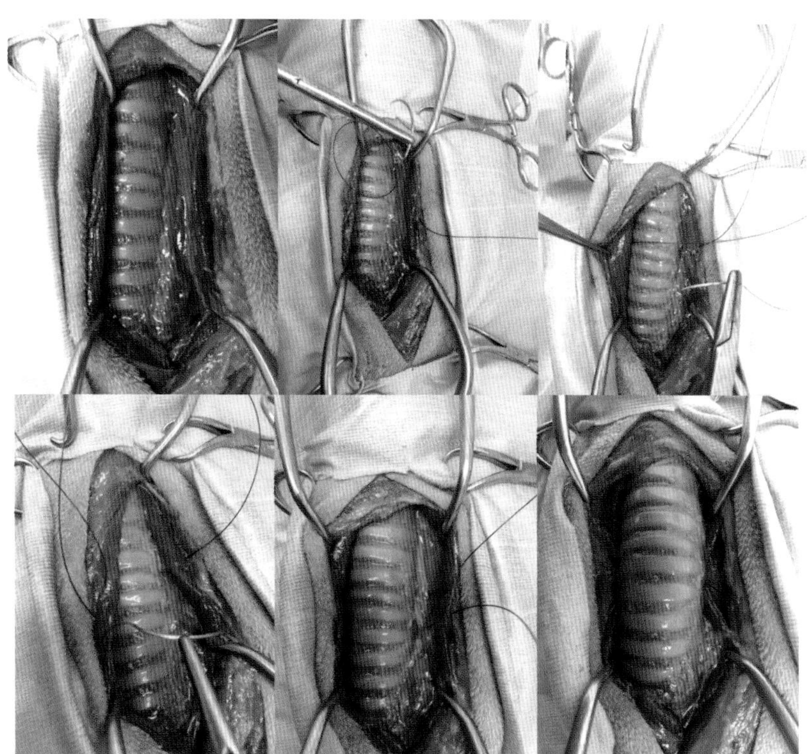

Fig. 7.56 Cadaver dissection showing mattress suture placement through the sternohyoid, dorsal to the trachea. Top left: paired sternohyoid muscles visible. Top middle: suture placed through the sternohyoid muscle. Top right: suture placement dorsal to the trachea. Bottom left: the needle is reversed and suture passed again through the sternohyoid muscle. Bottom middle: the suture has been placed ventral to the trachea again and back through the sternohyoid. Bottom right: once the mattress suture is tied, the sternohyoid muscle is pulled or 'nipped in' dorsal to the trachea, causing slight elevation in the trachea. The excessive dissection of the trachea in this cadaver is for illustrative purpose only and is not necessary when performing a permanent tracheostomy.

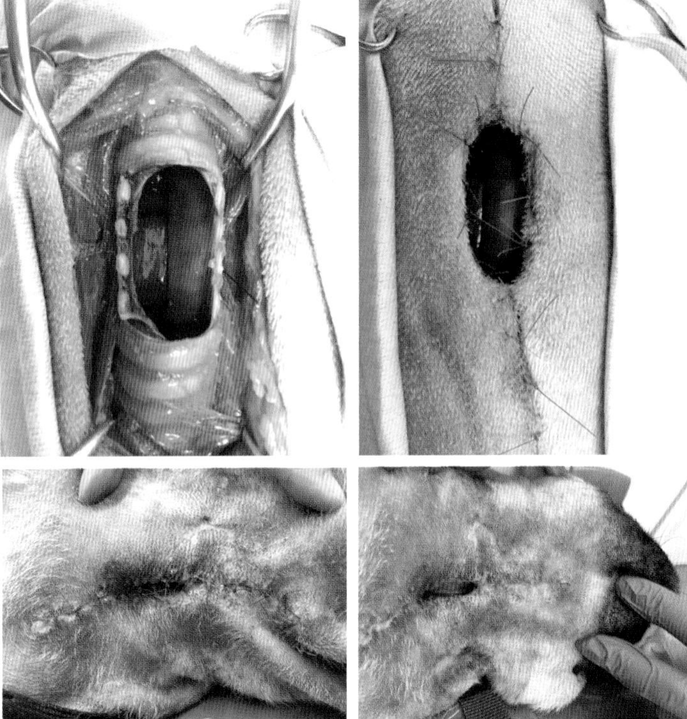

Fig. 7.57 Top left: cadaver dissection showing resection of the ventral aspect of four tracheal rings. Top right: cadaver dissection showing direct apposition of tracheal mucosa to skin using simple interrupted non-absorbable sutures. Bottom left: ten days post-surgery in a pug prior to suture removal. Bottom right: ten days post-surgery in a pug, post-suture removal. The excessive dissection of the trachea in this cadaver is for illustrative purpose only and is not necessary when performing a permanent tracheostomy.

- The mucosa is then incised separately in an 'H'-shaped incision and the tracheal mucosa reflected laterally towards the skin. This can, however, be challenging and often the mucosa is inadvertently incised whilst removing the cartilage.
- A simple interrupted suture pattern of 1.5 metric non-absorbable suture is used to appose the mucosa to the skin. Suture bites are placed approximately 2 mm apart (Fig. 7.57).

Complications of permanent tracheostomy include formation of mucus plugs, stenosis of the stoma site (if the stoma site is made too small), granulation tissue and collapse of the trachea (if the stoma site is made too large). Stoma management is important, and owners should be well informed of this. In some patients, it may be necessary to clip the hair around the stoma site to prevent obstruction of the stoma and irritation of the tracheal mucosa. Animals will need to wear a harness rather than a neck lead, and swimming should be avoided. In some animals, a second surgery may be required to remove any excess skin folds around the neck that are obstructing the stoma site. Whilst this is a simple surgery involving resection of skin alone, judgement of how much skin to resect and where to resect can be challenging. This surgery can be performed under the same anaesthetic as the permanent tracheostomy. However, at surgery, the patient is positioned in dorsal recumbency and the effect of gravity on the skin folds can prevent accurate assessment of the amount of skin to be resected. Assessing the animal when awake and walking is often more accurate. Temporary stay sutures in the skin around the neck can be placed following permanent tracheostomy surgery. Umbilical tape placed dorsally to the neck and through these stay sutures can assist in temporarily moving the excess skin away from the stoma site.

7.5.5 Tracheal collapse

Tracheal collapse is a progressive, irreversible condition of the lower airways, commonly associated with a 'goose honk' cough. Degeneration of the tracheal cartilage rings occurs, leading to a dorsoventral flattening of the trachea and laxity of the dorsal tracheal membrane. Dogs with tracheal collapse have reduced glycosaminoglycan, glycoprotein and chondroitin sulphate content of the hyaline cartilage, resulting in reduced water content of the cartilage (Dallman et al., 1988). Secondary factors involved in the development of clinical signs include airway irritants, chronic bronchitis, laryngeal paralysis, respiratory tract infection, obesity and tracheal inflammation (Maggiore, 2014). Tracheal collapse can be localised to either the cervical or thoracic trachea or can be generalised. Concurrent bronchomalacia is also reported in dogs with tracheal collapse, most commonly seen in the right middle and left cranial bronchi (Moritz et al., 2004).

Tracheal collapse is commonly reported in toy and small-breed dogs, including the Yorkshire terrier, miniature poodle, Chihuahua, Pomeranian and pug. As many as 25% of affected dogs are symptomatic by

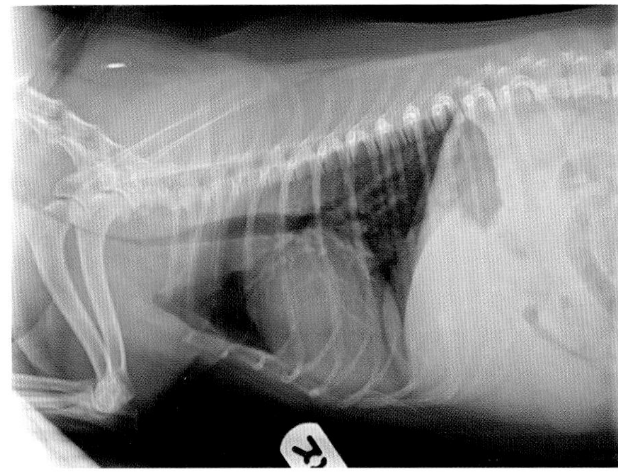

Fig. 7.58 Right lateral thoracic radiograph showing collapse of the cervical and cranial thoracic trachea.

approximately 6 months, although the majority remain asymptomatic until later in life. Dogs with tracheal collapse present with a dry, harsh cough, often triggered by excitement or exercise. They can also present with tachypnoea, respiratory distress, exercise intolerance, cyanosis and syncope.

Thoracic and cervical radiography (Fig. 7.58) should be used with caution in the diagnosis of tracheal collapse. As tracheal collapse is a dynamic process, not all cases will be diagnosed by radiography alone. Both inspiratory and expiratory lateral and dorsoventral radiographs should be taken, to increase the chance of demonstrating collapse. If available, fluoroscopy would be advantageous in capturing the entire respiratory phase, therefore increasing accuracy of diagnosis. Bronchoscopy has been considered the gold standard diagnostic tool. Direct observation allows classification of the severity and examination of the bronchi. A bronchoalveolar lavage (BAL) can also be performed. Tracheal collapse is graded from I to IV (Fig. 7.59; Tangner and Hobson, 1982). A 25, 50, 75 and 100% loss of luminal diameter is identified with grade I, II, III and IV tracheal collapse, respectively.

Treatment

Control of the environmental and secondary aspects of tracheal collapse is crucial to management. This includes control of obesity, inhaled irritants, respiratory infection and congestive heart failure. The use of a harness rather than a neck collar is also advised.

Approximately 71–93% of cases of tracheal collapse respond well to medical management (White and Williams, 1994). Antitussive therapy includes diphenoxylate hydrochloride and atropine (Lomotil, Amdipharm Mercury; 0.2–0.5 mg/kg BID), and butorphanol (0.5–1 mg/kg BID–QID). Glucocorticoid therapy may also be used, with caution. This is administered as either a tapering low-dose prednisolone (0.5 mg/kg PO BID) or an inhalational steroid such as fluticasone (125–250 g BID). Bronchodilators, such as theophylline (15–20 mg/kg BID–SID), may also be beneficial (Tappin, 2016).

Surgery is indicated for those cases that do not respond well to any form of medical management and environmental control. It is important to assess the trachea thoroughly prior to surgery for the presence of infection, bronchus collapse and congestive heart failure. All these would be contraindications to surgery. It is important to understand that no surgical procedure will cure tracheal collapse, and continued medical management in conjunction with surgical management is often needed. Patient selection is critical. Only dogs with severe collapse (grade II and higher) should be considered for surgery (Sun et al., 2008).

Both extra- and intra-luminal prostheses are available for surgical management of tracheal collapse. The former involves placement of external prosthetic support to the collapsing portion of the trachea using polypropylene rings or spirals (Fig. 7.60). C-shaped prostheses are placed via a ventral midline approach to the trachea, avoiding the thyroid arteries and recurrent laryngeal nerve. Complications associated with extraluminal tracheal rings are noted frequently and include laryngeal paralysis (due to iatrogenic nerve damage), tracheal necrosis, pneumonia, infection, coughing, dyspnoea and loosening/migration of implants. A survival time of 4 years and 6 months following placement of extra-luminal tracheal rings has been reported (Becker et al., 2012). In that study, there was no difference in survival of patients that had intrathoracic

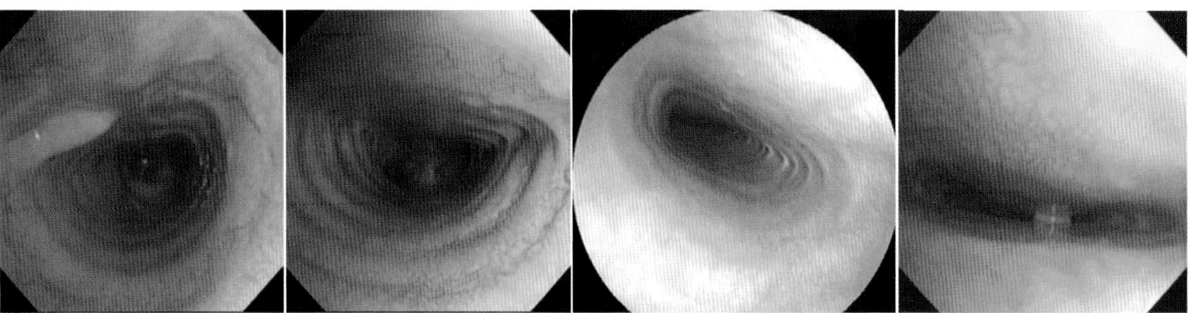

Fig. 7.59 Bronchoscopic images of grades I–IV (left to right) tracheal collapse. (From Tappin (2016); reprinted with permission.)

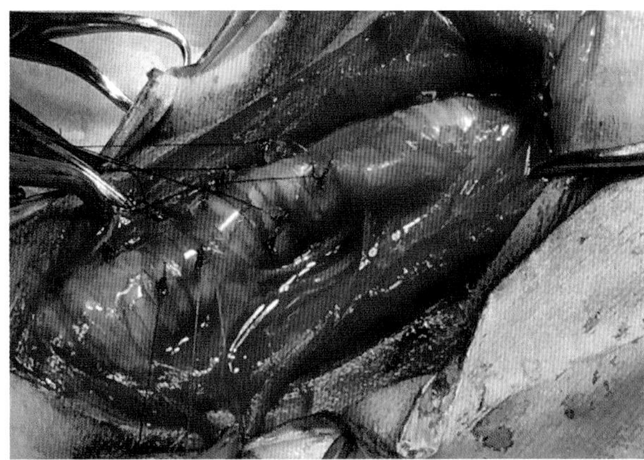

Fig. 7.60 Extra-luminal polypropylene ring placement for surgical management of tracheal collapse. (Image courtesy of Dr Carolyn Burton.)

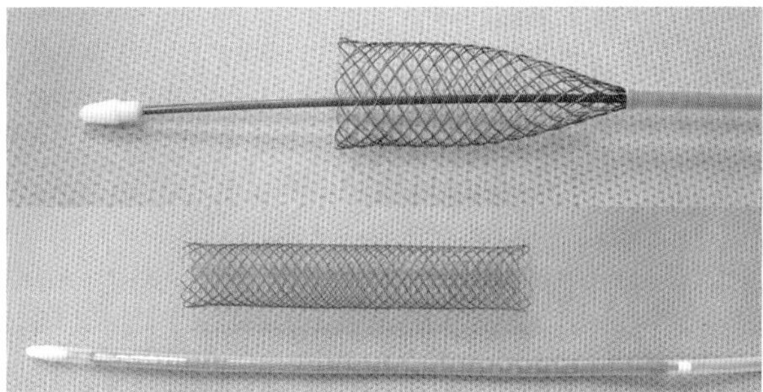

Fig. 7.61 Self-expanding nitinol stent. (From Tappin (2016); reprinted with permission.)

tracheal collapse vs cervical tracheal collapse. With an intra-luminal prosthesis, self-expanding stents, most commonly nitinol (made from nickel and titanium), are inserted under fluoroscopic guidance directly into tracheal lumen (Figs. 7.61, 7.62). The stents become fully integrated and covered with tracheal mucosa (Fig. 7.63). Correct sizing of the stents in terms of length and diameter is critical. Sizing of tracheal stents is achieved through thoracic radiography performed under peak inflation pressure of 20 cm of water. A marker catheter is placed in the oesophagus allowing a measurement to be taken. The tracheal stent should ideally be positioned 10 mm caudal to the cricoid cartilage and 10 mm cranial to the tracheal bifurcation. A phenomenon known as 'stent shortening' is noted when placing tracheal stents. To allow for this, stents are selected with a diameter 10–20% wider than measured on the radiograph, preventing shortening when the stents expand during placement. With stents that are too small, migration can occur. Overlarge stents can cause pressure necrosis. Similar to the extra-luminal prosthetic rings, stent placement does not cure tracheal collapse; continued long-term medical management is required. Complications associated with stent placement include selection of the wrong size of stent, fracture of the stent and continued coughing and formation of excessive granulation tissue within the tracheal lumen (associated with excessive movement of the stent).

In summary, extra- or intra-luminal prosthesis are reserved for only the most severe cases of tracheal collapse that are unresponsive to medical management. In up to 93% of cases, medical management alone can result in a successful outcome (White and Williams, 1994).

7.5.6 Tracheal trauma/tear

External injuries to the trachea include blunt penetrating traumas, for example bites, choke chains or road traffic accidents. Over-inflation of an endotracheal cuff during endotracheal intubation can also cause ischaemic necrosis of the tracheal mucosa.

Diagnosis of a tracheal tear is often achieved through cervical and thoracic radiography. The precise location of the tear can be identified through tracheoscopy. Tracheal tears often result in a pneumomediastinum and subcutaneous emphysema (Fig. 7.64). Small lacerations may resolve without intervention, but larger lacerations will require surgery (Fig. 7.65). It is important to decide whether a portion of the traumatised trachea needs to be resected or whether debridement and primary repair is possible. If resection is not required, the cartilage and mucosa are debrided and realigned and sutured with monofilament absorbable suture. If greater than 35% of the tracheal circumference is denuded of mucosa, then resection and anastomosis should be considered.

Anaesthesia management prior to surgery should be considered. With cervical tears, the endotracheal tube can often be passed beyond the tracheal tear and surgery can be performed with the endotracheal tube *in situ*. Should resection and anastomosis be required, a sterile endotracheal tube will need to be placed into the trachea by the surgeon through the site of resection and anastomosis at the time of surgery. In cases such as tracheal resection, the biggest challenge is often the pre-, peri- and postoperative management performed by the anaesthesia team. To maximise the success of these challenging cases, referral to a specialist centre may be indicated.

Step by step: primary repair of a cervical tracheal tear

- A ventral cervical midline approach through the skin and subcutaneous tissues is made, and the sternohyoid muscles are separated at their midline to expose the ventral trachea and the tracheal tear.
- Monofilament sutures are pre-placed around the cartilage ring proximal and distal to the tear (Fig. 7.65).

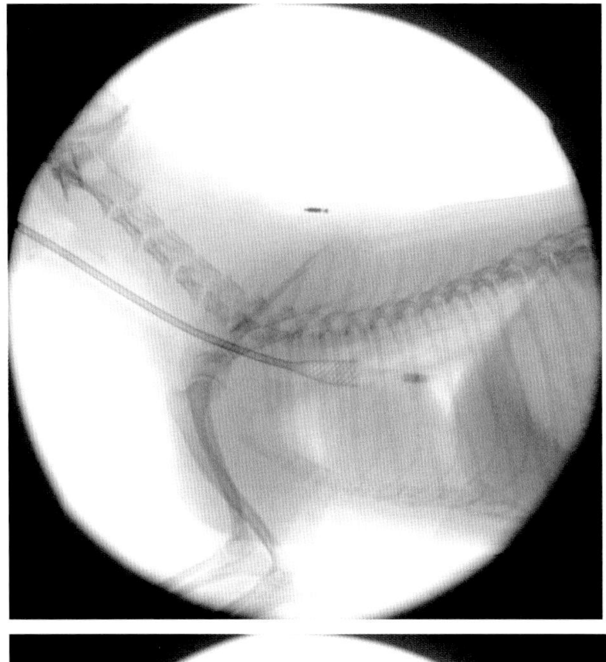

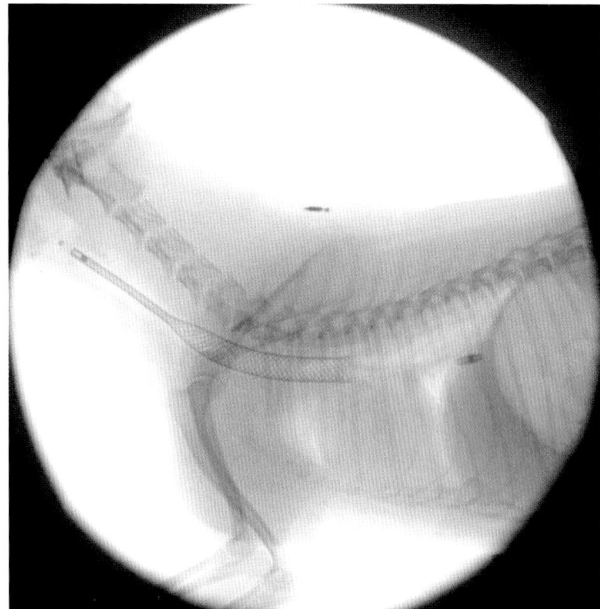

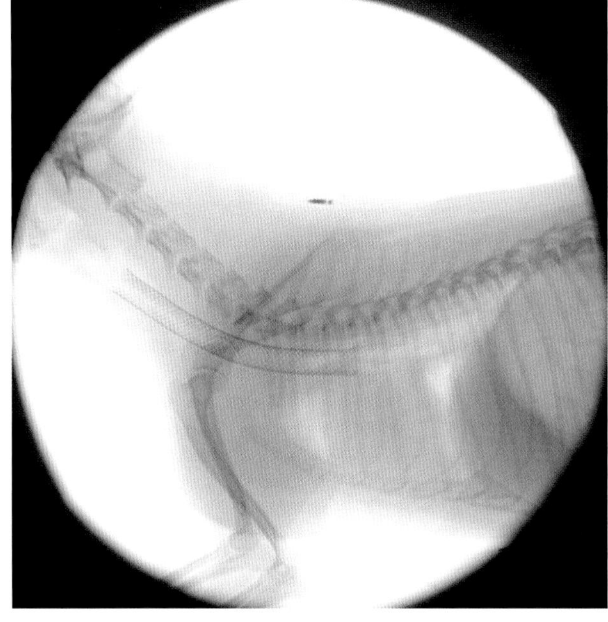

Fig. 7.62 Insertion of the self-expanding nitinol stent into the trachea under fluoroscopy. (From Tappin (2016); reprinted with permission.)

Care should be taken not to penetrate the endotracheal tube during suture placement.

- Only once all the sutures have been pre-placed are they tied.

7.5.7 Tracheal stenosis

Tracheal stenosis is usually a complication of tracheal surgery, endotracheal tube pressure or trauma. Treatment can include bougienage, laser excision of webs, stenting and resection and anastomosis. However, it may not be appropriate to perform resection/anastomosis on a trachea that has already had previous anastomosis surgery. Referral would be advised for these challenging cases.

7.5.8 Tracheal avulsion and pseudo-airway

Intrathoracic tracheal rupture can result in formation of a pseudo-airway. The rupture heals by second-intention healing, and granulation tissue and fibrosis become

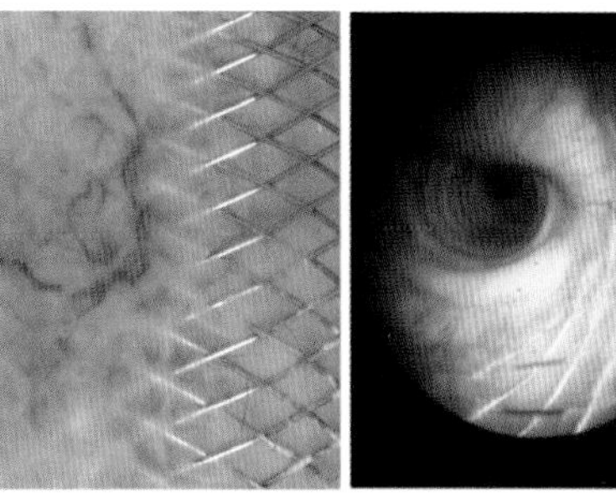

Fig. 7.63 An integrated tracheal stent covered by tracheal mucosa.

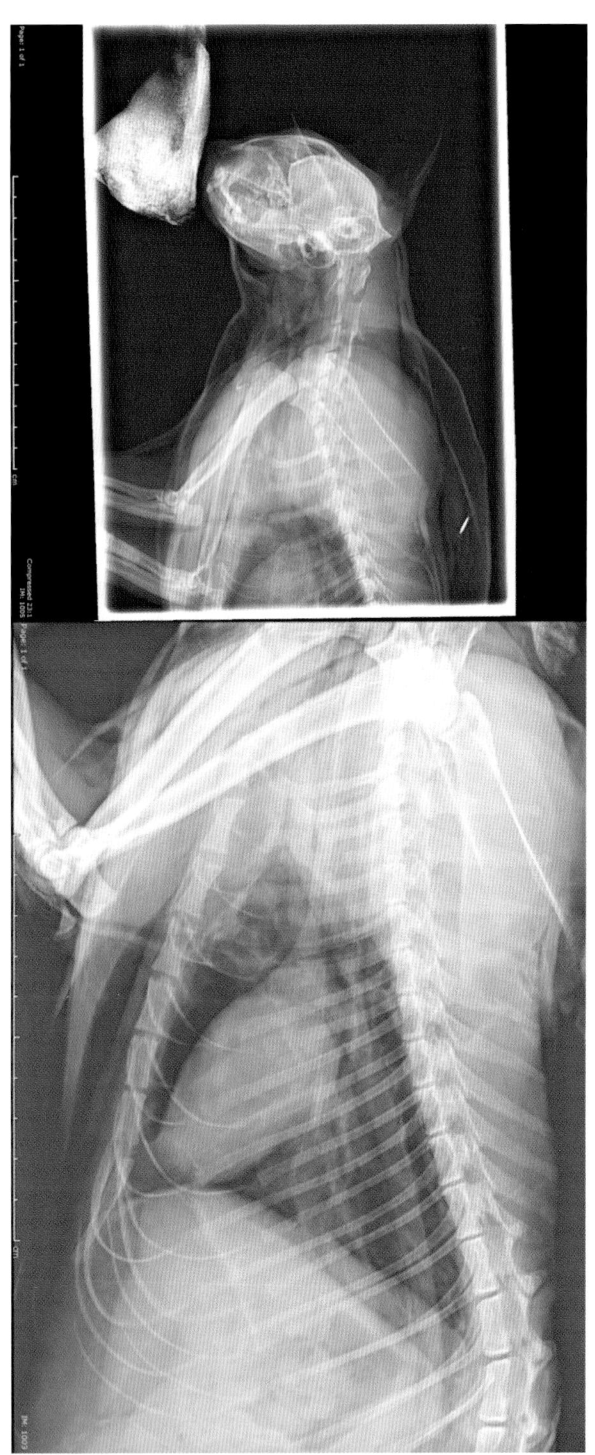

Fig. 7.64 Lateral cervical and lateral thoracic radiographs of a cat showing pneumomediastinum and subcutaneous emphysema as a result of a cervical tracheal tear. These radiographs were taken with the cat conscious and restrained with sandbags.

evident. Intrathoracic tracheal resection and anastomosis is required for treatment.

7.5.9 Tracheal foreign bodies

Although tracheal foreign bodies are uncommon, it is important to be aware of their management. Maintenance of an adequate oxygen supply can be challenging, and a male canine urinary catheter may be useful in bypassing the foreign body in order to supply oxygen. In situations where long, grabbing forceps have failed to remove the foreign body, inflation of a Foley catheter distal to the foreign body and subsequent dislodgement whilst pulling proximally may help. Fluoroscopically assisted removal of tracheal foreign bodies has also been reported.

7.5.10 Tracheal neoplasia

Tracheal neoplasms are rare in the dog and cat. Reported primary tumours include osteochondroma, osteosarcoma, chondroma, chondrosarcoma, leiomyoma, extramedullary plasmacytoma, mast cell tumour, adenocarcinoma, lymphoma and squamous cell carcinoma (Withrow, 2013). Clinical signs are consistent with airway obstruction, including cough, dyspnoea and collapse. Treatment recommendations and prognosis depend on tumour type. Tracheobronchoscopy is helpful in obtaining biopsy samples for diagnosis and for debulking tumours obstructing the airway. Resection with anastomosis is typically the treatment of choice for obstructive, solitary lesions, with lymphoma being a notable exception. Benign tracheal tumours include granulomatous disease from *Onchocerca* spp. and *Spirocerca lupi*. Management of these challenging cases may be best achieved in the referral setting.

7.5.11 Tracheal resection and anastomosis

The amount of trachea that can be resected depends mainly on the age of the patient and therefore the rigidity of the trachea. Tension at the anastomosis site is the most challenging intra-operative hurdle, and judgement as to how much trachea can be successfully resected is gained with experience. Tension can be partially alleviated by cautiously freeing up the trachea cranially and caudally and by using tension sutures. Tension sutures are placed as circumferential sutures from approximately two tracheal rings proximal and two tracheal rings distal to the anastomosis site. These sutures take the tension off the primary repair. One must be cautious regarding the segmental blood supply of the trachea, as damage to this can cause tracheal necrosis. The primary repair is sutured with a series of appositional sutures which are pre-placed around the circumference of the trachea before tying (Figs. 7.66, 7.67, 7.68). Depending on the location of the pathology, tracheal resection and anastomosis can be performed in both the cervical and thoracic trachea. A fully trained anaesthesia and surgical team are required for these surgeries.

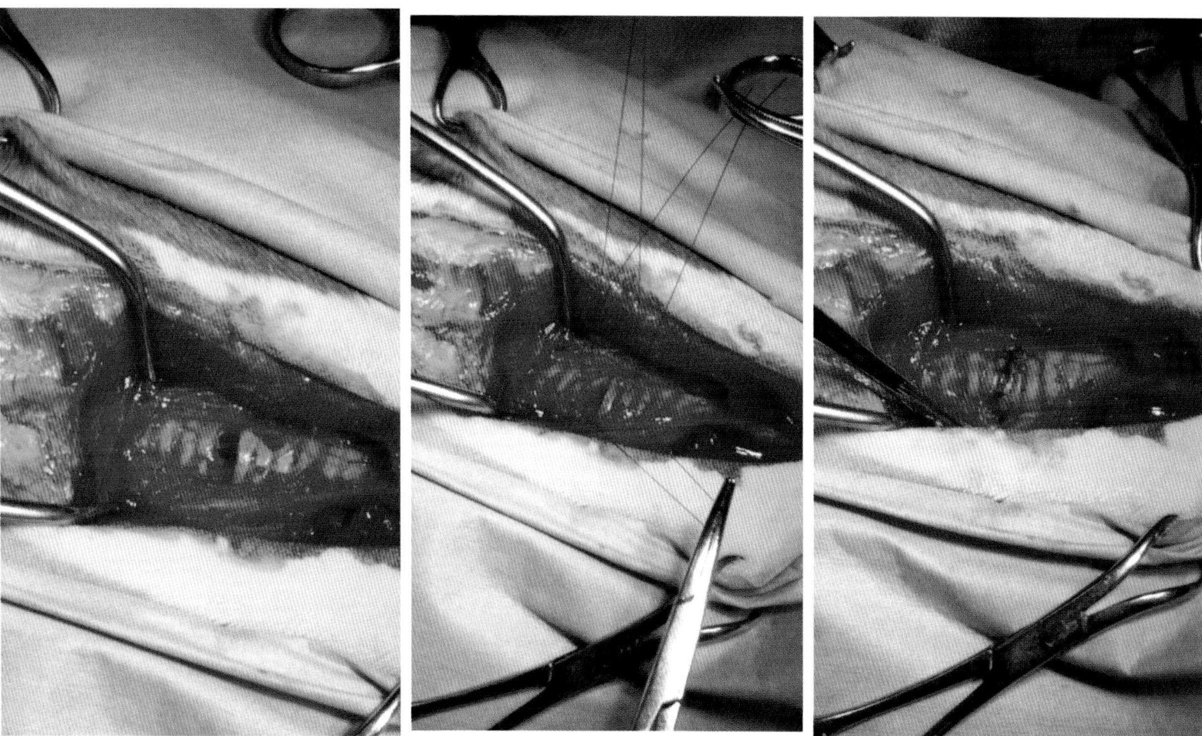

Fig. 7.65 Intra-operative photograph of a cervical tracheal tear in a cat. The tear is sutured with pre-placed simple interrupted absorbable sutures around the most proximal and most distal cartilage ring.

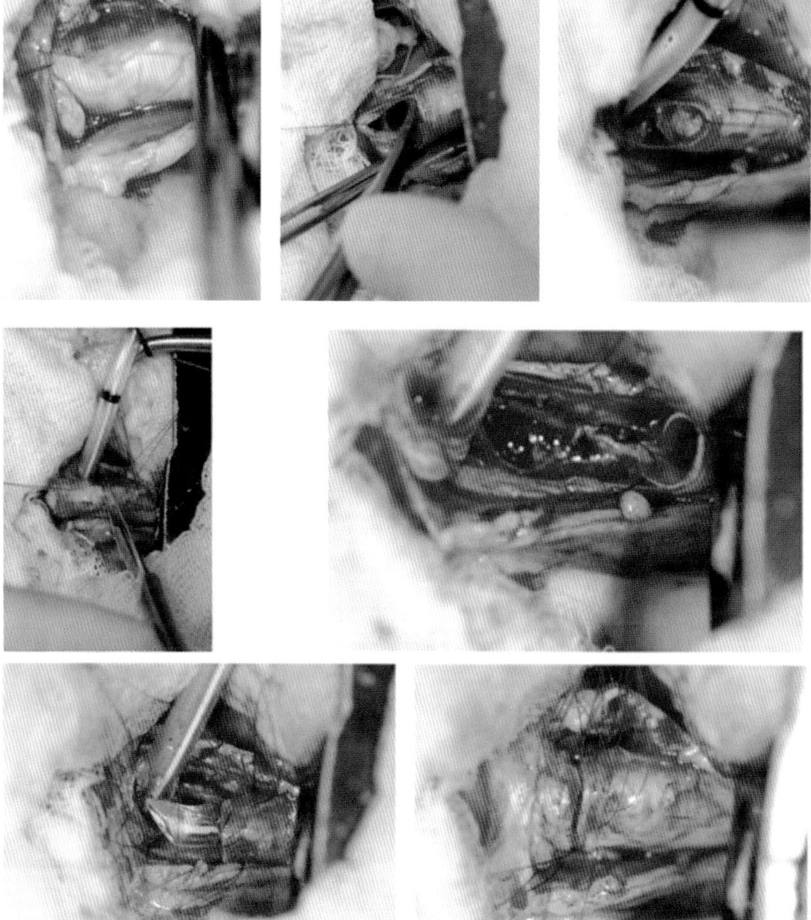

Fig. 7.66 Left: right 4th intercostal thoracotomy with ligation of the azygos vein and incision into the mediastinum to locate the thoracic trachea. Middle: a stay suture is placed two tracheal rings distal to the site of pathology (in this case a tracheal squamous cell carcinoma) and an incision is made into the trachea. Right: a sterile endotracheal tube is placed intra-operatively to maintain a patent airway. (Images courtesy of Dr Carolyn Burton.)

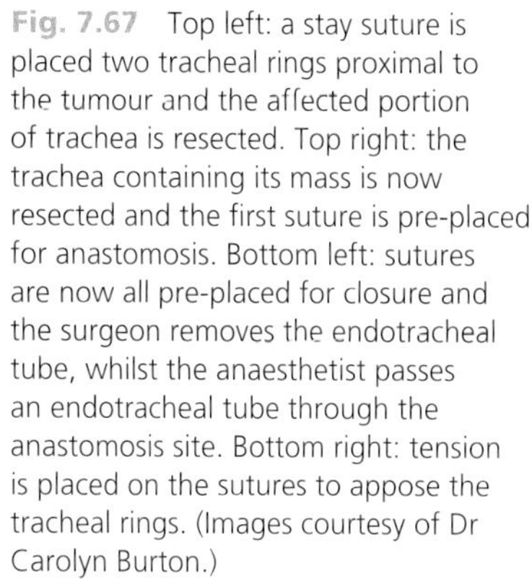

Fig. 7.67 Top left: a stay suture is placed two tracheal rings proximal to the tumour and the affected portion of trachea is resected. Top right: the trachea containing its mass is now resected and the first suture is pre-placed for anastomosis. Bottom left: sutures are now all pre-placed for closure and the surgeon removes the endotracheal tube, whilst the anaesthetist passes an endotracheal tube through the anastomosis site. Bottom right: tension is placed on the sutures to appose the tracheal rings. (Images courtesy of Dr Carolyn Burton.)

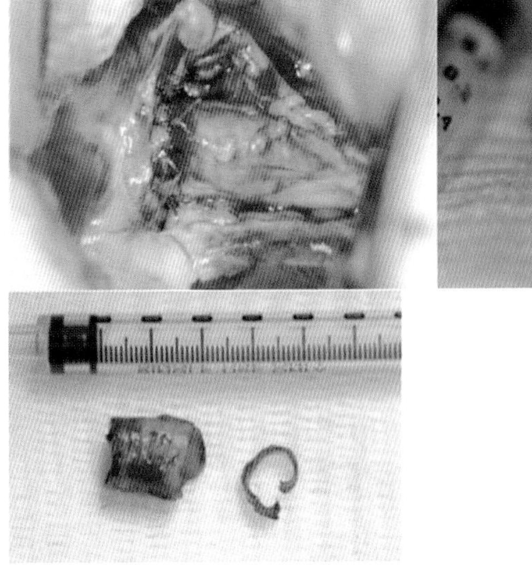
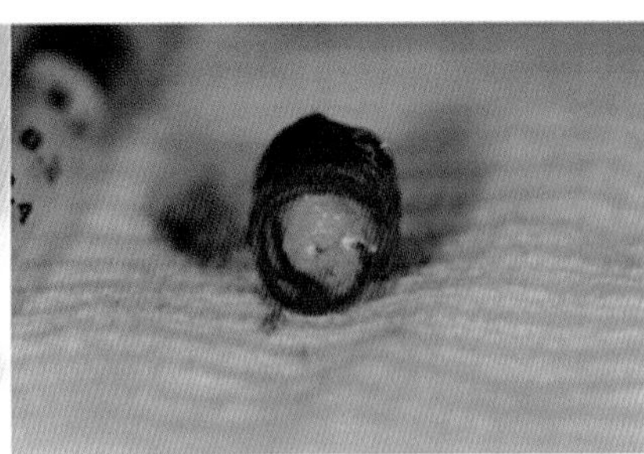

Fig.7.68 Top left: the sutures are tied and the anastomosis is complete. Top right and bottom: the resected trachea containing the squamous cell carcinoma. (Images courtesy of Dr Carolyn Burton.)

References

Adams, W.M., Bjorling, D.E., McAnulty, J.E., Green, E.M., Forrest, L.J. and Vail, D.M. (2005) Outcome of accelerated radiotherapy alone or accelerated radiotherapy followed by exenteration of the nasal cavity in dogs with intranasal neoplasia: 53 cases (1990–2002). *Journal of the American Veterinary Medical Association* 227, 936–941.

Adams, W.M., Miller, P.E., Vail, D.M., Forrest, L.J. and MacEwen, E.G. (1998) An accelerated technique for irradiation of malignant canine nasal and paranasal sinus tumours. *Veterinary Radiology & Ultrasound* 39, 475–481.

Barrs, V.R. and Talbot, J.J. (2014) Feline aspergillosis. *Veterinary Clinics of North America: Small Animal Practice* 44, 51–73.

Becker, W.M., Beal, M., Stanley, B.J. and Hauptman, J.G. (2012) Survival after surgery for tracheal collapse and the effect of intrathoracic collapse on survival. *Veterinary Surgery* 41, 501–506.

Bexfield, N.H., Stell, A.J., Gear, R.N. and Dobson, J.M. (2008) Photodynamic therapy of superficial nasal planum squamous cell carcinomas in cats: 55 cases. *Journal of Veterinary Internal Medicine* 22, 1385–1389.

Dallman, M.J., McClure, R.C. and Brown, E.M. (1988) Histochemical study of normal and collapsed tracheas in dogs. *American Journal of Veterinary Research* 49, 2117–21125.

Davidson, A., Komtebedde, J., Pappagianis, D. and Hector, R. (1992) Treatment of nasal aspergillosis with topical clotrimazole. *ACVIM Forum 10th Proceedings*. San Diego, California.

Day, M.J., Penhale, W.J., Eger, C.E., Shaw, S.E., Kabay, M.J., Robinson, W.F., Huxtable, C.R., Mills, J. N. and Wyburn, R.S. (1986) Disseminated aspergillosis in dogs. *Australian Veterinary Journal* 63, 55–59.

de Vos, J.P., Burm, A.G. and Focker, B.P. (2004) Results from the treatment of advanced stage squamous cell carcinoma of the nasal planum in cats, using a combination of intralesional carboplatin and superficial radiotherapy: a pilot study. *Veterinary Compendium Oncology* 2, 75–81.

Fasanella, F.J., Shivley, J.M., Wardlaw, J.L. and Givaruangsawat, S. (2010) Brachycephalic airway obstructive syndrome in dogs: 90 cases (1991–2008). *Journal of the American Veterinary Medical Association* 237, 1048–1051.

Fidel, J.L., Egger, E., Blattmann, H., Oberhansli, F. and Kaser-Hotz, B. (2001) Proton irradiation of feline nasal planum squamous cell carcinomas using an accelerated protocol. *Veterinary Radiology & Ultrasound* 42, 569–575.

Findji, L. and Dupre, G. (2009) Folded flap palatoplasty for treatment of elongated soft palates in 55 dogs. *European Journal of Companion Animal Practice* 19, 1–8.

Gallegos, J., Schmiedt, C.W. and McAnulty, J.F. (2007) Cosmetic rostral nasal reconstruction after nasal planum and premaxilla resection: technique and results in two dogs. *Veterinary Surgery* 36, 669–674.

Garcia, M.E., Caballero, J., Cruzado, M., Andrino, M., Gonzalez-Cabo, J.F. and Blanco, J.L. (2001) The value of the determination of anti-Aspergillus IgG in the serodiagnosis of canine aspergillosis: comparison with galactomannan detection. *Journal of Veterinary Medicine B Infectious Diseases of Veterinary Public Health* 48, 743–750.

Goodfellow, M., Hayes, A., Murphy, S. and Brearley, M. (2006) A retrospective study of (90) Strontium plesiotherapy for feline squamous cell carcinoma of the nasal planum. *Journal of Feline Medicine and Surgery* 8, 169–176.

Haimel, G. and Dupre, G. (2015) Brachycephalic airway syndrome: a comparative study between pugs and French bulldogs. *Journal of Small Animal Practice* 56, 714–719.

Hammond, G.M., Gordon, I.K., Theon, A.P. and Kent, M.S. (2007) Evaluation of strontium Sr 90 for the treatment of superficial squamous cell carcinoma of the nasal planum in cats: 49 cases (1990–2006). *Journal of the American Veterinary Medical Association* 231, 736–741.

Harris, B.J., Lourenco, B.N., Dobson, J.M. and Herrtage, M.E. (2014) Diagnostic accuracy of three biopsy techniques in 117 dogs with intra-nasal neoplasia. *Journal of Small Animal Practice* 55, 219–224.

Henderson, S.M., Bradley, K., Day, M.J., Tasker, S., Caney, S.M., Hotston Moore, A. and Gruffydd-Jones, T.J. (2004) Investigation of nasal disease in the cat – a retrospective study of 77 cases. *Journal of Feline Medicine and Surgery* 6, 245–257.

Henry, C.J., Brewer Jr. W.G., Tyler, J.W., Brawner, W.R.,

Henderson, R.A., Hankes, G.H. and Royer, N. (1998) Survival in dogs with nasal adenocarcinoma: 64 cases (1981–1995). *Journal of Veterinary Internal Medicine* 12, 436–439.

Jakubiak, M.J., Siedlecki, C.T., Zenger, E., Matteucci, M.L., Bruskiewicz, K.A., Rohn, D.A. and Bergman, P.J. (2005) Laryngeal, laryngotracheal, and tracheal masses in cats: 27 cases (1998–2003). *Journal of the American Animal Hospital Association* 41, 310–316.

Jeffery, N.D., Talbot, C.E., Smith, P.M. and Bacon, N.J. (2006) Acquired idiopathic laryngeal paralysis as a prominent feature of generalised neuromuscular disease in 39 dogs. *Veterinary Record* 158, 17.

Koch D.A., Arnold S., Hubler, M. and Montavon, P.M. (2003) Brachycephalic syndrome in dogs. *Compendium of Continuing Education for the Practicing Veterinarian* 25, 48–55.

Laing, E.J. and Binnington, A.G. (1988) Surgical therapy of canine nasal tumors: A retrospective study (1982–1986). *Canadian Veterinary Journal* 29, 809–813.

Lana, S.E., Ogilvie, G.K., Withrow, S.J., Straw, R.C. and Rogers, K.S. (1997) Feline cutaneous squamous cell carcinoma of the nasal planum and the pinnae: 61 cases. *Journal of the American Animal Hospital Association* 33, 329–332.

Lascelles, B.D., Parry, A.T., Stidworthy, M.F., Dobson, J.M. and White, R.A. (2000) Squamous cell carcinoma of the nasal planum in 17 dogs. *Veterinary Record* 147, 473–476.

Legendre, A.M., Rohrbach, B.W., Toal, R.L., Rinaldi, M.G., Grace, L.L. and Jones, J.B. (1996) Treatment of blastomycosis with itraconazole in 112 dogs. *Journal of Veterinary Internal Medicine* 10, 365–371.

Leonard, H.C. (1960) Collapse of the larynx and adjacent structures in the dog. *Journal of the American Veterinary Medical Association* 137, 360–363.

Macy, D.W. and Reynolds, H.A. (1981) The incidence, characteristics and clinical management of skin tumours in cats. *Journal of the Americal Animal Hospital Associiation* 17, 1026–1034.

Madewell, B.R., Priester, W.A., Gillette, E.L. and Snyder, S.P. (1976) Neoplasms of the nasal passages and paranasal sinuses in domesticated animals as reported by 13 veterinary colleges. *American Journal of Veterinary Research* 37, 851–856.

Maggiore, A.D. (2014) Tracheal and airway collapse in dogs. *Veterinary Clinics of North America: Small Animal Practice* 44, 117–127.

Mathews, K.G., Davidson, A.P., Koblik, P.D., Richardson, E.F., Komtebedde, J., Pappagianis, D., Hector, R.F. and Kass, P.H. (1998) Comparison of topical administration of clotrimazole through surgically placed versus nonsurgically placed catheters for treatment of nasal aspergillosis in dogs: 60 cases (1990–1996). *Journal of the American Veterinary Medical Association* 213, 501–506.

Moritz, A., Schneider, M. and Bauer, N. (2004) Management of advanced tracheal collapse in dogs using intraluminal self-expanding biliary wallstents. *Journal of Veterinary Internal Medicine* 18, 31–42.

Mukaratirwa, S., van der Linde-Sipman, J.S. and Gruys, E. (2001) Feline nasal and paranasal sinus tumours: clinicopathological study, histomorphological description and diagnostic immunohistochemistry of 123 cases. *Journal of Feline Medicine and Surgery* 3, 235–245.

Nelissen, P. and White, R.A. (2012) Arytenoid lateralization for management of combined laryngeal paralysis and laryngeal collapse in small dogs. *Veterinary Surgery* 41, 261–265.

Nicholson, I. and Baines, S. (2012) Complications associated with temporary tracheostomy tubes in 42 dogs (1998–2007). *Journal of Small Animal Practice* 53, 108–114.

Oechtering, G.U., Pohl, S., Schlueter, C. and Schuenemann, R. (2016) A novel approach to brachycephalic syndrome. 2. Laser-assisted turbinectomy (LATE). *Veterinary Surgery* 45, 173–181.

Patnaik, A.K., Lieberman, P.H., Erlandson, R.A. and Liu, S.K. (1984) Canine sinonasal skeletal neoplasms: chondrosarcomas and osteosarcomas. *Veterinary Pathology* 21, 475–482.

Peeters, D. and Clercx, C. (2007) Update on canine sinonasal aspergillosis. *Veterinary Clinics of North America: Small Animal Practice* 37, 901–916.

Peeters, D., Day, M.J. and Clercx, C. (2005) An immunohistochemical study of canine nasal aspergillosis. *Journal of Companion Pathology* 132, 283–288.

Plickert, H.D., Tichy, A. and Hirt, R.A. (2014) Characteristics of canine nasal discharge related to intranasal diseases: a retrospective study of 105 cases. *Journal of Small Animal Practice* 55, 145–152.

Poncet, C.M., Dupre, G.P., Freiche, V.G., Estrada, M.M., Poubanne, Y.A. and Bouvy, B.M. (2005) Prevalence of gastrointestinal tract lesions in 73 brachycephalic dogs with upper respiratory syndrome. *Journal of Small Animal Practice* 46, 273–279.

Poncet, C.M., Dupre, G.P., Freiche, V.G. and Bouvy, B.M. (2006) Long-term results of upper respiratory syndrome surgery and gastrointestinal tract medical treatment in 51 brachycephalic dogs. *Journal of Small Animal Practice* 47, 137–142.

Rassnick, K.M., Goldkamp, C.E., Erb, H.N., Scrivani, P.V., Njaa, B.L., Gieger, T.L., Turek, M.M., McNiel, E.A., Proulx, D.R., Chun, R., Mauldin, G.E., Phillips, B.S. and Kristal, O. (2006) Evaluation of factors associated with survival in dogs with untreated nasal carcinomas: 139 cases (1993–2003). *Journal of the American Veterinary Medical Association* 229, 401–406.

Rogers, K.S., Helman, R.G. and Walker, M.A. (1995) Squamous cell carcinoma of the canine nasal planum: eight cases (1988–1994). *Journal of the American Animal Hospital Association* 31, 373–378.

Saunders, J.H. and van Bree, H. (2003) Comparison of radiography and computed tomography for the diagnosis of canine nasal aspergillosis. *Veterinary Radiology & Ultrasound* 44, 414–419.

Schuenemann, R. and Oechtering, C. (2014) Inside the brachycephalic nose: conchal regrowth and mucosal contact points after laser-assisted turbinectomy. *Journal of the American Animal Hospital Association* 50, 237–246.

Schuller, S. and Clercx, C. (2007) Long-term outcomes in dogs with sinonasal aspergillosis treated with intranasal infusions of enilconazole. *Journal of the American Animal Hospital Association* 43, 33–38.

Sharp, N.J. and Sullivan, M. (1986) Treatment of canine nasal aspergillosis with systemic ketoconazole and topical enilconazole. *Veterinary Record* 118, 560–561.

Sharp, N., Harvey, C. and Sullivan, M. (1991) Canine nasal aspergillosis and penicillosis. *Compendium on Continuing Education for the Practicing Veterinarian* 13, 41–47.

Sissener, T.R., Bacon, N.J., Friend, E., Anderson, D.M. and White R.A. (2006) Combined clotrimazole irrigation and depot therapy for canine nasal aspergillosis. *Journal of Small Animal Practice* 47, 312–315.

Stanley, B.J., Hauptman, J.G., Fritz, M.C., Rosenstein, D.S. and Kinns, J. (2010) Esophageal dysfunction in dogs with idiopathic laryngeal paralysis: a controlled cohort study. *Veterinary Surgery* 39, 139–149.

Sun, F., Uson, J., Ezquerra, J., Crisostomo, V., Luis, L. and Maynar, M. (2008) Endotracheal stenting therapy in dogs with tracheal collapse. *Veterinary Journal* 175, 186–193.

Tangner, C.H. and Hobson, H. (1982) A retrospective study of 20 surgically managed cases of collapsed trachea. *Veterinary Surgery* 11, 146–149.

Tappin, S.W. (2016) Canine tracheal collapse. *Journal of Small Animal Practice* 57, 9–17.

Tasker, S., Knottenbelt, C.M., Munro, E.A., Stonehewer, J., Simpson, J.W. and Mackin, A.J. (1999). Aetiology and diagnosis of persistent nasal disease in the dog: a retrospective study of 42 cases. *Journal of Small Animal Practice* 40, 473–478.

Taylor, S.S., Harvey, A.M., Barr, F.J., Moore, A.H. and Day, M.J. (2009) Laryngeal disease in cats: a retrospective study of 35 cases. *Journal of Feline Medicine and Surgery* 11, 954–962.

Ter Haar, G. and Hampel, R. (2015) Combined rostrolateral rhinotomy for removal of rostral nasal septum squamous cell carcinoma: Long-term outcome in 10 dogs. *Veterinary Surgery* 44, 843–851.

Theon, A.P., Madewell, B.R., Harb, M.F. and Dungworth, D.L. (1993) Megavoltage irradiation of neoplasms of the nasal and paranasal cavities in 77 dogs. *Journal of the American Veterinary Medical Association* 202, 1469–1475.

Theon, A.P., Peaston, A.E., Madewell, B.R. and Dungworth, D.L. (1994) Irradiation of nonlymphoproliferative neoplasms of the nasal cavity and paranasal sinuses in 16 cats. *Journal of the American Veterinary Medical Association* 204, 78–83.

Thieman, K.M., Krahwinkel, D.J., Sims, M.H. and Shelton, G.D. (2010) Histopathological confirmation of polyneuropathy in 11 dogs with laryngeal paralysis. *Journal of the American Animal Hospital Association* 46, 161–167.

Tomsa, K., Glaus, T.M., Zimmer, C. and Greene, C.E. (2003) Fungal rhinitis and sinusitis in three cats. *Journal of the American Veterinary Medical Association* 222, 1380–1384.

Torrez, C.V. and Hunt, G.B. (2006) Results of surgical correction of abnormalities associated with brachycephalic airway obstruction syndrome in dogs in Australia. *Journal of Small Animal Practice* 47, 150–154.

White, R.A. (2009) Canine laryngeal surgery: time to rethink? *Veterinary Surgery* 38, 432–433.

White, R.N. (2012) Surgical management of laryngeal collapse associated with brachycephalic airway obstruction syndrome in dogs. *Journal of Small Animal Practice* 53, 44–50.

White, R.A. and Williams, J.M. (1994) Tracheal collapse in the dog – is there really a role for surgery? A survey of 100 cases. *Journal of Small Animal Practice* 35, 191–196.

Whitney, B.L., Broussard, J. and Stefanacci, J.D. (2005) Four cats with fungal rhinitis. *Journal of Feline Medicine and Surgery* 7, 53–58.

Withrow, S.J. (2013) Tumours of the respiratory system. In: Withrow, S.J, Vail, D.M. and Page, R.L. (eds) *Withrow & MacEwen's Small Animal Clinical Oncology*. Elsevier/Saunders, Philadelphia, Pennsylania, pp. 432–462.

Case 7.1

A 5-year-old Labrador retriever presents with a mucopurulent nasal discharge. Occasional blood specks on the floor have also been noted by the owner.

- What further clinical history is important in reaching a diagnosis?
- What further clinical examination do you wish to perform?

On further discussion with the owner, you discover that the nasal discharge has been present for approximately 6 months and is unilateral. On examination, there is no evidence of nasal depigmentation. Nasal airflow, assessed by cotton wool, appears symmetrical. No pain on sinus or nasal percussion could be elicited and there was no evidence of lymphadenopathy.

- What are your differentials at this stage?
- What diagnostic procedures would you like to perform?

The owner was well informed that neoplasia, aspergillosis and inflammatory rhinitis could not be excluded. Due to the chronicity of clinical signs, a nasal foreign body was less likely at this stage. Systemic diseases resulting in epistaxis were also possible differentials, including coagulopathies, hypertension, polycythaemia and hyperviscosity syndrome. Biochemistry, haematology and clotting profiles were all unremarkable. The dog was normotensive.

Intra-oral radiographs raised suspicion of an area of radiolucency within the nostril and, following discussion with the owner, the dog was referred for advanced imaging and computed tomography (CT) was performed (Fig. 7.69).

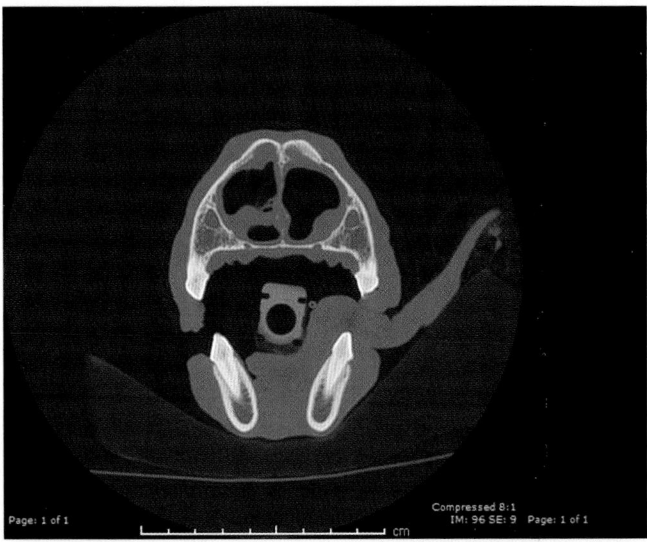

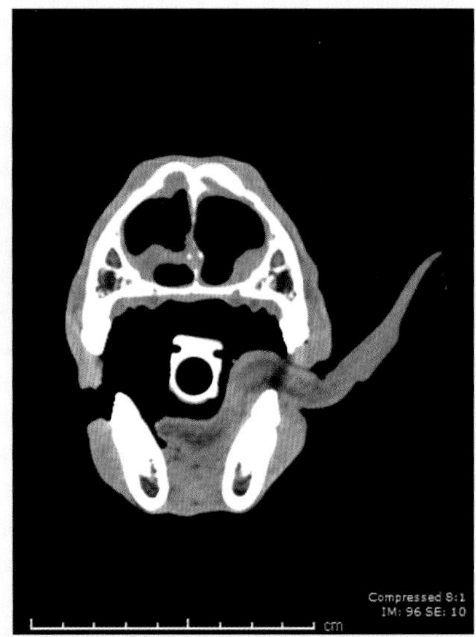

Fig. 7.69 Transverse CT scan showing bilateral nasal turbinate destruction. Left: bone window. Right: soft tissue window.

- What is the most likely diagnosis based on the images presented?
- What is the next step to confirming this diagnosis?

The CT scan showed significant nasal turbinate destruction, and aspergillosis was suspected. A rhinoscopy confirmed the presence of nasal plaques, and biopsy and culture of these plaques confirmed the diagnosis of aspergillosis.

- What treatment options are available to the owner?
- What is the reported success rate of each of these treatment options?
- What are the contraindications to each of the treatment options?

The dog received a 1-hour 1% clotrimazole soak followed by trephination of the frontal sinus and deposition of clotrimazole cream into each frontal sinus. Every two weeks, clotrimazole deposition into the frontal sinus was repeated. Following the fourth treatment, full resolution of clinical signs was achieved.

Case 7.2

History

A 12-month-old English bulldog presents with two episodes of cyanosis following exercise over the last 3 months. A 5-month history of regurgitation was also noted, with an increase in frequency over the last 3 weeks. An intermittent cough and lethargy is reported over the last 3 days.

Clinical examination

Examination revealed tachypnoea (35/min) and dyspnoea. Intermittent regurgitation was noted. Thoracic auscultation revealed harsh lung sounds and crackles bilaterally. Cardiac auscultation was unremarkable. The dog was pyrexic at 40.3°C. All other clinical findings were unremarkable.

- What are your thoughts regarding the underlying aetiology of the exercise intolerance and cyanosis?
- What is the most likely aetiology of the regurgitation?
- What is the likely cause of the pyrexia?
- What is required for immediate management of the dog?
- What is required for long-term management of the dog?

Immediate management

The dog was placed on nasal oxygen and an IV catheter was placed. Acepromazine was administered (0.01 mg/kg IV) and the air-conditioning set to cool. Cold towels were placed on the skin and an external fan positioned accordingly.

Intravenous broad-spectrum antibiotics and IV omeprazole were administered. Once stabilised, a conscious thoracic DV radiograph confirmed aspiration pneumonia (Fig. 7.70). The dog was hospitalised on IV antibiotics for 48 hours and his respiratory rate and pattern normalised. The dog was discharged on oral antibiotics and omeprazole.

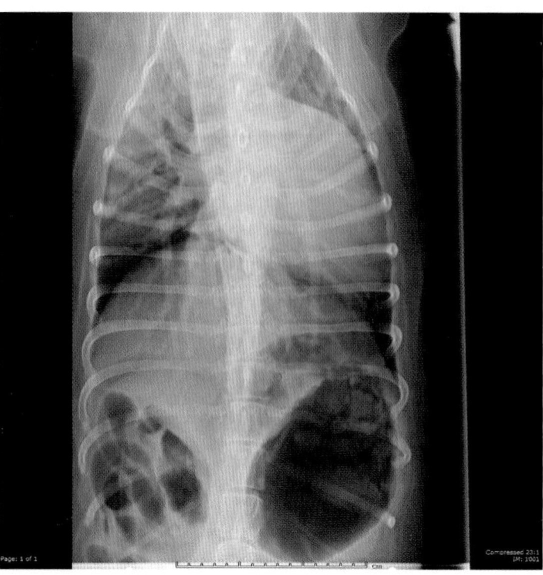

Fig 7.70 Dorsoventral thoracic radiograph showing evidence of aspiration pneumonia in the right cranial lung lobe.

Long-term management

Two weeks following medical management for aspiration pneumonia, the dog was re-admitted for BOAS surgery. Thoracic radiographs prior to surgery were unremarkable. Nasoplasty, folded-flap palatoplasty and laryngeal saccule resection were performed, and the dog was discharged the following day with 4 weeks of omeprazole.

Three months later, there were no further episodes of dyspnoea or cyanosis but the dog still had daily episodes of regurgitation. A repeat thoracic radiograph (Fig. 7.71) and a fluoroscopy study (Fig. 7.72) showed the dog had a hiatal hernia. The dog had surgery the following day, where a hiatal hernia was confirmed (Fig. 7.73). Plication of the phrenico-oesophageal ligament, oesophagopexy and gastropexy were performed to correct the type I sliding hiatal hernia. The dog went on to make a full recovery with no further episodes of regurgitation.

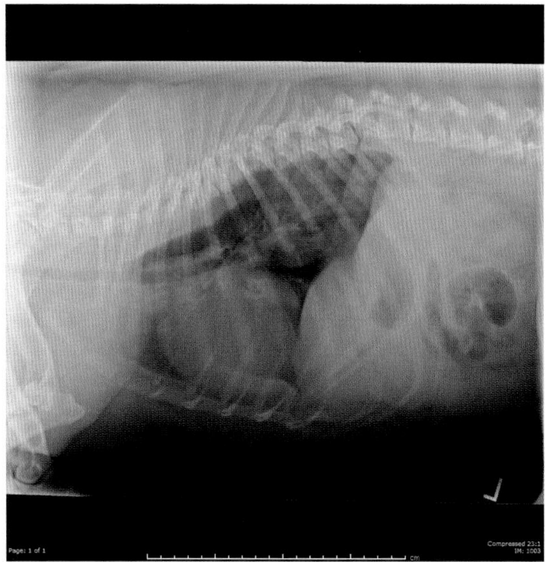

Fig 7.71 Thoracic radiograph showing evidence of a suspected hiatal hernia.

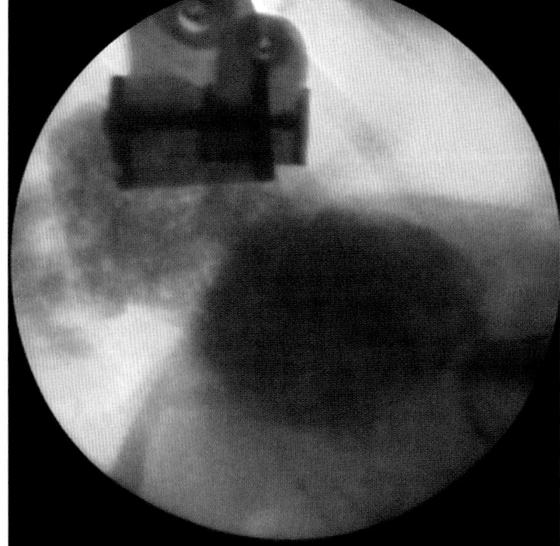

Fig 7.72 Fluoroscopic image showing the cardia of the stomach cranial to the diaphragm, confirming a hiatal hernia.

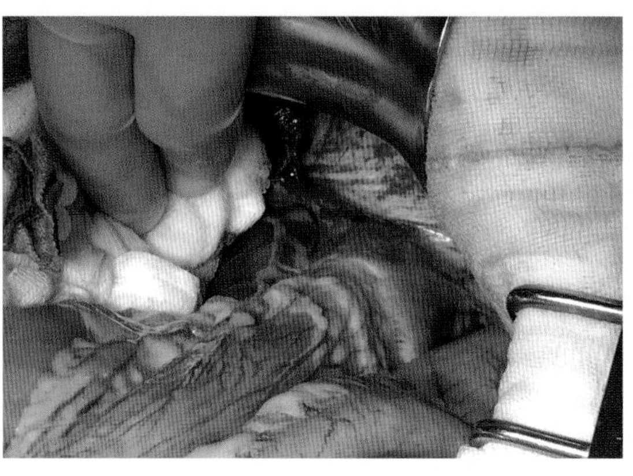

Fig 7.73 Intra-operative photograph showing the oesophageal hiatus following caudal traction of the oesophagus and subsequent reduction of the hiatal hernia.

Surgery of the abdominal cavity

8

Kelly L. Bowlt Blacklock

Chapter summary

8.1 Approach to the abdominal cavity

Key points

- A rigorous sign-in and sign-out checklist is essential for all surgeries, particularly those involving the abdominal or thoracic cavity.
- The ventral midline approach is almost exclusively used for abdominal surgery.
- Closure of the ventral midline requires incorporation of the strength-holding external rectus fascia.
- Suture failure occurs most commonly at the knot: tight, square knots are mandatory.
- Both simple interrupted and simple continuous suture patterns are acceptable for midline laparotomy closure.

8.1.1 Complications of abdominal surgery

Surgical complications occur in every hospital and to every surgeon, resulting in increased patient morbidity/mortality, increased cost and increased stress for everyone involved. Complications can arise due to clinician error or unforeseen circumstances: the former can be addressed by the use of guidelines to improve surgical safety. The World Health Organization (WHO) addresses the safety of surgical care via the 'Safe Surgery Saves Lives' campaign (www.who.int/patientsafety/safesurgery/en/), inspired by the checklists used by airline pilots to reduce error. Surgeons should familiarise themselves with the content of this campaign and the current literature in reducing surgical complications (Gasson, 2011; Gawande, 2009; Tivers, 2011, 2015). Compliance with a surgical checklist significantly decreases the frequency and severity of postoperative complications in veterinary hospitals (Bergstrom et al., 2016). Since 2008, the Animal Health Trust has used a modified surgical safety checklist for all patients undergoing procedures in theatre, with the aim of reducing harm in the perioperative setting (explanatory notes available at www.aht.org.uk/patientsafetyfirst) (Fig. 8.1).

AHT Surgical Safety Checklist

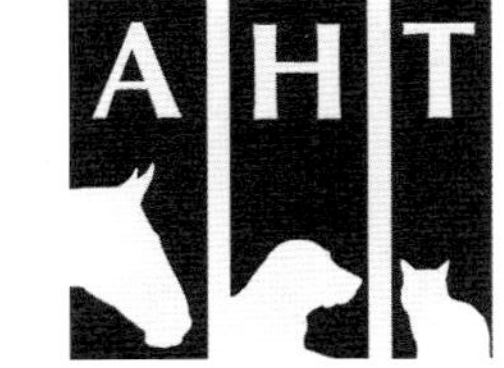

SIGN IN (To be read out loud)

Before induction of anaesthesia aesthesia

Has the patient had their identity confirmed, procedure verified and consent checked?

- ☐ Yes

Is the surgical site marked?

- ☐ Yes/not applicable

Is the anaesthesia machine and medication check complete?

- ☐ Yes

Does the patient have a:

Known allergy?

☐ No ☐ Yes

Difficulty airway/aspiration risk?

☐ No ☐ Yes

Risk of >15% blood loss

- ☐ No
- ☐ Yes and adequate IV access/fluids planned
- ☐ Patient position in theatre known?
- ☐ Antibiotics at induction? Yes / NA
- ☐ Estimated surgery time is ....
- ☐ Team discusses perioperative plan & designates roles
- ☐ Any concerns?

TIME OUT (To be read out loud)

Before start of surgical intervention For example, skin incision

Surgeon, Anaesthetist and Theatre Practitioner verbally confirm:

- ☐ What is the patient's name?
- ☐ Procedure, site and position are confirmed?

Anticipated critical events:

Surgeon:

- ☐ How much blood loss is anticipated?
- ☐ Are there any specific equipment requirements or special investigations?
- ☐ Are there any critical or unexpected steps you want the team to know about?

Anaesthetist:

- ☐ Are there any patient specific concerns?
- ☐ What is the patient's ASA grade?
- ☐ What monitoring equipment and other specific levels of support are required, e.g. blood?

Nurse/ODP:

- ☐ Has the sterility of the instrumentation been confirmed (including indicator results)
- ☐ Are there any equipment issues or concerns?

Has the surgical site infection (SSI) bundle been undertaken?

- ☐ Yes/not applicable
- Antibiotic prophylaxis within the last 60 mins
- Patient warming (state temperature)
- Hair removal
- Antisepsis

Is essential imaging displayed?

- ☐ Yes/not applicable

SIGN OUT (to be read out loud)

Before any member of the team leaves the operating room

Theatre Practitioner verbally confirms with the team:

- ☐ Has the name of the procedure been recorded?
- ☐ Has it been confirmed that instruments, swabs and sharps counts are complete (or not applicable)?
- ☐ Have the specimens been labelled (including patient name)?
- ☐ Have any equipment problems been identified that need to be addressed?

Surgeon, Anaesthetist and Theatre Practitioner:

- ☐ What is the key concerns for recovery and management of this patient?

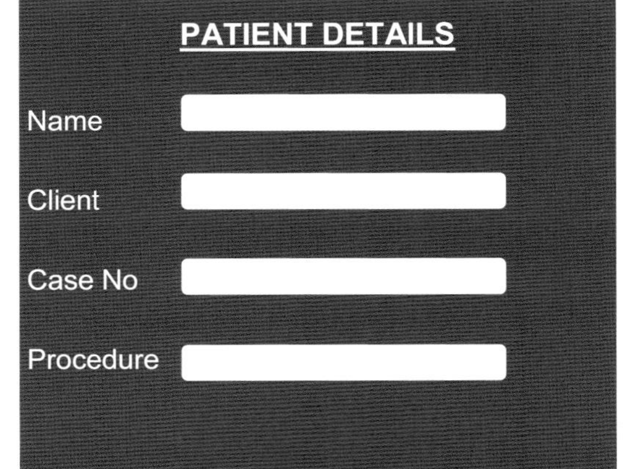

Fig. 8.1 A modified surgical safety checklist for all patients undergoing procedures in theatre. (Copyright Animal Health Trust.)

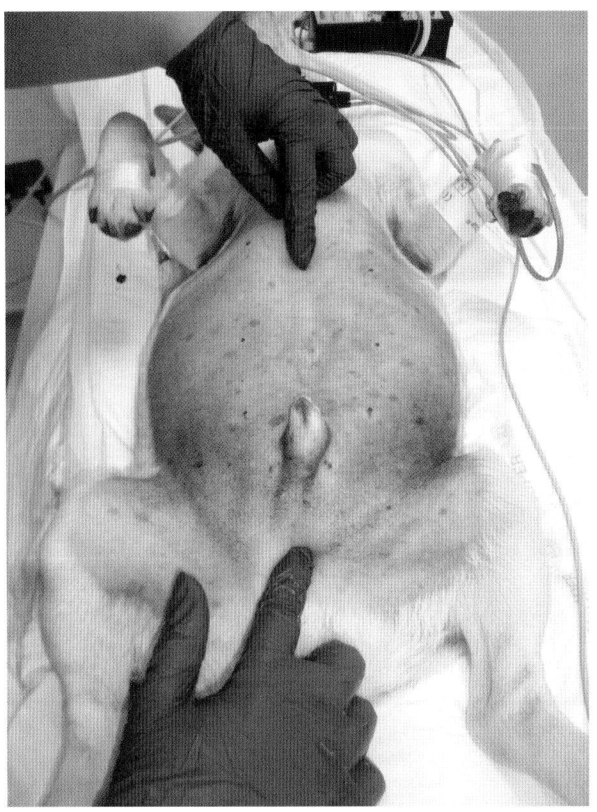

Fig. 8.2 For an exploratory laparotomy, the incision should extend from the xiphoid to the pubis, as shown, in order to allow complete exposure of the abdomen without excessive pressure during retraction.

As for every surgical procedure, informed client consent should be acquired: this involves a full and frank discussion about the diagnosis, potential complications of surgery/treatment, likely outcomes, additional/alternative treatment options and estimated costs involved.

8.1.2 Ventral midline approach to the abdomen

Almost without exception, the approach to the abdominal cavity should be via the ventral midline. This approach ensures anatomical familiarity and is associated with decreased postoperative pain compared with a flank approach. For an exploratory laparotomy, the incision should extend from the xiphoid to the pubis in order to allow complete exposure of the abdomen without excessive pressure during retraction (Fig. 8.2).

The skin is clipped and aseptically prepared, the prepuce is lavaged (the author's institution uses 0.05% chlorhexidine gluconate in sterile water) and the surgical site is draped (Fig. 8.3a,b). After the skin is incised, the incision is continued through the subcutaneous fat (addressing small bleeding vessels as encountered with sutures, artery clamps, mono- or bipolar diathermy, etc.) on to the linea alba. In the male dog, the

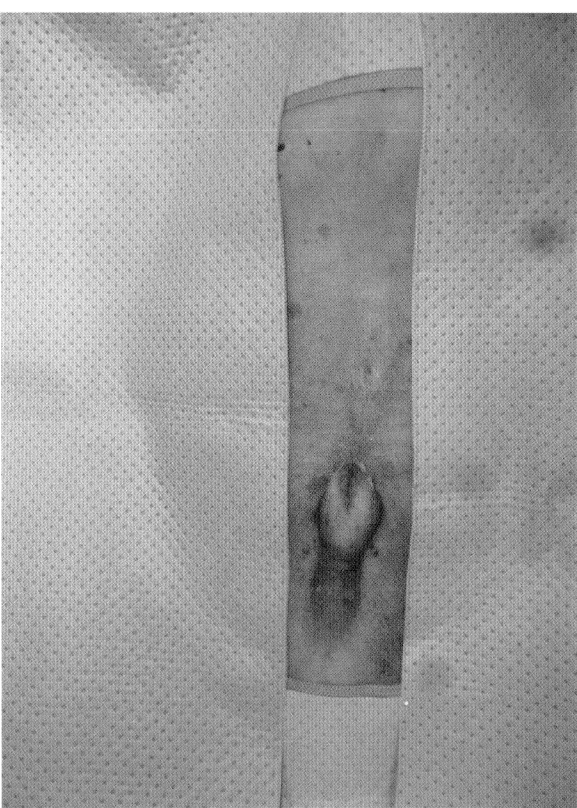

Fig. 8.3a The skin is clipped and aseptically prepared, the prepuce is lavaged and the surgical site is draped.

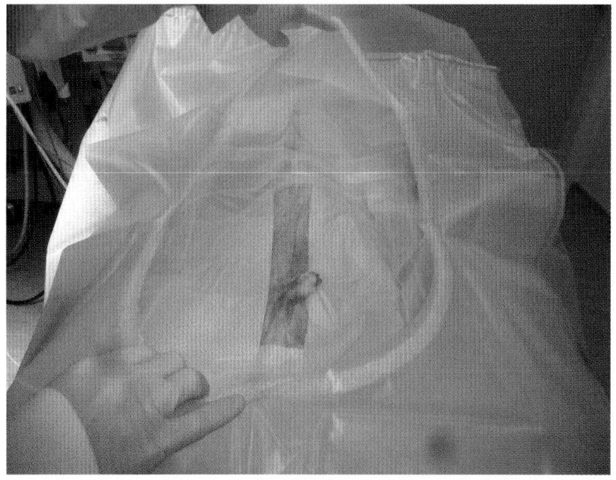

Fig. 8.3b Where large volumes of fluid are anticipated (e.g. in cases of septic peritonitis), Caesarean drapes can be useful in keeping the patient, table and theatre floor dry and uncontaminated.

skin incision continues paramedian to one side of the prepuce and preputial muscles, and vessels are divided to allow the penis to be reflected laterally and the linea alba exposed on the midline (Fig. 8.4). The linea alba is elevated and a stab incision made full thickness into the abdomen, with the belly of the blade pointing away from the abdominal cavity (Fig. 8.5). The linea alba is then opened along its entire length using Mayo scissors; during this part of the approach, the surgeon's hand

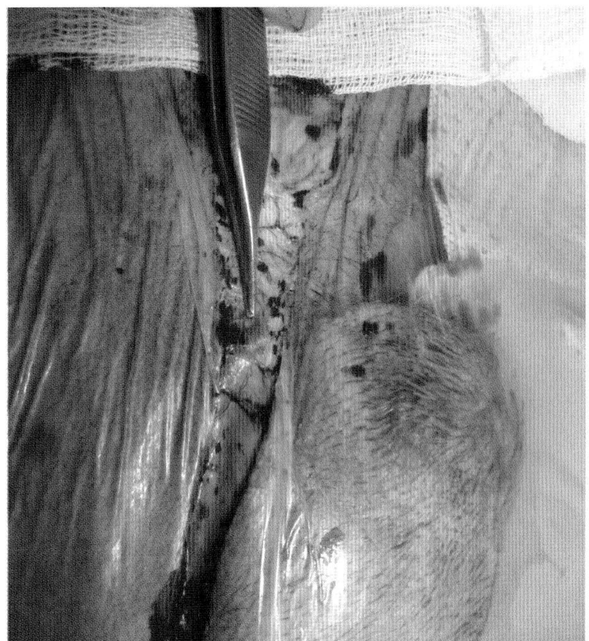

Fig. 8.4 In the male dog, the skin incision continues paramedian to one side of the prepuce, and preputial muscles and vessels identified as shown. These are divided to allow the penis to be reflected laterally and the linea alba exposed on the midline.

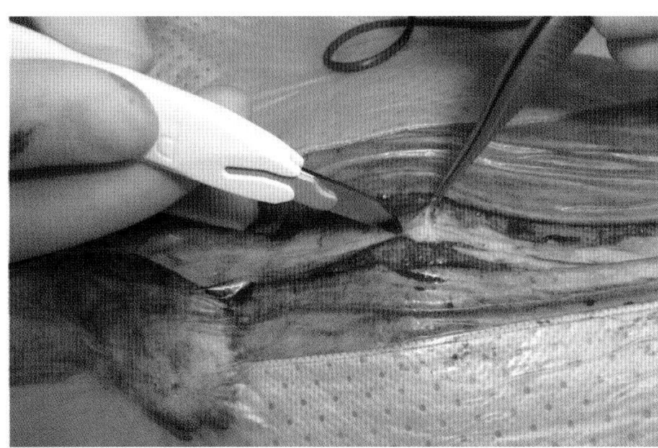

Fig. 8.5 The linea alba is elevated and a stab incision made full thickness into the abdomen, with the belly of the blade pointing away from the abdominal cavity.

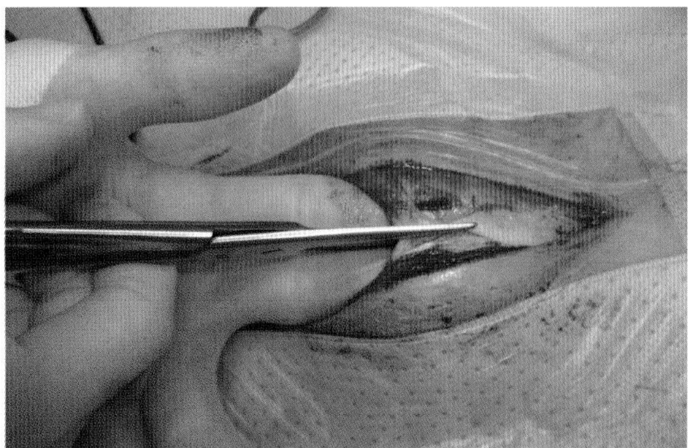

Fig. 8.6 The linea alba is opened along its entire length using Mayo scissors; during this part of the approach, the surgeon's hand should lie under the lower jaw of the scissors to protect the underlying abdominal viscera and to identify any adhesions that may be present near the midline before they are inadvertently cut.

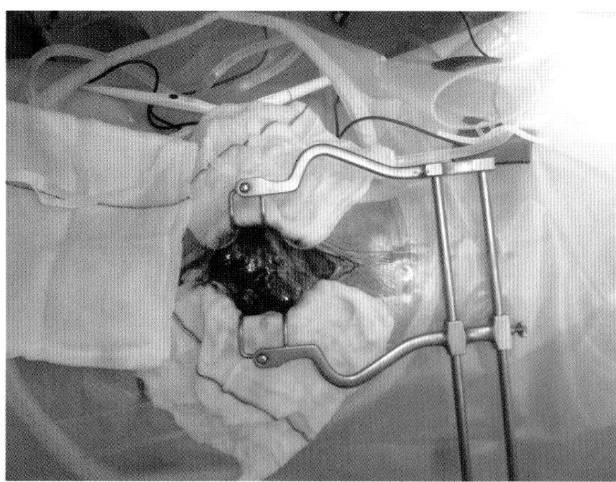

Fig. 8.7a Once the abdomen is fully opened, retractors should be inserted, with the wound edges protected by moist laparotomy swabs.

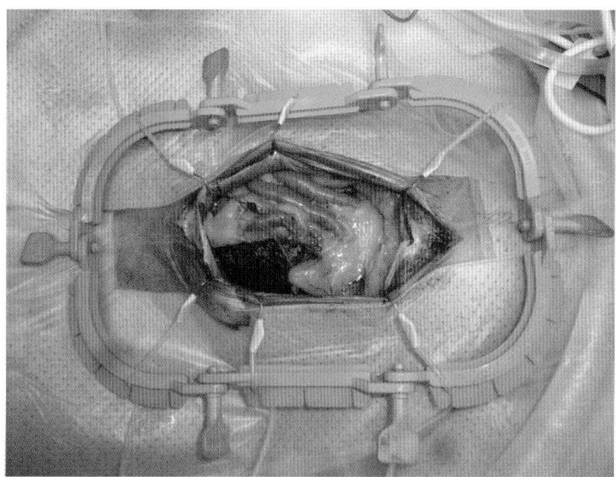

Fig. 8.7b In small dogs or cats, ring retractors are particularly useful to aid abdominal retraction.

should lie under the lower jaw of the scissors to protect the underlying abdominal viscera and to identify any adhesions that may be present to the midline before they are inadvertently cut (Fig. 8.6). Once the abdomen is fully opened, retractors should be inserted, with the wound edges protected by moist laparotomy swabs. In small dogs or cats, ring retractors are particularly useful (Fig. 8.7a,b). Falciform fat can be removed to improve visualisation if required: diathermy or suturing of the cranial vasculature is required (Fig. 8.8).

Once the abdominal procedure has been completed, the retractors are removed and all sharps and swabs accounted for (Figs. 8.1, 8.9a,b). Kit and gloves are changed before closure if there is contamination/infection or neoplasia intra-abdominally. The choice of suture material used for closure is particularly important in patients with prolonged wound healing, wound infection or those who are severely catabolic (Smeak, 2012). The author prefers polydioxanone for closure of the linea alba. Suture failure occurs most commonly at

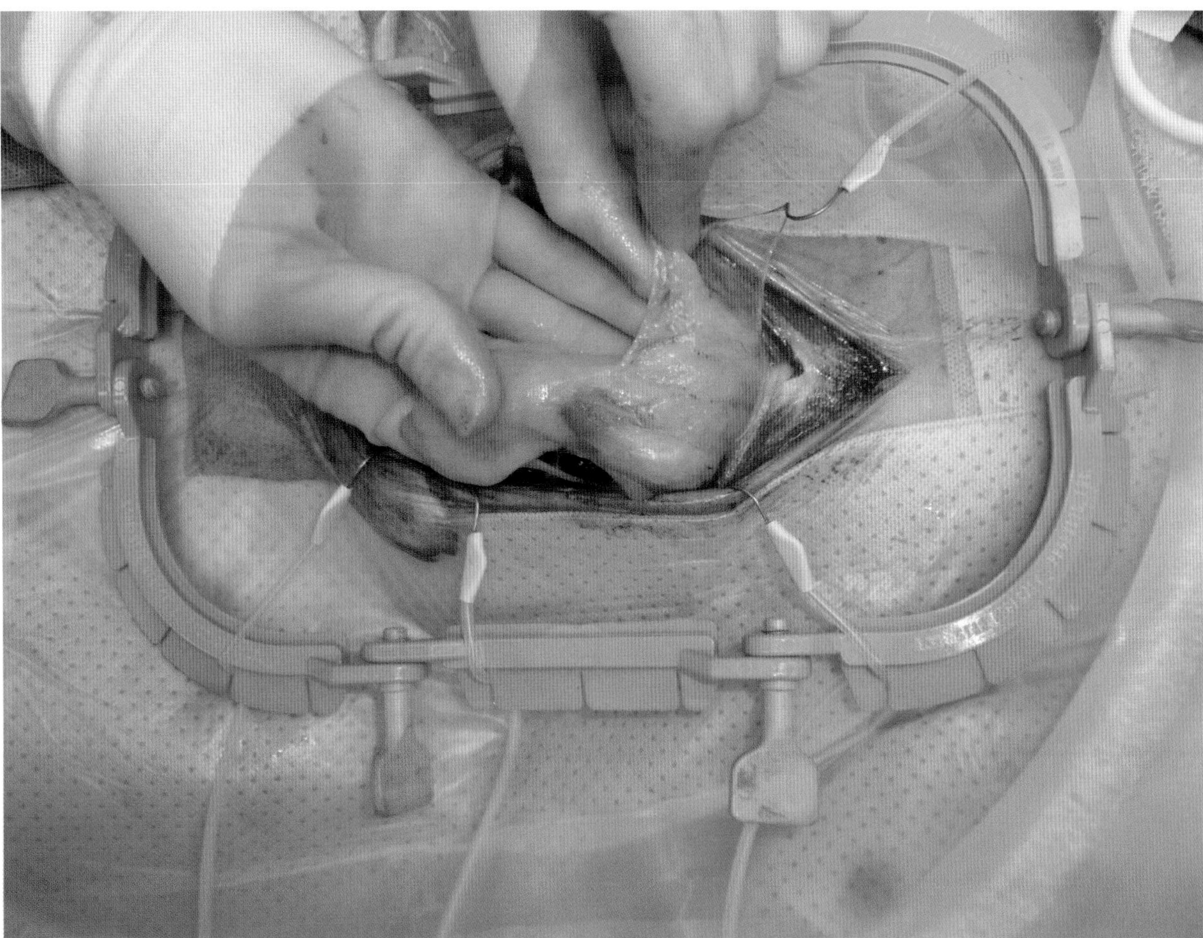

Fig. 8.8 The falciform fat is shown here and can be removed to improve visualisation if required.

the knot, and therefore a tight square knot is imperative (Rosin and Robinson, 1989). Closure of the abdomen in a simple continuous or simple interrupted pattern does not have any significance in the likelihood of developing an incisional hernia, provided all knots are tight and square, and at least 5 mm of healthy strength-holding

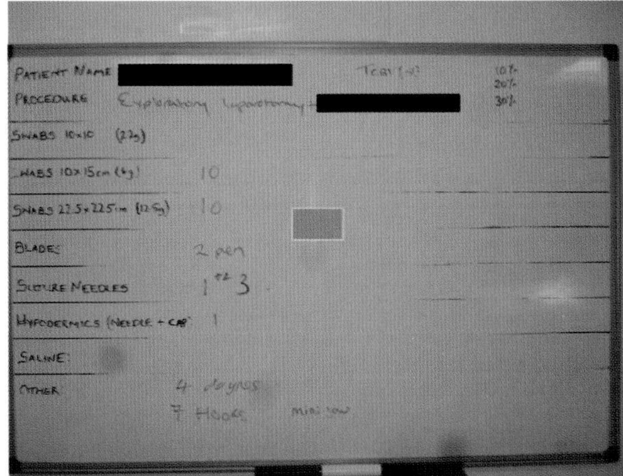

Fig. 8.9a Surgical whiteboard containing instrument, sharps and swab counts. Confidential information is concealed. Where >10% blood loss is anticipated, total circulating blood volume (TCBV) is calculated along with the volume equivalent for 10, 20 and 30% blood loss.

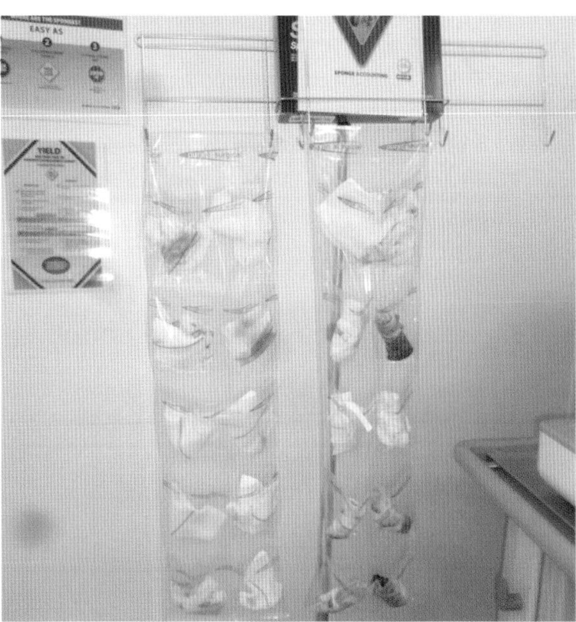

Fig. 8.9b Swabs are issued in counts of ten. Before abdominal closure, surgery is briefly paused and all swabs are visually accounted for by all staff present in theatre. No missing swab pouches should be present. Failure to fill every pouch with a swab results in surgical closure of the abdomen being suspended until that swab is located. Swabs with radiopaque markers are mandatory for surgery of any cavity; those without markers should not be used.

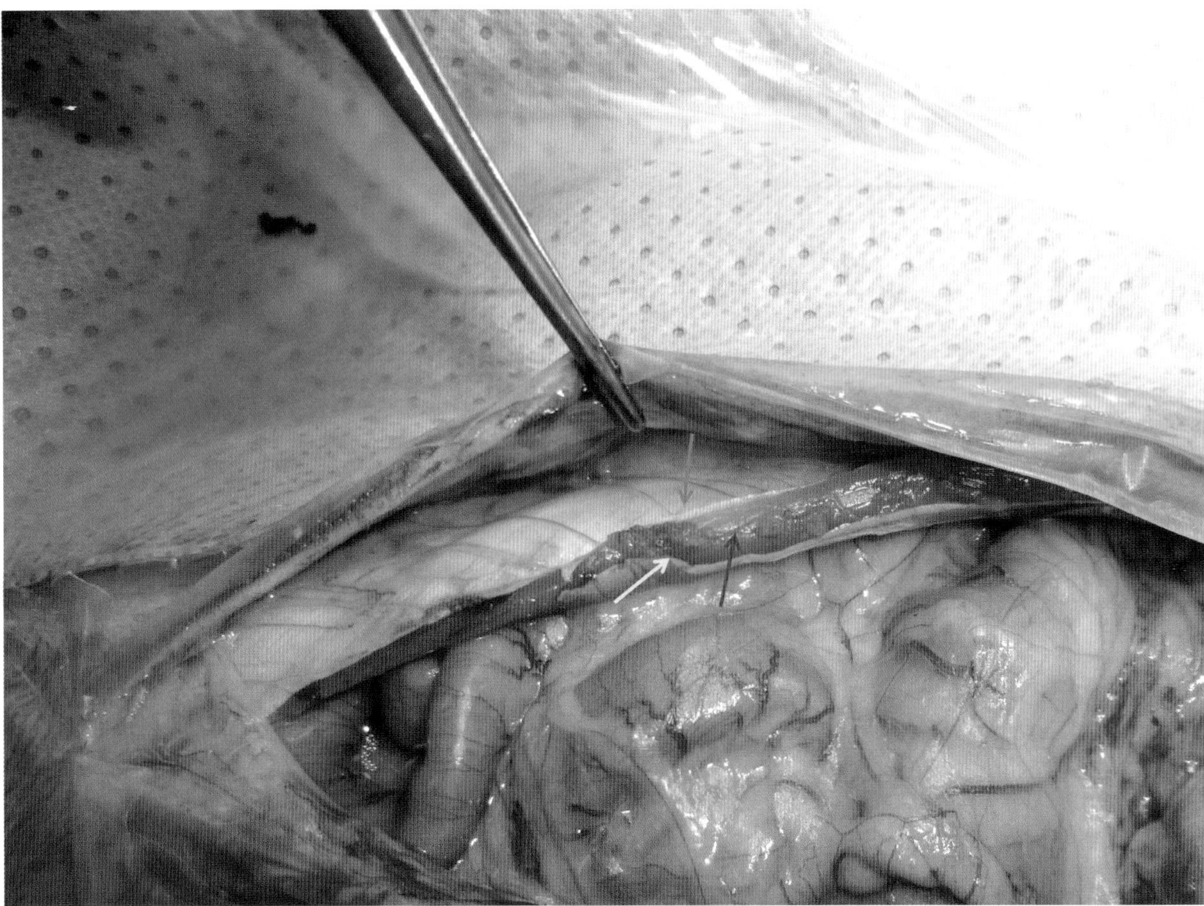

Fig. 8.10 The strength-holding layer of the abdominal wall is the external rectus fascia (blue arrow), which must be included in the closure. The peritoneum and muscle are shown (yellow and red arrows, respectively).

layer (the external rectus fascia, Fig. 8.10) is included (Smeak, 2012). If a simple continuous pattern is used, the suture line can be finished with a square knot (with an extra one or two square throws at the beginning and end (Rosin and Robinson, 1989) or an Aberdeen knot (4+1 throws with a 3 mm ear (Schaaf et al., 2009)). Fat and skin are closed routinely.

8.1.3 Other approaches to the abdomen

The flank approach to the abdomen is almost never indicated: access to dorsally located organs is perfectly satisfactory via the ventral midline, but access to both ovaries and the entire uterus is limited (Smeak, 2012). An example of the rare requirement for a flank approach might include laparoscopically assisted prophylactic gastropexy (Rivier et al., 2011). Alternatively, an inguinal approach has been described as a minimally invasive approach to the urinary bladder, which can be useful on occasion (Bray et al., 2009). If the flank approach is required, the external abdominal oblique, internal abdominal oblique and transversus abdominis are traversed and are all bluntly split along the direction of their fibres. Each individual muscle is closed separately.

The majority (96%) of UK veterinary surgeons perform feline ovariohysterectomy via a flank approach, which is associated with a greater incidence of postoperative wound discharge and pain compared with a midline approach (Coe et al., 2006; Grint et al., 2017; Oliveira et al., 2014). The flank approach is also described for ovariohysterectomy in the dog.

A paracostal and combined midline and paracostal approach have been described, supposedly to allow increased exposure to cranial abdominal organs. This is very rarely required and results in increased postoperative pain compared with a ventral midline approach (Bellenger, 2003).

8.2 Abdominal hernias

Key points

- An abdominal hernia is any full-thickness defect or weakness in the abdominal wall (hernia ring) that may allow protrusion of viscera (hernia contents), usually into a hernia sac.

- Hernias may be congenital, degenerative, incisional or traumatic in origin.
- Abdominal organs contained within the hernia may be viable/reducible, incarcerated or strangulated.
- Common sites for abdominal hernias include paracostal, dorsolateral, inguinal, cranial pubic, femoral, umbilical, ventral and scrotal.
- The nature of herniated contents can be determined using radiography, ultrasound, CT, MRI, etc.
- Multiple hernias in different anatomical locations are not uncommon.
- Prognosis for uncomplicated hernias is excellent; prognosis for those involving strangulated viscera depends on the individual patient.

Introduction

An abdominal hernia is any full-thickness defect or weakness in the abdominal wall (hernia ring) that may allow protrusion of viscera (hernia contents) (Smeak, 2012). Atraumatic hernia contents may be contained within a hernia sac. Hernias may be congenital, degenerative, incisional or traumatic in origin.

Abdominal organs contained within the hernia may be viable / reducible, incarcerated or strangulated. Incarceration or strangulation is more likely with small defects surrounded by an inelastic hernia ring (Smeak, 2012). Hollow organs (e.g. uterus, intestines, bladder) which are incarcerated suffer from altered function secondary to luminal obstruction; this may require immediate stabilisation of the patient and urgent surgical correction of the incarcerated viscera. Strangulated viscera have occluded arterial and / or venous circulation, which can result in tissue necrosis, bacterial translocation, release of vasoactive substances, blood cell autolysis and severe cardiopulmonary effects (Brady and Otto, 2001; Smeak, 2012). Rapid release of vasoactive substances into the systemic circulation during attempted surgical reduction of the strangulated hernia can result in sudden death under anaesthesia, and therefore *en bloc* resection of the devitalised tissue is required before resection / repair of the hernia ring.

'Loss of domain' of the body wall can be seen, particularly in chronic hernias. This may result in difficulty in obtaining primary closure of the defect following reduction of the hernia contents. In such circumstances, prosthetic implants, autogenous flaps or fascial relaxing incisions may be required (Smeak, 2012). Forced closure of the abdomen may result in wound dehiscence, raised intra-abdominal pressure (and abdominal compartment syndrome, which can seriously impede blood supply to abdominal viscera) or impairment of ventilation (secondary to diaphragm restriction) (Islam, 2008).

Common sites for abdominal hernias include paracostal, dorsolateral, inguinal, cranial pubic, femoral, umbilical, ventral and scrotal (Smeak, 2012). Because of the potential heritable nature of congenital or acquired hernias, neutering should be recommended in all patients.

Diagnosis

Patients with abdominal wall hernias present with a palpable mass, which may or may not be reducible. Clinical signs associated with entrapped viscera may also be apparent: for example, gastrointestinal strangulation or incarceration and obstruction may cause vomiting, abdominal pain, depression, cardiovascular collapse, shock, systemic inflammatory response syndrome (SIRS), etc. (Kirby and Jones, 1988). Bladder entrapment may cause stranguria, abdominal pain, dysuria, etc. The nature of herniated contents can be determined using radiography, ultrasound, CT, MRI, etc. Patients should be thoroughly examined for evidence of any other defects or congenital abnormalities. Multiple hernias in different anatomical locations are not uncommon.

Surgery

Preoperative cardiovascular stabilisation may be required if incarceration or strangulation is present. The goals of surgery are detailed in Table 8.1. Sufficient surgical exposure is required to assess hernia contents: if abdominal trauma or visceral strangulation is apparent, the ventral midline approach is indicated. If the hernia is uncomplicated, an approach can be made directly over the hernial ring. Potential complications associated with abdominal hernias are detailed in Table 8.2.

Postoperative management

Postoperative management for acute traumatic hernias (not involving evisceration) is as for any elective abdominal surgery, including nutritional management, pain management, exercise restriction, prevention of wound interference, routine wound care etc.

Prognosis

The prognosis for uncomplicated umbilical hernias is excellent and postoperative care requirements are usually limited to appropriate wound management and analgesia. The prognosis for hernias containing strangulated viscera or omphalocoeles will depend on the individual patient and extent / type of organs involved. The prognosis for uncomplicated inguinal hernias is

Table 8.1 Goals for uncomplicated abdominal herniorrhaphy.

Preoperative goals
Client education and informed consent
Patient cardiovascular and respiratory stabilisation
Understanding of the viscera (and its viability) involved in the herniation
Understanding of any co-morbidities or injuries
Smooth, rapid induction of anaesthesia
Thorough understanding of regional anatomy
Aseptic preparation of the patient
Surgical goals
Adherence to Halsted's principles
Ensure viability of entrapped hernia contents
Reduction of herniated tissue and resection of damaged tissue
Anatomic closure of the defect
Removal of redundant hernia sac tissue and closure of the sac
Abdominal closure of viable tissue without undue tension
Postoperative goals
Thorough evaluation and control of the patient postoperatively
Monitoring and early treatment for any complications

Table 8.2 Summary of potential complications associated with repair of abdominal hernias.

Perioperative complications
Anaesthetic complications
Haemorrhage
Visceral injury/strangulation
Inability to close the abdominal wall in chronic hernias
Complications arising secondary to resection of strangulated viscera
Early postoperative complications
Infection/abscessation
Pain
Seroma
Haematoma
Hypoventilation
Sudden cardiac arrest
Reperfusion injury
Wound dehiscence and evisceration
Abdominal compartment syndrome
Peritonitis/sepsis
Complications arising secondary to resection of strangulated viscera
Scrotal dermatitis or scrotal swelling (in case of scrotal hernia)
Late postoperative complications
Hernia recurrence
Infection of implants

excellent and postoperative care requirements are usually limited to appropriate wound management, analgesia and exercise restriction (to decrease oedema/seroma formation). The prognosis for hernias containing strangulated viscera will depend on the individual patient and extent/type of organs involved. Vomiting for 2–6 days is predictive of non-viable small intestine, which is more likely in intact dogs younger than 2 years (Waters et al., 1993). The prevalence of postoperative complications and the mortality rate is 17% and 3% respectively (Waters et al., 1993). The prognosis for incisional hernias is good to excellent. Aggressive medical and surgical treatment of patients with evisceration can also result in a good outcome (Gower et al., 2009).

8.2.1 Umbilical hernia

Congenital umbilical hernia is the most common abdominal hernia in small animals (Robinson, 1977; Ruble and Hird, 1993), and is inheritable, resulting from failure of fusion of the rectus abdominis muscle and fascia after normal return of the midgut from the umbilical cord at six weeks of gestation (Klein and Hertzler, 1981; Robinson, 1977). Neutering should be recommended. Concurrent congenital abnormalities are not uncommon, such as cryptorchidism (Bellenger, 1996), fucosidosis (Taylor et al., 1987), other hernias (e.g. scrotal, diaphragmatic, PPDH), sternal defects, cardiac abnormalities (Bellah et al., 1989a,b), hypospadia and imperforate anus (Klein and Hertzler, 1981). Therefore, the patient should be thoroughly examined for other defects before proceeding to surgery.

Omphalocoeles are large umbilical hernias with overlying skin defects which allow protrusion or extrusion of abdominal viscera from the abdominal cavity. Surgery should be attempted as soon as possible to minimise the risk of visceral damage (Smeak, 2012).

Most small umbilical hernias contain falciform fat and result in no clinical problems for the patient (Smeak, 2012). Healthy puppies with defects less than 2 mm in size can be treated conservatively in the first instance: closure of the defect can occur up to 6 months of age (Smeak, 2012). Current recommendations are to perform surgical closure of inelastic hernia rings with a diameter equal to that of the small intestines because of the theoretical increased risk of visceral strangulation (Smeak, 2012). Smaller or larger defects can also be closed or managed conservatively.

Surgical closure of an uncomplicated umbilical hernia begins with a skin incision directly over the herniation, and the hernia sac is dissected free and removed. Usually, no debridement of the rectus sheath is required and closure is routine. Excess skin can be removed if required. In hernias containing abdominal organs, the hernia ring should be enlarged along the linea alba to return the viscera to the abdomen.

Strangulated or damaged viscera should be removed and adhesions broken down before routine abdominal closure.

In the rare case where primary abdominal closure is not possible, advice should be sought from a surgical specialist. The abdominal wall can be reconstructed using implants (e.g. small intestinal submucosa (Clarke et al., 1996) or prosthetic mesh) or autologous reconstruction (e.g. fascia-relaxing incisions (Smeak, 2012), cranial sartorius muscle flap (Weinstein et al., 1989), external abdominal oblique myofascial flap (Alexander et al., 1991)).

8.2.2 Inguinal hernia

Inguinal hernia describes herniation of abdominal contents directly through the inguinal ring. Congenital inguinal hernias are uncommon and may be concurrent with umbilical hernias: they are more common in male dogs (Smeak, 2012) and may resolve by 12 weeks of age (Fox, 1963). Acquired inguinal hernias are more common in middle-aged, intact bitches (Bellenger, 1996; Waters et al., 1993), particularly those in oestrus or during pregnancy (Waters et al., 1993). Obesity contributes to the development of acquired inguinal hernias (Smeak, 2012). The pathogenesis and heritability of congenital and acquired inguinal hernias is unclear, so affected animals should not be bred from at this time (Fox, 1963). Inguinal hernias may also be traumatic in origin (Smeak, 2012).

The internal inguinal ring is bordered medially by the rectus abdominis muscle, cranially by the internal abdominal oblique muscle and caudolaterally by the inguinal ligament. The external inguinal ring is bordered by the aponeurosis of the external abdominal oblique muscle. The genitofemoral nerve, artery and vein and external pudendal vessels pass through the canal. Both inguinal rings should be carefully palpated because bilateral hernias are seen in 17% of patients (Waters et al., 1993).

Inguinal hernias are best repaired at the time of diagnosis (Smeak, 2012). Surgical closure of an uncomplicated inguinal hernia begins with a skin incision directly over the herniation, and the hernia sac is dissected free and removed. Fat and omentum are the most common hernia contents (Waters et al., 1993). No debridement of the hernia ring is required and the repair is routine, ensuring no neurological or vascular entrapment. In hernias containing abdominal organs, a ventral midline approach should be made initially to allow abdominal exploration, inspection of the contralateral ring and repair of the viscera as required (Waters et al., 1993). The hernia ring itself is then repaired extra-abdominally. Where the uterus is herniated, ovariohysterectomy or hysterotomy should be considered after 7 weeks of gestation; before this time, the uterus can be replaced to its abdominal location if it is not incarcerated (Smeak, 2012).

In the rare case where primary abdominal closure is not possible, advice should be sought from a surgical specialist. Reconstruction can be performed with implants or autologous tissue.

8.2.3 Scrotal hernia

Scrotal hernias are rare, and result from abdominal organs passing through the vaginal ring and into the vaginal process (Smeak, 2012). Strangulation of hernial contents is more common with scrotal hernias compared to other abdominal hernias (Waters et al., 1993). The pathogenesis and heritability of scrotal hernias is unknown. The contralateral side should be carefully inspected. Ectopic testes are reported in up to 33% of dogs with inguinal hernia (Waters et al., 1993).

Surgical repair is indicated as soon as possible because of the high risk of strangulation (Smeak, 2012). In reducible hernias the incision is made over the inguinal ring, which is then repaired, avoiding vital structures. The surgeon should leave the caudal aspect of the external inguinal ring open just sufficiently to allow passage of the genital artery/vein/nerve, external pudendal vessels/nerves and, if castration is not being performed (not advised), the spermatic cord. Bilateral castration is advisable because of the potential heritability of hernias, increased risk of testicular tumours and increased risk of recurrence (Pendergrass and Hayes, 1975). Similar to inguinal hernias, scrotal hernias containing strangulated viscera are approached through the ventral midline to resect and repair the tissues as required; repair of the hernia ring is performed extra-abdominally. Scrotal ablation may be required to minimise dead space.

8.2.4 Femoral hernia

Femoral hernias are rare, and are similar in appearance to inguinal hernia. Knowledge of the regional anatomy and protection of the neurovascular structures is essential: referral to a specialist is advised.

8.2.5 Traumatic hernia

Traumatic abdominal hernias are usually caused by blunt trauma (Waldron et al., 1986) and their contents are more likely to form adhesions because of the lack of a hernial sac (Smeak, 2012). Up to 75% of patients have significant concurrent traumatic injuries (Smeak, 2012) and hernias can form through fractures (Dom and Olmstead, 1976). Strangulation is more likely with traumatic hernias (Crowe, 1988).

Patients with traumatic hernia are challenging to manage, and the hernias themselves can be variable in their extent (e.g. a hernia could involve both the inguinal hernia and femoral canals), necessitating special repair techniques and the requirement for prosthetic implants if tissue damage prevents adequate suture holding. The urgent advice of a surgical specialist should be sought on a case-by-case basis.

8.2.6 Incisional hernia

Incisional hernias occur secondary to dehiscence of a previous surgical site and may occur acutely (within 7 days postoperatively) or more chronically. Risk factors for the development of incisional hernia are detailed in Table 8.3. An impending incisional hernia can be strongly suspected within 5 days of surgery if wound oedema, inflammation and serosanguinous fluid leakage is apparent (Smeak, 2012).

The patient should be examined meticulously and further investigation (e.g. imaging) performed because evisceration (herniation and skin defect) will often result in rapid organ mutilation, which can be fatal. For this reason, immediate repair is indicated if a hernia is identified. If evisceration has occurred, the abdomen should be bandaged and the patient stabilised before surgical intervention at the earliest opportunity. To repair an incisional hernia, the entire surgical line should be re-opened and explored (Fig. 8.11a–d). Debridement of the hernial ring is contraindicated unless necrosis is apparent. Strangulated viscera should be resected and repaired. Closure of the abdominal wall should be tension free and requires inclusion of the strength-holding external rectus sheath in the suture line.

Chronic hernias usually do not result in evisceration, and therefore where the hernial contents are reducible

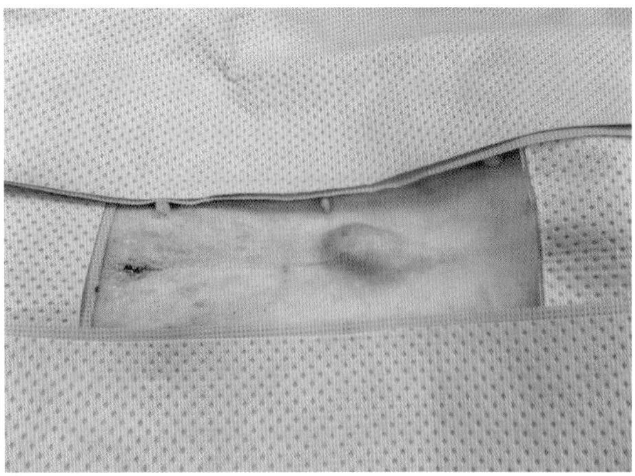

Fig. 8.11a A small incisional hernia at the cranial edge of a midline laparotomy wound, which is 6 months old. The skin is intact.

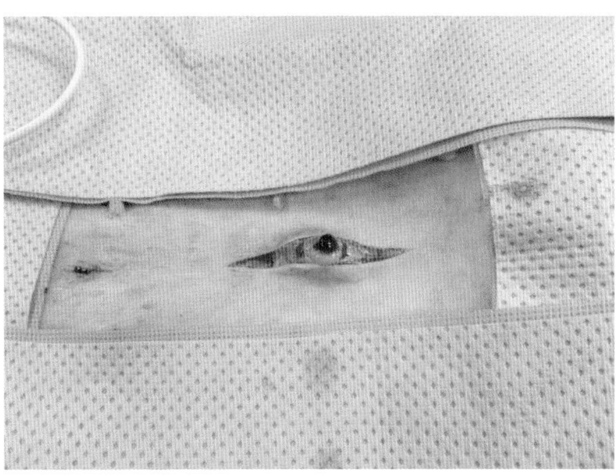

Fig. 8.11b The skin is incised directly over the hernia.

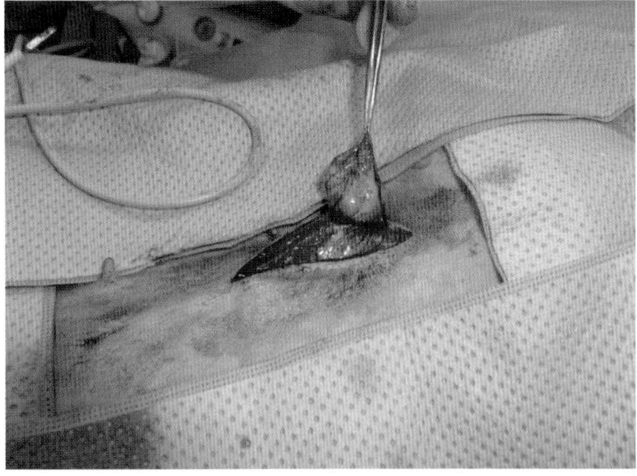

Fig. 8.11c The hernial sac is dissected out.

Table 8.3 Risk factors for the development of incisional hernia.

Surgeon (most common cause of acute hernias)
Tissue (e.g. fat, omentum) trapped between wound edges
Unhealthy tissue at wound site
Incorrect suture selection or suture/knot failure
Poor suture placement (e.g. through peritoneum, rather than the strength-holding external rectus fascia)
Excessive wound tension or traumatic tissue handling
Patient
Elevated intra-abdominal pressure: pain, abdominal distention, coughing, vomiting, straining, etc.
Infection (most common cause of chronic hernia)
Steroid treatment or Cushing's syndrome
Obesity
Hypoproteinaemia
Carer
Poor postoperative care
Excessive exercise
Allowing patient interference with the wound
Poor compliance with medical management (e.g. antibiotics)

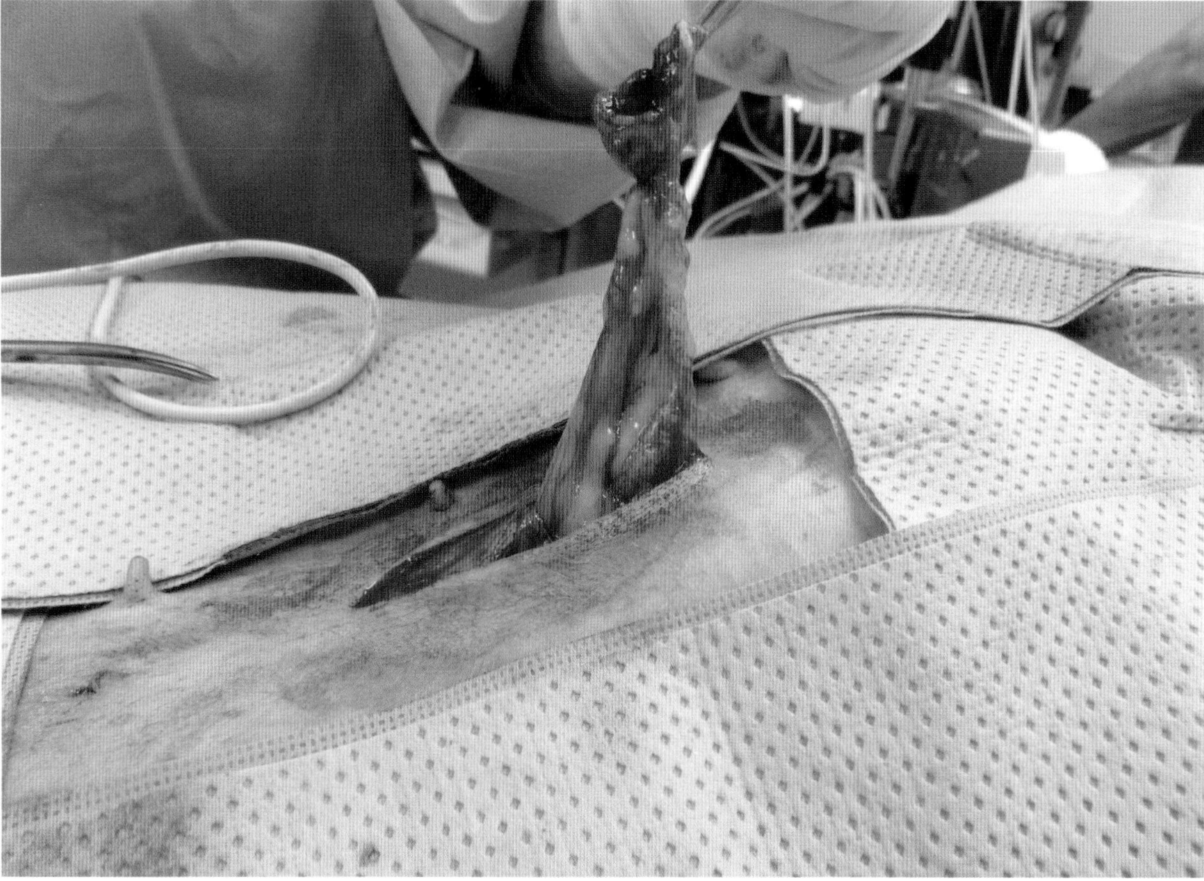

Fig. 8.11d The hernia contains omentum only, which will be resected. Abdominal closure will proceed routinely, ensuring the strength-holding external rectus fascia is included in the closure.

and the hernial ring is large, surgical repair can be scheduled electively. The approach is over the original incision site. Strangulated viscera should be resected and repaired. Simple closure of the chronic hernial ring often results in recurrence (Smeak, 2012), and identification of the strength-holding external rectus sheath within the scar tissue can be challenging. Additionally, loss of domain can ensure that primary closure results in elevated intra-abdominal pressure, which can result in increased likelihood of wound dehiscence, development of potentially fatal abdominal compartment syndrome and impairment of ventilation. Closure using prosthetic implants or autologous repairs (e.g. cranial sartorius muscle flap (Weinstein et al., 1989)) or external abdominal oblique myofascial flap (Alexander et al., 1991) may be indicated.

8.3 Diaphragmatic hernia

Key points

- Diaphragmatic hernia can be traumatic or congenital in origin.
- Traumatic diaphragmatic hernia can result in respiratory and cardiac compromise, alongside visceral entrapment and strangulation.
- Surgery should be performed urgently in traumatic cases of diaphragmatic hernia with gastric entrapment and tympany, ongoing haemorrhage or hypovolaemia, or severe/relentless abdominal pain.
- Preoperative cardiovascular stabilisation is imperative.
- Traumatic diaphragmatic hernias are repaired by primary apposition of the defect edges; postoperative complications occur in 50% of patients; survival to discharge is up to 89%.
- PPDH is congenital in origin.
- Conservative treatment with monitoring can be recommended for asymptomatic PPDH patients.
- Symptomatic PPDH patients should undergo surgery: cats and dogs have a survival rate of 86 and 82–100%, respectively. Complications can be seen in up to 78% of patients.

Introduction

The diaphragm is the musculotendinous separation between the thoracic and abdominal organs and assists in ventilation and movement of lymphatic fluid (Hunt and Johnson, 2012). Diaphragmatic hernia is the disruption of the diaphragm that allows abdominal organs to migrate into the thorax.

Two types of diaphragmatic hernias occur in the dog and cat:

- traumatic – usually following a road traffic accident (RTA)
- congenital – most commonly PPDH.

8.3.1 Traumatic diaphragmatic hernia

Pathophysiology

Traumatic diaphragmatic hernia usually occurs secondary to RTAs (in up to 85% of cases (Gibson et al., 2005; Wilson et al., 1971)), but may also be a result of falling, an unknown or penetrating trauma or a dog attack (Gibson et al., 2005). The diaphragmatic rupture occurs along the fibre orientation of the costal musculature (radial tear, seen in 45% of cases), the muscular attachment to the ribs (circumferential tear, seen in 23% of cases) or a combination of both (Sullivan and Reid, 1990). Abdominal organs can herniate into the thorax: the liver is the most commonly herniated organ, but the stomach, uterus, omentum, small/large intestine, spleen and pancreas can also be involved (Sullivan and Reid, 1990).

Traumatic diaphragmatic hernias may be acute or chronic upon presentation (Minihan et al., 2004; Schmiedt et al., 2003). The most common clinical signs include tachypnoea (up to 79.4%), dyspnoea (41.1%), muffled heart sounds (29.4%) and vomiting (11.7%) (Schmiedt et al., 2003). Other clinical findings include anorexia, diarrhoea, open-mouth breathing, cyanosis, cachexia, icterus, increased or decreased lung sounds, exercise intolerance, shock, cardiac arrhythmia, pale mucous membranes and hypothermia (Minihan et al., 2004; Schmiedt et al., 2003). Up to 27 and 33.3% of patients have concurrent soft tissue or orthopaedic injuries, respectively (e.g. urinary bladder rupture or fractures) (Gibson et al., 2005).

Respiratory compromise occurs secondary to loss of the mechanical function of the diaphragm, pleural space-occupying effect of abdominal organs (plus associated air or fluid accumulation), compression and atelectasis of lung lobes, or ventilatory impairment (e.g. as a result of concurrent rib fractures, intercostal muscle damage, pulmonary contusion, pain, etc.) (Worth and Machon, 2005). This results in significant hypoventilation and alveolar ventilation–perfusion mismatch, leading to potentially life-threatening hypoxia.

Cardiac arrhythmias have been reported in 12% of dogs with traumatic diaphragmatic hernias, resulting in the death of one-third of those patients (Boudrieau and Muir, 1987). Cardiac arrythmia occurs because herniation of abdominal viscera may compress the thoracic caudal vena cava, decreasing venous return and reducing cardiac output. Additionally, traumatic myocarditis (Reiss et al., 2002), poor oxygen delivery and hypovolaemic shock can also affect cardiac function.

The abdominal organs herniated into the thoracic cavity can become entrapped and strangulated, leading to accumulation of transudate, adhesion formation and visceral torsion, perforation or necrosis (Minihan et al., 2004). Resection of affected tissue is required in such patients.

Diagnosis

Not all patients with traumatic diaphragmatic hernia present with a history of RTA or respiratory compromise. In such patients, failure to initially identify a diaphragmatic hernia is not uncommon (Wilson et al., 1971) and it may be identified some years later (Minihan et al., 2004). All patients presenting following a traumatic episode should undergo detailed imaging of the thoracic and abdominal cavities, even in the absence of clinical signs of injury to these sites.

Radiography is the initial imaging modality of choice for patients with diaphragmatic hernia (Sullivan and Lee, 1989), but only achieves a diagnosis in 70% of cases (Minihan et al., 2004). Pre-oxygenation and minimal restraint is recommended. Compromised patients can deteriorate with the stress of handling and positioning for radiography, and therefore appropriate stabilisation for shock and respiratory compromise should take place beforehand. Radiographic findings include partial loss of the normal line of the diaphragm (seen in up to 97% of patients; Minihan et al., 2004; Sullivan and Lee, 1989), herniation of small intestine or other viscera (up to 61 and 35%, respectively; Sullivan and Lee, 1989), obscured or displaced cardiac silhouette, lung collapse, rib fractures and pleural fluid (Fig. 8.12a–c).

Contrast studies can be performed, but are rarely indicated (Hunt and Johnson, 2012).

Ultrasound examination can document organ herniation and loss of the diaphragmatic line in 90% of patients (Minihan et al., 2004). Cardiovascular stabilisation, pre-oxygenation and minimal restraint are advised. Advanced imaging (e.g. CT) can also diagnose diaphragmatic hernia, but has the disadvantage that general anaesthesia is required.

Treatment

Surgical timing

The treatment of choice for traumatic diaphragmatic hernia is surgical repair. Historically, clinicians advocated delaying surgery because of a reported increase in

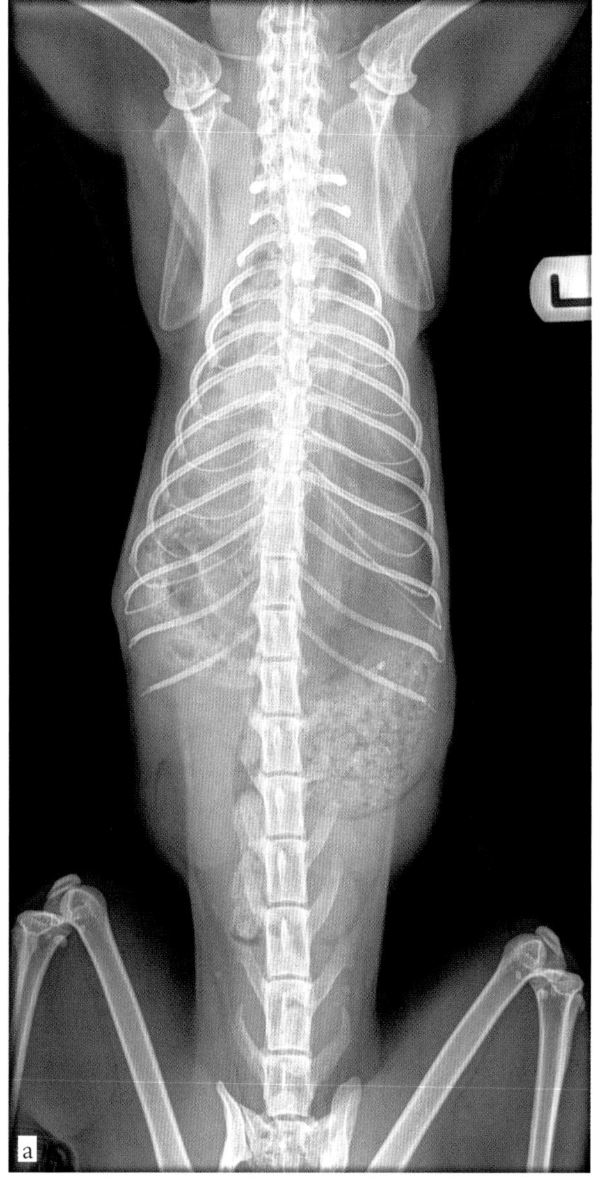

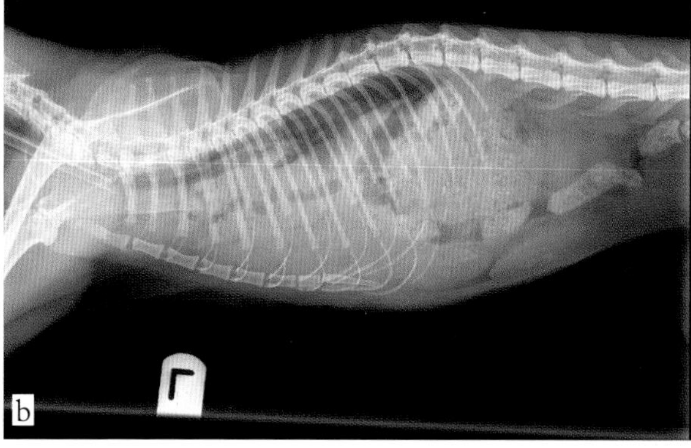

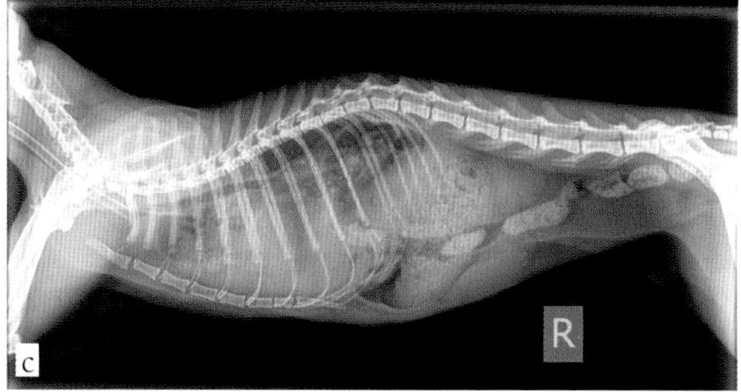

Fig. 8.12a–c Traumatic diaphragmatic hernia. Dorsoventral (Fig. 8.12a), left lateral (Fig. 8.12b) and right lateral (Fig. 8.12c) radiographs of the thorax and abdomen of a skeletally mature cat, showing loss of the diaphragmatic outline bilaterally. The abdominal cavity contains only the descending colon, some small intestine, spleen, stomach, kidneys and urinary bladder. The majority of the small and large intestines and the liver are displaced in the thoracic cavity. The stomach is moderately to severely distended with food and gas, and appears still to be intra-abdominal. There is pleural effusion and displaced abdominal organs causing border effacement of the cardiac silhouette and dorsal displacement of the trachea and lung lobes. Compression atelectasis of the lung lobes is evidenced by air bronchograms, soft tissue opacity and decreased lung lobe size. There is no evidence of fracture or subluxation of the spine, or fracture of other bony structures included in the radiographs.

mortality (33%) in patients undergoing surgery within 24 hours of trauma (Boudrieau and Muir, 1987). The same study that reported these findings also showed an increase in mortality (62.5%) in patients undergoing surgery after one year (Boudrieau and Muir, 1987). Recent larger studies have disproved this (Downs and Bjorling, 1987): early surgical intervention (within 24 hours) for acute diaphragmatic hernias and repair of chronic hernia are both associated with good perioperative survival rates (89.1 and 79%, respectively; Gibson et al., 2005; Minihan et al., 2004). Therefore, timing of surgery should be based on the extent of cardiopulmonary dysfunction, respiratory compromise and organ entrapment. As soon as the patient is sufficiently stable for anaesthesia, surgery should be performed. Surgery should be performed urgently in cases with gastric entrapment and tympany (which can cause life-threatening lung compression), ongoing haemorrhage and hypovolaemia (suggestive of hepatic/splenic involvement) or severe/relentless abdominal pain (suggestive of visceral strangulation). Diaphragmatic hernia repair has a higher priority than definitive fracture repair, so any concurrent orthopaedic injuries may have to be addressed during subsequent surgeries. Appropriate analgesia and immobilisation (e.g. Robert Jones bandages) should be provided until definitive orthopaedic repair.

Perioperative care

Patients with traumatic diaphragmatic hernias represent a significant anaesthetic risk and should be stabilised as much as possible before surgery. Detailed discussion of cardiorespiratory stabilisation is beyond the scope of this chapter. Adequate volume replacement is required for hypovolaemic shock: isotonic crystalloids, hypertonic saline, colloids, blood products and combinations of these fluids are all commonly used. Patients with respiratory compromise (e.g. tachypnoea, dyspnoea, cyanosis, orthopnoea) should be provided with oxygen via face mask, oxygen cage, nasal prongs, nasal catheters, flow-by, etc. Significant pneumothorax should be addressed to aid ventilation, and gastric decompression should be performed if the stomach is trapped. Regular monitoring, assessment and modification of the treatment plan is essential for critically ill patients.

Patients with traumatic diaphragmatic hernia should receive generous multimodal analgesia, judicious premedication, pre-oxygenation and a rapid, smooth induction. Rapid control of airway and ventilation via an endotracheal tube is required, along with intermittent positive-pressure ventilation (IPPV). High inspiratory pressure (>20 cmH_20) should be avoided, to reduce the risk of re-expansion pulmonary oedema (Hunt and Johnson, 2012).

The provision of antibiotics depends on the individual patient, surgical duration and potential for intra-operative contamination. Clostridial bacteria can occur in incarcerated liver lobes and may cause release of toxins into the circulation after the lobes are repositioned (Hunt and Johnson, 2012): patients with liver or biliary tract herniation should receive prophylactic antibiosis.

Once anaesthetised, the patient should be placed in dorsal recumbency with the table tilted such that the head is elevated (Fig. 8.13). Patients with a predominantly unilateral hernia may benefit from the affected side being tilted downwards to reduce compression of the functional lung (Garson et al., 1980). The ventral thorax and abdomen should be clipped and aseptically prepared. The clip should extend laterally over the thorax to allow positioning of a chest drain.

Surgery

Goals for uncomplicated herniorrhaphy are listed in Table 8.4. Traumatic diaphragmatic rupture is repaired via a midline laparotomy from xiphoid to pubis. This can be extended into a caudal sternotomy if wider access is required, but is rarely indicated and is associated with greater postoperative morbidity and pain (Worth and Machon, 2005). The falciform ligament should be excised to improve exposure, using diathermy or ligatures around the vasculature located near the xiphoid. Retractors are essential for good visualisation; in the cat, a ring retractor is particularly useful. The entire diaphragm should be inspected, because multiple rents can be apparent in traumatic hernias (Garson et al., 1980). Many herniated abdominal contents can be repositioned using gentle traction, taking particular care with herniated liver and spleen, which can become congested and friable.

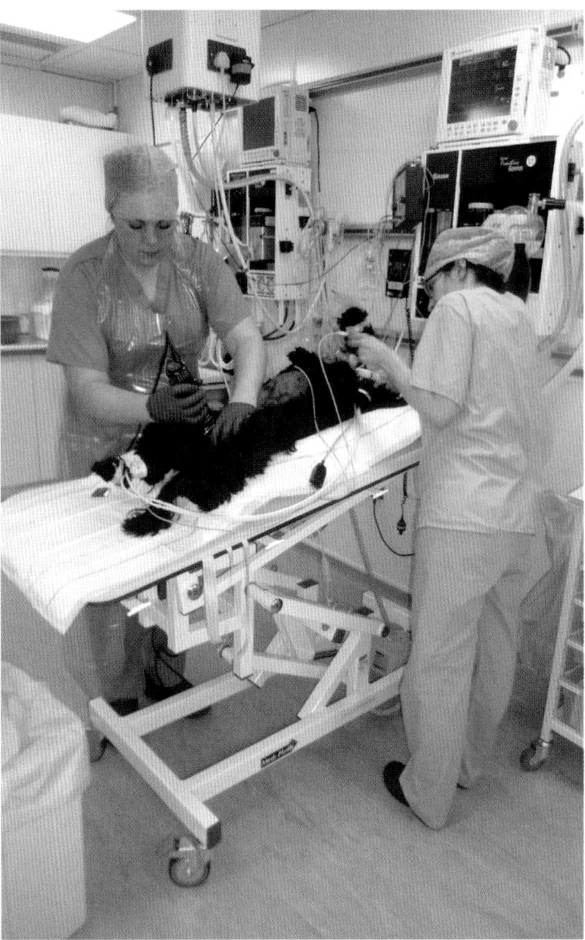

Fig. 8.13 Once anaesthetised, the patient with diaphragmatic hernia should be placed in dorsal recumbency, with the table tilted such that the head is elevated.

Table 8.4 Goals for uncomplicated diaphragmatic herniorrhaphy.

Preoperative goals
Client education and informed consent
Patient cardiovascular and respiratory stabilisation
Understanding of the viscera involved in the herniation
Understanding of any co-morbidities or injuries
Smooth, rapid induction to anaesthesia and establishment of airway access for ventilation
Thorough understanding of regional anatomy
Aseptic preparation of the patient
Surgical goals
Adherence to Halsted's principles
Reduction of herniated tissue and removal of adhesions or damaged tissue
Anatomic closure of the defect
Placement of a chest drain and evacuation of the chest sufficiently to allow ventilation
Abdominal closure without undue tension
Postoperative goals
Thorough evaluation and control of the patient postoperatively
Monitoring and early treatment for any complications

A malleable retractor can be helpful in such circumstances. If hernia contents are irreducible, then the hernial ring should be enlarged, avoiding the phrenic vessels, phrenic nerves and caudal vena cava. Any intrathoracic adhesions should be broken down under direct observation using blunt (in cases of more recent fibrinous adhesions) or sharp (in cases of more mature adhesions) dissection. Occasionally, mature adhesion formation will require transection of viscera (e.g. lung, liver, omentum, etc.), and the surgeon must be capable of performing surgery on a variety of organs. The thoracic and abdominal viscera should all be inspected for viability and a thoracostomy tube placed (see this volume, Chapter 9 for further details). There is debate regarding the need to debride the edges of the rent; currently, recommendations are to perform simple closure because debridement risks iatrogenic trauma, increasing the size of the defect and decreasing the holding power of the sutures (Hunt and Johnson, 2012; Worth and Machon, 2005). Closure of tissue margins of recent traumatic hernias is relatively easy: suture closure should proceed in a dorsal to ventral direction, using an absorbable monofilament synthetic material (e.g. polydioxanone or polyglyconate) in a continuous pattern (Hunt and Johnson, 2012). With circumferential tears, the diaphragm can be approximated to the thoracic wall using circumcostal sutures. Rarely, chronic diaphragmatic hernia may atrophy such that primary closure with sutures is not possible: such cases should be referred to a specialist surgeon and closure options may include autologous tissue (e.g. omentum (Bright and Thacker, 1982), muscle (Helphrey, 1982), liver (Neville and Clowes, 1954), fascia) or synthetic/natural implants (e.g. mesh, porcine submucosa or silicon rubber tubing (Hunt and Johnson, 2012)). In a recent study of 34 dogs and 16 cats with chronic diaphragmatic hernias, all rents were closed primarily (Minihan et al., 2004).

Closure of the linea alba is routine. The thoracostomy tube should remain open and IPPV continued until the abdomen is closed and the thoracic cavity has been gently evacuated of air/fluid (see note on re-expansion pulmonary oedema). Chronic hernias may rarely be accompanied by contraction of the abdominal volume secondary to displacement of abdominal viscera (Worth and Machon, 2005).

A postoperative radiograph is indicated if there are concerns about persistent pneumothorax, pleural effusion, collapsed lung lobes or chest tube positioning (Hunt and Johnson, 2012).

Postoperative care

Postoperatively, the patient's cardiovascular and respiratory status should be monitored closely. The patient should be provided with intravenous fluid therapy (as required until (s)he is eating and drinking), generous multimodal analgesia (as determined by regular pain scoring and including intrapleural bupivacaine via the thoracostomy tube) and oxygen if necessary. Postoperative antibiotics are unnecessary, unless the liver has been herniated or injured or a hollow abdominal organ perforated (Hunt and Johnson, 2012). The thoracostomy tube is removed when no air and less than 2 ml/kg/24 h of fluid is evacuated – in most cases, this occurs within hours of surgery. Potential complications are seen in Table 8.5.

Reperfusion injury occurs when blood supply returns to hitherto strangulated abdominal organs, releasing toxic by-products of anaerobic metabolism (e.g. unbuffered acids, potassium and lysosomal

Table 8.5 Summary of potential complications associated with repair of diaphragmatic hernia.

Surgical complications
Anaesthetic complications
Haemorrhage
Visceral injury/strangulation
Inability to close the hernia rent or abdominal wall in chronic hernias
Iatrogenic trauma to the phrenic nerves, vessels or caudal vena cava
Complications arising secondary to resection of adherent viscera
Early postoperative complications
Infection
Pain
Seroma
Haematoma
Tachypnoea
Hypoventilation
Hypoxia
Respiratory acidosis (secondary to pain-associated inadequate ventilation)
Ventilation–perfusion abnormalities
Sudden cardiac arrest
Reperfusion injury
Ascites
Re-expansion pulmonary oedema
Pulmonary oedema
Pneumothorax
Haemothorax
Wound dehiscence and evisceration
Abdominal compartment syndrome
Transient megaoesophagus and oesophagitis
Gastric ulceration
Late postoperative complications
Hernia recurrence
Hiatal hernia
Rupture, strangulation or obstruction of the gastrointestinal tract
Infection of implants

enzymes) (Worth and Machon, 2005). Re-expansion pulmonary oedema is a common cause of postoperative death in cats, and occurs when atelectatic lungs are re-expanded, especially if the atelectasis is chronic (Boudrieau and Muir, 1987; Downs and Bjorling, 1987; Garson et al., 1980). Clinical signs precede radiographic changes and the prognosis is guarded. Treatment may include haemodynamic support, oxygen, diuretics, bronchodilators and positive end-expiratory pressure ventilation (Hunt and Johnson, 2012). Occurrence of re-expansion pulmonary oedema can be minimised by ensuring that IPPV pressures do not exceed 15–20 cmH_2O and by avoiding high airway inflation pressures to evacuate the chest of air prior to closure. Instead, the chest should be gently evacuated of air until the patient is ventilating easily (i.e. not necessarily until negative pressure is achieved), and then the pneumothorax alleviated gradually over the following 8–12 hours (Worth and Machon, 2005).

Abdominal compartment syndrome may occur in patients with chronic hernia secondary to 'loss of domain', and the advice of a surgical specialist should be sought at an early stage in such cases. Increased intra-abdominal pressure can result in decreased visceral perfusion, acidosis, decreased renal function, decreased cardiac output (leading to hypotension), decreased ventilation (leading to hypoxia) and increased intracranial pressure (Hunt and Johnson, 2012).

Measurement of intra-abdominal pressure (IAP) can be performed via an indwelling urinary catheter: patients with IAP 5–10 mmHg should be monitored; patients with IAP 11–20 mmHg should receive medical treatment (analgesia, evacuation of any intraperitoneal or intra-luminal contents); patients with IAP >20 mmHg and unresponsive to medical management should undergo surgical decompression (Hunt and Johnson, 2012). Surgical options to increase abdominal space and decrease IAP include the use of surgical mesh, removal of viscera (e.g. splenectomy), diaphragmatic advancement, relaxing incisions in the external rectus sheath or a staged closure of the abdomen (Hunt and Johnson, 2012): these procedures should be performed by a surgical specialist in a multi-disciplinary hospital.

Prognosis

Approximately 15% of patients with diaphragmatic hernia die before presentation (Hunt and Johnson, 2012). Although surgical repair of traumatic diaphragmatic herniation is commonly performed in general practice, referral to a hospital with a dedicated anaesthetist, means to measure airway pressures and intensively monitor and treat patients is optimal. Patients with traumatic diaphragmatic hernia are challenging: acutely traumatised patients often have several co-morbidities; chronic cases can require extensive visceral resection secondary to adhesions or result in difficulty with abdominal closure due to 'loss of domain'. Recent advances in surgical and anaesthetic management of patients have contributed to improved survival within referral hospitals. Survival to discharge is currently reported at up to 89% (Gibson et al., 2005; Minihan et al., 2004; Schmiedt et al., 2003), with similar results reported for dogs and cats, acute and chronic hernias, and patients undergoing surgery within 12 and 24 hours. Postoperative complications occur in up to 50% of patients (Schmiedt et al., 2003). A single case report exists detailing multiple acquired portosystemic shunt in a cat secondary to chronic diaphragmatic rupture, clinical signs of which resolved within 1 year of herniorrhapy (Barfield et al., 2015a,b).

8.3.2 Peritoneo-pericardial diaphragmatic hernia (PPDH)

Pathophysiology

PPDH occurs secondary to a failure in development of the transverse septum of the diaphragm (Noden and de Lahunta, 1985), resulting in herniation of abdominal viscera into the pericardial sac. Despite the congenital nature of PPDH, patients may be asymptomatic for years and the condition may remain undiagnosed or be identified incidentally (Evans and Biery, 1980). Where clinical signs are present, they may be secondary to indirect lung compression, visceral obstruction or strangulation, chylothorax or cardiac tamponade and right-sided heart failure (Corfield et al., 2009; Hunt and Johnson, 2012; Schmiedt et al., 2009). The patient should be thoroughly examined to identify any concurrent sternal or abdominal wall defects, which are seen in up to 57.1% of dogs and 23.3% of cats (Bellah et al., 1989a,b ; Burns et al., 2013). Rarely, intracardiac defects can also be present.

Diagnosis

Physical examination may be unremarkable, or heart sounds may be muffled or abnormally placed. PPDH can be diagnosed using radiography or ultrasonography. Radiography shows an enlarged, oval/rounded cardiac silhouette (filled with soft tissue/fat opacity, or gas/faeces-filled bowel) with a dorsally displaced trachea. The diaphragmatic border is discontinuous. Contrast studies are rarely indicated and are generally unhelpful (Evans and Biery, 1980). Ultrasound examination via the right fifth intercostal space or trans-abdominally will aid in identifying the hernial contents, and has the advantage that it can be performed on conscious animals if clinical signs are severe (Hay et al., 1989).

Surgery

Conservative treatment with monitoring can be recommended for asymptomatic patients (Burns et al., 2013). Where surgical correction is required, analgesia, anaesthesia and stabilisation is as for traumatic diaphragmatic hernia. Surgical goals are shown in this volume, section 8.3.1. Surgery is via a ventral midline laparotomy (from xiphoid to pubis). The viscera are returned to the abdomen, adhesions are removed and any damaged or diseased tissue is resected. Small defects are closed with a simple continuous pattern of monofilament absorbable material (e.g. polydioxanone or polyglyconate), beginning dorsally as for traumatic diaphragmatic hernias. The pericardial sac should be drained immediately after hernia closure. Large defects are uncommon and can be repaired using flaps or grafts, taking care to avoid the phrenic nerves (Hunt and Johnson, 2012). Most patients do not require a thoracostomy tube, and postoperative care is similar to that for traumatic diaphragmatic hernia.

Prognosis

Prognosis for the surgical management of PPDH is good, assuming there are no concurrent intracardiac defects (Bellah et al., 1989a,b). Clinical signs associated with PPDH resolve in 85.3% of surgically treated patients (Burns et al., 2013). Cats have a survival rate of around 86% (Reimer et al., 2004) and dogs 82–100% (Bellah et al., 1989a,b; Evans and Biery, 1980). Potential complications in addition to those seen in Table 8.5 include hyperthermia, partial blindness (in the cat), metaplastic transformation of liver into sarcoma, refractory pneumothorax, cough, constrictive pericarditis and development of pericardial cysts (Hunt and Johnson, 2012; Murphy et al., 2014; Linton et al., 2016). Complications can be seen in up to 78% of patients, particularly cats (Reimer et al., 2004).

8.4 Septic peritonitis

Key points

- Septic peritonitis is characterised by inflammation of the peritoneum secondary to bacterial contamination.
- The gastrointestinal tract is a source of septic peritonitis in up to 75% of cases.
- Septic peritonitis is usually polymicrobial.
- The mortality rate in patients is 37–85%.
- Clinical signs can be variable.
- Abdominocentesis is the single most useful diagnostic test.
- Surgery depends on the source of the peritonitis. Gastrointestinal perforation usually necessitates resection–anastomosis, serosal patching and omentalisation.
- Copious abdominal lavage should be performed.
- The abdomen can be closed primarily, or managed with closed or open drainage.
- Patients require individualised intensive care postoperatively.

Introduction and pathophysiology

Septic peritonitis is a potentially fatal condition, characterised by inflammation of the peritoneum secondary to bacterial contamination (Hosgood and Salisbury, 1988). The gastrointestinal tract is the most common source: this is the case in up to 80% and 47% of cases in the dog and cat, respectively (Adams et al., 2014; Costello et al., 2004; Hosgood and Salisbury, 1988).

Up to 12% of dogs undergoing gastrointestinal surgery suffer from enteric wound dehiscence 3–9 days postoperatively (Shales et al., 2005). Increased risk for ingesta leakage and decreased survival is seen in patients undergoing a greater number of enteric procedures (Wylie and Hosgood, 1994), following trauma (Allen and Schertel, 1992; Ralphs et al., 2003) or in the presence of preoperative septic peritonitis, low preoperative serum albumin and plasma protein concentrations, and intra-operative hypotension (Grimes et al., 2011). The increased bacterial load and higher proportion of anaerobic bacteria present in the distal gastrointestinal tract are responsible for increased mortality associated with large intestinal perforation, which can approach 100% (Toombs et al., 1986). For this reason, alternatives to full-thickness intestinal biopsy (e.g. endoscopic biopsy) should be pursued preferentially wherever possible and large intestinal biopsy should be avoided. Other causes of gastrointestinal-related septic peritonitis include perforation secondary to gastric dilation volvulus, foreign bodies, ulcers, trauma, intussusception, neoplasia (Kirby, 2012), iatrogenic injury (Kirby, 2012) and leakage of feeding tubes (Elliott et al., 2000).

Other causes of septic peritonitis can result from perforation of the urogenital tract (seen in 21.4% of all cases, usually pyometra; Kenney et al., 1987; Wheaton et al., 1989); hepatobiliary system (9.5% of cases, and often secondarily infected with *Clostridium* spp.; Bentley et al., 2007; Hosgood and Salisbury, 1988); perforated abscess (e.g. sublumbar abscess secondary to a migrating foreign body, or pancreatic abscess; Hosgood and Salisbury, 1988); or as a complication of peritoneal dialysis (Hosgood and Salisbury, 1988).

Septic peritonitis is usually polymicrobial, with *E. coli* predomination, but other organisms involved may include staphylococci, streptococci, *Enterococcus* spp., *Enterobacter* spp., *Klebsiella* spp., *Clostridium* spp. and *Bacteroides fragilis* (Kirby, 2012). Early mortality is increased by Gram-negative aerobic organisms and the resultant high levels of endotoxin (e.g. α-haemolysin) which are absorbed into the systemic circulation: this is seen particularly with *E. coli* (Johnson et al., 1997). These endotoxins are toxic to mammalian cells, decrease intraperitoneal pH, lyse intraperitoneal erythrocytes and decrease viable peritoneal leucocytes.

Clinical signs in patients with septic peritonitis can be variable and may include those signs described in Table 8.6. A history of recent gastrointestinal surgery should raise a high index of suspicion for postoperative septic peritonitis.

Diagnosis

Abdominal radiographs (Fig. 8.14a,b) are often performed in the first instance. In cases with septic peritonitis, loss of serosal detail may indicate the presence of free abdominal fluid; this is also seen as a normal finding in young or thin animals. Free abdominal gas is normal following recent abdominal surgery, but otherwise is indicative of gastrointestinal perforation, gas-producing organisms or penetrating abdominal trauma. If neoplasia is suspected, three-view inflated thoracic radiographs should be considered preoperatively to aid in determining metastatic status. Double effusions (e.g. pleural and peritoneal) are associated with a 3.3-fold increased risk of death and may be a sequela to disseminated intravascular coagulation (Steyn and Wittum, 1993). Contrast studies are rarely indicated; barium should always be avoided because leakage into the peritoneum is associated with increased mortality (Cochran et al., 1963). CT can also be used, where available.

Abdominal ultrasound (Fig. 8.15a–d) is extremely useful in the diagnosis of septic peritonitis, because it will permit detection of small volumes of free abdominal fluid which can be aspirated. The underlying cause

Table 8.6 Potential clinical signs associated with septic peritonitis.

Abdomen
Abdominal enlargement (which may cause tachypnoea due to diaphragmatic compression, pleural effusion and pain)
Abdominal pain (seen in only 62% of cats (Costello et al., 2004))
Lack of bowel sounds (reflecting ileus (Tivers, 2011))

Dehydration and/or hypovolaemia

Demeanour
Depression, malaise, collapse

Gastrointestinal
Anorexia, vomiting, diarrhoea

Genitourinary tract
Vaginal/preputial discharge
Pyuria/haematuria
Abnormal hindlimb gait

Polyuria/polydipsia

Icterus

SIRS/sepsis
In the early stages of the disease, the patient may have a hyperdynamic pulse, fast capillary refill time, tachycardia, pyrexia and injected mucous membranes
As hypovolaemia and vasodilation progress, patients develop severe tachycardia, weak pulse, prolonged capillary refill time, hypothermia and pale mucous membranes. White blood cell counts may be high or low (>19,500 or <5000 cells/μl in the cat; >18,000 or <5000 cells/μl in the dog (Kirby, 2012)), typically with an increased proportion of band neutrophils (>5%) and toxic changes
Severe cases may develop fulminant septic shock and/or disseminated intravascular coagulation (DIC)

Temperature:
Patients may be hypo-, hyper- or normothermic
Cats are more commonly hypothermic (Kirby, 2012)

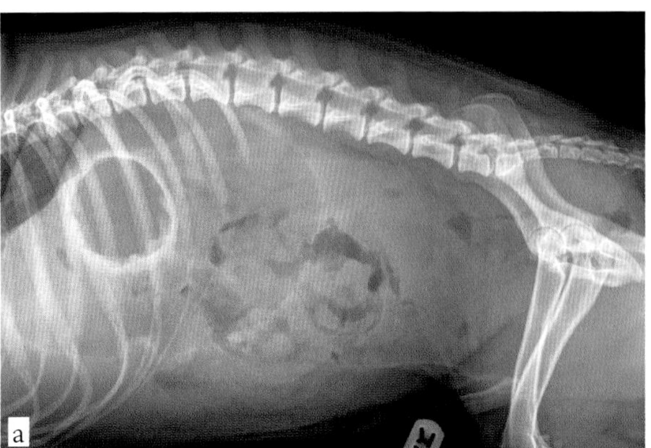

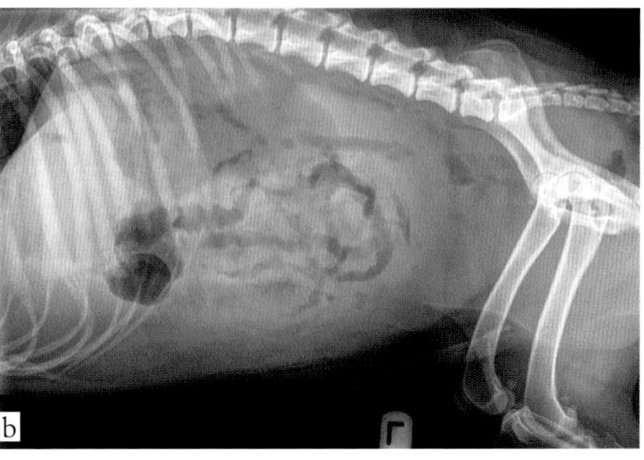

Fig. 8.14a,b Right (Fig. 8.14a) and left (Fig. 8.14b) lateral abdominal radiographs of a dog, showing loss of serosal detail and corrugation of the intestinal tract.

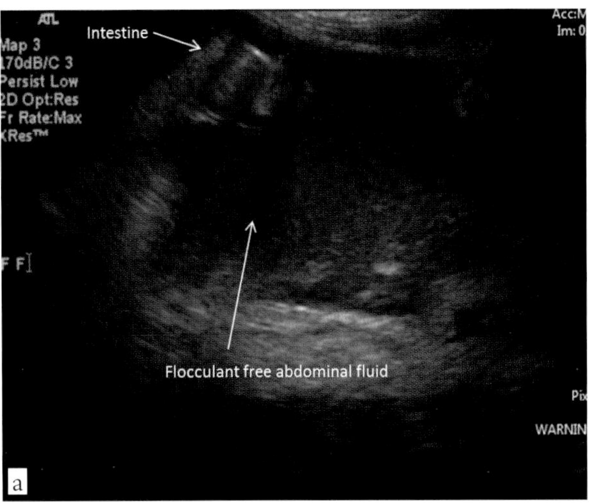

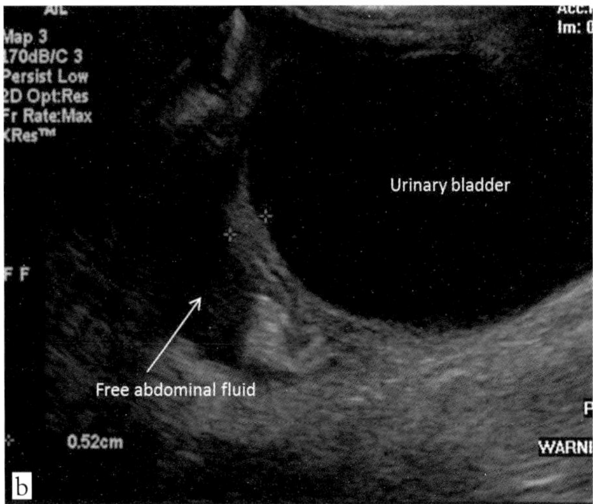

Fig. 8.15a,b Ultrasound images of the patient in Fig. 8.14 showing a large volume of echogenic free abdominal fluid. The free fluid was aspirated under ultrasound guidance and examined microscopically in-house (Fig. 8.16).

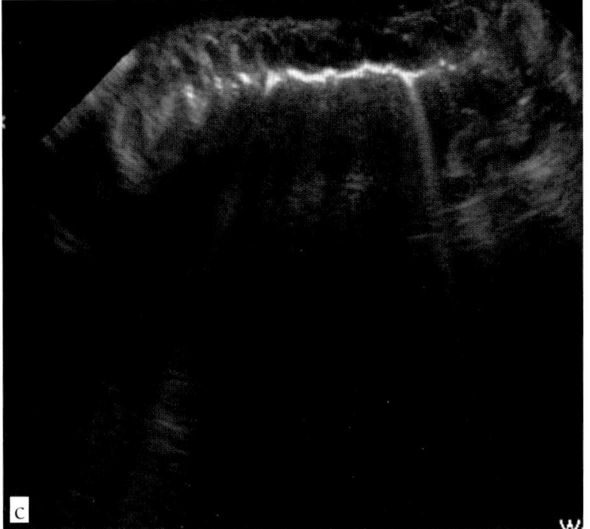

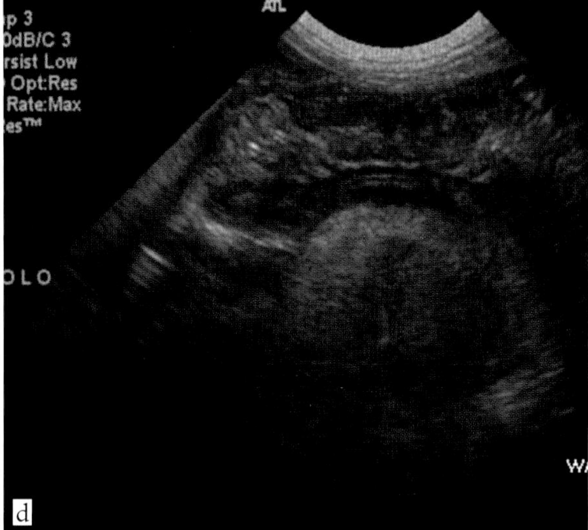

Fig. 8.15c,d Ultrasound images of the patient in Fig. 8.14. Corrugation of the small and large intestine is seen.

of the peritoneal effusions can also be determined, as can the presence/absence of pancreatitis.

Abdominocentesis (usually ultrasound guided) is the single most useful diagnostic test for septic peritonitis; a butterfly catheter is passed into the fluid which is collected for analysis, giving an overall accuracy of 82.9% (Crowe, 1984). Diagnostic peritoneal lavage increases diagnostic accuracy to 94.6% (Crowe, 1984), but is rarely required where ultrasound-guided abdominocentesis is available. Evaluation and interpretation (gross, cytological, biochemical and microbiological) of peritoneal fluid is essential; results suggestive of septic peritonitis are illustrated in Table 8.7. Cytology (Diff-Quik and/or Gram stain, Fig. 8.16) is the most useful test and is up to 87% accurate (Levin et al., 2004); it should be performed urgently (often in-house). Chemical analysis of abdominal fluid is of very limited use, because blood-to-peritoneal fluid lactate and glucose concentrations in normal dogs 4 days after exploratory laparotomy

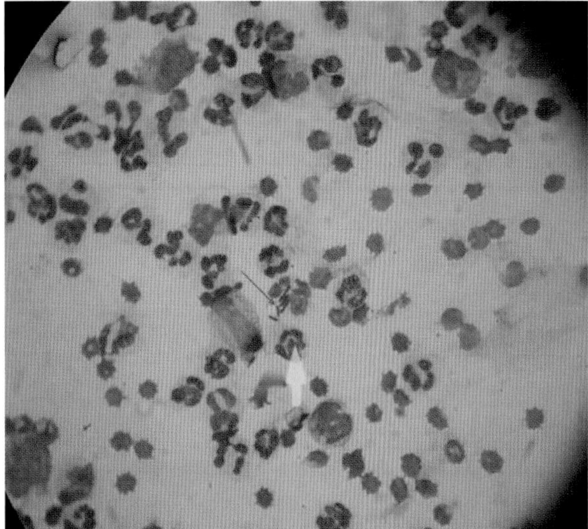

Fig. 8.16 In-house cytological assessment of free abdominal fluid obtained via ultrasound-guided abdominocentesis, air-dried on a slide and stained with Diff-Quik, shows rods within a degenerate neutrophil, diagnostic of septic peritonitis.

Table 8.7 Results of peritoneal fluid analysis suggestive of septic peritonitis.

Cytology is the single most useful analysis that can be performed
Gross appearance: clear, serosanguinous, turbid, purulent, green (bile), food/faeces
Cytology: toxic and degenerate neutrophils, intracellular bacteria, vegetable material
Fluid analysis (Kirby, 2012):
total protein >3 g/μl
nucleated cell count >5000/μl (note that no cell count can reliably differentiate between a normal postoperative response and septic peritonitis)
presence of plant material
peritoneal fluid creatinine or bilirubin concentration higher than that in the serum (suggestive of uro-abdomen or free intraperitoneal bile, respectively)
peritoneal fluid pH <7.35
blood-to-peritoneal fluid glucose difference >1.12 mmol/l*
peritoneal fluid glucose concentration <2.75 mmol/l*
peritoneal fluid lactate concentration >2 mmol/l higher than in the blood*

*may not be reliable indicators of septic peritonitis in postoperative patients (Szabo et al., 2011).

mirror those of patients with septic peritonitis (Szabo et al., 2011). The inoculation of blood culture bottles with abdominal fluid greatly increases the success of culture (Laroche and Harding, 1998).

Treatment

Preoperative management

Animals with septic peritonitis represent a significant anaesthetic risk and should be stabilised as much as possible before surgery. Detailed discussion of cardiorespiratory stabilisation is beyond the scope of this chapter. Adequate volume replacement is required for hypovolaemic shock: isotonic crystalloids, hypertonic saline, colloids, blood products and combinations of these fluids are all commonly used. Patients with increased respiratory rate or effort (secondary to ascites) should be provided with oxygen via face mask, oxygen cage, nasal prongs, nasal catheters, flow-by, etc. Regular monitoring, assessment and modification of the treatment plan are essential for critically ill patients. Patients with septic peritonitis should receive generous multimodal analgesia, judicious premedication, pre-oxygenation and a rapid, smooth anaesthetic induction. If ascites is severe and impinging on ventilation, the table should be tilted such that the head is elevated. The ventral abdomen should be widely clipped and aseptically prepared.

The provision of antibiotics (guided by Gram staining) is indicated as soon as peritoneal fluid samples have been obtained for aerobic and anaerobic culture and sensitivity. Bactericidal antibiotics effective against Gram-positive and -negative aerobes and anaerobes are recommended. Currently, good initial empirical choices include clavulanic amoxicillin (20 mg/kg IV q6 h) or a second-generation cephalosporin (20 mg/kg IV q6 h) and metronidazole (10 mg/kg IV q12 h). Fluoroquinolones should be avoided unless indicated by sensitivity results: their use may increase bacterial resistance and less than 52% of isolates found in cases of septic peritonitis are sensitive to fluoroquinolones (Lee et al., 2000). Currently, appropriate empirical antibiotics are only provided to 52.6% of dogs with septic peritonitis and this is more likely to occur where previous antibiotics have been administered or recent abdominal surgery has been performed (Dickinson et al., 2015). Current evidence in veterinary practice has not demonstrated a clear benefit for certain antimicrobial choices, so recommendations are based on expected sensitivities and tissue penetration (Dickinson et al., 2015). Antimicrobials should be initiated as soon as possible and their use should be modified, if required, once sensitivity results become available. In humans with septic peritonitis, antibiotics are recommended for 5–7 days in most cases; where pancreatic necrosis or *Staphylococcus aureus* is apparent, antibiotics should be provided for 2–3 weeks (Blot and DeWaele, 2005). Similar studies on antibiotic selection and duration of use in veterinary patients are lacking.

Surgery

The goals of surgery are detailed in Table 8.8. The surgical management of each individual depends largely

Table 8.8 Goals for surgical treatment of septic peritonitis.

Preoperative goals
Client education and informed consent
Patient cardiovascular and respiratory stabilisation
Understanding of the viscera involved
Understanding of any co-morbidities or injuries
Smooth, rapid induction of anaesthesia
Thorough understanding of regional anatomy
Aseptic preparation of the patient

Surgical goals
Adherence to Halsted's principles
Elimination of source of contamination/infection
Prevention of continued leakage
Reduction of bacterial load, foreign material and inflammatory mediators
Provision of postoperative nutritional support if required (e.g. oesophageal feeding tube)

Postoperative goals
Thorough evaluation and control of the patient postoperatively
Monitoring and early treatment for any complications

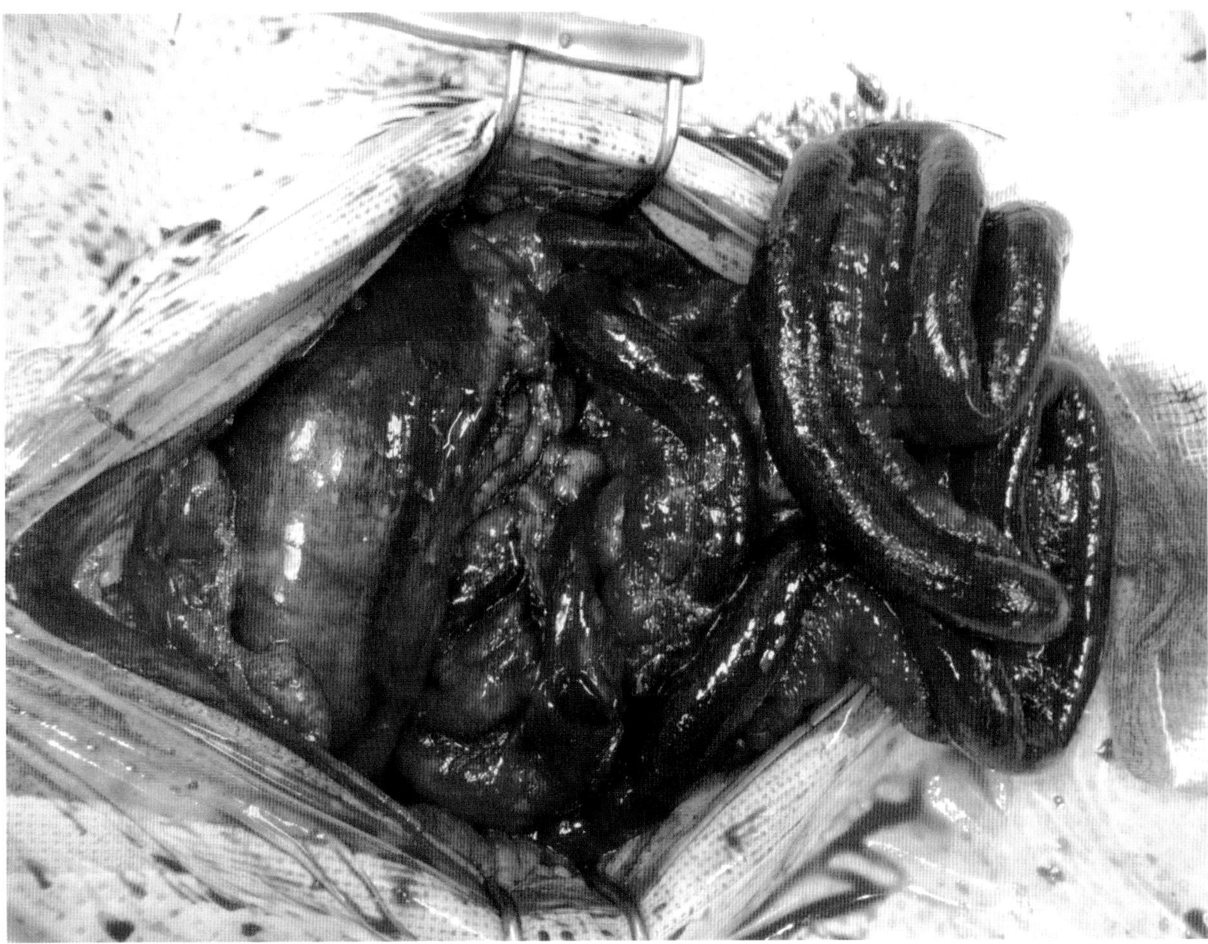

Fig. 8.17a Gross appearance of the abdomen in a dog undergoing surgery for septic peritonitis.

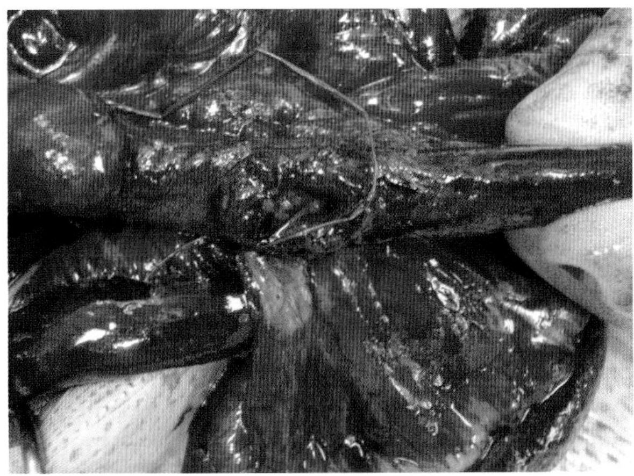

Fig. 8.17b The entire gastrointestinal tract has been examined and a perforation in the mid-jejunum located.

on the source of the contamination/infection: further details can be found in the individual chapters associated with each abdominal organ. In all cases, a ventral midline approach is required from xiphoid to pubis (using local anaesthetic techniques) to permit full and systematic examination of the entire abdomen (Fig. 8.17a,b). Abdominal retractors, suction, diathermy and copious quantities of body-temperature sterile saline or Hartmann's are basic essential requirements. Laparoscopic treatment of septic peritonitis is not currently recommended (Kirby, 2012). Where previous gastrointestinal surgery has been performed, the entire gastrointestinal tract should be thoroughly examined. The site of dehiscence should be isolated from the remainder of the abdomen with moist laparotomy swabs and the leakage addressed using the following techniques (see this volume, Chapter 3 on GI surgery for more detailed descriptions).

For resection-anastomosis of the leaking site, sutures or staples are equally reliable closure methods. Closure of any hollow organ must be followed by leak testing. For canine jejunum, saline volumes of 16.3–19 ml (digital occlusion) and 12.1–14.8 ml (Doyen occlusion) can be used to achieve intra-luminal pressure of 34 cm water (pressure apparent during a peristaltic wave) during leak testing of a 10 cm segment containing a closed biopsy site (Saile et al., 2010). Similar studies in the cat or for other hollow organs are lacking.

Serosal patching is prudent, because preoperative peritonitis significantly increases the risk of postoperative enteric wound dehiscence (Crowe, 1984; Grimes et al., 2011).

of surgical complications in dogs and cats by the use of surgical safety checklist. *Veterinary Surgery* 5, 571–576.

Blot, S. and DeWaele, J.J. (2005) Critical issues in the clinical management of complicated intra-abdominal infections. *Drugs* 65, 1611–1621.

Boudrieau, R.J. and Muir, W.W. (1987) Pathophysiology of traumatic diaphragmatic hernia in dogs. *Compendium* 9, 379–385.

Brady, C.A. and Otto, C.M. (2001) Systemic inflammatory response syndrome, sepsis and multiple organ dysfunction. *Veterinary Clinics of North America: Small Animal Practice* 6, 1147–1162.

Bray, J.P., Doyle, R.S. and Burton, C.A. (2009) Minimally invasive inguinal approach for tube cystotomy. *Veterinary Surgery* 3, 411–416.

Bright, R.M. and Thacker, H.L. (1982) The formation of an omental pedicle flap and its experimental use in the repair of a diaphragmatic rent in the dog. *Journal of the American Animal Hospital Association* 18, 283–289.

Buote, N.J. and Havig, M.E. (2013) The use of vacuum-assisted closure in the management of septic peritonitis in six dogs. *Journal of the American Animal Hospital Association* 48, 164–171.

Burns, C.G., Bergh, M.S. and McLoughlin, M.A. (2013) Surgical and nonsurgical treatment of peritoneo-pericardial diaphragmatic hernia in dogs and cats: 58 cases (1999–2008). *Journal of the American Veterinary Medical Association* 242, 643–650.

Bush, M., Carno, M.A., St. Germaine, L. and Hoffmann, D.E. (2016) The effect of time until surgical intervention on survival in dogs with secondary septic peritonitis. *Canadian Veterinary Journal* 57, 1267–1273.

Campbell, S.J., Marks, S.L., Yoshimoto, S.K., Riel, D.L. and Fascetti, A.J. (2006) Complications and outcomes of one-step low-profile gastrostomy devices for long-term enteral feeding in dogs and cats. *Journal of the American Animal Hospital Association* 42, 197–206.

Cioffi, K.M., Schmiedt, C.W., Cornell, K.K. and Radlinsky, M.G. (2012) Retrospective evaluation of vacuum-assisted peritoneal drainage for the treatment of septic peritonitis in dogs and cats: 8 cases (2003–2010). *Journal of Veterinary Emergency and Critical Care* 22, 601–609.

Clarke, K.M., Lantz, G.C., Salisbury, S.K., Badylak, S.F., Hiles, M.C. and Voytik, S.L. (1996) Intestine submucosa and polypropylene mesh for abdominal wall repair in dogs. *Journal of Surgical Research* 60, 107–114.

Cochran, D.Q., Almond, C.H. and Shucart, W.A. (1963) An experimental study of the effects of barium and intestinal contents on the peritoneal cavity. *American Journal of Roentgenology Radium Therapy and Nuclear Medicine* 89, 883–887.

Coe, R.J., Grint, N.J., Tivers, M. and Holt, P.E. (2006) Comparison of flank and midline approaches to ovariohysterectomy of cats. *Veterinary Record* 159, 309–313.

Corfield, G.S., Read, R.A., Nicholls, P.K. and Lester, N. (2007) Gall bladder torsion and rupture in a dog. *Australian Veterinary Journal* 85, 226–231.

Cortellini, S., Seth, M. and Kellett-Gregory, L.M. (2015) Plasma lactate concentrations in septic peritonitis: a retrospective study of 83 dogs (2007–2012). *Journal of Veterinary Emergency and Critical Care* 25, 288–295.

Costello, M.F., Drobatz, K.J., Aronson, L.R. and King, L.G. (2004) Underlying cause, pathophysiologic abnormalities, and response to treatment in cats with septic peritonitis: 51 cases (1990–2001). *Journal of the American Veterinary Medical Association* 225, 897–902.

Crowe, D.T. (1984) Diagnostic abdominal paracentesis techniques: clinical evaluation in 129 dogs and cats. *Journal of the American Animal Hospital Association* 20, 223–226.

Crowe, D.T. (1988) Dealing with visceral injuries of the cranial abdomen. *Veterinary Medicine* 83, 682–683.

Dickinson, A.E., Summers, J.F., Wignal, J., Boag, A.K. and Keir, I.K. (2015) Impact of appropriate empirical antimicrobial therapy on outcome of dogs with septic peritonitis. *Journal of Veterinary Emergency and Critical Care* 25, 152–159.

Dom, A.S. and Olmstead, M.L. (1976) Herniation of the urinary bladder through the pubic symphysis in a dog. *Journal of the American Veterinary Medical Association* 168, 688–689.

Downs, M.C. and Bjorling, D.E. (1987) Traumatic diaphragmatic hernias: A review of 1674 cases [abstract]. *Veterinary Surgery* 16, 87.

Elliott, D.A., Riel, D.L. and Rogers, Q.R. (2000) Complications and outcomes associated with use of gastrostomy tubes for nutritional management of dogs with renal failure: 56 cases (1994–1999). *Journal of the American Veterinary Medical Association* 217, 1337–1342.

Evans, S.M. and Biery, D.N. (1980) Congenital peritoneopericardial diaphramatic hernia in the dog and cat: a literature review and 17 additional case histories. *Veterinary Radiology* 21, 108–110.

Fox, M.W. (1963) Inherited inguinal hernia and midline defects in the dog. *Journal of the American Veterinary Medical Association* 143, 602–604.

Garson, H.L., Dodman, N.H. and Baker, G.J. (1980) Diaphragmatic hernia: Analysis of fifty-six cases in dogs and cats. *Journal of Small Animal Practice* 21, 469–481.

Gasson, J. (2011) Reducing surgical complications using a safety checklist. *Veterinary Record* 169, 503.

Gawande, A. (2009) *The Checklist Manifesto: How to get things right*, 1st edn. Henry Holt and Company, New York, New York.

Gibson, T.W.G., Brisson, B.A. and Sears, W. (2005) Perioperative survival rates after surgery for diaphragmatic hernia in dogs and cats: 92 cases (1990–2002). *Journal of the American Veterinary Medical Association* 227, 105–109.

Gower, S.B., Weisse, C.W. and Brown, D.C. (2009) Major abdominal evisceration injuries in dogs and cats: 12 cases (1998–2008). *Journal of the American Veterinary Medical Association* 234, 1566–1572.

Grimes, J.A., Schmiedt, C.W., Cornell, K.K. and Radlinsky, M.G. (2011) Identification of risk factors for septic peritonitis and failure to survive following gastrointestinal surgery in dogs. *Journal of the American Veterinary Medical Association* 38, 486–494.

Grint, N.J., Murison, P.J., Coe, R.J. and Waterman Pearson, A.E. (2017) Assessment of the influence of surgical technique on postoperative pain and wound tenderness in cats following ovariohysterectomy. *Journal of Feline Medicine and Surgery* 8, 15–21.

Guieu, L.V.S., Bersenas, A.M., Brisson, B.A., Holowaychuk, M.K., Ammersbach, M.N., Beaufrere, H., Fujita, H. and

Weese, J.S. (2016) Evaluation of peripheral blood and abdominal fluid variables as predictors of intestinal surgical site failure in dogs with septic peritonitis following celiotomy and the placement of closed-suction abdominal drains. *Journal of the American Veterinary Medical Association* 249, 515–525.

Hay, W.H., Woodfield, J.A. and Moon, M.A. (1989) Clinical, echocardiographic and radiographic findings of peritoneopericardial diaphragmatic hernia in two dogs and a cat. *Journal of the American Veterinary Medical Association* 195, 1245–1248.

Hayes, H.M. and Pendergrass, T.W. (1976) Canine testicular tumours: epidemiological features of 410 dogs. *International Journal of Cancer* 18, 482–487.

Helphrey, M.L. (1982) Abdominal flap graft for repair of chronic diaphragmatic hernia in the dog. *Journal of the American Veterinary Medical Association* 181, 791–793.

Hosgood, G. and Salisbury, S.K. (1988) Generalised peritonitis in dogs: 50 cases (1975–1986). *Journal of the American Veterinary Medical Association* 193, 1488–1450.

Hunt, G.B. and Johnson, K.A (2012) Diaphragmatic hernias. In: Tobias, K.M. and Johnston, S. (eds) *Veterinary Surgery: Small Animal*. Elsevier Saunders, St. Louis, Missouri, pp. 1380–1390.

Islam, S. (2008) Clinical care outcomes in abdominal wall defects. *Current Opinion in Pediatrics* 3, 305–310.

Johnson, C.C., Baldessarre, J. and Levison, M.E. (1997) Peritonitis: update on pathophysiology, clinical manifestations, and management. *Clinical Infectious Diseases* 24, 1035–1045.

Kenney, K.J., Matthiesen, D.T., Brown, N.O. and Bradley, R.L. (1987) Pyometra in cats: 183 cases (1979–1984). *Journal of the American Veterinary Medical Association* 191, 1130–1132.

King, L.G. (1994) Postoperative complications and prognostic indicators in dogs and cats with septic peritonitis: 23 cases (1989–1992). *Journal of the American Veterinary Medical Association* 204, 407–414.

Kirby, B.M. (2012) Peritoneum and retroperitoneum. In: Tobias, K.M. and Johnston, S. (eds) *Veterinary Surgery: Small Animal*. Elsevier Saunders, St. Louis, Missouri, pp. 1391–1423.

Kirby, R. and Jones, B.D. (1988) Gastrointestinal emergencies: acute vomiting. *Seminars in Veterinary Medicine and Surgery (Small Animal)* 3, 256–264.

Klein, M.D. and Hertzler, J.H. (1981) Congenital defects of the abdominal wall. *Surgery Gynecology Obstetrics* 152, 805–808.

Lanz, O.I., Ellison, G.W., Bellah, J.R., Weichman, G. and VanGilder, J. (2001) Surgical treatment of septic peritonitis without abdominal drainage in 28 dogs. *Journal of the American Animal Hospital Association* 37, 89–92.

Laroche M. and Harding G. (1998) Primary and secondary peritonitis: an update. *European Journal of Clinical Microbiology & Infectious Diseases* 17, 542–550.

Lee, J.A., Otto, C.M. and King, L.G. (2000) Septic peritonitis and antibiotic therapy in dogs: A retrospective study of 23 cases (1998–1999). In: *Proceedings Seventh International Veterinary Emergency and Critical Care Symposium*. Omnipress, Madison, Wisconsin, p. 987.

Levin, G.M., Bonczynski, J.J., Ludwig, L.L., Barton, L.J. and Loar, A.S. (2004) Lactate as a diagnostic test for septic peritoneal effusion in dogs and cats. *Journal of the American Animal Hospital Association* 40, 364–371.

Linton, M., Tong, L., Simon, A., Buffa, E., McGregor, R., Labruyere, J. and Foster, D. (2016) Hepatic fibrosarcoma incarcerated in a peritoneopericardial diaphragmatic hernia in a cat. *Journal of Feline Medicine and Surgery Open Reports* 2, 1–7.

Minihan, A.C., Berg, J. and Evans, K.L. (2004) Chronic diaphragmatic hernia in 34 dogs and 16 cats. *Journal of the American Animal Hospital Association* 50, 51–63.

Murphy, L.A., Russell, N.J., Dulake, M.I. and Nakamura, R.K. (2014) Constrictive pericarditis following surgical repair of a peritoneopericardial diaphragmatic hernia in a cat. *Journal of Feline Medicine and Surgery* 16, 708–712.

Neville, W.E. and Clowes, G.H. Jr (1954) Congenital absence of hemidiaphragm and use of a lobe of liver in its surgical correction. *AMA Archives of Surgery* 69, 282–290.

Noden, D.M. and de Lahunta, A. (1985) *The Embryology of Domestic Animals: Developmental Mechanisms and Malformations*. Williams and Wilkins, Baltimore, Wisconsin, pp. 276–277.

Oliveira, J.P., Mencalha, R., Sousa, C.A., Abidu-Figueiredo, M. and Jorge, S.F. (2014) Pain assessment in cats undergoing ovariohysterectomy by midline or lateral celiotomy through use of a previously validated multidimensional composite pain scale. *Acta Chirurgica Brasileira* 29, 633–638.

Orton, E.C. (1986) Enteral hyperalimentation administered via needle catheter-jejunostomy as an adjunct to cranial abdominal surgery. *Journal of the American Veterinary Medical Association* 188, 1406–1411.

Pendergrass, T.W. and Hayes H.M. (1975) Cryptorchidism and related defects in dogs: epidemiologic comparisons with man. *Teratology* 12, 51–55.

Ralphs, S.C., Jessen, C.R. and Lipowitz, A.J. (2003) Risk factors for leakage following intestinal anastomosis in dogs and cats: 115 cases (1991–2000). *Journal of the American Veterinary Medical Association* 223, 73–77.

Reimer, S.B., Kyles, A.E., Filipowicz, D.E. and Gregory, C.R. (2004) Long-term outcome of cats treated conservatively or surgically for peritoneopericardial diaphragmatic hernia: 66 cases (1987–2002). *Journal of the American Veterinary Medical Association* 224, 728–732.

Reiss, A.J., McKiernan, B.C. and Wingfield, W.E. (2002) Myocardial injury secondary to blunt thoracic trauma in dogs: Incidence and pathophysiology *Compendium on Continuing Education for the Practising Veterinarian* 24, 934–941.

Rivier, P., Furneaux, R. and Viguier, E. (2011). Combined laparoscopic ovariectomy and laparoscopic-assisted gastropexy in dogs susceptible to gastric dilatation-volvulus. *Canadian Veterinary Journal* 52, 62–66.

Robinson, R. (1977) Genetic aspects of umbilical hernia incidence in cats and dogs. *Veterinary Record* 100, 9–10.

Rogers C.L., Gibson, C., Mitchell, S.L., Keating, J.H. and Rozanski, E.A. (2009) Disseminated candidiasis secondary to fungal and bacterial peritonitis in a young dog. *Journal of Veterinary Emergency and Critical Care* 19, 193–198.

Rosin, E. and Robinson, G.M. (1989) Knot security of suture materials. *Veterinary Surgery* 18, 269–273.

Ruble, R.P. and Hird, D.W. (1993) Congenital abnormalities in immature dogs from a pet store: 253 cases (1987–1988). *Journal of the American Veterinary Medical Association* 202, 633–636.

Saile, K., Boothe, H.W. and Boothe, D.M. (2010) Saline volume necessary to achieve predetermined intraluminal pressures during leak testing of small intestinal biopsy sites in the dog. *Veterinary Surgery* 39, 900–903.

Schaaf, O., Glyde, M. and Day, R.E. (2009) A secure Aberdeen knot: in vitro assessment of knot security in plasma and fat. *Journal of Small Animal Practice* 50, 415–421.

Schmiedt, C.W., Tobias, K.M. and Stevenson, M.A. (2003) Traumatic diaphragmatic hernia in cats: 34 cases (1991-2001). *Journal of the American Veterinary Medical Association* 222, 1237–1240.

Schmiedt, C.W., Wasabaugh, K.F., Rao, D.B. and Stephien, R.L. (2009) Chylothorax associated with a congenital peritoneopericardial diaphragmatic hernia in a dog. *Journal of the American Animal Hospital Association* 45, 134–137.

Seim, H.B. (1995) Management of peritonitis. In: Bonagura, J.D. (ed.) *Kirk's Current Veterinary Therapy XII*. Elsevier Saunders, Philadelphia, Pennsylvania, pp. 764–770.

Shales, C.J., Warren, J., Anderson, D.M., Baines, S.J. and White, R.A.S. (2005) Complications following full-thickness small intestinal biopsy in 66 dogs: a retrospective study. *Journal of Small Animal Practice* 46, 317–321.

Smeak, D.D. (2012) Abdominal wall reconstruction and hernias. In: Tobias, K.M. and Johnston, S. (eds) *Veterinary Surgery: Small Animal*. Elsevier Saunders, St. Louis, Missouri, pp. 1353–1379.

Staatz, A.J., Monnet, E. and Seim, H.B. (2002) Open peritoneal drainage versus primary closure for the treatment of septic peritonitis in dogs and cats: 42 cases (1993–1999). *Veterinary Surgery* 31, 174–180.

Steyn P.F. and Wittum, T.E. (1993) Radiographic, epidemiologic, and clinical aspects of simultaneous pleural and peritoneal effusions in dogs and cats: 48 cases (1982–1991). *Journal of the American Veterinary Medical Association* 202, 307–312.

Sullivan, M. and Lee, R. (1989) Radiological features of 80 cases of diaphragmatic rupture. *Journal of Small Animal Practice* 30, 561–566.

Sullivan, M. and Reid, J. (1990) Management of 60 cases of diaphragmatic ruptures. *Journal of Small Animal Practice* 31, 423-430.

Szabo, S.D., Jermyn, K., Neel, J. and Mathews, K.G. (2011) Evaluation of postcoeliotomy peritoneal drain fluid volume, cytology, and blood-to-peritoneal fluid lactate and glucose differences in normal dogs. *Veterinary Surgery* 40, 444–449.

Taylor, R.M., Farrow, B.R.H. and Healy, P.J. (1987) Canine fucosidosis: clinical findings. *Journal of Small Animal Practice* 28, 291–293.

Tennant, B. and Willoughby, K. (1993) The use of enteral nutrition in small animal medicine. *Compendium Continuing Education Practitioner Vet* 15, 1054–1059.

Tivers, M. (2011) Reducing surgical complications. *Veterinary Record* 169, 334–335.

Tivers, M. (2015) Reducing error and improving patient safety. *Veterinary Record* 177, 436–437.

Toombs, J.P., Collins L.G., Graves G.M., Crowe D.T. and Caywood D.D. (1986) Colonic perforation in corticosteroid treated dogs. *Journal of the American Veterinary Medical Association* 188, 145–150.

Waldron, D.R., Hedlund, C.S. and Pechman, R. (1986) Abdominal hernias in dogs and cats: a review of 24 cases. *Journal of the American Animal Hospital Association* 22, 817–820.

Waters, D.J., Roy, R.G. and Stone, E.A. (1993) A retrospective study of inguinal hernia in 35 dogs. *Veterinary Surgery* 22, 44–49.

Weinstein, M.J., Pavletic, M.M., Boudrieau, R.J. and Engler, S.J. (1989) Cranial sartorius muscle flap in the dog. *Veterinary Surgery* 18, 286–291.

Wheaton, L.G., Johnson, A.L., Parker, A.J. and Kneller, S.K. (1989) Results and complications of surgical treatment of pyometra: a review of 80 cases. *Journal of the American Animal Hospital Association* 25, 563–567.

Wilson, G.P., Newton, C.D. and Burt, J.K. (1971) A review of 116 diaphragmatic hernias in dogs and cats. *Journal of the American Veterinary Medical Association* 159, 1142–1145.

Woolfson, J.M. and Dulisch, M.L. (1986) Open abdominal drainage in the treatment of generalised peritonitis in 25 dogs and cats. *Veterinary Surgery* 15, 27–32.

Worth, A.J. and Machon, R.G. (2005) Traumatic diaphragmatic herniation: Pathophysiology and management. *Compendium* 27, 178–190.

Wylie, K.B. and Hosgood, G. (1994) Mortality and morbidity of small and large intestinal surgery in dogs and cats: 74 cases (1980–1982). *Journal of the American Animal Hospital Association* 30, 469–474.

Case 8.1

History and presentation

A 3-year-old male neutered Border collie presented as an emergency for assessment two days following duodenal enterectomy for a linear foreign body. Foreign bodies had been removed on multiple occasions previously. The dog is currently receiving clavulanic amoxicillin and meloxicam. There is no other significant history.

On presentation, he is collapsed, but responsive. Major body systems assessment shows:

- Mucous membranes are pale.
- Capillary refill time is less than 1 second.
- Heart rate and pulse rate are synchronous; tachcardia (180 bpm); pulse quality is poor; no cardiac arrhythmias or murmurs.
- Respiratory rate is 50 bpm and lung sounds are normal bilaterally.
- Abdominal palpation is painful.
- The previous laparotomy site appears normal for this stage in healing.
- Neurological examination is within normal limits.
- Orthopaedic examination is within normal limits.

Problem list

- Collapse.
- Mucous membranes are pale.
- Brisk capillary refill time.
- Tachcardia (180 bpm); pulse quality is poor.
- Tachypnoea (50 bpm).
- Clinical signs of shock.
- Abdominal palpation is painful.
- Recent gastrointestinal surgery.

Plan

- Emergency blood panel: PCV/TS, urea, creatinine, lactate, electrolytes, blood gas analysis.
- Cardiovascular stabilisation, including fluid boluses of crystalloids (10 ml/kg over 15 minutes initially and reassess clinical examination; shock doses are up to 60–90 ml/kg; consider colloids if required), oxygenation.
- Provide appropriate analgesia (opioids would be suitable, e.g. methadone).
- Thoracic imaging (radiographs and ultrasound with minimal restraint).

Investigation

Emergency blood panel results showed elevated lactate, urea, creatinine, PCV and TS. Electrolytes were normal. Blood gas analysis was consistent with a metabolic acidosis.

Methadone (0.2 mg/kg IV) was provided. Mask oxygenation was provided. Two 10 ml/kg boluses of Hartmann's were provided over 20 minutes, following which heart rate was 100 bpm and pulse quality improved.

Abdominal ultrasound identified a large volume of free abdominal fluid, and abdominocentesis showed large numbers of intracellular rods, consistent with septic peritonitis. A sample was submitted for aerobic and anaerobic culture.

Surgery

Additional crystalloid fluid therapy and oxygenation were administered, and repeat blood sampling showed a reduction in previously elevated parameters. The patient was anaesthetised and ventilated and a midline laparotomy was performed. Significant free abdominal fluid was encountered and removed by suction. The previous enterotomy site was leaking and there was significant abdominal contamination and adhesions (Figs. 8.18, 8.19, 8.20). The leaking site was resected *en bloc* and a sutured end-to-end anastomosis was performed, using 3-0 Monocryl in a continuous pattern. The site was leak-tested to confirm that no leakage was present. Kit and gloves were changed. The mesenteric rent was repaired and a serosal patch and omentalisation performed (Fig. 8.21). The abdomen was copiously lavaged with body-temperature sterile saline. An active suction drain (Jackson–Pratt) was placed in the abdominal cavity, and a gastrostomy tube was also placed. The linea alba, subcutaneous fat and skin were closed routinely. Local anaesthetic was infused into the wound site.

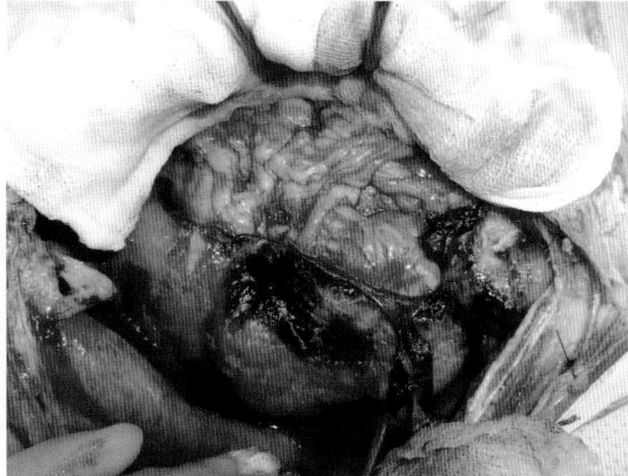

Fig. 8.18 Significant adhesions were encountered in the gastrointestinal tract.

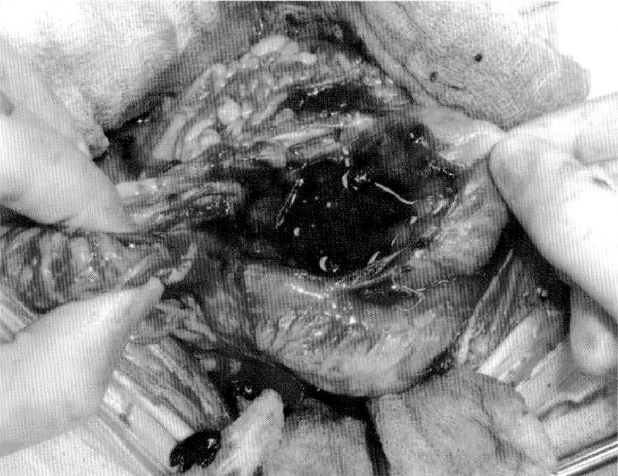

Fig. 8.19 A large volume of free abdominal fluid was removed, originating from the region of the previous enterotomy site.

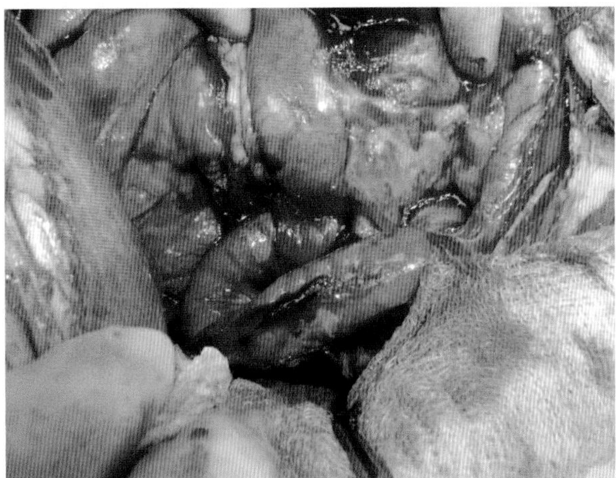

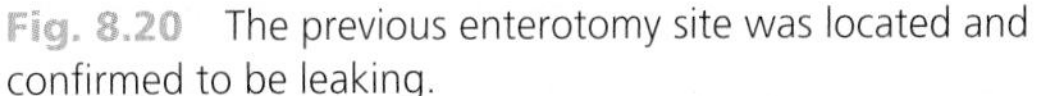

Fig. 8.20 The previous enterotomy site was located and confirmed to be leaking.

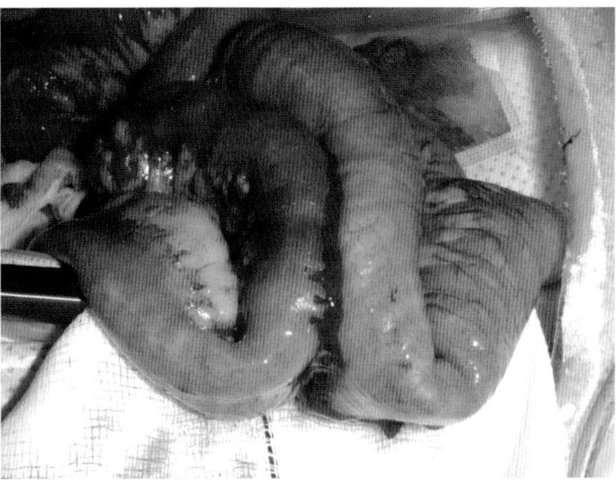

Fig. 8.21 Following leak-testing of the anastomotic site, serosal patching was performed.

Postoperative care

- Pain scores were documented every 2 hours, and methadone (0.2 mg/kg IV) provided as required. A ketamine and lidocaine infusion was administered for 24 hours. Paracetamol was given twice daily for 1 week.
- Intravenous crystalloids were provided at maintenance rates (2 ml/kg/h).
- The abdominal drain was ordered to be aseptically evacuated every 4 hours. The drain was removed 48 hours postoperatively, when fluid production decreased to <1 ml/kg/24 h.
- Antibiotics (clavulanic amoxycillin, 20 mg/kg IV TID) were provided postoperatively, whilst bacterial culture and sensitivity was pending.
- Enteral nutrition was provided via the gastrostomy tube following surgery. In this case, the patient was much improved clinically once recovered from anaesthesia and began to eat and drink the following day. The intravenous fluids were discontinued 48 hours postoperatively.
- The patient was discharged 72 hours postoperatively with oral paracetamol and clavulanic amoxicillin, and instructions for strict room rest with short lead walks for toileting purposes only. The buster collar and protective vest were to remain in place for a fortnight in order to prevent interference with the gastrostomy tube. The gastrostomy tube was scheduled for removal 14 days after placement.

Unfortunately, the dog re-presented again as an emergency ten days after discharge because he had eaten his gastrostomy tube. Physical examination was generally within normal limits.

Abdominal radiography showed that the tube has been chewed into numerous smaller pieces, some of which were in the large intestine (Fig. 8.22).

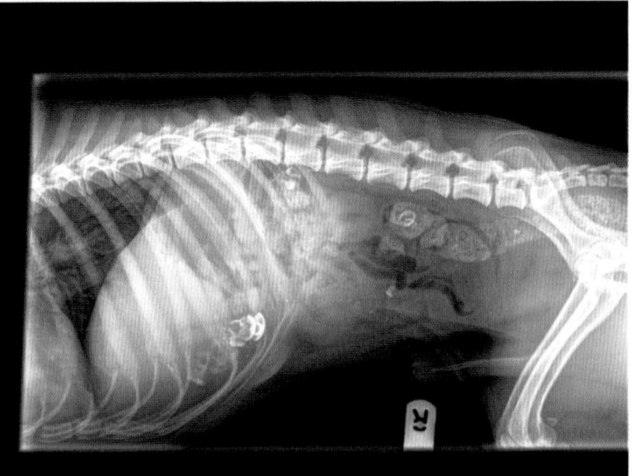

Fig. 8.22 Right lateral abdominal radiograph of a dog 13 days following gastrostomy tube placement. The dog has interfered with the tube.

Abdominal ultrasound scan did not identify any free abdominal fluid, which would be suggestive of gastrointestinal leakage.

The patient was managed conservatively overnight, and repeat radiographs the following day showed that the components of the tube within the stomach had remained there. They were removed endoscopically and the patient was discharged the following day.

His owners were advised that it is imperative that he is not permitted to scavenge at home or outdoors. If his scavenging is very difficult to control whilst out walking, it might be worthwhile his wearing a basket muzzle.

The patient recovered uneventfully and has not re-presented for gastrointestinal foreign body to date.

Case 8.2

History and presentation

A 2-year-old male neutered domestic shorthaired cat presented as an emergency following a road traffic accident 30 minutes ago. There is no other significant history.

On presentation, he is quiet, alert and responsive. Major body systems assessment shows:

- Mucous membranes are pale pink.
- Capillary refill time is 1 second.
- Heart rate and pulse rate are synchronous (160 bpm); pulse quality is good; no cardiac arrhythmias or murmurs.
- Respiratory rate is 50 bpm and lung sounds are dull bilaterally.
- Abdominal palpation is within normal limits and comfortable.
- There are no visible skin wounds.
- Neurological examination is within normal limits.
- Orthopaedic examination is within normal limits.

Problem list

- Increased respiratory rate and dull lung sounds.
- Recent road traffic accident.

Note that there was no evidence of cardiovascular compromise in this case.

Plan

- Pre-oxygenation.
- Emergency blood panel: PCV/TS, urea, creatinine, lactate, electrolytes, blood gas analysis.
- Provide analgesia (opioids would be suitable, e.g. morphine, methadone).
- Thoracic radiographs (with minimal restraint). If appropriate and required, sedation could be achieved with ketamine plus midazolam, for example. Alternatively, general anaesthesia might be an option.

Investigation

Emergency blood panel results were all within normal limits.

Thoracic radiographs (Fig. 8.23) showed pleural effusion and abdominal organs displaced into the thoracic cavity, causing border effacement of the cardiac silhouette and dorsal displacement of the trachea and lung lobes. The diaphragmatic border is obscured.

Imaging of the abdomen (radiography and ultrasound) showed no trauma or damage to the viscera remaining in the abdomen. The urinary bladder was intact.

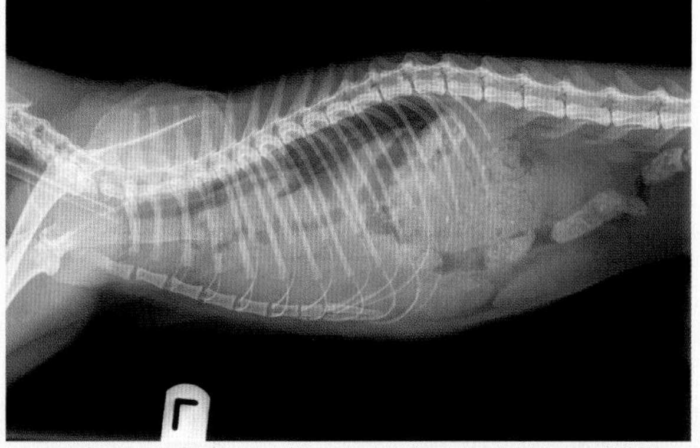

Fig. 8.23 Left lateral thoracic and abdominal radiograph, consistent with a diagnosis of diaphragmatic hernia.

Surgery

Informed client consent was obtained. The patient was anaesthetised and ventilated. The table was tilted to elevate the head and thorax. A midline laparotomy was performed. During surgery, a simple acute radial tear of the diaphragm was identified (Fig. 8.24). The herniated organs were readily replaced into the abdominal cavity. Further inspection of the abdomen identified haemorrhage in the right retroperitoneal region (Fig. 8.25). No other damage could be identified. No surgical intervention was required in this site. A thoracostomy tube was placed and left open. Closure of the radial tear was performed, beginning dorsally and progressing ventrally, using 3-0 polydioxanone (Fig. 8.26). The linea alba, subcutaneous fat and skin were closed routinely. Local anaesthetic was infused into

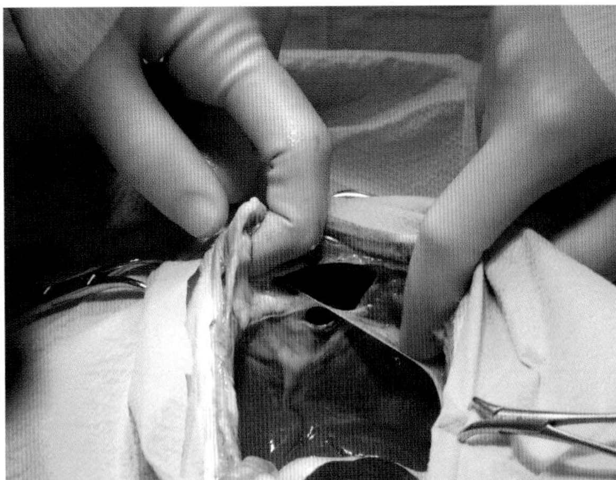

Fig. 8.24 Simple acute radial tear of the diaphragm in a cat following an RTA, viewed via a midline laparotomy.

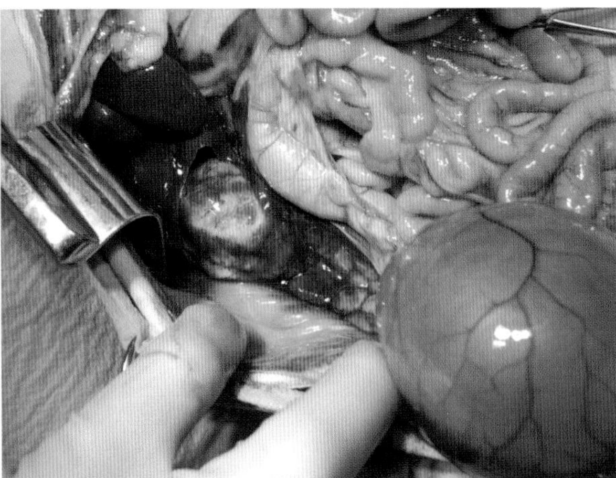

Fig. 8.25 It is imperative that the viscera of the thorax and abdomen are inspected, particularly where trauma has been reported. In this patient, there is evidence of haemorrhage and bruising of the right retroperitoneum.

the wound site. The thoracic cavity was gently evacuated until the patient was able to ventilate satisfactorily. The chest drain was closed. Antibiotics were not provided intra-operatively.

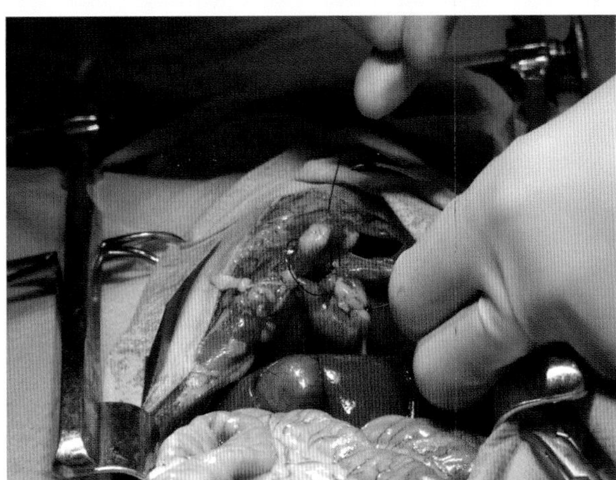

Fig. 8.26 Closure of the radial tear has begun dorsally and is progressing ventrally, using a monofilament absorbable suture material (polydioxanone).

Postoperative care

- Pain scores and multimodal analgesia (systemic opioids, local anaesthetic into the thoracostomy tube, non-steroidal anti-inflammatories) were provided every 2–4 hours.
- Intravenous crystalloids were provided at maintenance rates (2 ml/kg/h).
- The thoracostomy tube was ordered to be aseptically evacuated if respiratory rate or effort increased, but this was not required and the drain was removed 24 hours postoperatively.
- Antibiotics were not provided postoperatively.
- The patient was bright and alert once recovered from anaesthesia, and began to eat and drink the following day. The intravenous fluids were discontinued.
- Haematuria became apparent, presumed to be secondary to the haemorrhage associated with trauma of the right kidney. Repeated blood samples (urea, creatinine, electrolytes) remained within normal limits. Ultrasound examination of the kidney remained within normal limits. The haematuria resolved after 3 days.
- The patient was discharged after resolution of the haematuria, with instructions for room rest to allow wound healing and non-steroidal anti-inflammatory medication.
- There were no postoperative complications and the patient made an uneventful recovery.

Case 8.3

History and presentation

A 4-year old male neutered cocker spaniel presented for investigation of a lifelong history of exercise intolerance. He had been vomiting intermittently for the last two weeks. There is no other significant history.

On presentation, he is bright, alert and responsive. Physical examination was unremarkable.

Problem list

- exercise intolerance (lifelong)
- 2-week history of vomiting.

Plan

- routine serum biochemistry and haematology
- abdominal and thoracic imaging (radiography in the first instance, followed by ultrasonography if required).

Investigation

Blood results were all within normal limits.

Thoracic radiographs (Figs. 8.27, 8.28, 8.29) showed that the heart was obscured and the trachea dramatically elevated by soft tissue opacities extending into the thorax from the cranial abdomen, crossing the diaphragm line. These include gas-filled (but not over-distended) pylorus and soft tissue opacity ventrally suggesting liver ± splenic tail. Cranial abdominal viscera were displaced accordingly. No thoracic effusion was seen.

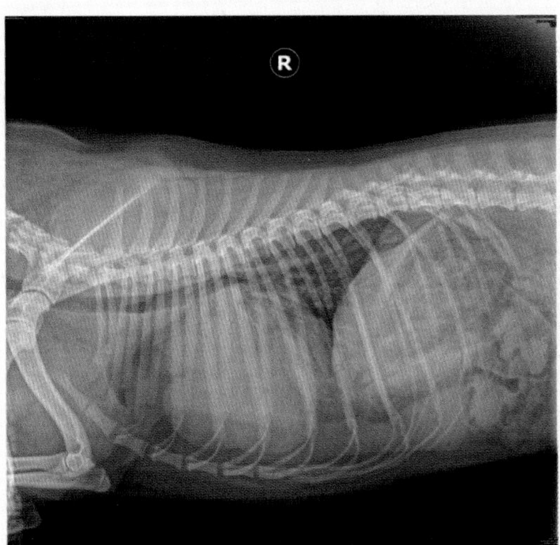

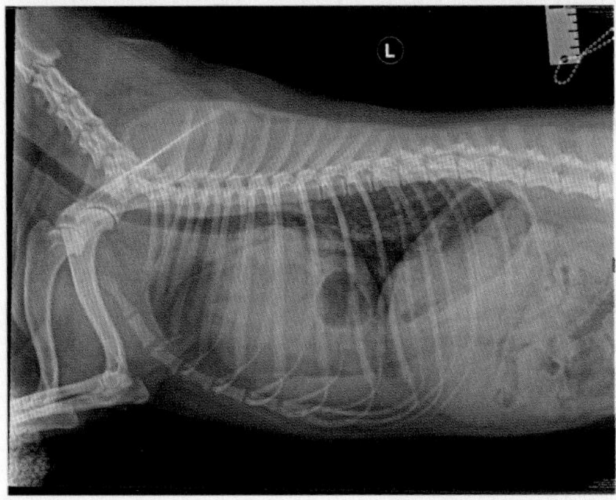

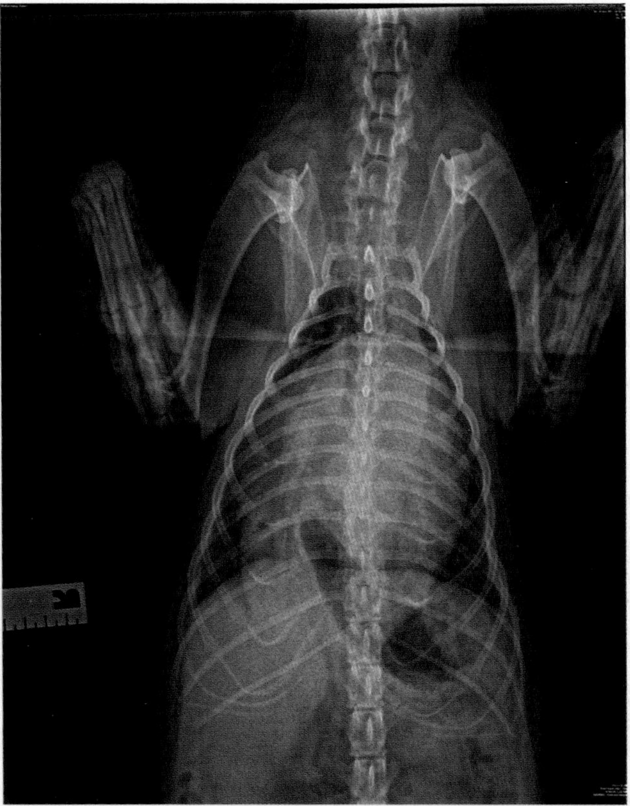

Figs. 8.27, 8.28, 8.29 Right and left lateral, and dorsoventral thoracic radiographs of a 4-year-old neutered male cocker spaniel, consistent with a diagnosis of PPDH. (Copyright RSPCA Putney.)

Surgery

Informed client consent was obtained. The patient was anaesthetised and ventilated. The table was tilted to elevate the head and thorax. A midline laparotomy was performed. During surgery, a PPDH was identified. The organs herniated into the pericardium included small intestines and spleen (Figs. 8.30, 8.31). These were readily reduced into the abdomen and were not compromised. Further inspection of the abdominal viscera was unremarkable. No other defects could be identified. Closure of the PPDH was performed, beginning dorsally and progressing ventrally, using 2-0 polydioxanone (Figs. 8.32, 8.33, 8.34). Before complete closure of the pericardium, an intravenous catheter was placed across the diaphragm into the pericardium (Figs. 8.35, 8.36). The pericardium was closed and air evacuated via the

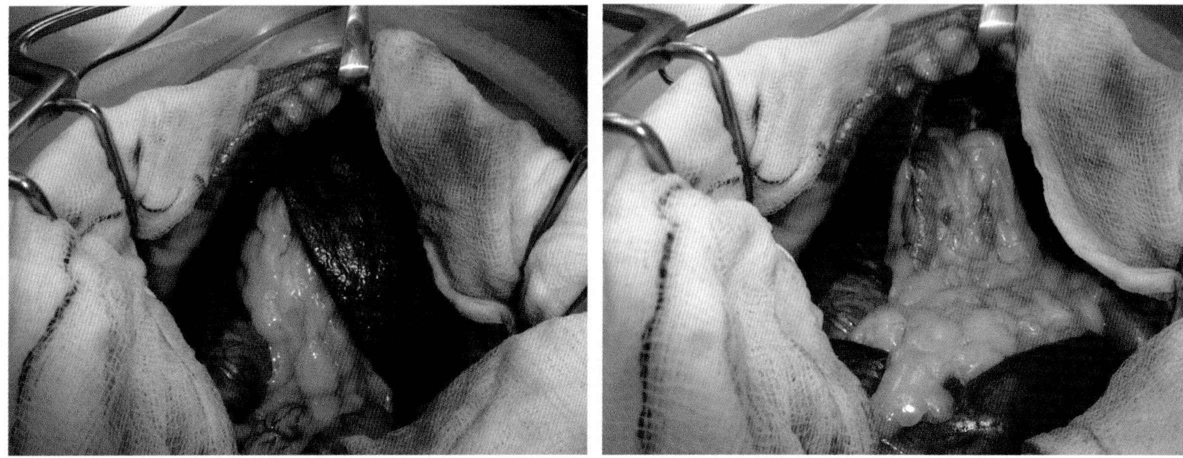

Figs. 8.30, 8.31 A midline laparotomy was performed. During surgery, a PPDH was identified. The organs herniated into the pericardium included small intestines and spleen.

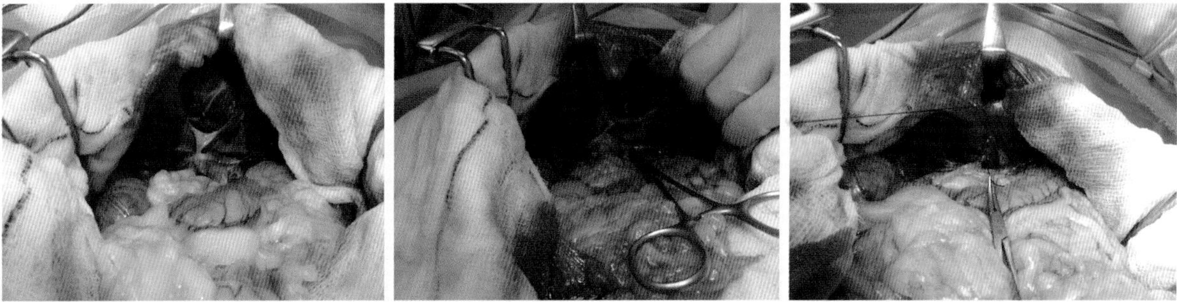

Figs. 8.32, 8.33, 8.34 Closure of the PPDH was performed, beginning dorsally and progressing ventrally, using 2-0 polydioxanone.

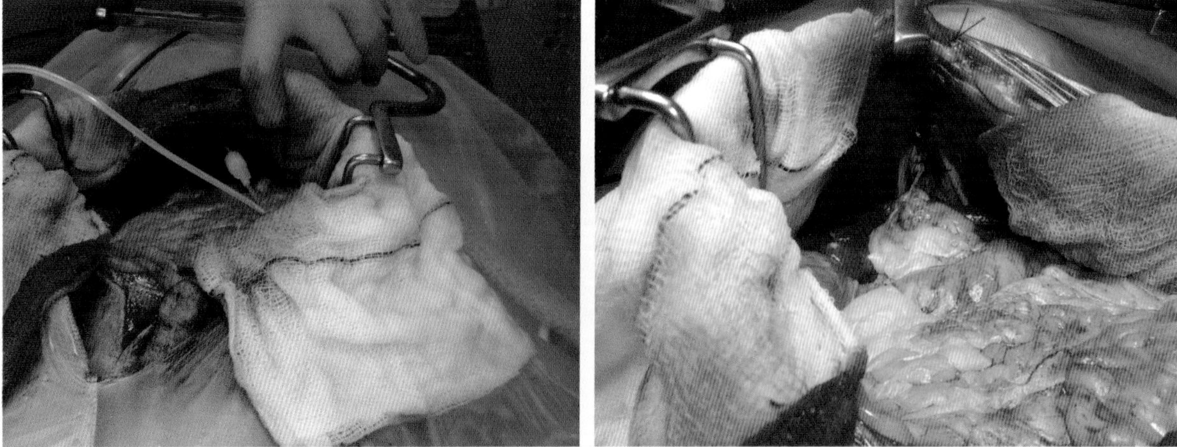

Figs. 8.35, 8.36 Before complete closure of the pericardium, an intravenous catheter was placed across the diaphragm into the pericardium. The pericardium was closed and air evacuated via the trans-diaphragmatic catheter, which was then removed.

trans-diaphragmatic catheter, which was then removed. The linea alba, subcutaneous fat and skin were closed routinely. Local anaesthetic was infused into the wound site. Antibiotics were not provided intra-operatively.

Postoperative care

- Pain scores and multimodal analgesia (systemic opioids, non-steroidal anti-inflammatories) were provided every 2–4 hours.
- Intravenous crystalloids were provided at maintenance rates (2 ml/kg/h) until the patient was eating.
- Antibiotics were not provided postoperatively.
- The patient was bright and alert once recovered from anaesthesia, and began to eat and drink the following day. The intravenous fluids were discontinued.
- There were no postoperative complications and the patient made an uneventful recovery. The vomiting and exercise intolerance resolved.

Surgery of the thoracic cavity

9

Kelly L. Bowlt Blacklock

Chapter summary

9.1 Approach to the thoracic cavity

Key points

- A rigorous sign-in and sign-out checklist is essential for all surgeries, particularly those involving the abdominal or thoracic cavity (Bergstrom et al., 2016; Gasson, 2011; Gawande, 2009).
- Intercostal thoracotomy is the preferable approach to the thoracic cavity, if clinically appropriate.
- Potential postoperative complications may include haemorrhage, infection, osteomyelitis, seroma formation, ipsilateral forelimb lameness, wound complications and rib fractures.
- Postoperative complications are more common following median sternotomy than intercostal thoracotomy.
- Other approaches to the thoracic cavity (e.g. rib resection, trans-sternal and trans-diaphragmatic thoracotomies) are rarely indicated.

9.1.1 Complications of thoracic surgery

Surgical complications occur in every hospital and to every surgeon, resulting in increased patient morbidity/mortality, cost and stress for everyone involved. Complications can arise due to clinician error or unforeseen circumstances: the former can be addressed by the use of guidelines to improve surgical safety. The World Health Organization (WHO) addresses the safety of surgical care via the 'Safe Surgery Saves Lives' campaign (www.who.int/patientsafety/safesurgery/en/), inspired by the checklists used by airline pilots to reduce error. Surgeons should familiarise themselves with the content of this campaign and the current literature in reducing surgical complications (Tivers, 2011; Tivers, 2015).

As for every surgical procedure, informed client consent should be acquired: this involves a full and frank discussion about the diagnosis, potential complications of surgery/treatment, likely outcomes, additional/alternative treatment options and estimated costs involved. It is beyond the realms of this chapter to discuss the frequently complicated requirements for critical care, analgesia, anaesthesia and ventilation of a patient undergoing thoracotomy. A multi-disciplinary approach to diagnostics and pre-/postoperative care, combined with a multimodal analgesia protocol (intravenous analgesics, intercostal nerve blocks, intrapleural catheters, local anaesthetic wound infiltration, etc.) is essential and the veterinary surgeon caring for such patients must be well versed in these fields. If any concerns exist, advice should be sought from a board-certified veterinary anaesthetist and/or surgeon. Referral to a specialist surgeon and anaesthetist should be offered and encouraged for patients requiring thoracotomy procedures if possible.

Postoperative complications are reported in around 39% of patients undergoing both intercostal thoracotomy and median sternotomy (Tattersall and Welsh, 2006), being up to 71% for median sternotomy and 23% for intercostal thoracotomy (Tattersall and Welsh, 2006). Half of dogs undergoing median sternotomy have postoperative pain (Ringwald and Birchard, 1989); however, a study directly comparing postoperative pain scores among patients undergoing median sternotomy and intercostal thoracotomy is lacking. Wound complications are significantly more common following median sternotomy (Tattersall and Welsh, 2006). Additional complications of median sternotomy include instability, which causes severe postoperative pain, prolonged recovery and seroma formation (Hunt, 2012). For this reason, sternebrae should be sectioned longitudinally without being broken, and the manubrium and xiphoid should be left intact if possible. If the skin wound remains closed, the seroma should be managed conservatively; if dehiscence is encountered, open wound management should be pursued (the author utilises vacuum-assisted closure in such cases) and the increased potential for infection (including osteomyelitis) should be considered.

Other potential complications following thoracotomy include seroma formation (11–22%), wound discharge/dehiscence/infection (4–8%), osteomyelitis (1–11%), displaced/fractured sternebrae (3%), fractured ribs (2%), haemorrhage and ipsilateral thoracic limb lameness (1–4%) and neurological deficits (Burton and White, 1996; Moores, 2016a,b; Tattersall and Welsh, 2006).

A list of potential advantages and disadvantages to performing lateral intercostal thoracotomy versus median sternotomy is given in Table 9.1. Intercostal thoracotomy is the author's approach of choice for most thoracotomy procedures, with the exception of genuine exploratory thoracotomies (e.g. pyothorax unresponsive to medical management where access to both hemithoraces is required) or mediastinal masses (e.g. thymoma). In most cases, preoperative imaging (e.g. CT, radiography, ultrasound) can sufficiently aid in diagnosis and identify the site of the lesion to permit an intercostal approach. The location varies, depending on the target structure. Intercostal thoracotomy would be the approach of choice for lung lobectomy; ligation of patent ductus arteriosus, persistent right aortic arch or thoracic duct; and surgery of the right heart, pericardium, vena cava, azygous vein, oesophagus and mediastinum. In one study, median sternotomy was the preferred approach for pyothorax (85%) and penetrating thoracic injuries (66%); intercostal thoracotomy was the preferred approach for all other diseases (Tattersall and Welsh, 2006).

9.1.2 Lateral intercostal thoracotomy

The patient is positioned in lateral recumbency and the forelimbs secured cranially (Fig. 9.1). An intercostal

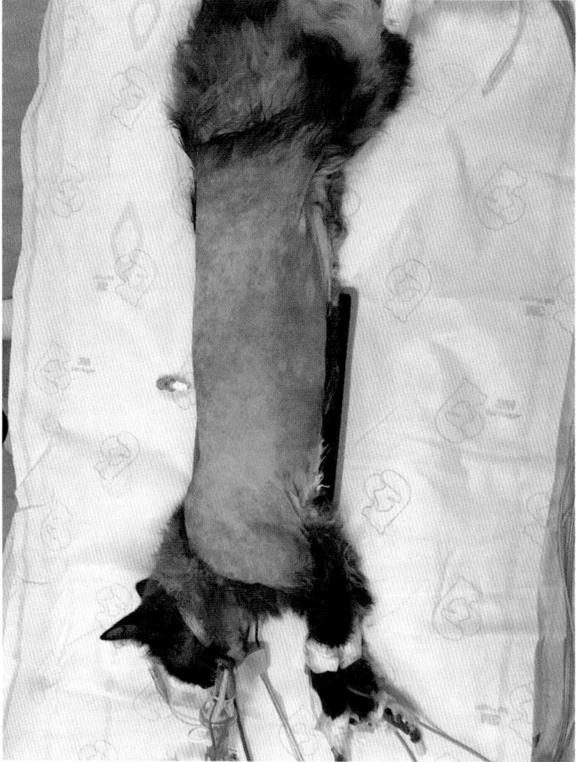

Fig. 9.1 A 5-year-old MN domestic shorthaired cat under general anaesthesia and positioned in lateral recumbency with the forelimbs secured cranially in preparation for left intercostal thoracotomy.

Table 9.1 Potential advantages and disadvantages of median sternotomy versus lateral intercostal thoracotomy in the dog and cat.

	Median sternotomy	Lateral intercostal thoracotomy
Advantages	Can examine both hemithoraces	Patient usually requires less postoperative analgesia
Disadvantages	Complications seen in up to 71% of patients Patient usually requires more postoperative analgesia Increased risk of wound complications Potential risk of osteomyelitis Potential requirements for non-absorbable material for sternotomy closure Dorsal access to the great vessels, pulmonary hilus and thoracic duct is limited	Complications seen in up to 23% of patients Exploration of the thoracic cavity is limited to one-third of the ipsilateral thoracic cavity directly underneath the thoracotomy site Potential risk of rib fracture Potential risk of ipsilateral forelimb lameness or neurological deficits

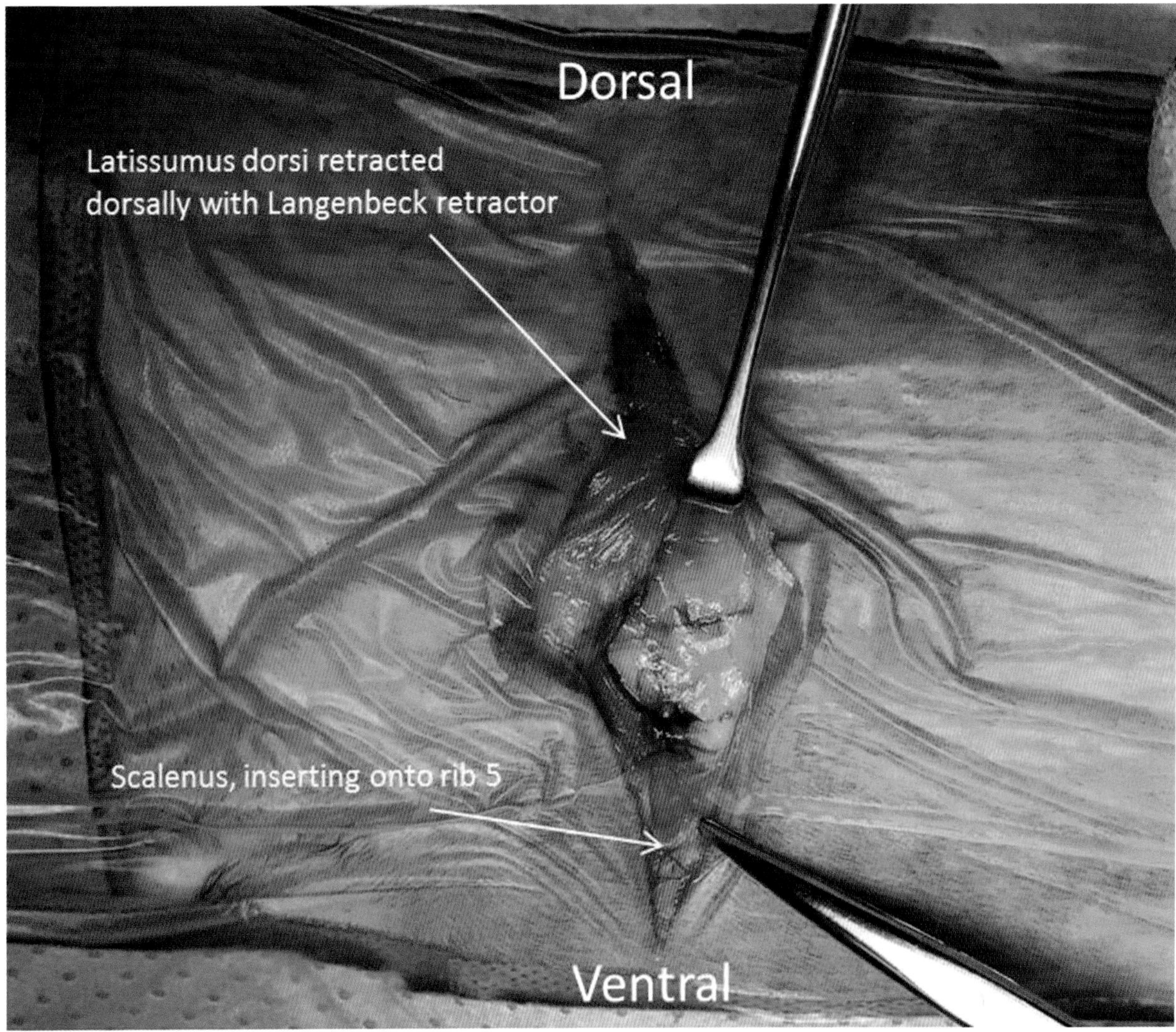

Fig. 9.2 To proceed with intercostal thoracotomy, a skin incision is made at the appropriate level in a dorsoventral direction from the hypaxial musculature to the sternum, and the subcutaneous tissue is incised down to the latissimus dorsi muscle. The latissimus dorsi is undermined and retracted dorsally using Langenbeck retractors. The scalenus muscle can be seen ventrally attaching to the fifth rib, and is incised to expose the underlying serratus ventralis muscle.

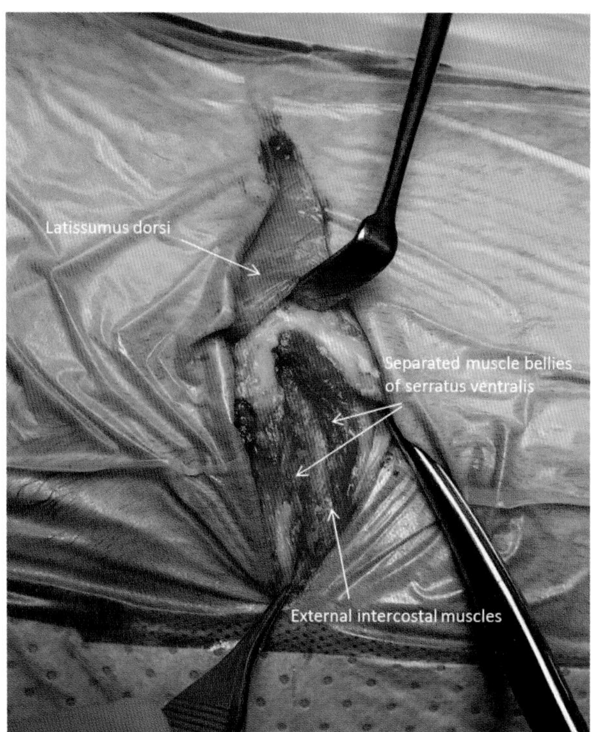

Fig. 9.3 The serratus ventralis muscle is separated between two muscle bellies. Deep to the serratus ventralis muscle lie the external and internal intercostal muscles and the pleura, which are transected using Metzenbaum scissors midway between the ribs to avoid damage to the neurovascular bundles.

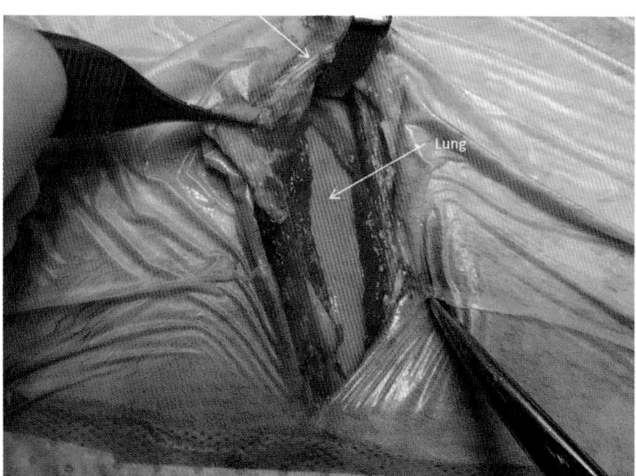

Fig. 9.4 The incision through the external and internal intercostal muscles and the pleura is continued, taking care to ensure any adhesions are identified before the incision is progressed.

nerve block should be performed using bupivacaine injected just caudal to the ribs, in the dorsal third, at the level of the proposed surgical site and including two ribs cranially and caudally (i.e. five rib spaces in total). A skin incision is made at the appropriate level in a dorsoventral direction from the hypaxial musculature to the sternum, and the subcutaneous tissue is incised down to the latissimus dorsi. The latissimus dorsi is undermined and retracted dorsally using Langenbeck retractors (Fig. 9.2). The advantages of leaving the latissimus dorsi intact are a more rapid closure, and reduced postoperative pain and lameness (Radlinsky, 2012).

Slightly reduced access to the thoracic cavity results, especially dorsally, but this rarely has clinical implications and incision of the latissimus dorsi muscle parallel to the intercostal incision can be performed if necessary. At this stage, identification of the correct intercostal space is achieved, either by counting ribs caudally from the J-shaped first rib, or by identifying the fifth rib from attachments of the caudal end of the scalenus muscle and the cranial end of the external abdominal oblique muscle. The scalenus or external abdominal oblique muscle is incised and the deeper serratus ventralis muscle is separated between two muscle bellies (Fig. 9.3). Deep to the serratus ventralis muscle lies the external and internal intercostal muscles and the pleura, which are transected using Metzenbaum scissors midway between the ribs to avoid damage to the neurovascular bundles (sited caudal to the rib). Care should be taken when puncturing the pleura to identify and avoid any adhesions between pleura and lung. This incision should not continue ventrally beyond the internal thoracic vessels (which lie laterally and parallel to the sternum, and can be identified by palpation) and dorsally beyond the costochondral junction (otherwise epaxial muscle and intercostal arterial damage may ensue) (Fig. 9.4). Saline-soaked laparotomy swabs should be inserted to protect the wound edges, if there is sufficient room, and Finochietto rib retractors inserted and retracted gently.

After the intrathoracic procedure is completed, a thoracostomy tube is placed and the thoracotomy wound closed using pre-placed circumcostal polydioxanone sutures (Figs. 9.5, 9.6). The author prefers to pass sutures using the swaged end of the needle (rather

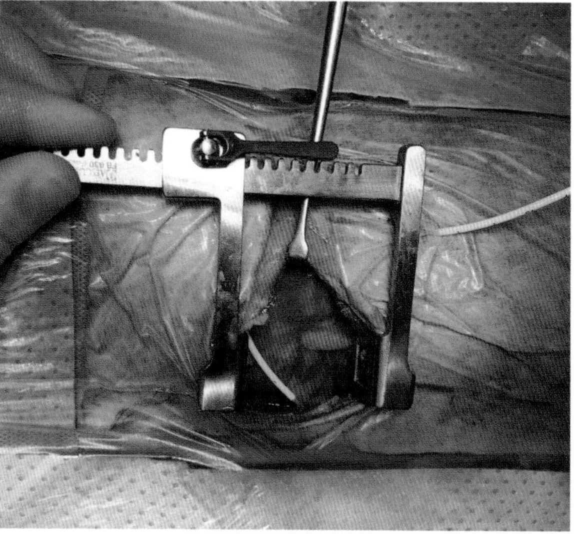

Fig. 9.5 Following completion of the intrathoracic procedure, a thoracostomy tube is placed.

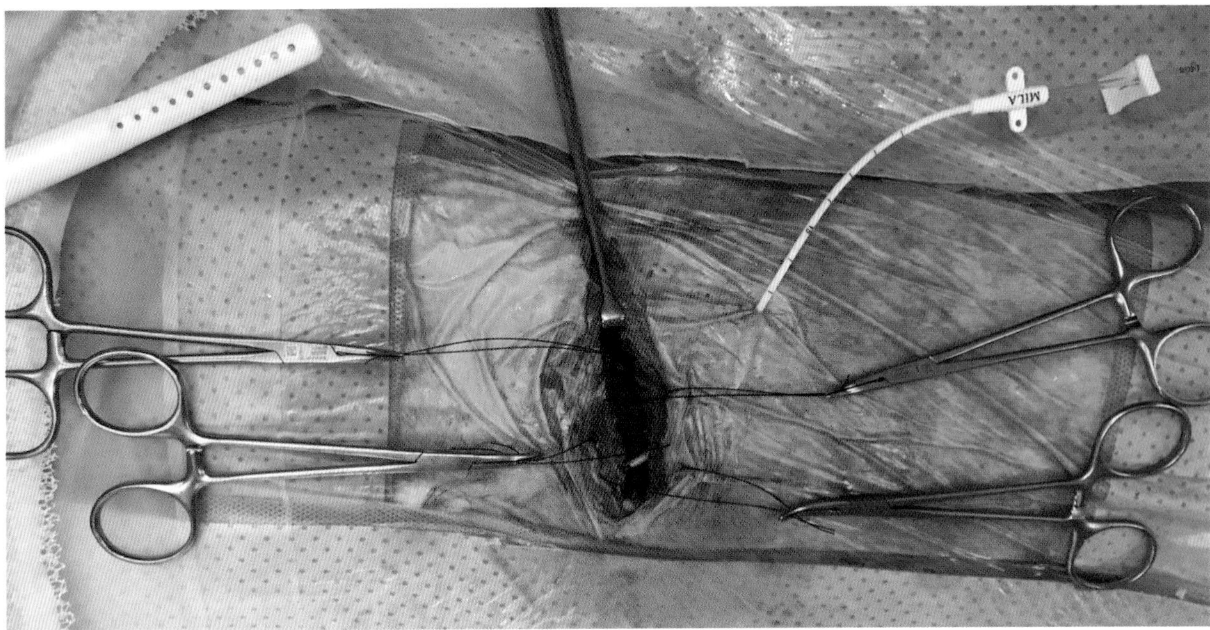

Fig. 9.6 The thoracotomy wound closed using pre-placed circumcostal polydioxanone sutures.

than the needle tip), which may be more likely to avoid damage to neurovascular structures or lung parenchyma (Radlinsky, 2012). The aim of these sutures is to maintain anatomic rib position and reduce tension on the soft tissue repair, not to appose or immobilise the ribs: excessive tension may result in rib fractures (Hunt, 2012). In larger dogs (22–29 kg), transcostal sutures have been reported in one study to result in less pain during the first 24 hours postoperatively, presumably because of the reduced incidence of nerve entrapment compared with circumcostal closure techniques (Rooney et al., 2004). Apposition of the intercostal muscles is unnecessary. The serratus ventralis and scalenus or external abdominal oblique muscles are apposed using an absorbable monofilament suture, and the latissimus dorsi is released and apposed ventrally (Fig. 9.7). Subcutis and skin closure is routine.

9.1.3 Median sternotomy

Median sternotomy is the approach of choice for patients requiring an exploratory thoracotomy with access to both hemithoraces (e.g. pyothorax unresponsive to medical management with extensive, bilateral

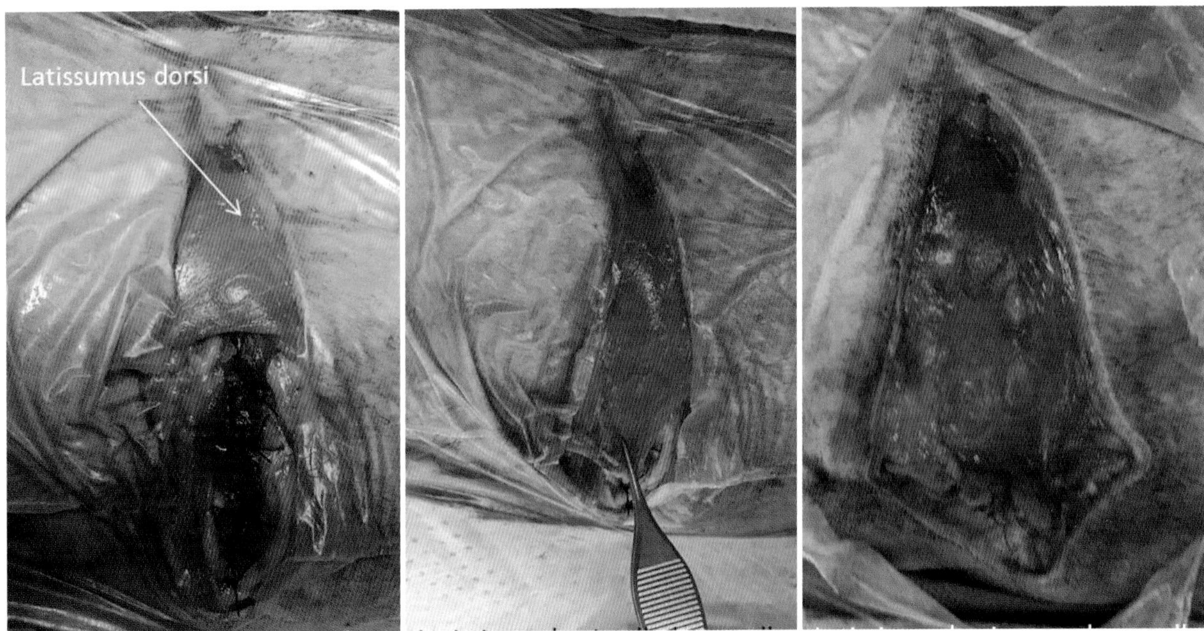

Fig. 9.7 The serratus ventralis and scalenus or external abdominal oblique muscles are apposed using an absorbable monofilament suture and the latissimus dorsi is released and apposed ventrally. Subcutis and skin closure is routine.

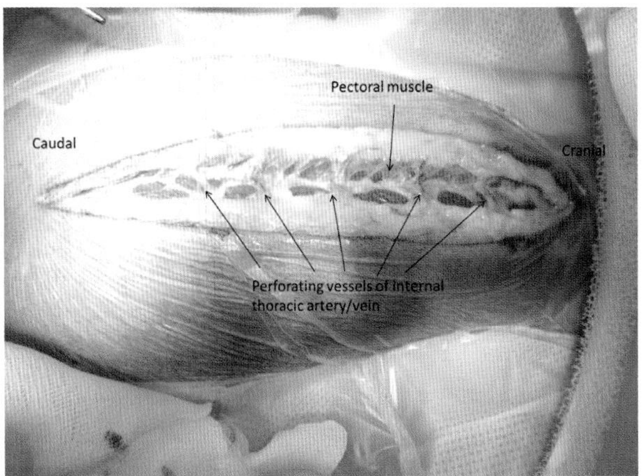

Fig. 9.8 After surgical clipping and aseptic preparation, the skin incision is made from the manubrium to the xiphoid on the midline.

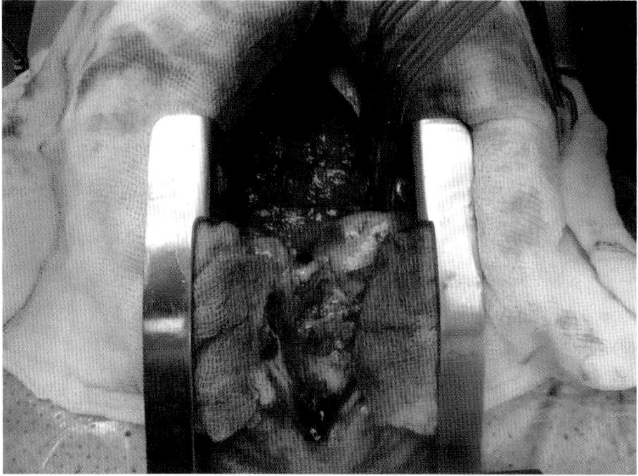

Fig. 9.10 Moist laparotomy swabs are laid over the wound edges and Finochetto rib retractors placed to retract the cut sternum, allowing access to the thoracic cavity.

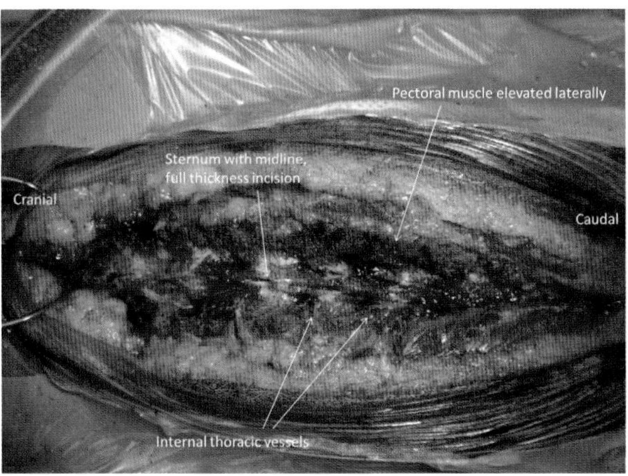

Fig. 9.9 An oscillating saw is used on the midline to cut full thickness through the sternum, keeping the manubrium and xiphoid intact.

lesions reported on CT) or to access mediastinal structures. The patient is positioned in dorsal recumbency with the forelimbs secured cranially. After surgical clipping and aseptic preparation, the skin incision is made from the manubrium to the xiphoid on the midline (Fig. 9.8). The pectoral muscles are slightly elevated to increase exposure of the sternum, taking care to avoid cutting the perforating branches of the internal thoracic artery and vein associated with each sternebra. Electocautery is helpful at this stage. An oscillating saw is used on the midline to cut full thickness through the sternum, keeping the manubrium and xiphoid intact (Fig. 9.9). This will reduce motion of the two halves of the sternum postoperatively (Radlinsky, 2012), decreasing pain and seroma formation. In order to access both hemithoraces, the mediastinum must be perforated at the dorsal aspect of the sternum. Moist laparotomy swabs are laid over the wound edges and Finochetto rib retractors placed to retract the cut sternum, allowing access to the thoracic cavity (Fig. 9.10).

A thoracostomy tube should be placed after the intrathoracic procedure is completed. Closure of the sternotomy is achieved using figure-of-eight (Davis et al., 2006) stainless steel wire or suture (e.g. polydioxanone or polypropylene) (Fig. 9.11). The author uses polydioxanone in patients under 30 kg: one study investigated sternotomy closure in greyhounds and found that sterna closed with polydioxanone or stainless steel wire has similar mechanical properties (Gines et al., 2011).

Heavier dogs may benefit from the use of polydioxanone, but mechanical testing of polydioxanone on dogs heavier than 30 kg has not been performed. The advantage of polydioxanone is its absorbable nature, although one study (Pelsue et al., 2002) demonstrated that sternotomies closed with wire showed a trend towards being more stable and had significantly less displacement on radiographic evaluation at 28 days. All sterna closed with wire examined histopathologically showed evidence of chondral or osteochondral bridging, while sterna closed with suture only showed fibrous union. Significant differences were not observed

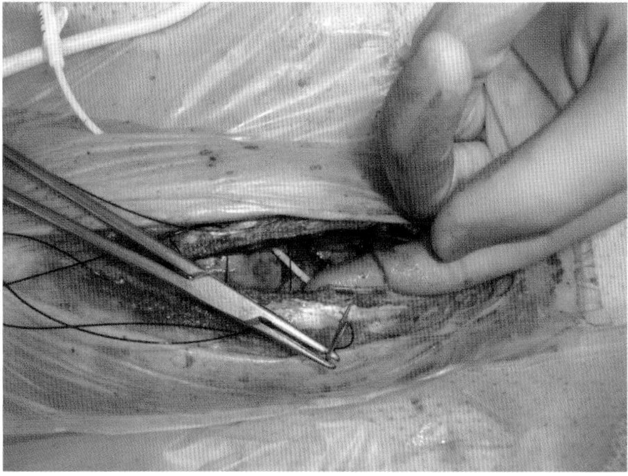

Fig. 9.11 Closure of the sternotomy is achieved using figure-of-eight stainless steel wire or suture (e.g. polydioxanone or polypropylene). The author prefers to pass the needle with the swaged end first.

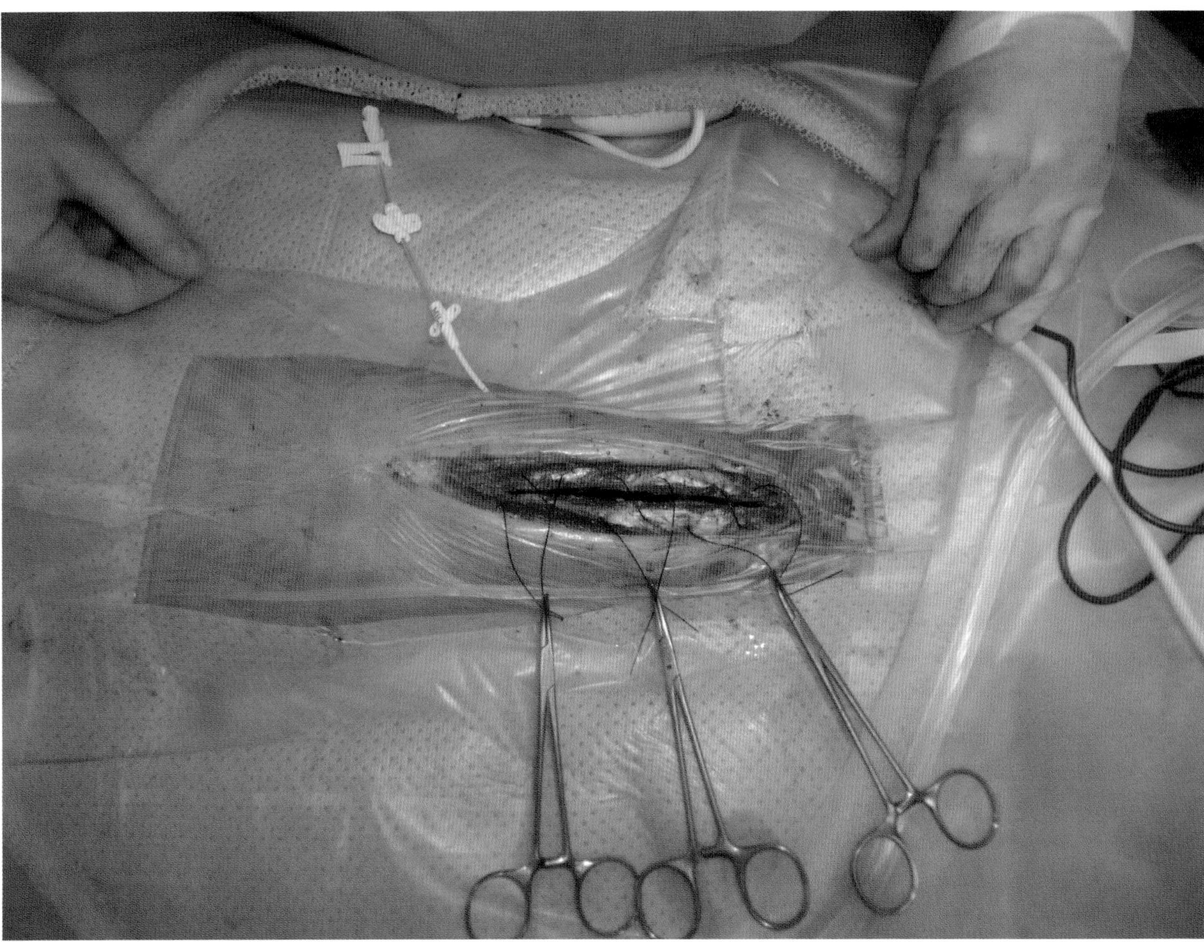

Fig. 9.12 Sutures or wires used for median sternotomy closure are pre-placed.

in degree of postoperative pain or wound complication rates (Pelsue et al., 2002). Sutures or wires are pre-placed (Fig. 9.12). Traction on the middle suture as those at either end are tied is recommended in order to maximise compression between the sternotomy edges (Fig. 9.13). The pectoral muscles are reapposed with an absorbable monofilament suture (Fig. 9.14) and a wound-soaker catheter should be placed for the provision of local anaesthetic, if appropriate to do so (Fig. 9.15) (Abelson et al., 2009). The subcutis and skin are closed routinely.

9.1.4 Thoracoscopy

Thoracoscopy has been described for treating numerous conditions, including thoracic duct ligation,

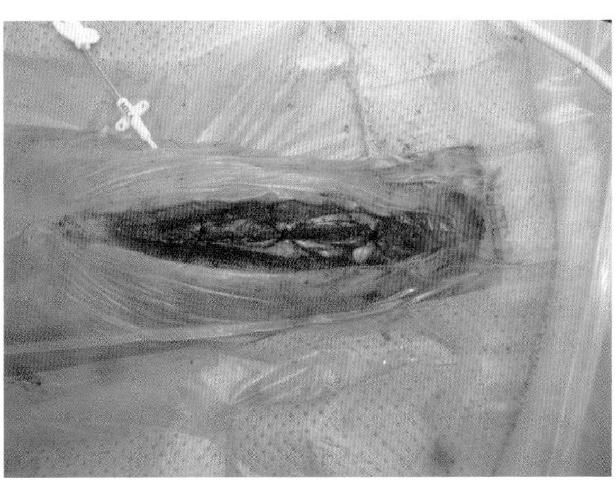

Fig. 9.13 Traction on the middle suture as those at either end are tied is recommended in order to maximise compression between the sternotomy edges.

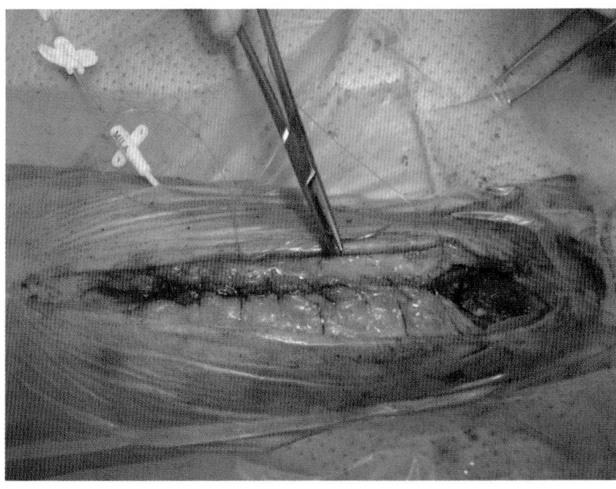

Fig. 9.14 Following sternotomy closure, the pectoral muscles are reapposed with an absorbable monofilament suture.

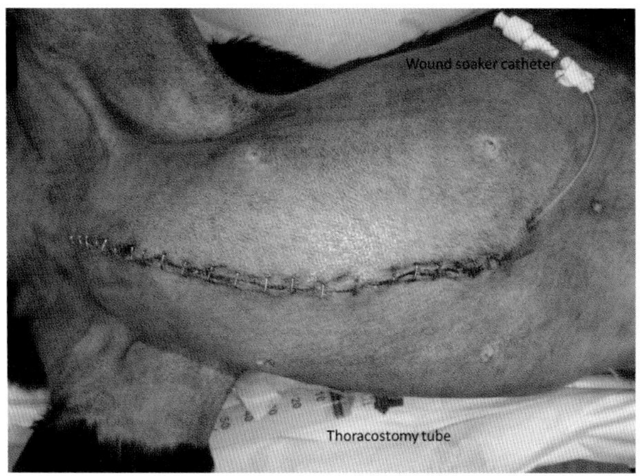

Fig. 9.15 A wound soaker catheter should be placed for the provision of local anaesthetic, if appropriate to do so.

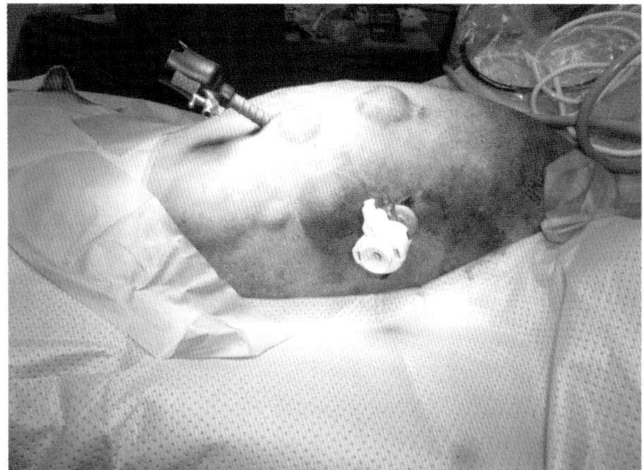

Fig. 9.16 Thoracoscopy portal placement in an adult dog for biopsy of a mediastinal mass lesion. The dog is in dorsal recumbency. The black and green port is placed trans-diaphragmatically to allow positioning of the camera into the thoracic cavity. The white and blue portal is positioned intercostally to permit passage of instruments into the thoracic cavity. The cutaneous masses visible are large lipomas, which were not removed at the time of surgery.

pericardectomy, correction of persistent right aortic arch and lung lobectomy (Dupre, et al., 2001; Jackson et al., 1999; MacPhail et al., 2001; Radlinsky et al., 2002). It is also useful for collecting biopsies of intrathoracic lesions (Figs. 9.16, 9.17, 9.18). Potential complications are the same as for thoracotomy, although morbidity is considered to be lower (Radlinsky, 2012). Lack of visualisation is reported and requires conversion to an open approach or one-lung ventilation (Kudnig et al., 2006). Port site metastasis is reported (Brisson et al., 2006).

9.1.5 Other thoracotomy approaches

Other thoracotomy approaches have been described, but are rarely indicated. Median sternotomy can be combined with a cranial laparotomy if abdominal exposure is also required (Radlinsky, 2012). Rib resection, trans-sternal and trans-diaphragmatic thoracotomies have all been described, but are rarely used.

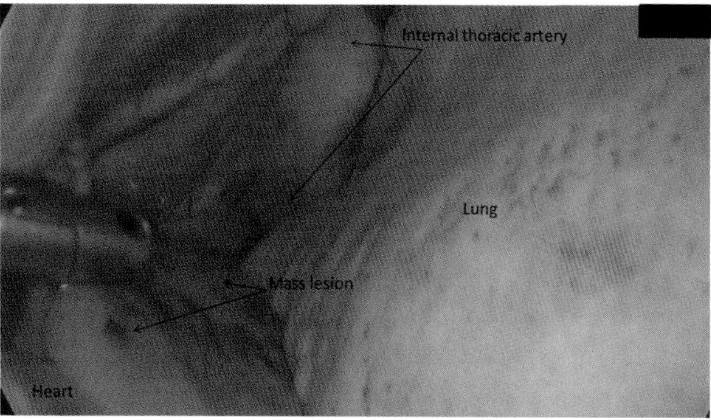

Fig. 9.17 Intra-operative view of a thoracoscopic procedure via a trans-diaphragmatic camera, looking cranially.

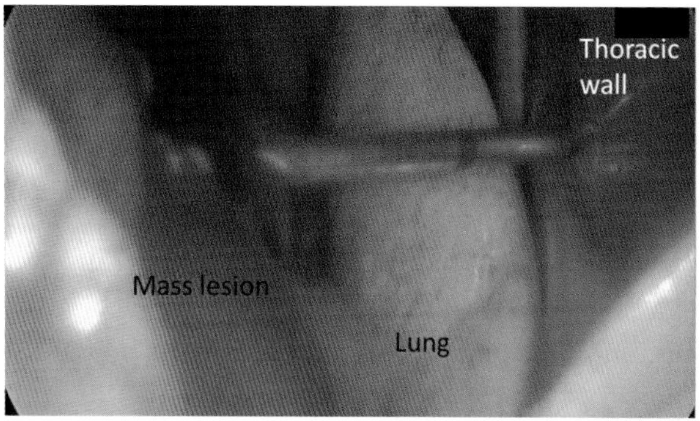

Fig. 9.18 Intra-operative view of a thoracoscopically guided biopsy of an invasive mediastinal mass lesion.

9.2 Surgical techniques

9.2.1 Thoracic drainage

Key points

- Thoracic drainage can be performed via thoracocentesis or following placement of thoracostomy tubes.
- The small-bore, wire-guided catheters can be placed following administration of local anaesthetic, with the patient conscious or sedated. Trochar tubes must only be placed with the patient under general anaesthetic.
- Compared with trochar drains, small-gauge, wire-guided catheters are associated with fewer insertional and infectious complications and are considered more comfortable for the patient.
- Complications associated with thoracostomy tubes are seen in 22% of patients.
- Radiographs following chest tube placement are mandatory to ensure correct placement.
- Animals with thoracostomy tubes should never be

left unattended and must wear an Elizabethan collar and a body stocking until the tubes are removed.
- Thoracic drainage consists of thoracocentesis or thoracostomy tube placement (either trochar tubes or small-gauge, wire-guided catheters).

Thoracocentesis

Thoracocentesis is used for both diagnostic evaluation and therapeutic purposes. Indications for immediate thoracocentesis include dyspnoea and dull/absent lung sounds suggestive of air, fluid or soft tissue accumulation within the pleural space. Fluid collected should be placed in ethylenediaminetetraacetic acid (EDTA) and plain tubes for cytological, biochemical and bacteriological analysis. Volumes of air/fluid yielded should be recorded. Mass lesions should be aspirated for cytological analysis, ideally under ultrasound guidance.

Thoracocentesis can be performed with the patient in sternal or lateral recumbency. In the emergency patient, appropriate stabilisation and oxygen administration may be required and the thoracocentesis should be performed in the position in which the patient can most readily ventilate. One or both hemithoraces are clipped and aseptically prepared, and a needle passed aseptically into the thoracic cavity in the 4th–7th intercostal space. Fluid will settle in the most dependent part of the chest, and air in the least dependent part, which may influence the thoracocentesis site. A butterfly catheter, over-the-needle catheter or hypodermic needle can be used and should be connected to a three-way tap, extension set and syringe (Fig. 9.19).

Potential complications following thoracocentesis include iatrogenic intrathoracic or abdominal damage, laceration of the intercostal vessels, pyothorax and insufficient pleural drainage (Moores, 2016a,b). To decrease the risk of lung lobe laceration, flexible tubing is included between the syringe and needle (Crowe, 1983) and the bevelled edge of the needle is positioned parallel to the intrathoracic wall: this can be achieved by facing the bevelled edge towards the lung and angling the needle at 45° (Kolata, 1981). To avoid the intercostal vessels (located on the caudal edge of the ribs), the needle should be positioned midway between the ribs. Where the thoracic wall is thick, the animal is agitated or there is a high likelihood of repeated thoracocentesis being required, due consideration should be given to the preferential placement of a thoracostomy tube.

Thoracostomy tubes

Thoracostomy tubes consist of trochar tubes and small-gauge, wire-guided catheters (Fig. 9.20a–c). They should be considered for patients that require repeated thoracocentesis and for every patient following thoracotomy. Some texts encourage the modification of tubes by the placement of additional fenestrations (Radlinsky, 2012), but in the author's opinion, this is unnecessary where commercial tubes are utilised and may damage the tube or facilitate breakage.

Trochar tubes and small-gauge, wire-guided catheters can be used for all clinical situations in all sizes of patient. Trochar tubes are associated with greater pain due to their large diameter (Moores, 2016a,b). Complications encountered with thoracostomy tubes are seen in 22% of patients and include inability to place the tube, improper tube placement, problems with tube maintenance, iatrogenic intrathoracic or abdominal drainage, insufficient pleural drainage, pyothorax, haemothorax, pleural effusion and pneumothorax (Marques et al., 2009; Moores, 2016a,b; Tattersall and Welsh, 2006). In one study looking at the small-gauge, wire-guided catheter, the most common complication reported was failure of the catheter to drain as a result of kinking or malpositioning. Obstruction of the drain by fluid or fibrin clot was not encountered, despite the fact that many of the drains were used to manage

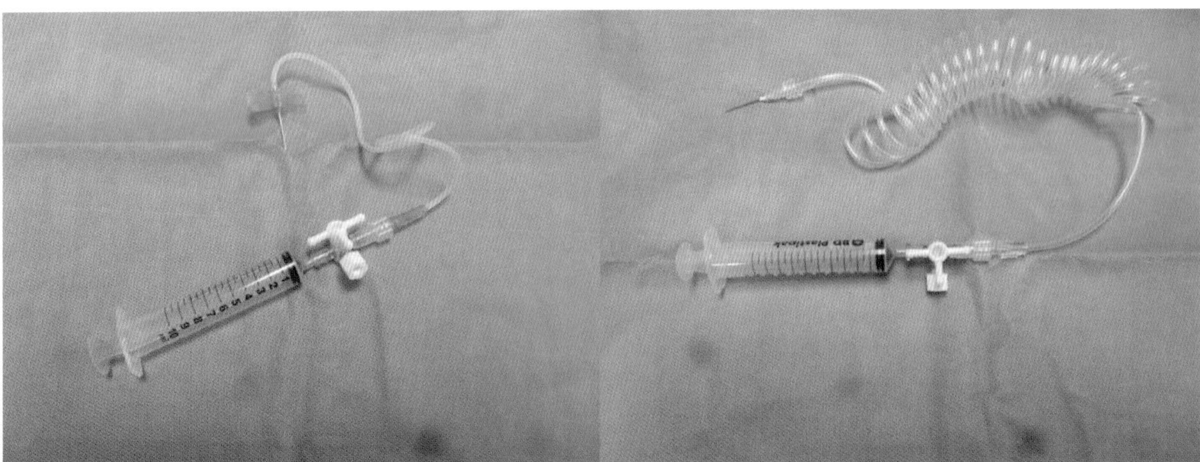

Fig. 9.19 In order to perform thoracocentesis, a butterfly catheter, over-the-needle catheter or hypodermic needle can be used and should be connected to a three-way tap, extension set and syringe.

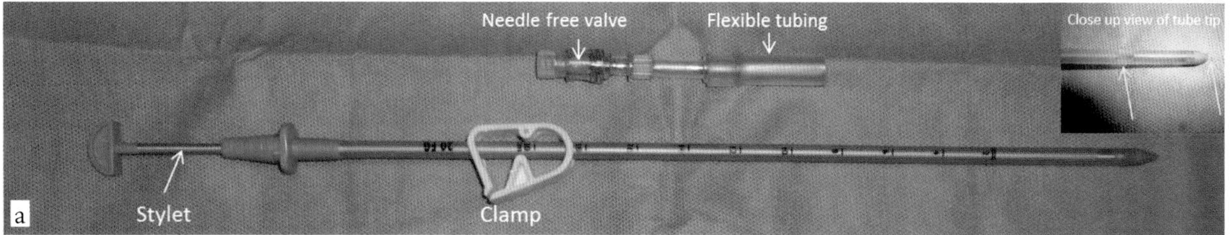

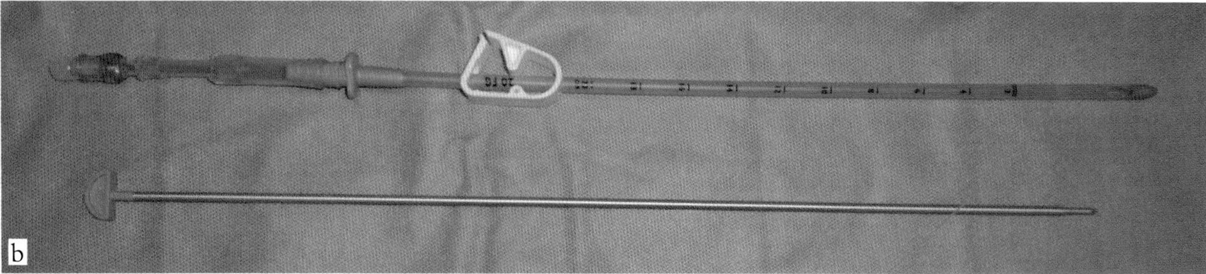

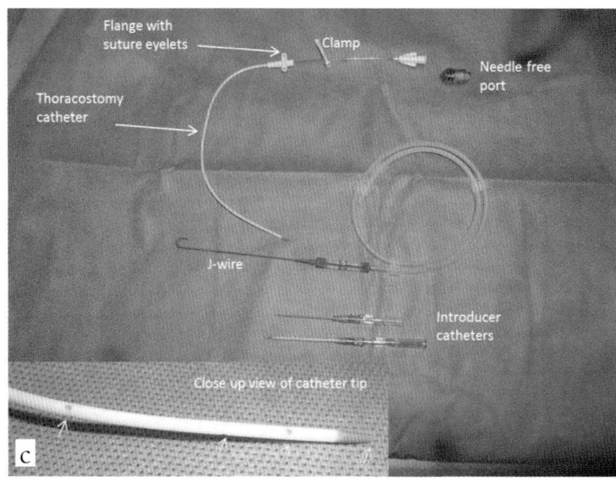

Fig. 9.20a–c Thoracostomy tubes consist of trochar tubes and small-gauge, wire-guided catheters.

pyothorax (Valtolina and Adamantos, 2009). None of the patients reported in this study developed pyothorax as a tube-related complication and, in humans, lower infection rates are seen when tubes of smaller bore are preferentially selected over those with a large bore (Moores, 2016a,b).

It is imperative that patients are appropriately nursed to minimise the risk of complications. Animals with a thoracostomy tube should never be left unattended and must wear an appropriately sized rigid Elizabethan collar at all times. Additionally, the tube should be covered with a body stocking to prevent patient interference, minimise environmental contamination and reduce the risk of dislodgement by catching on kennel doors, etc. Tubes should be regularly inspected for signs of infection and should only be handled following scrupulous hand hygiene and whilst wearing gloves. Ports should be cleansed with alcohol wipes before drainage or fluid instillation.

Following tube placement, all patients should undergo thoracic radiography to confirm proper placement (i.e. all fenestrations are in the pleural space, the tip does not extend cranial to the manubrium, the tube is not kinked, etc.). If repositioning is performed, radiographs must be repeated. The decision to place uni- or bilateral drains depends on the clinical requirement. The author often places one drain and reassesses the patient clinically and radiographically before placing a second drain if the contralateral hemithorax has not been adequately evacuated. If any doubt exists, a second drain should be placed because it can readily be removed if later deemed to be surplus to requirements.

A thoracostomy tube can be placed with the patient in sternal or lateral recumbency. Placement of the large-bore trochar drain requires general anaesthesia with local anaesthetic. The small-gauge, wire-guided catheter can be placed with the patient conscious or sedated, using local anaesthetic before placement. The latter may be more appropriate in an emergency patient where general anaesthesia is undesirable. One or both hemithoraces are clipped and aseptically prepared in preparation for tube placement, and local anaesthetic (lidocaine) is infused into the appropriate interspace just behind the rib and dorsal to the proposed site of tube/catheter placement. The two interspaces caudally and cranially are infused likewise. Potential complications

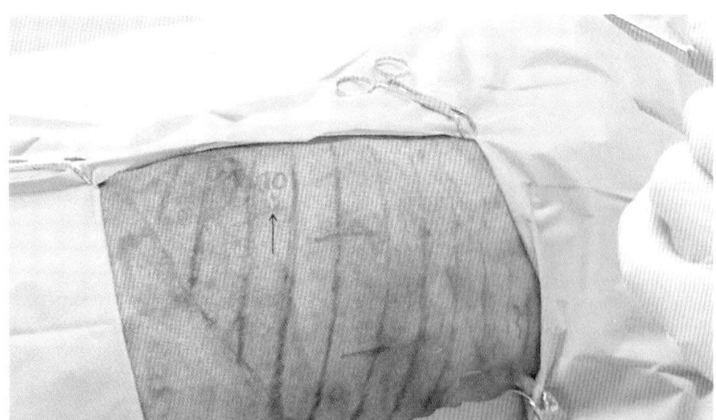

Fig. 9.21 To place a trochar drain, a stab incision is made into the skin in the proximal third of the thoracic wall at the level of the 10th intercostal space (arrow). (Image courtesy of Georg Haimel.)

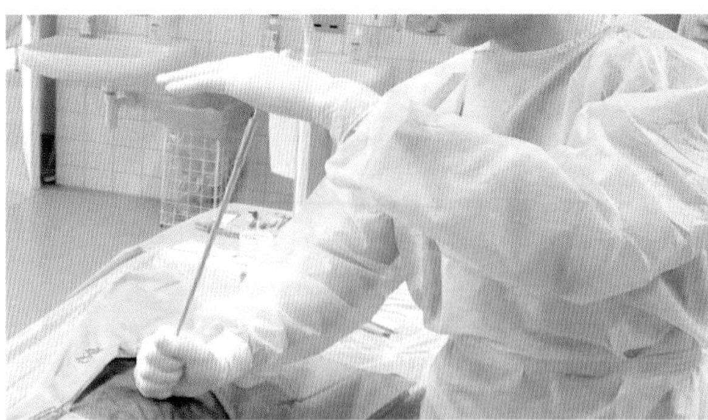

Fig. 9.23 The trochar tube is angled perpendicular to the body wall and held in one fist, with the distance between the fist and skin being approximately the thickness of the thoracic wall. Firm pressure is applied to the stylet until the tube penetrates the thoracic cavity. (Image courtesy of Georg Haimel.)

might include haemorrhage if the intercostal vasculature is damaged. After tube placement, local anaesthetic (bupivacaine) should be regularly instilled into the chest cavity via the thoracostomy tube.

To place a trochar tube, the tube is measured to avoid entering the most cranial portion of the thorax/mediastinum. A skin tunnel is required with large-bore tubes: this will collapse upon tube removal and act as a one-way valve, preventing pneumothorax developing. In order to achieve this, a skin incision is made over the 10th rib and the trochar drain tunnelled subcutaneously and cranioventrally, to the 7th–8th intercostal space (Figs. 9.21, 9.22). The trochar tube is angled perpendicular to the body wall and held in one fist, with the distance between the fist and skin being approximately the thickness of the thoracic wall. Firm pressure is applied to the stylet until the tube penetrates the thoracic cavity (Fig. 9.23); the purpose of the fist is to act as a buffer, preventing excessive advancement of the stylet into the thoracic cavity. The tube is redirected towards the contralateral shoulder and the tube advanced off the stylet (Fig. 9.24). The clamp is closed and appropriate connectors attached to allow drainage of the chest. The tube is secured to avoid dislodgement or extrathoracic migration of fenestrations using a Chinese finger trap suture (Fig. 9.25) and the thoracic cavity is drained (Fig. 9.26). Post-placement radiographs are imperative (Fig. 9.27).

To place a small-gauge, wire-guided catheter, the Seldinger technique is used. The skin is clipped and aseptically prepared. A small skin incision is made at the level of the 9th intercostal space. The introducer catheter is inserted into the thoracic cavity midway between the ribs: no subcutaneous tunnelling is required because of the catheter's small bore (Fig. 9.28). The introducer is advanced fully into the thorax over the stylet and the stylet is removed. The J-wire is threaded through the catheter and advanced approximately 12–20 cm, or until resistance is felt (Fig. 9.29). The introducer is removed, leaving the guidewire in place (Fig. 9.30). The small-bore catheter is then advanced over the guidewire into the thoracic cavity and the guidewire removed (Fig. 9.31). A needle-free valve is attached to the end of the catheter and the catheter secured using the eyelets on the flange (Fig. 9.32). Post-placement radiographs are imperative (Fig. 9.33).

Removal of the chest tube will depend on the clinical parameters of the individual patient. As a general rule, tubes are removed when air production is almost zero and when fluid production is less than 2 ml/kg/

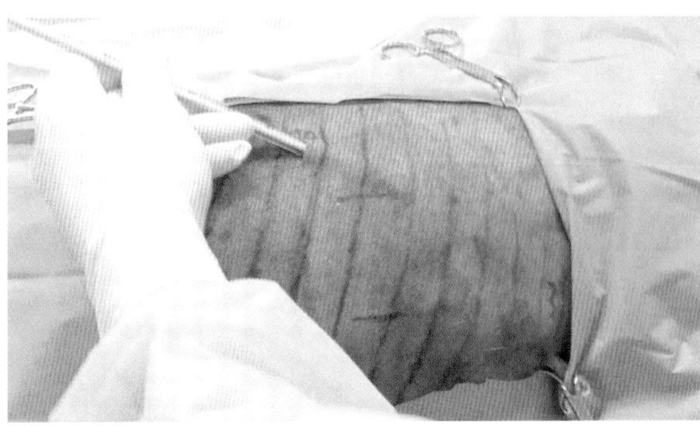

Fig. 9.22 The trochar drain is tunnelled subcutaneously and cranioventrally for a distance of 2–3 rib spaces. (Image courtesy of Georg Haimel.)

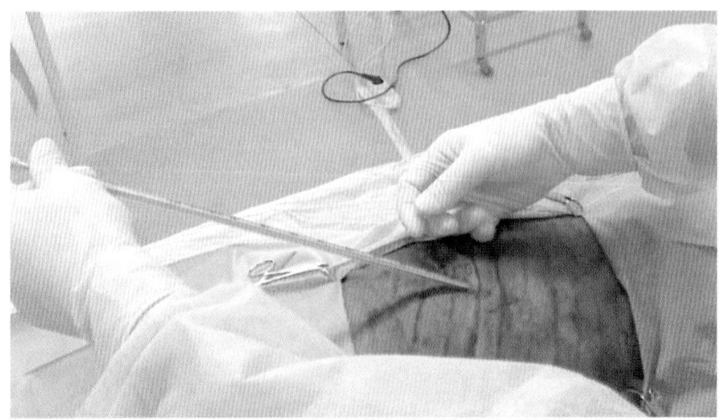

Fig. 9.24 The trochar tube is redirected towards the contralateral shoulder and the tube advanced off the stylet. (Image courtesy Georg Haimel.)

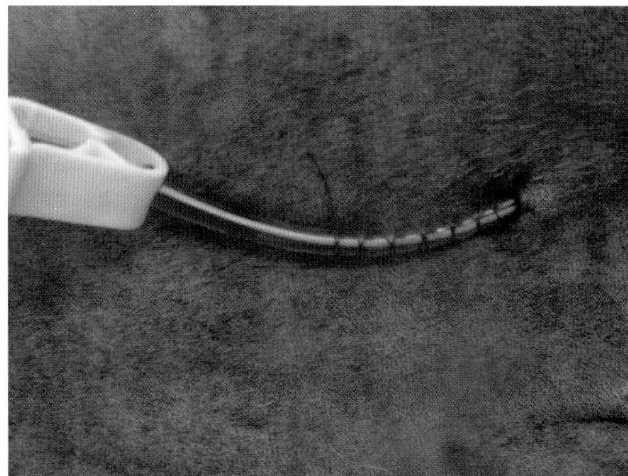

Fig. 9.25 The trochar thoracostomy tube is secured to avoid dislodgement or extrathoracic migration of fenestrations, using a Chinese finger trap suture.

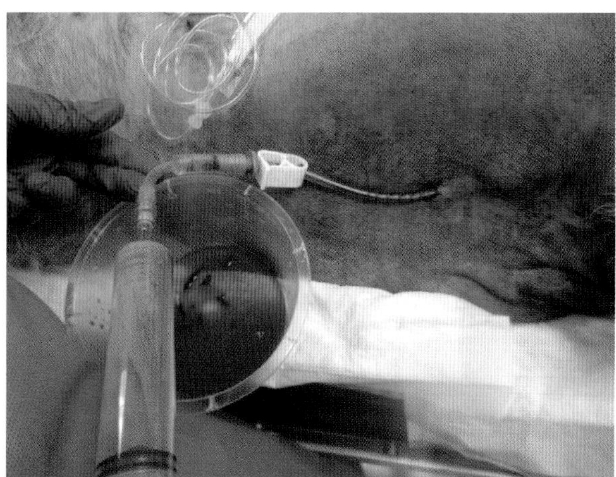

Fig. 9.26 The thoracic cavity is aseptically drained.

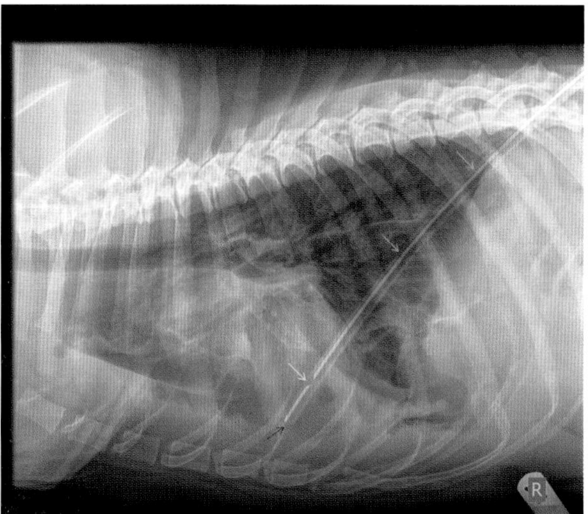

Fig. 9.27 Following thoracotomy tube placement, radiographs are imperative to ensure that the tube is appropriately sited and not kinked. The red and yellow arrows show the sites of the terminal and side openings of the thoracostomy tube, respectively. The green and blue arrows show the site of entry of the thoracostomy tube into the thoracic cavity and skin, respectively.

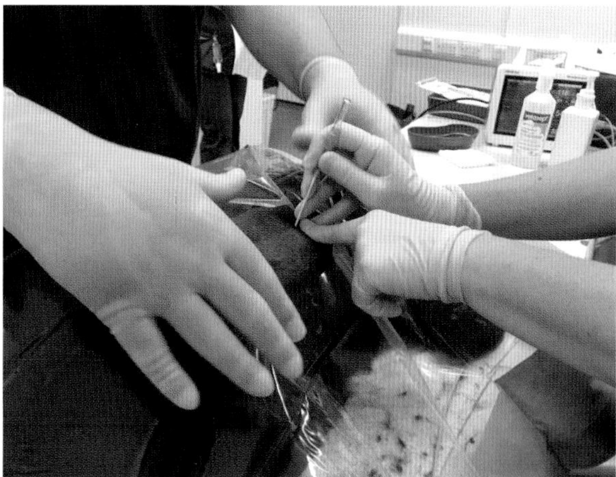

Fig. 9.28 To place a small-gauge, wire-guided catheter, a small skin incision is made at the level of the 9th intercostal space. The introducer catheter is inserted into the thoracic cavity midway between the ribs. The introducer is advanced fully into the thorax over the stylet and the stylet is removed.

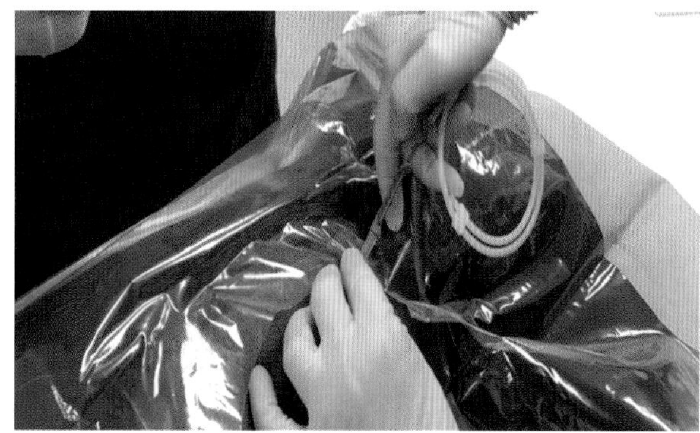

Fig. 9.29 The J-wire is threaded through the catheter and advanced approximately 12–20 cm, or until resistance is felt.

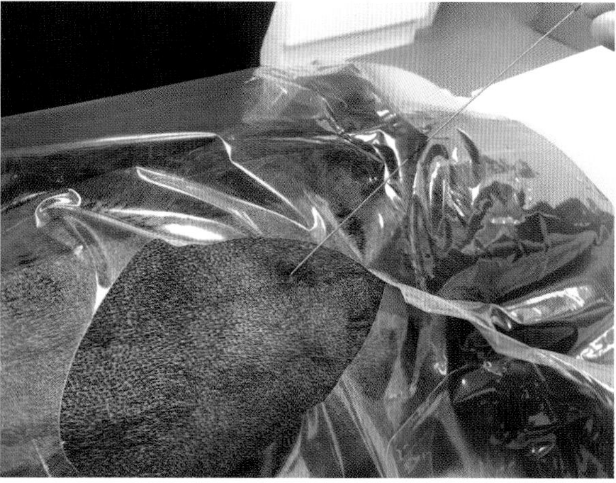

Fig. 9.30 The introducer is removed, leaving the guidewire in place.

day. However, a recent study has shown that the tube may be removed when fluid production is greater than this, providing other clinical parameters are taken into account (Marques et al., 2009). To remove tubes, the sutures are removed and the drain gently and steadily

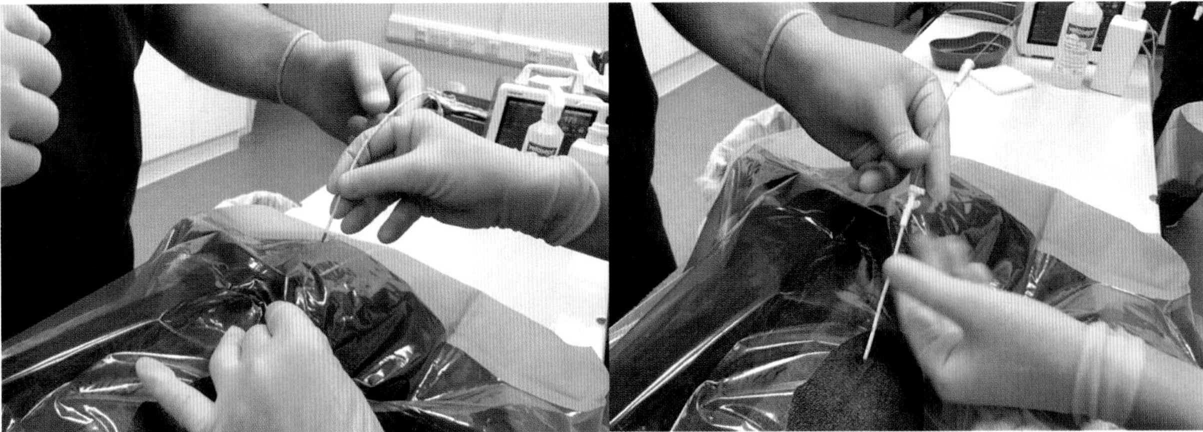

Fig. 9.31 The small-bore catheter is advanced over the guidewire into the thoracic cavity and the guidewire removed.

extracted. The author covers the skin site with a film dressing if a trochar drain has been removed. No sutures are required.

9.2.2 Lung lobectomy

Key points

- Lung lobectomy is indicated for conditions of the lungs such as cysts, bullae, blebs, broncho-oesophageal fistula, consolidated lung lobe/abscess, bronchiectasis, lung laceration, lung lobe torsion and neoplasia.
- Accurate diagnostic evaluation is imperative preoperatively, and assistance should be sought from specialist imagers, anaesthetists and surgeons.
- Lung lobectomy can be performed by hand or using staplers. The advantage of staplers is the reduced surgical time and minimal leakage; the disadvantage is increased cost.
- Following lung lobectomy, the site must be assessed for leakage of air by flooding the thoracic cavity with saline.
- If lung lobectomy is undertaken for neoplasia, the wound edges must be protected from seeding and kit/gloves should be changed before closure.
- Dogs can survive loss of 50% of their total lung volume, but loss of >75% is fatal and acute pulmonary hypertension occurs after acute restriction of >60% of pulmonary arterial outflow.
- Because the left and right lungs comprise 42 and 58% of lung tissue, respectively, excision of the left lung is possible if the right lung is healthy.

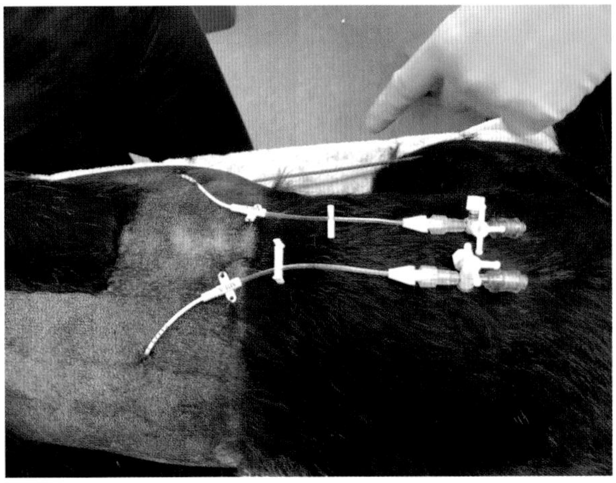

Fig. 9.32 A needle-free valve is attached to the end of the catheter and the catheter secured using the eyelets on the flange.

Lung lobectomy is indicated for conditions of the lungs such as cysts, bullae, blebs, broncho-oesophageal fistula, consolidated lung lobe/abscess, bronchiectasis, lung laceration, lung lobe torsion and neoplasia. Accurate diagnostic evaluation is imperative preoperatively, and

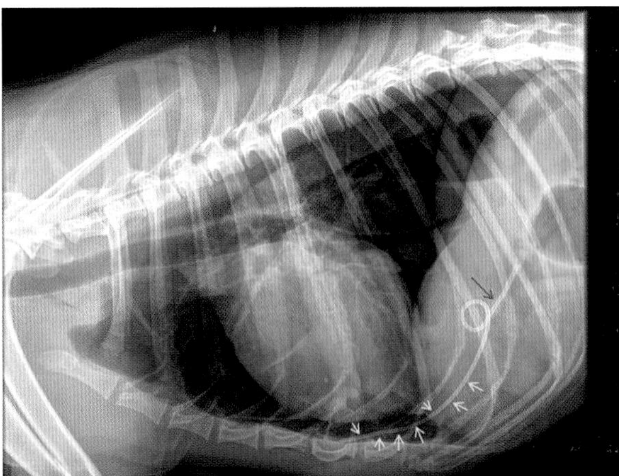

Fig. 9.33 Post-placement radiographs are imperative following placement of all thoracostomy tubes. The skin is entered at the level of the red arrow. The multiple fenestrations are marked by the yellow arrows. The loop identified on the radiograph is not uncommon in small-bore catheters and the catheter should be functional. Kinked catheters require replacement.

Table 9.2 Potential complications of lung lobectomy (Brissot, 2016).

Potential complication	Comments
Bronchopleural fistula	Can be seen up to 3 weeks postoperatively and requires emergency surgical re-exploration
Perioperative failure to achieve an airtight suture line	
Haemorrhage	Double transfixing ligation of all vessels is indicated. Consider individually suturing large vessels before stapling. *En bloc* stapling of the hilus should be performed with a vascular stapler (e.g. TA30 V3) (Brissot, 2016)
Airway obstruction	Ensure lung manipulation is minimised until complete cross-clamping of the bronchus is achieved distal to the proposed resection site (LaRue et al., 1987)
Intra-operative pleural contamination	
Postoperative subcutaneous emphysema	Usually resolves spontaneously if localised. If generalised, can disrupt the vascular supply to the skin (Brissot, 2016)
Postoperative cardiac complications, including arrhythmia	Supraventricular tachycardia most commonly observed, seen in 25–75% of patients undergoing lobectomy/pneumonectomy (Liptak et al., 2004)
Acute respiratory distress syndrome	Secondary to inflammation and increased vascular permeability. Often fatal (Ave et al., 2004)
Pulmonary oedema	
Respiratory insufficiency	Risk is greater when right pneumonectomy is performed (Liptak et al., 2004)
Mediastinal shift	May result in regurgitation, which can be successfully managed medically (Liptak et al., 2004)
Acute anaphylactic shock	Reported after lung lobectomy in a patient with heartworm (Carter et al., 2011)
Portal site metastasis	Protect the surgical wound (Brisson et al., 2006)

assistance should be sought from specialist imagers, anaesthetists and surgeons. Referral should be offered if appropriate. Potential complications associated with lung lobectomy are shown in Table 9.2.

Partial lung lobectomy is the removal of the distal two-thirds or less of the lung, and can be performed via an intercostal thoracotomy, median sternotomy or thoracoscopic approach. Partial lung lobectomy can be performed by hand or using staplers. The advantage of staplers is that lobectomy can be completed rapidly and leakage is infrequent; the disadvantages are their size (which may be too large in very small patients) and cost. Following completion of the procedure the site must be tested for leakage, which is performed by flooding the thoracic cavity with body-temperature sterile saline and examining the resection site during inspiration. Leaks are controlled by a few interrupted absorbable monofilament sutures.

To perform partial lung lobectomy by hand, the site to be removed is identified and crushing forceps placed at the level of the proposed resection, allowing adequate gross margins, depending on the diagnosis. Two rows of continuous overlapping sutures are placed 2 mm proximal to the forceps using an absorbable monofilament suture. If large bronchi or blood vessels are identified, these are ligated individually. The lung is transected proximal to the forceps and the edge of the lung is oversewn and observed for leakage. Where neoplasia is suspected, kit and gloves should be changed before wound closure to minimise contamination.

To perform a stapled partial lung lobectomy, a thoraco-abdominal stapler with a staple leg length of 2.5 mm is used. Staplers which incorporate a double or triple row of staggered staplers are acceptable; the author prefers to use a vascular stapler. The stapler is positioned proximal to the lesion and deployed. The lobe is transected distal to the stapler and observed for leakage. In small patients, a linear cutting stapler is useful: this deploys two or three staggered rows of staples either side of a cutting blade, and can be easier to manoeuvre and position than a thoraco-abdominal stapler (Figs. 9.34, 9.35, 9.36).

A total lung lobectomy is preferentially performed through a lateral intercostal approach, if possible. During caudal lung lobectomy, the pulmonary ligament must be transected to mobilise the lobe; this runs from the caudal edge of the hilus to the mediastinal pleura. Stapling is the methodology of choice, being more rapid than suture ligation and with minimal complications (Monnet, 2018a). The author prefers to use a vascular stapler (usually 3.5 mm), which delivers three staggered rows of staples and will occlude the vessels and bronchus when placed across the hilus. Ensure all other tissue is excluded. Non-crushing clamps are

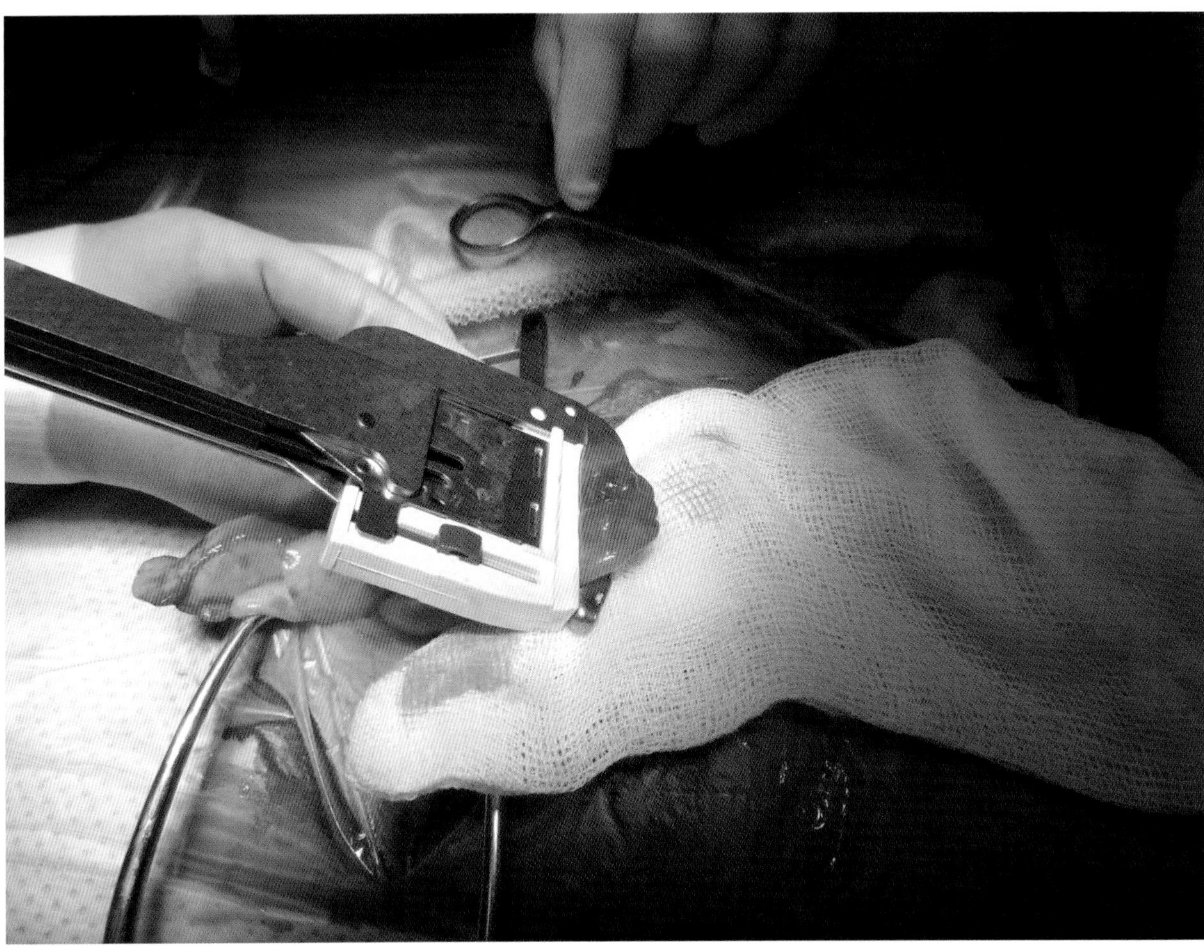

Fig. 9.34 Placement of a thoraco-abdominal stapler for a partial lung lobectomy via an intercostal approach, as treatment for a ruptured bulla causing pneumothorax. The lung will be resected distal to the stapler using a scalpel blade.

positioned distal to the stapler and the lung transected proximal to the clamp, which avoids any contamination from lung contents. The lung lobe is released from the stapler and tested for leakage. Some leakage may occur through the B-shaped staples, and additional sutures can be placed if required.

To perform total lung lobectomy by hand, the hilus is isolated and the pulmonary artery triple ligated (with transfixing suture) and divided, followed by the pulmonary vein. The bronchus is clamped with two Satinsky forceps and a horizontal mattress suture placed proximal to the clamps and tied. The bronchus is transected between the clamps and the end oversewn with a simple continuous pattern. The site is leak tested.

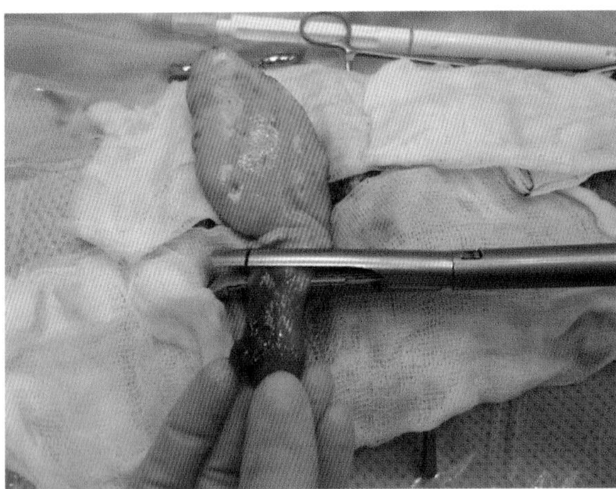

Fig. 9.35 Use of a linear cutting stapler to perform partial lung lobectomy in a small dog with a lung laceration secondary to a thoracic dog bite.

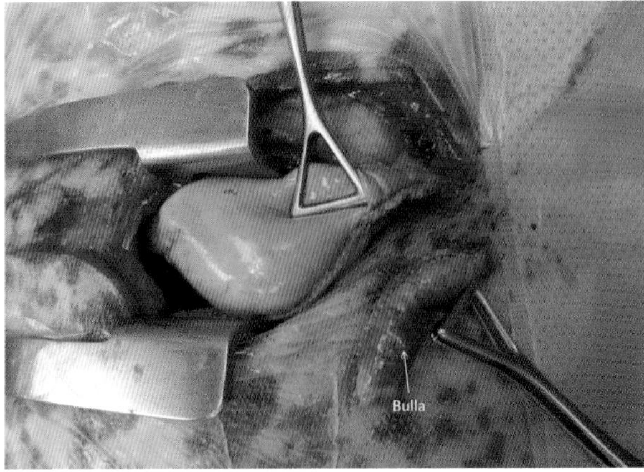

Fig. 9.36 Image following deployment of a linear cutter to perform a partial lung lobectomy for resection of a small bulla in a dog. Staplers are positioned proximal and distal to the resection site.

Pneumonectomy is required for disease processes affecting one lung where the contralateral lung is normal. Dogs can survive loss of 50% of their total lung volume, but loss of >75% is fatal and acute pulmonary hypertension occurs after acute restriction of >60% of pulmonary arterial outflow (Brugarolas and Takita, 1973; Tronc et al., 1999). Because the left and right lungs comprise 42 and 58% of lung tissue respectively, excision of the left lung is possible if the right lung is healthy. Right-sided pneumonectomy may be possible if the disease process has resulted in an insidious decline in right lung function, but is fatal if performed acutely (Liptak et al., 2004; Monnet, 2018a). Referral must be sought for such cases – surgery and aftercare can be challenging. Approach is via an intercostal thoracotomy, and the same sequence of vessel and bronchus ligation is performed as for total lung lobectomy.

9.2.3 Pericardectomy

Key points

- Pericardectomy is indicated for conditions such as pericardial effusion causing tamponade or chylothorax.
- Pericardectomy can be performed via a median sternotomy or a right intercostal thoracotomy. Alternatively, thoracoscopic pericardectomy can be performed.

Pericardectomy is indicated for conditions such as pericardial effusion causing tamponade (where it may be curative in idiopathic cases and palliative in neoplastic cases) or chylothorax. It is imperative that samples are submitted for histopathological and bacteriological analysis.

Pericardectomy can be performed via a median sternotomy or a right intercostal thoracotomy. A transdiaphragmatic subxiphoid open approach has been described (Monnet, 2018b), but results in limited visualisation and should be avoided.

To perform a subtotal pericardectomy, an incision is made into the pericardium and any pericardial effusion removed using suction. The pericardium is removed ventral to both phrenic nerves, ideally using bipolar sealing technology to facilitate haemostasis. The sternopericardial ligament is transected and the pericardium removed. The wound edges should be protected with saline-soaked swabs to prevent contamination with neoplastic cells during pericardial removal. In oncology patients, kit and gloves are changed before routine thoracostomy tube placement and wound closure.

Thoracoscopic pericardectomy has been successfully described: a subxiphoid camera port is placed, along with two instrument portals (positioned in the right and left 7th interspaces, or the right 4th and 7th interspaces). Removal of a pericardial window (3×3 cm) using bipolar sealing technology will suffice. Single lung ventilation is not required. Protection of the wound edges (e.g. with specimen retrieval bags) is recommended in neoplastic cases.

Potential complications of pericardectomy include haemorrhage, cardiac tamponade, phrenic nerve injury, cardiac herniation and recurrence of pericardial effusion.

9.3 Specific diseases of the thoracic cavity

9.3.1 Patent ductus arteriosus

Key points

- Patent ductus arteriosus (PDA) is one of the most common congenital cardiac defects seen in the dog.
- If pressure in the left heart is higher than the right, blood will flow from systemic to pulmonary circulations ('left to right').
- If pulmonary hypertension has developed, blood flow will reverse and travel from the pulmonary to the systemic circulations ('right to left') (Arora, 2001; Cote and Ettinger, 2001).
- Closure of PDA can be achieved via an open approach and surgical ligation or, preferably, by a cardiologist via percutaneous placement of embolisation coils or Amplatzer ductal occluders.

Patent ductus arteriosus is one of the most common congenital cardiac defects in the dog (Buchanan, 1999; Schrope, 2015) and is also seen in the cat, albeit with a lower prevalence (Jones and Buchanan, 1981). It is a complex, polygenic threshold trait with a graded phenotypic expression (Patterson et al., 1971) and for which a female sex predisposition has been described (Schrope, 2015). Many breeds have been documented as predisposed, including keeshonds, poodles, Maltese, bichon frises, Yorkshire terriers, cocker spaniels, Pekingese, collies, Shelties, pomeranians and Welsh corgis (Buchanan, 1999; Pelosi and Orton, 2018). Heritability has been demonstrated in breeds such as the poodle, Welsh corgi and Dutch stabyhoun (Den Toom et al., 2016; Pelosi and Orton, 2018; Oswald and Orton, 1993).

In utero, the ductus arteriosus carries blood from the pulmonary artery to the aorta, bypassing the still non-functional lungs. The ductus arteriosus closes within the first week of life by contraction of the ductus muscle, enabling normal blood flow through the lungs and aorta (Coceani and Baragatti, 2012; House and Ederstrom, 1968). In cases of PDA, the ductus fails to close: histological studies in dogs suggest that smooth muscle hypoplasia and asymmetry of the ductus tissue is the major cause of PDA (Buchanan and Patterson, 2003). The direction of blood flow in this resultant shunting vessel depends on left and right heart pressures. If pressure in the left heart is higher than in the right, blood will flow from systemic to pulmonary circulations ('left to right'). If pulmonary hypertension has developed, blood flow will reverse and travel from the pulmonary to the systemic circulation ('right to left'). This reversal occurs in 5% of dogs with PDA (Buchanan, 1999). Bidirectional flow has also been reported. If left untreated, most patients with PDA die within a year from progressive heart failure (Eyster et al., 1976).

Clinical signs

Clinical signs and imaging findings are summarised in Table 9.3. Patients with left-to-right PDA may be asymptomatic at first and then develop clinical signs associated with left-sided heart failure (Ackerman et al., 1978). Animals with right-to-left PDA have a very different clinical presentation, namely cyanosis. Electrocardiography is of limited use in achieving a diagnosis – the methodology of choice is echocardiography with Doppler or bubble study (Pelosi and Orton, 2018; Scurtu et al., 2016).

Treatment

Closure of PDA should be performed as soon as possible in patients with left-to-right shunt; any clinical signs of congestive heart failure should be addressed first with diuretics, and closure performed as soon as the patient is stable. Ductal occlusion in right-to-left shunt is contraindicated, but reasonable survivals have been reported following treatment for pulmonary hypertension (e.g. sildenafil) and polycythaemia (e.g. phlebotomy, hydroxyurea) (Scurtu et al., 2016; Kellum and Stepien (2007).

Closure of PDA can be achieved via an open approach and surgical ligation or, preferably, by a

Table 9.3 Clinical findings in patients with patient ductus arteriosus.

<table>
<tr><th></th><th>Clinical signs</th><th>Physical examination findings</th><th>Thoracic radiographic findings</th><th>Electrocardiography</th><th>Echocardiography</th></tr>
<tr><td rowspan="5">Left-to-right PDA</td><td>Exercise intolerance</td><td rowspan="3">Continuous murmur at the left heart base</td><td>Left atrial and ventricular enlargement</td><td>Tall R-waves (>2.5 mV) on lead II in some cases</td><td>Eccentric left ventricular hypertrophy</td></tr>
<tr><td>Stunted growth</td><td rowspan="2">Dilation of descending aorta on dorsoventral view</td><td>Atrial fibrillation</td><td>Dilation of the left atrium, ascending aorta and pulmonary artery</td></tr>
<tr><td>Cough</td><td rowspan="3">Supraventricular and ventricular ectopic beats</td><td>Visualisation of the PDA</td></tr>
<tr><td>Exertional tachypnoea</td><td rowspan="2">Hyperkinetic femoral pulses</td><td rowspan="2">Pulmonary vasculature enlargement</td><td>Increased aortic ejection velocity</td></tr>
<tr><td>Dyspnoea</td><td>Reverse turbulent flow in the pulmonary artery on Doppler</td></tr>
<tr><td rowspan="4">Right-to-left PDA</td><td>Exercise intolerance</td><td>Normal femoral pulses</td><td>Right heart enlargement</td><td rowspan="4">Right axis deviation and increased S-wave amplitude due to right ventricular hypertrophy</td><td>Right atrial dilation and right ventricle hypertrophy</td></tr>
<tr><td rowspan="2">Pelvic limb collapse</td><td rowspan="2">Brick-red mucous membranes due to polycythaemia</td><td rowspan="2">Marked dilation of the pulmonary artery</td><td>Visualisation of the PDA</td></tr>
<tr><td>Interventricular septal flattening</td></tr>
<tr><td>Differential cyanosis (more severe caudally)</td><td>No murmur, or a soft systolic murmur at the left heart base</td><td>Enlarged or tortuous pulmonary arteries</td><td>Dilated pulmonary artery</td></tr>
</table>

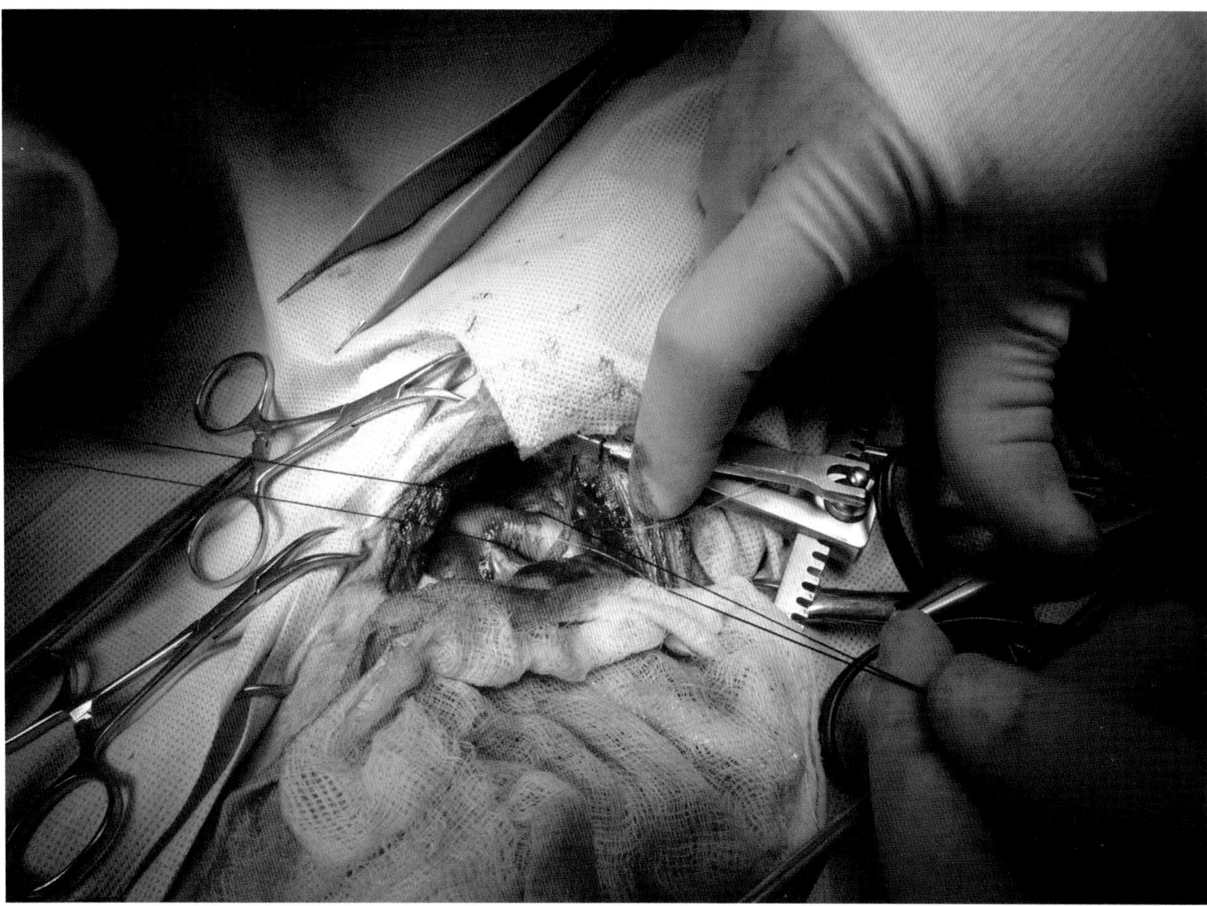

Fig. 9.37 Surgical ligation of PDA via a left intercostal approach. Non-absorbable ligatures (e.g. silk or polypropylene) are passed around the PDA and slowly tightened. (Image courtesy of Domingo Casamian Sorrosal.)

cardiologist via percutaneous placement of embolisation coils or Amplatzer ductal occluders.

Surgical ligation of PDA can be performed in patients over 8 weeks of age, and should be undertaken at the earliest opportunity following diagnosis. Even animals with severe secondary myocardial failure and mitral regurgitation will benefit from surgery (Pelosi and Orton, 2018). Open surgery is performed via a left 4th–5th intercostal thoracotomy (Fig. 9.37). The vagus nerve travels along the ventral border of the aorta and is a landmark for identification of PDA – the vagus nerve courses directly over and perpendicular to it. The vagus nerve is isolated and retracted dorsally with a suture. The PDA is isolated using blunt dissection with right-angled forceps. Non-absorbable ligatures (e.g. silk or polypropylene) are passed around the PDA and slowly tightened. The use of haemostatic clips has also been described, but is not advisable because of significant risk for residual ductal flow and recanalisation (Corti et al., 2000). Surgical mortality is 0–7%, and ductal occlusion is curative in the majority of cases when performed at an early age (Pelosi and Orton, 2018). Potential complications associated with open surgical ligation of a PDA include intra-operative haemorrhage, recanalisation of the ductus, recurrent laryngeal nerve injury, left atrial herniation and ductus aneurysmal rupture (Brockman, 2016). Residual flow secondary to incomplete surgical ligation or recanalisation has been reported in 21–53% of cases based on echocardiography, and 2–3% based on auscultation (Miller et al., 2005; Stanley et al., 2003).

Ductal occlusion can also be performed percutaneously via placement of an Amplatzer ductal occluder or embolisation coils (Faella and Hijazi, 2000; Snaps et al., 1995) (Fig. 9.38a–c). Serious complications (including death) are reduced with percutaneous occlusion (<1%) compared with the open approach (Gordon and Miller, 2005). Mild complications are rare, and include haematoma at the femoral arterial cut-down site and short-term lameness on the cut-down leg (Gordon and Miller, 2005).

Prognosis

A study of 316 patients undergoing Amplatzer placement for PDA occlusion showed that at 12-month follow-up, 100% of patients had complete ductal occlusion as documented by colour Doppler echocardiography (Faella and Hijazi, 2000). Complications were encountered in 15 patients, including one major complication

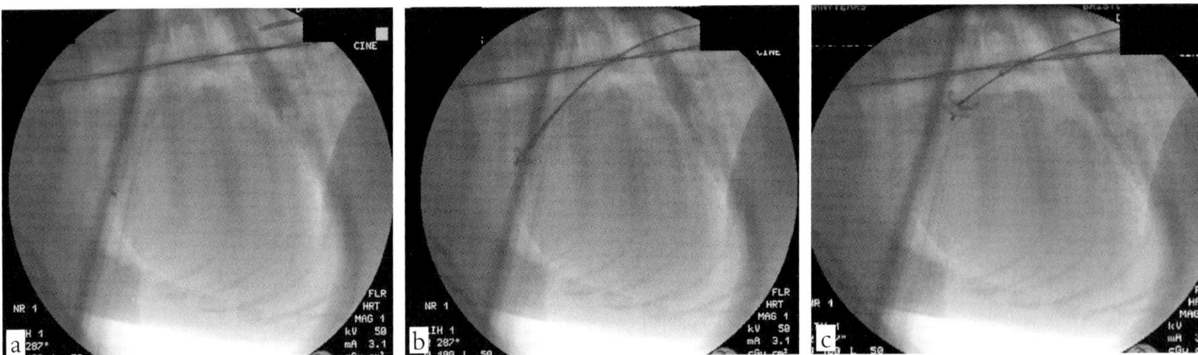

Fig. 9.38a–c Fluoroscopic images of PDA occlusion performed percutaneously via placement of an Amplatzer ductal occluder. Images are before (a), during (b) and following (c) Amplatzer deployment across the PDA. (Images courtesy of Domingo Casamian Sorrosal.)

due to device embolisation and subsequent death, six moderate complications and eight minor complications. The median fluoroscopy time was 12 min and the median total procedure time was 70 min. There have been no reported episodes of delayed device migration, endocarditis, thromboembolism, wire fracture or device disruption.

Coil embolisation results in <5% of dogs showing residual ductal flow 3 months postoperatively. These patients require an additional embolisation procedure, which is usually successful in achieving complete occlusion (Gordon and Miller, 2005). Recanalisation is not recognised in PDA coil embolisation. Potential complications of coil embolisation include accidental pulmonary artery embolisation (requiring no retrieval); accidental pulmonary artery embolisation (not typically associated with adverse effects in dogs); significant residual ductal flow requiring a second coil embolisation procedure; severe femoral artery haemorrhage; late pulmonary artery embolisation requiring a second procedure (surgical ligation); partial aortic deployment; and haemolysis (Gordon and Miller, 2005; Van Israel et al., 2001).

9.3.2 Persistent right aortic arch

Key points

- Persistent right aortic arch (PRAA) is the most common vascular ring anomaly in the dog and extends between the left pulmonary artery and the right aortic arch, encircling the oesophagus.
- PRAA may be present in 10% of dogs.
- Clinical signs of PRAA are consistent with oesophageal constriction and first become apparent at weaning.
- The treatment of choice is ligation and surgical division of the compressive left ligamentum arteriosum via either a left fourth intercostal thoracotomy or a thoracoscopic approach.

Persistent right aortic arch with left ligamentum arteriosum is a vascular anomaly of the thoracic great vessels, resulting in the oesophagus being encircled and constricted. PRAA is the most common (95%) vascular ring anomaly in dogs (Buchanan, 1968; Kyles, 2003). There are six primordial embryonic arches and a dorsal and ventral aorta. In the adult, arches 3, 4 and 6 remain in their original form. In PRAA, the right fourth arch, instead of the left, remains as the aorta. The ligamentum arteriosum extends between the left pulmonary artery and the right aortic arch, encircling the oesophagus, and may be patent in 10% of dogs (Ellison, 1980). It is important to clarify whether there is concurrent presence of a left cranial vena cava, because this prevents correction via a left lateral thoracotomy (Kyles and Huck, 2012).

Clinical signs

Clinical signs of PRAA are consistent with oesophageal constriction and first become apparent at weaning (Kyles, 2003). Signs include postprandial regurgitation, poor growth, malnourishment despite a good appetite and signs of aspiration pneumonia (e.g. coughing, pyrexia, dyspnoea). German shepherds and Irish setters are over-represented (Buchanan, 2003; Kyles, 2003). Affected animals should not be used for breeding.

Diagnosis

Diagnosis of PRAA is based on history, clinical findings and imaging (Table 9.4; Fig. 9.39).

Treatment

Medical management of PRAA is unrewarding because of progressive oesophageal dilation and regurgitation. Before surgery, malnourished animals should be fed liquid food from a height (or via a gastrostomy tube) and aspiration pneumonia should be treated. Patients are young, and therefore blood glucose levels should be monitored throughout surgery and in the postoperative period.

The treatment of choice is ligation and surgical

Table 9.4 Diagnostic tests and their results utilised in diagnosis of PRAA in the cat and dog.

Test	Findings
Serum biochemistry and haematology	Usually within normal limits, unless aspiration pneumonia or other co-morbidity present
Plain thoracic radiographs	Cranial oesophageal dilation; identification of right descending aorta (which may also cause left tracheal deviation); aspiration pneumonia
Barium contrast study	Cranial oesophageal dilation; oesophageal constriction at the level of the heart base
Angiography (MRI or CT)	Useful in identifying vascular ring anomaly
Oesophagoscopy	Aortic pulse on the right side of oesophagus; extra-luminal compression of oesophagus at level of heart base

division of the compressive left ligamentum arteriosum via either a left fourth intercostal thoracotomy or a thoracoscopic approach (Plesman et al., 2011; Fig. 9.40). Peri-oesophageal fibrous bands that form underneath the ligamentum arteriosum should also be divided: intra-operative oesophagoscopy and oesophageal balloon dilation should be performed to confirm that all extra-luminal oesophageal compression has been removed before routine closure of the thoracotomy site. Any oesophageal dilation should not be treated surgically.

Postoperative care

Patients should be fed liquid diets from an elevated position postoperatively. If minimal regurgitation is noted, the water content can be reduced gradually until solid food is offered. If solid food is tolerated with minimal regurgitation, the bowl can be lowered. Occasionally patients cannot tolerate the above protocol without regurgitating, and require lifelong liquid feeding from a height.

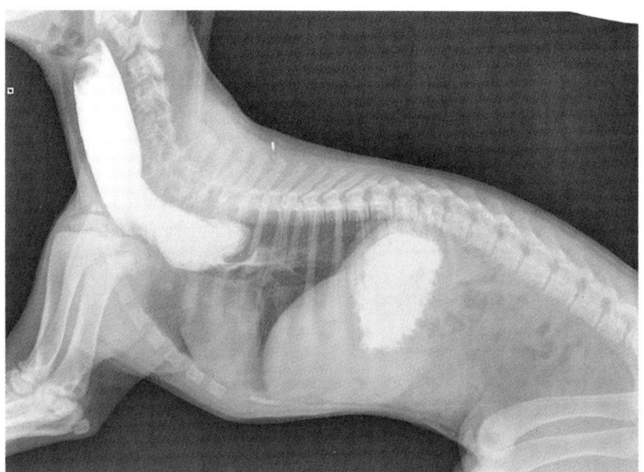

Fig. 9.39 Right lateral thoracic radiograph following a liquid barium swallow study in a 3-month-old large-breed dog. There is abrupt termination of the contrast at the level of the heart base, suggestive of a vascular ring anomaly, with oesophageal dilation oral to this region. MRI angiography confirmed this as a persistent right aortic arch (PRAA) with persistent left ductus arteriosus.

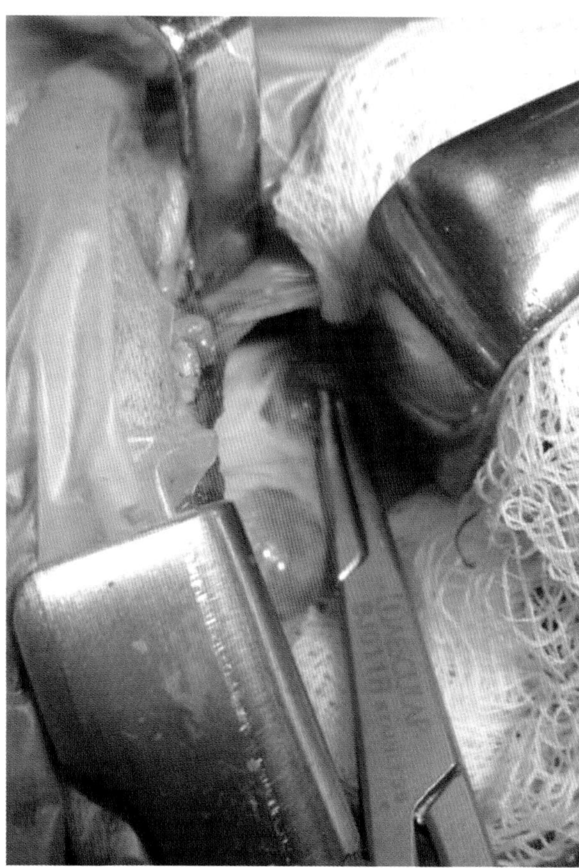

Fig. 9.40 Intra-operative image of a left fourth intercostal thoracotomy in a 3-month-old miniature schnauzer, showing a PRAA before ligation and division.

Prognosis

Postoperative prognosis depends on the presence of aspiration pneumonia and oesophageal dysmotility, and on the degree of oesophageal dilation and concurrent systemic debilitation. The most common complication is persistent regurgitation, but others include haemorrhage, oesophageal perforation, remnant fibrotic bands constricting the oesophagus, pain and perforation/penetration of the vascular structures or lungs (Isakow et al., 2000). Age at the time of surgery does not influence outcome (Krebs et al., 2014). Reported survival to discharge is 92–94%: outcome is considered excellent in 30–92% and good in 8–57% of patients (Krebs et al., 2014). Up to 13% of patients have a poor outcome, being daily regurgitation in spite of diet therapy (Krebs et al., 2014).

9.3.3 Pyothorax

Key points

- Pyothorax is development of purulent fluid within the pleural cavity, usually secondary to an infectious agent.
- Intrapleural infection is usually bacterial and mixed.
- Affected animals are often systemically extremely unwell, particularly cats.
- Non-surgical and surgical management has been described.
- In one study, a successful outcome was obtained in 86% of patients.
- The underlying cause is uncommonly identified.

Pyothorax is development of purulent fluid within the pleural cavity, usually secondary to an infectious agent (Tobias et al., 2012). Causes might include penetrating wounds from the external environment (e.g. cat bite) or penetration via the airways/oesophagus (e.g. inhaled grass seed or perforated oesophageal foreign body), haematogenous spread or extension of infection from neighbouring regions (e.g. discospondylitis, pneumonia, pulmonary abscessation). Pyothorax is always a potential complication following any thoracic surgery (Meakin et al., 2013).

Intrapleural infection is usually bacterial and mixed. Bacteria can be isolated from up to 92 and 96% of canine and feline pleural fluid samples, respectively (Walker et al., 2000). Samples from cats most commonly yield *Pasteurella*; samples from dogs more often yield *E. coli* (Walker et al., 2000).

Clinical signs

Affected animals are often systemically extremely unwell, particularly cats. Clinical signs include dyspnoea, tachpnoea, pyrexia, lethargy, cough, abnormal lung sounds, visible wounds/scars and variable signs of cardiovascular collapse/shock.

Investigation

Investigative tests used to diagnose pyothorax are detailed in Table 9.5 and Figs. 9.41, 9.42.

Treatment

In systemically unwell patients, stabilisation is indicated in the first instance. Patients may require intravenous crystalloids/colloids/dextrose, oxygen supplementation and/or warming, in addition to antibiotic provision.

Non-surgical management is indicated initially in most patients, with the exception of those with evidence of disease that would benefit from immediate surgery (e.g. a foreign body or lung lobe abscess identified on CT). Non-surgical management consists of uni- or bilateral thoracostomy tube placement in order to regularly lavage and evacuate the pleural space. In the author's opinion, repeat needle thoracocentesis is not an optimal treatment option because it is not effective for complete drainage of the pleural space, does not allow pleural lavage, carries a risk of lung laceration and is less well tolerated than a thoracostomy tube in the longer term. Prolonged courses (6 weeks) of a variety of antibiotics have been recommended as a first-line choice (Tobias et al., 2012): responsible

Table 9.5 Investigative tests described for the diagnosis of pyothorax.

Test	Findings
Haematology	Inflammatory leucogram, left shift, toxic neutrophils
Serum biochemistry	Hypoalbuminaemia, hyperglobulinaemia, hypoglycaemia, azotaemia
Thoracic radiography	Pleural effusion, mass lesion, pneumothorax, pleural thickening, focal interstitial/alveolar pattern
Thoracic CT	As for radiography, but may also include foreign body visualisation, lymph node enlargement, pericardial thickening, mediastinal effusion
Thoracic ultrasound	Pleural effusion, mass lesions, foreign material, fibrosing pleuritis
Thoracocentesis (gross)	Opaque and turbid
Thoracocentesis (cytology)	Nucleated cell counts >7000/μl, degenerate neutrophils with intracellular bacteria, sulphur granules (suggestive of *Nocardia* or *Actinomyces*)
Thoracocentesis (biochemical)	Protein >3.5 g/dl

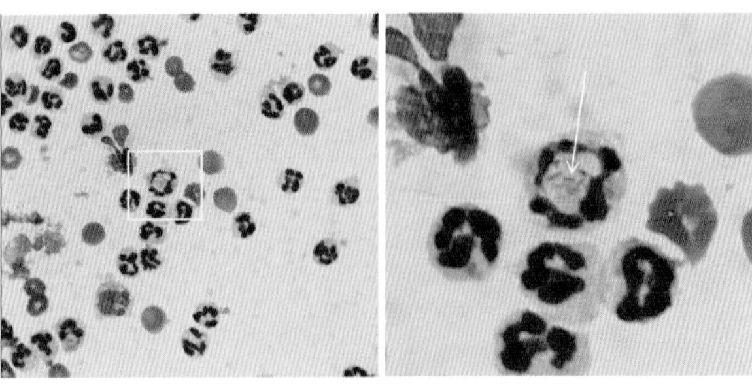

Fig. 9.41 Image of the cytological appearance of turbid fluid obtained via thoracocentesis. A large number of neutrophils are seen, with intracellular rods. Magnification of the area contained within the yellow box is shown to the right of the main image. Stain used is Diff-Quik, and magnification is ×100.

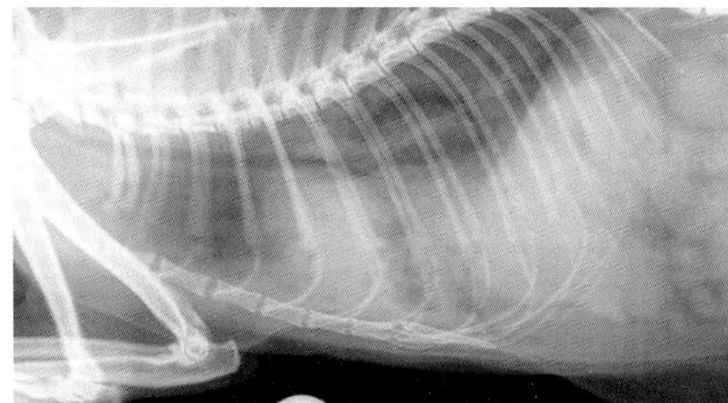

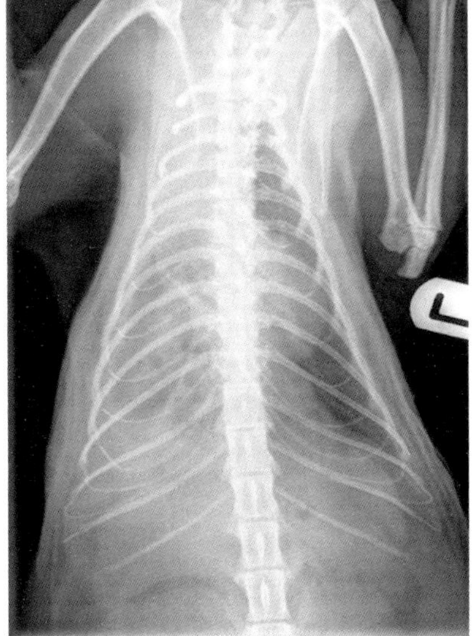

Fig. 9.42
Dorsoventral and right lateral thoracic radiographs of an 8-year-old female domestic shorthaired cat which presented for investigation of cardiovascular collapse and dyspnoea. Thoracic radiographs show a pleural effusion, worse on the right.

antibiotic stewardship should be practised at all times (ampicillin and metronidazole have been successfully used (Johnston and Martin, 2007)).

Trochar or small-bore thoracostomy tubes can be equally successful in managing pyothorax (Valtolina and Adamantos, 2009). The thoracic cavity is drained and then flushed with isotonic, body-temperature crystalloids every 8 hours. The author prefers to use 10–20 ml/kg boluses, which are instilled into the chest tube. The fluid is delivered slowly, with respiratory rate/effort monitored for compromise and, if there are concerns, fluid is removed and smaller boluses used subsequently. Once the fluid has been instilled, it is withdrawn and the volume retrieved is recorded. The installation is repeated until the fluid returned is as clear as it can be. The volume of fluid retrieved before lavage begins, and the total volume of lavage fluid required until it is returned clear, are recorded. When the volume of fluid retrieved before lavage is performed is minimal, the volume of lavage fluid required to flush the chest is minimal and the patient is clinically well, the author performs repeat thoracic radiographs at this stage and, if the radiographs show significant improvement in the pyothorax, the thoracostomy tubes can be removed. Some authors prefer to repeat cytology at this time: fluid returned after repeated, successful lavage should lack bacteria and should not contain degenerate neutrophils. Throughout treatment, packed cell volume, total protein, albumin and nutritional status should be monitored, particular in patients producing large volumes of exudate (Tobias et al., 2012).

Surgical management

Surgery is required if a lesion is identified on initial imaging which requires resection (i.e. a mediastinal or pulmonary lesion), if *Actinomyces* spp. is isolated or if non-surgical management has failed (persistent effusion beyond 3–7 days; Rooney and Monnet, 2002). Open surgical intervention is most commonly performed via a median sternotomy (Fig. 9.43). The lesion is resected or debrided as appropriate using staplers or vessel-sealing devices. Thoracic omentalisation has also been reported to be successful if indicated (Meakin et al., 2013; Fig. 9.44a–d).

Prognosis

In one study, which reported pyothorax in 36 dogs and 14 cats, a successful outcome was obtained in 86% of patients (Demetriou et al., 2002). The underlying cause was identified in only 18% of patients, and positive bacteriological cultures were obtained in 68.7% of samples (Demetriou et al., 2002).

In one small study (26 dogs), 25% and 78% of patients presenting with pyothorax were disease free one year following medical and surgical treatment respectively (Rooney and Monnet, 2002). Another study (15 dogs) reported 100% treatment success with no recurrence following medical management, provided cases were appropriately selected (i.e. no pulmonary or mediastinal masses) (Johnston and Martin, 2007). A larger study (46 dogs) investigated three cohorts: pyothorax treated with antimicrobial and thoracocentesis; pyothorax treated with thoracostomy tube, with and without pleural lavage and heparin; and pyothorax treated with thoracotomy and thoracostomy tube, with and without pleural lavage and heparin. In the respective groups, short-term survival was 29, 77 and 92%, and long-term survival was 29, 71 and 70% (Booth et al., 2010). Pleural lavage and heparin increased treatment success. Mortality rate is high (67%) for dogs that develop pyothorax as a complication of previous thoracotomy: methicillin-resistant and multidrug-resistant bacteria were commonly cultured (Meakin et al., 2013).

Overall survival in cats with pyothorax was around 48.8–66.1%, with a low recurrence rate (1/17, 5.8%) in survivors (Waddell et al., 2002).

Complications of pyothorax include death, sepsis, disseminated intravascular coagulation, recurrence, treatment failure, thoracostomy tube complications and surgical wound infection.

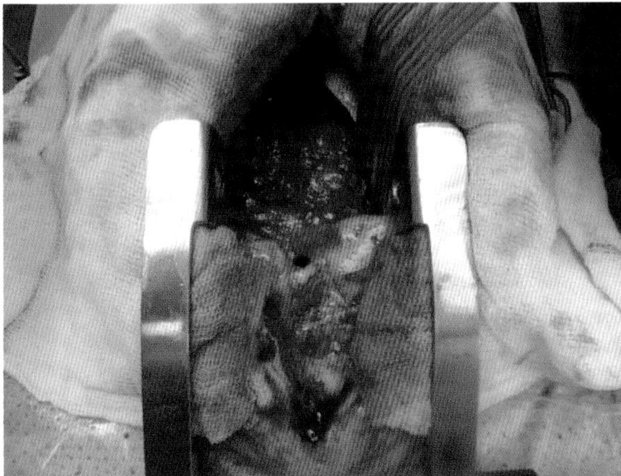

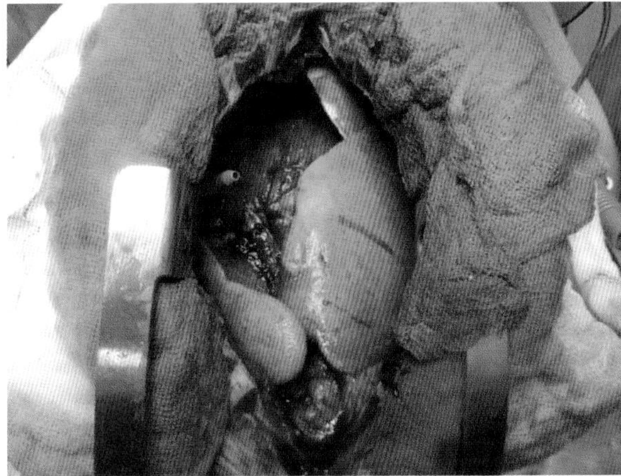

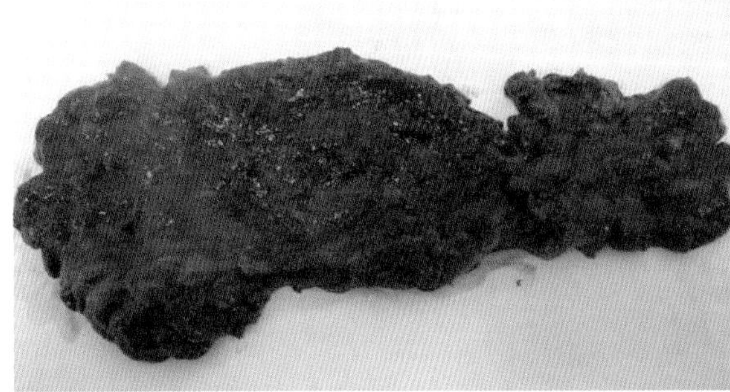

Fig. 9.43 Intra-operative photographs of a medium-sized mixed-breed dog undergoing exploratory thoracotomy (via sternotomy) for pyothorax which failed to resolve following medical management. The top photo shows the soft tissue appearance after entry into the thoracic cavity. The central photo shows the appearance of the thoracic cavity after resection of grossly diseased, necrotic and thickened tissue. The bottom photo highlights the necrotic and thickened tissue that was found diffusely throughout the thoracic cavity. Thoracic lavage continued postoperatively and the dog made an uneventful recovery.

9.3.4 Chylothorax

Key points

- Chylothorax is a failure of the intestinal lymph to drain normally via the thoracic duct into the venous circulation.
- Most cases of chylothorax are idiopathic.
- Numerous surgical techniques are reported for treatment of canine and feline chylothorax.
- Overall success following surgery is 4–90%.
- In all cases, surgery should be performed by an experienced specialist at a tertiary referral centre.

Chylothorax is a failure of the intestinal lymph to drain normally via the thoracic duct into the venous circulation. The thoracic duct returns lymph to the venous circulation from all regions of the body except the right thoracic limb, shoulder and cervical regions. It begins in the sublumbar region and terminates on the left external jugular vein or jugulosubclavian angle. In the caudal thorax, the thoracic duct is sited on the dorsolateral aorta, on the right side in the dog and the left in the cat. At this level, there are a huge number of variations among individuals in the course and number of thoracic duct branches.

Most cases of chylothorax are idiopathic, being associated with thoracic lymphangectasia, but reported underlying causes include mediastinally or heart-based masses (usually neoplastic), jugular vein/cranial vena cava thrombosis, diaphragmatic hernia, pericardial effusion, congenital abnormalities, lung lobe torsions, obstruction of cranial mediastinal veins and thoracic duct trauma. Any condition that increases cranial vena cava hydrostatic pressure can result in chylothorax formation by causing obstruction of the lymphaticovenous junctions and subsequent lymphangectasia. Where trauma is the cause, the thoracic duct is torn and usually heals spontaneously (Hodges et al., 1993). Afghan hounds and Siamese cats are predisposed to developing chylothorax (Fossum et al., 1986, 1991).

Clinical signs

Clinical signs are associated with pleural effusion (e.g. tachypnoea, dyspnoea, lethargy, cough, restrictive breathing pattern). Chronically affected animals may be emaciated.

Diagnosis

Thoracic radiographs are consistent with pleural effusion. Thoracocentesis yields a milky-coloured fluid (Fig. 9.45), and a definitive diagnosis is made by comparing triglyceride levels in paired pleural and serum samples (Table 9.6). Definitive diagnosis requires lymphangiography immediately before thoracic CT (or, less commonly, radiography), performed by injecting iohexol via ultrasound guidance into the popliteal or mesenteric lymph nodes (Kim et al., 2011; Millward et al., 2011; Fig. 9.46).

Treatment

Before treatment is instigated, a complete work-up is essential in order to rule out any underlying causes or

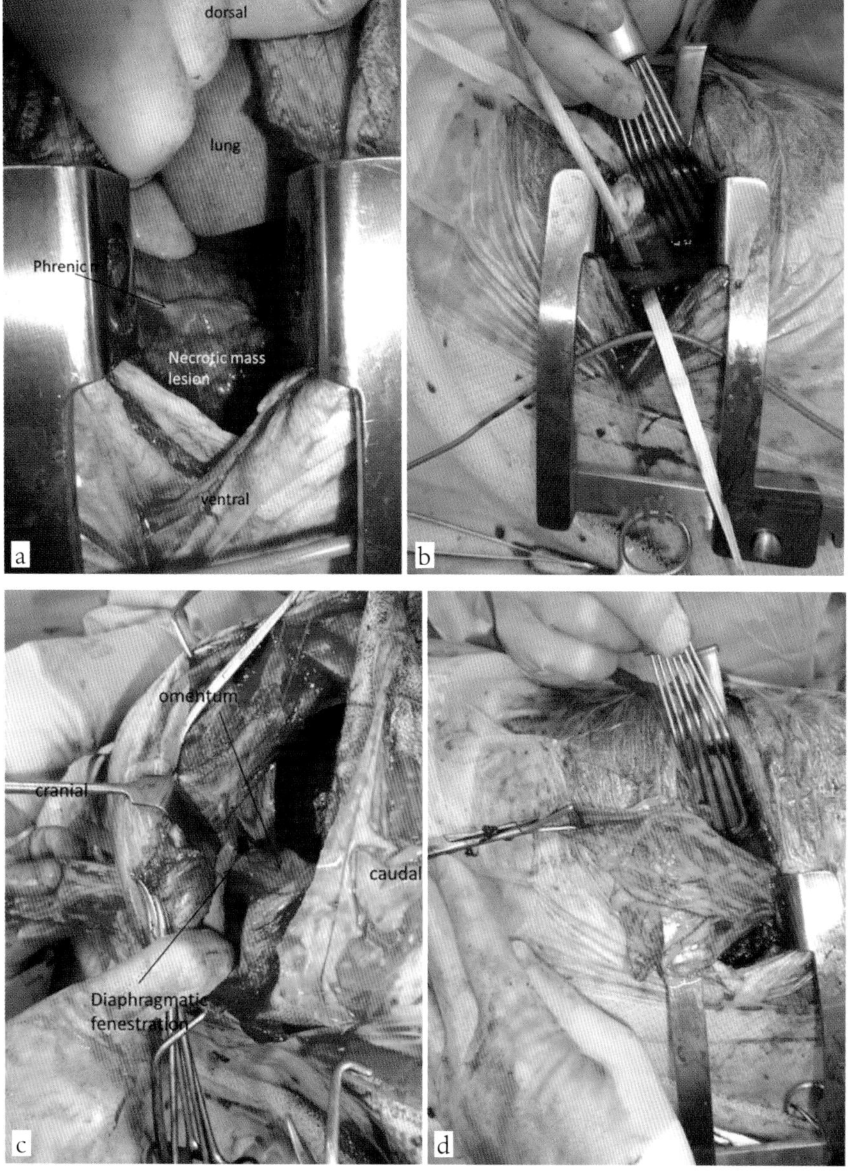

Fig. 9.44a–d Intra-operative photographs of a medium-sized dog undergoing intercostal thoracotomy for resection of a necrotic mass lesion (identified via CT) causing pyothorax. a. The mass is wrapped around the phrenic nerve. b. The phrenic nerve is dissected free of the mass and retracted in order to allow removal of the remainder of the mass. The decision was made to omentalise the thorax, because it was not possible to remove the entire mass completely due to extensive adhesions. c. is an Intra-operative view of a paracostal laparotomy approach to the omentum, which is introduced into the thoracic cavity via diaphragmatic fenestration. d. The omentum in the thoracic cavity. It will be secured in place, thoracic drains placed and the thoracic cavity routinely closed.

concurrent disease. This may consist of biochemistry, haematology, thoracic CT, abdominal imaging, echocardiography, pleural fluid cytology and bacterial culture.

Where no underlying abnormality is detected, treatment includes medical or surgical options. Medical management consists of a low-fat diet and rutin to reduce chylous effusion by decreasing leakage of the lymphatics, increasing protein removal and augmenting macrophage numbers and phagocytosis (Thompson et al., 1999). Intermittent thoracocentesis may be required. Large-scale clinical trials are lacking.

The most common surgical therapy for chylothorax involves identification and ligation of all branches of the thoracic duct, which encourages formation of new anastomoses between the lymphatic and venous systems. Concurrent pericardectomy is recommended to decrease right-sided pressure, which facilitates anastomotic development. Alternative techniques reported are shown in Table 9.7. In all cases, surgery should be performed by a specialist at a tertiary referral centre.

Thoracic duct ligation and pericardectomy can be performed either open or thoracoscopically. For open surgery, a 10th intercostal thoracotomy is performed (right-sided in the dog, left-sided in the cat). Methylene blue is injected into either the ileocaecal (via a paracostal approach) or popliteal lymph node, or an intestinal lymphatic is cannulated and methylene blue injected. The thoracic duct will become coloured, and all branches are dissected free from the aorta and parietal pleura as far caudally in the thoracic cavity as possible, where the number of branches is likely to be fewer. The branches are ligated or clipped, and repeat lymphangiography performed fluoroscopically to confirm that no patent branches remain. Alternatively, *en bloc* ligation of all structures dorsal to the aorta and ventral to the sympathetic trunk (including the azygous vein)

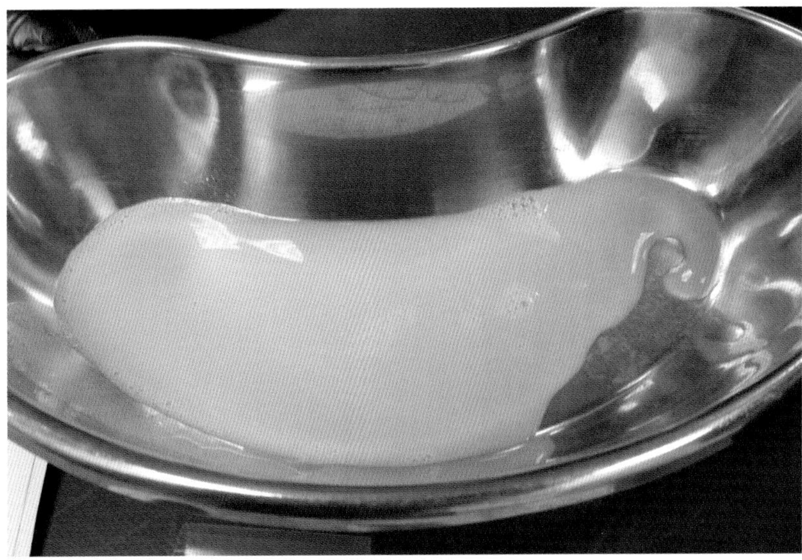

Fig. 9.45 Chylous fluid obtained via thoracocentesis in a 5-year-old domestic shorthair cat with radiographic evidence of pleural effusion.

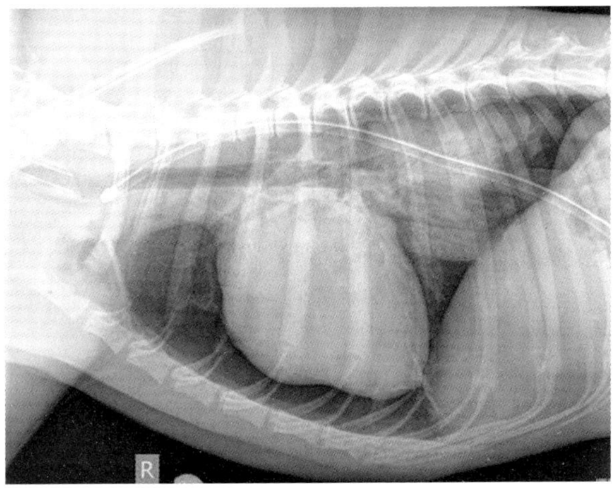

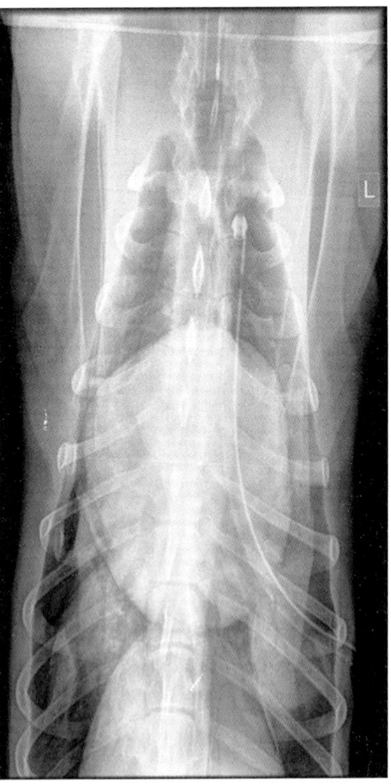

Fig. 9.46 Dorsoventral and right lateral thoracic radiographs of a 10-year-old greyhound. There is increased radiolucency and absence of pulmonary vasculature in the periphery of the thoracic cavity (indicative of lung lobar retraction), dorsal elevation of the cardiac silhouette and increased parenchymal radiopacity (indicative of atelectasis), suggestive of pneumothorax.

has been reported. Overall success following surgery is 40–90% (Allman et al., 2010; Fossum et al., 2004).

Potential surgical complications include pyothorax, wound complications, haemorrhage, recurrence of chylothorax, complications associated with the use of methylene blue (e.g. acute renal failure, Heinz body anaemia), lung lobe torsion and persistent non-chylous effusions (Tobias et al., 2012).

9.3.5 Pneumothorax

Key points

- Pneumothorax is characterised by a rapid, shallow breathing pattern (hypoventilation) with reduced/absent lung sounds.
- Most commonly, pneumothorax is diagnosed radiographically in a stabilised patient.
- Thoracocentesis should be performed initially and thoracostomy tubes placed if repeated thoracocentesis is required, or if negative pressure cannot be achieved.
- Surgery is indicated in patients with significant wounds, failure of the pneumothorax to resolve after 5 days of intermittent/continuous suction or an abnormality seen on radiography/CT.

Pneumothorax can occur for several reasons (Table 9.8) and is characterised by a rapid, shallow breathing pattern (hypoventilation) with reduced/absent lung sounds. Patients presenting following traumatic episodes may show orthopaedic/neurological injuries and/or wounds/bruising.

Tension pneumothorax is very uncommon, and develops from a closed pneumothorax where soft tissue acting as a one-way valve allows air to enter the

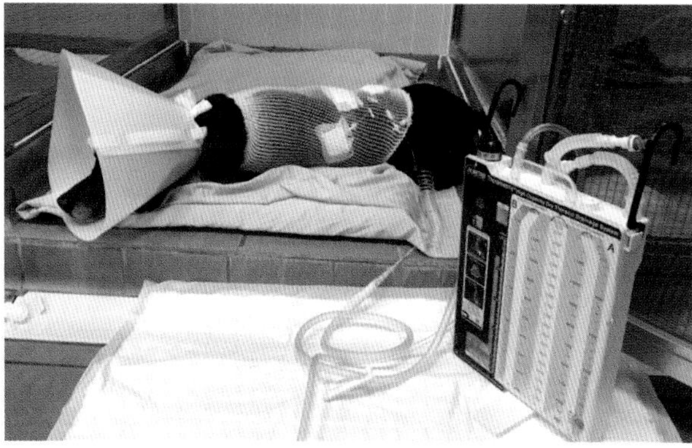

Fig. 9.47 If air reaccumulates rapidly following thoracic drainage for pneumothorax, or negative pressure cannot be reached, continuous suction should be used. This 7-year-old Labrador has bilateral thoracic drains connected to a high-capacity continuous thoracic drainage unit. Surgery was required for removal of a large ruptured bulla, which was the cause of the pneumothorax. Following partial lung lobectomy, the pneumothorax resolved.

pleural space during inspiration, but not to exit during expiration. This results in supra-atmospheric pressure, which severely compromises ventilation and venous return,and leads to death within minutes. Radiography of the thorax will reveal a large volume of pleural air visible. Increased pleural pressure will result in marked lobar collapse, mediastinal shift to the right and a flattened left hemidiaphragm.

Diagnosis

Most commonly, pneumothorax is diagnosed radiographically in a stabilised patient. Where required, thoracocentesis can be used as a therapeutic and diagnostic aid. Radiographic signs consistent with pneumothorax include: increased radiolucency and absence of pulmonary vasculature in the periphery of the thoracic cavity (indicative of lung lobar retraction), dorsal elevation of the cardiac silhouette, increased parenchymal radiopacity (indicative of atelectasis) and pneumomediastinum (Fig. 9.46). CT is superior for detecting blebs and bullae associated with spontaneous pneumothorax (Au et al., 2006).

Treatment

Thoracocentesis should be performed initially, and thoracostomy tubes placed if repeated thoracocentesis is required or if negative pressure cannot be achieved. Once the thoracostomy tubes are placed, the chest should be evacuated regularly (every 2–4 hours initially, or more often if required) and the volume of air yielded recorded. Typically, the volume produced declines over days and the thoracostomy tubes can be removed once air production is nil. If air reaccumulates rapidly, or negative pressure cannot be reached, continuous suction should be used (Fig. 9.47). Surgery is indicated in patients with significant wounds, failure of the pneumothorax to resolve after 5 days of intermittent/continuous suction or an abnormality seen on radiography/CT (e.g. foreign body, mass, abscess, bulla.; Figs. 9.48, 9.49). The approach will be dictated by accurate localisation of the surgical lesion. Other techniques described for the treatment of pneumothorax include autologous blood patch pleurodesis (Merbl

Table 9.6 Diagnostic tests described for the diagnosis of chylothorax.

Gross appearance	Milky white ± pink tone
Fluid type	Modified transudate: protein >2.5 g/dl
Cytology	Initially, lymphocytes and non-degenerate neutrophils predominate (6000–7000 nucleated cells/μl). Later, degenerate neutrophils predominate
Sudan black	Detection of chylomicrons
Biochemistry (test of choice)	In chyle, serum triglycerides are higher and cholesterol lower compared with serum
Ether clearance test	Chylous fluid will clear when potassium hydroxide and ether are added

Table 9.7 Surgical options available for treatment of canine and feline chylothorax.

Thoracic duct ligation
Pericardectomy
Thoracic duct glue embolisation
Thoracoscopic thoracic duct ligation
Pleuroperitoneal drainage
Pleural omentalisation
Pleurodesis
Cysterna chyli ablation
Decortication
Percutaneous drainage (e.g. PleuralPort)

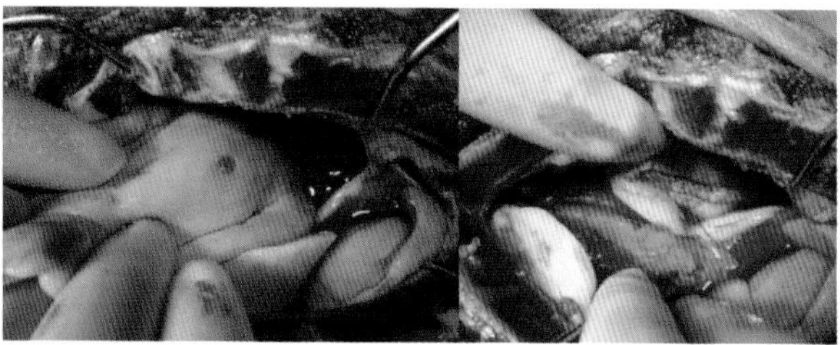

Fig. 9.48 Median sternotomy in a medium-breed dog for exploratory thoracotomy. The dog presented with pneumothorax which failed to resolve with repeated drainage. Thoracic CT showed bilateral bullae, which can be seen intra-operatively on the left photograph. Partial lung lobectomies were required to remove the bullae, performed using staplers. The staple line can be seen in the right photo and was leak tested before sternotomy closure. The pneumothorax resolved postoperatively. As an alternative to median sternotomy, bilateral intercostal approaches might be appropriate.

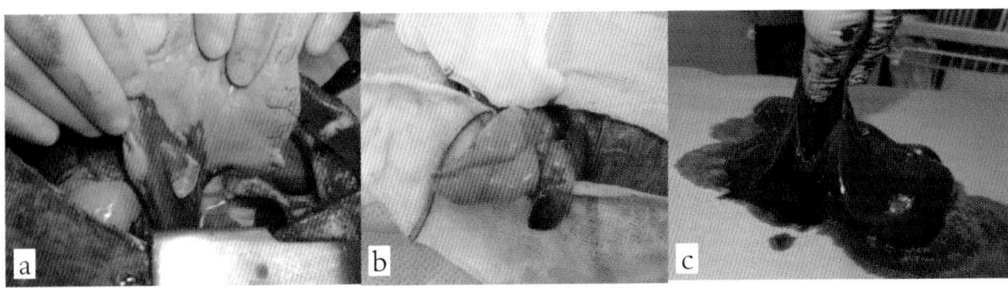

Fig. 9.49 Causes of pneumothorax. a. Intra-operative photograph of a bulla in a dog. b. Intra-operative photograph of a lung laceration following a thoracic bite in a cat. c. Resected lung tissue.

et al., 2010) and placement of a PleuralPort (Cahalane and Flanders, 2012).

Prognosis

Outcome following surgical and non-surgical management of pneumothorax has been reported in 64 dogs within referral settings (a similar study has not been undertaken in first-opinion practice; Puerto et al., 2002): dogs that underwent surgery had significantly lower recurrence (1/30) and mortality (4/33) rates compared with those treated non-surgically (6/12 and 8/15, respectively). Postoperative complications may include recurrent pneumothorax, haemorrhage, pyothorax, pneumonia, sepsis, reflux oesophagitis and wound complications (Tobias et al., 2012).

In the cat, spontaneous pneumothorax is almost exclusively associated with lung disease (e.g. inflammatory airway disease, neoplasia, heartworm, lungworm, abscessation; Mooney et al., 2012). In this study, 8/12 cats managed with thoracocentesis and 10/16 managed with observation alone survived to discharge, compared with 1/5 that underwent thoracotomy (Mooney et al., 2012).

9.3.6 Thymoma

Key points

- Diagnosis of thymoma is via thoracic imaging in the first instance.
- It is imperative to differentiate between thymoma and lymphoma; flow cytometry is often required.
- Treatment of choice for thymoma is resection via median sternotomy.
- Surgical excision of thymoma is associated with a median survival of 1825 days in cats and 790 days in dogs.

Mediastinal mass lesions in dogs are most commonly thymoma (incidence); in cats, lymphoma is more common (Reichle and Wisner, 2000). Other differentials might include sarcomas (osteo-, fibro-, histiocytic or undifferentiated), neuroendocrine tumours, carcinomas, granulomas, mesothelioma, abscesses, teratomas, mast cell tumours, lipomas and heart-based tumours (Radlinsky, 2012). Clinical signs are detailed in Table 9.9 and Fig. 9.50.

Diagnosis

Diagnosis of thymoma is via thoracic imaging in the first instance, which will identify a soft tissue opacity in the mediastinum (Fig. 9.51). Advanced imaging (e.g. CT) is recommended to ascertain the extent of the lesion and the presence of other pathology. However, using preoperative CT to determine the presence of caval invasion is not 100% accurate (Yoon et al., 2004) – ultimately, the extent of invasion may not be known until surgery is attempted. Neighbouring structures which may be involved within the mass include cranial

Table 9.8 Reported causes of pneumothorax in the cat and dog.

Penetration of thoracic wall	Fight/bite wounds, stab/gunshot wounds, blunt trauma
Penetration of oesophagus	Oesophageal foreign bodies
Penetration of airways	Foreign bodies, blunt trauma
Iatrogenic	Following thoracocentesis/thoracostomy tube, thoracotomy, mechanical ventilation, tracheal intubation
Primary spontaneous	The lung is the cause of the leak, but there is no clinical evidence of pulmonary disease. In this case, pneumothorax is secondary to rupture of pulmonary blebs (local accumulations of air within the visceral pleura) or bullae (confluent alveoli). This condition has been reported most commonly in large, deep chested breeds of dog. The aetiology of the pulmonary blebs and bullae are unknown in dogs.
Secondary spontaneous	The lung is the cause of the leak, with clinical evidence of pulmonary disease e.g. bacterial pneumonia, chronic obstructive lung diseases, asthma, tuberculosis, fungal granuloma, neoplasia, ruptured pulmonary abscesses, heartworm thromboembolism (causing bronchopleural communications).

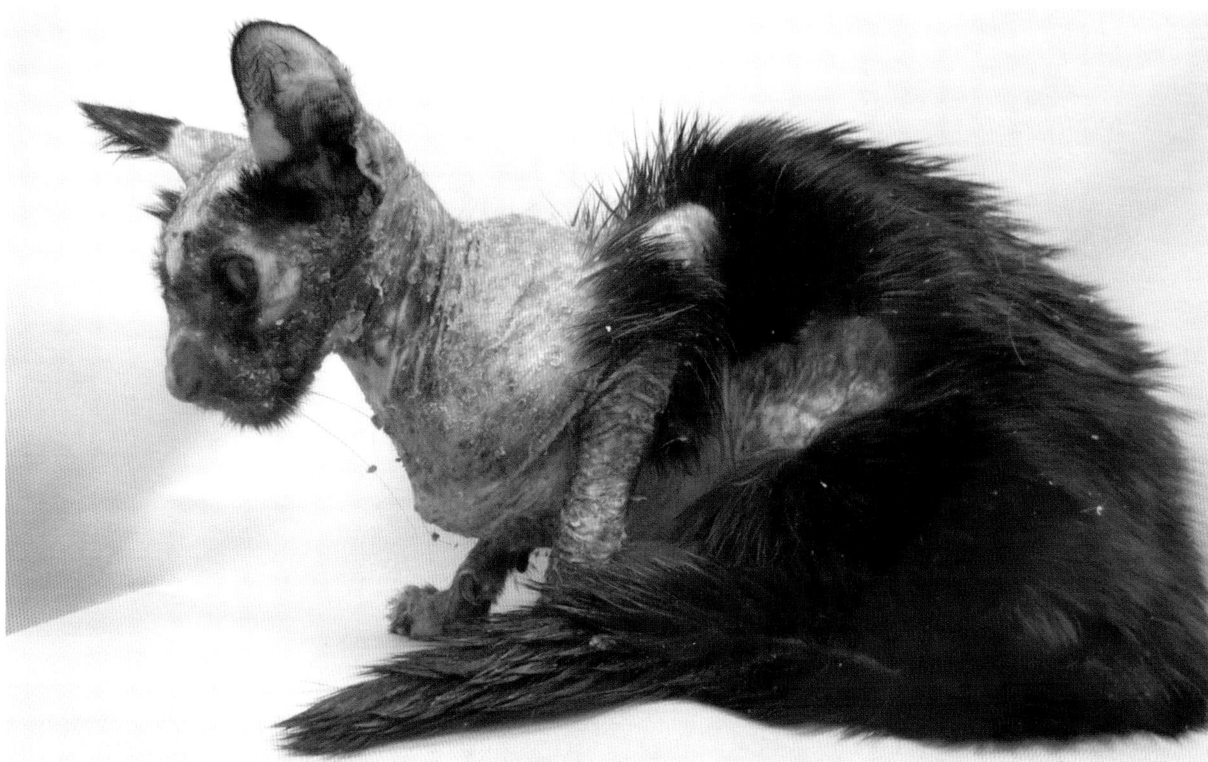

Fig. 9.50 Cat with exfoliative dermatitis associated with a thymoma. (Image courtesy of Daniela Murgia.)

vena cava, internal thoracic artery, axillary vein and phrenic nerve.

It is important to differentiate between thymoma and lymphoma preoperatively: surgery is the initial treatment of choice for the former, whilst chemotherapy is used for the latter. There is no clinically exploitable relationship between the CT appearance and histological characterisation of the mass (Yoon et al., 2004). Tumour samples can be procured via fine needle aspiration or needle biopsy, preferably under ultrasound guidance to avoid both vascular damage and sampling any cystic areas. Both thymoma and lymphoma exfoliate large numbers of lymphocytes, making diagnosis by fine needle aspiration challenging. Therefore, flow cytometry is often employed to differentiate between the two tumour types.

Table 9.9 Clinical signs of thymoma in the dog and cat.

Space-occupying lesion	Weakness Anorexia Lethargy Cough Dyspnoea Vomiting Regurgitation Decreased thoracic compliance
Cranial vena cava compression	Pleural effusion Oedema of the head, neck and forelimbs
Paraneoplastic signs	Myasthenia gravis (17% dogs), causing megaoesophagus and regurgitation, aspiration pneumonia, PUPD, weakness Hypercalcaemia Feline exfoliative dermatitis Polymyositis Myocarditis Granulocytopenia T-cell lymphocytosis Granular cell proliferation

Treatment

Preoperative treatment may include treatment of hypercalcaemia, aspiration pneumonia (secondary to megaoesophagus) or myasthenia gravis.

Thymoma is resected via a median sternotomy using vessel-sealing devices (Fig. 9.52). All excised tissue should be submitted for histopathological analysis. Thoracoscopic resection of smaller, non-invasive thymoma has been described in two dogs (Meyhew and Friedberg, 2008).

Complications

Complications of surgery include haemorrhage, infection, those associated with a sternotomy wound (e.g. seroma, dehiscence), hypocalcaemia, aspiration pneumonia, persistent myasthenia gravis, tumour recurrence and cardiac arrest (Zitz et al., 2008). Surgical

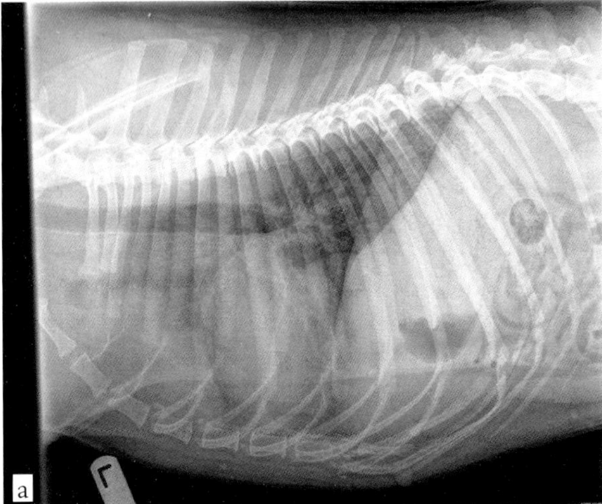

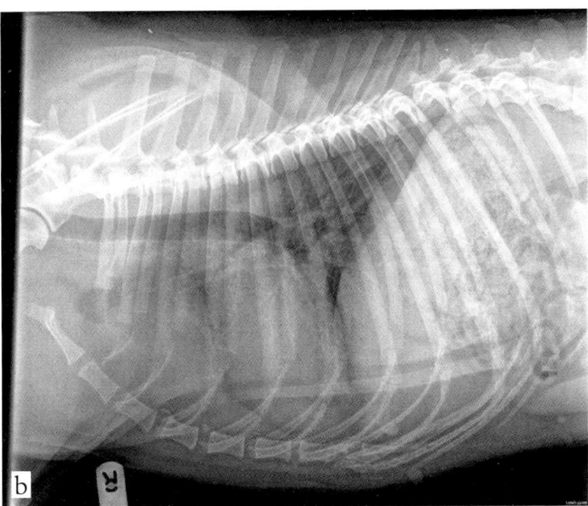

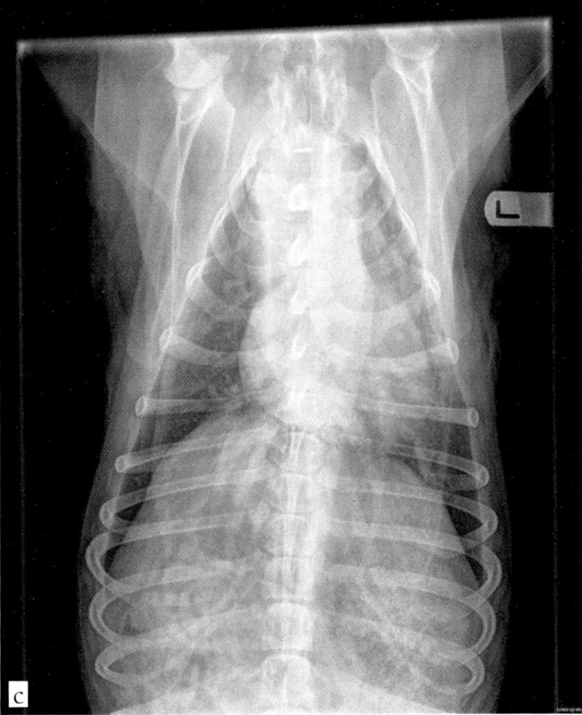

Fig. 9.51a–c. Left, right and dorsoventral thoracic radiographs of a 9-year-old boxer, presented for investigation of hypercalcaemia. A large soft tissue mass is seen occupying the cranioventral thorax; it shows ventral broad-base margins with the sternum. It is localised within the cranial mediastinum (mediastinal widening on the DV view) and causes a mass effect displacing the cardiac silhouette caudally. The trachea is not dorsally displaced. There is an equivocal minimal volume of mediastinal–pleural effusion in the ventral aspect of the thorax, superimposed over the cardiac silhouette.

excision of thymoma is associated with a median survival of 1825 and 790 days in the cat and dog, respectively (Zitz et al., 2008). Survival is shorter in dogs with high-grade tumours, secondary tumours, megaoesophagus, aspiration pneumonia or mass invasion. Radiation therapy should also be considered for patients with thymoma: the advice of an oncologist and surgeon should be sought before treating a patient with thymoma.

9.3.7 Lung lobe torsion

Lung lobe torsion has been reported in both the dog and cat, but the cause is poorly understood. Torsion may occur spontaneously, as a sequel to partial collapse of the lung lobe, or secondary to thoracic pathology (e.g. chylothorax, trauma, neoplasia, diaphragmatic hernia; Monnet, 2018a). Large, deep-chested dogs are predisposed and the right middle or left cranial lobe is most commonly affected (Monnet, 2018a; Neath et al., 2000). In the pug, torsion most commonly occurs in the left cranial lung lobe, which is the most common site of bronchial collapse (De Lorenzi et al., 2009). Venous, lymphatic and bronchial obstruction occurs, leading to lung congestion and necrosis.

Clinical findings

Dogs with lung lobe torsion may have acute or chronic presentation and can be variably clinically unwell. Clinical signs might be non-specific, related to the local and systemic effects of the torsion. Clinical signs and physical examination findings may include dyspnoea, tachpnoea, lethargy, coughing, anorexia, weight loss, pyrexia and dull lung sounds (secondary to pulmonary effusion, usually serosanguinous or chyle). Haematological results can show neutrophilia, left shift and anaemia. Cytological examination of the fluid does not show evidence of sepsis.

Diagnosis

Diagnosis of lung lobe torsion is achieved via thoracic radiographs, which show a consolidated lung lobe. Findings suspicious for a lung lobe torsion include air bronchogram, emphysematous lobe, irregular/narrowed/displaced bronchus, mediastinal shift and dorsal tracheal displacement (Fig. 9.53). CT is

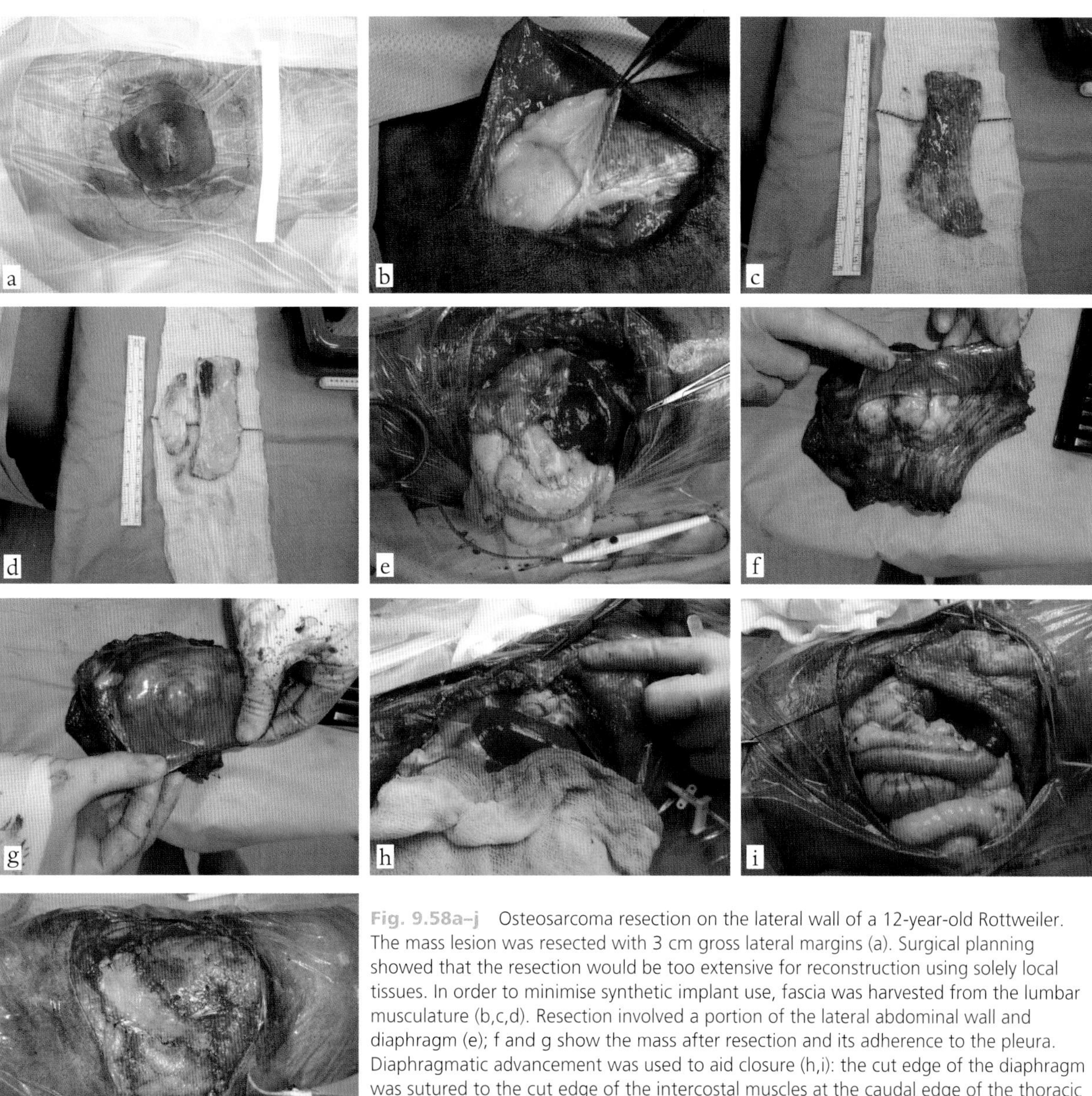

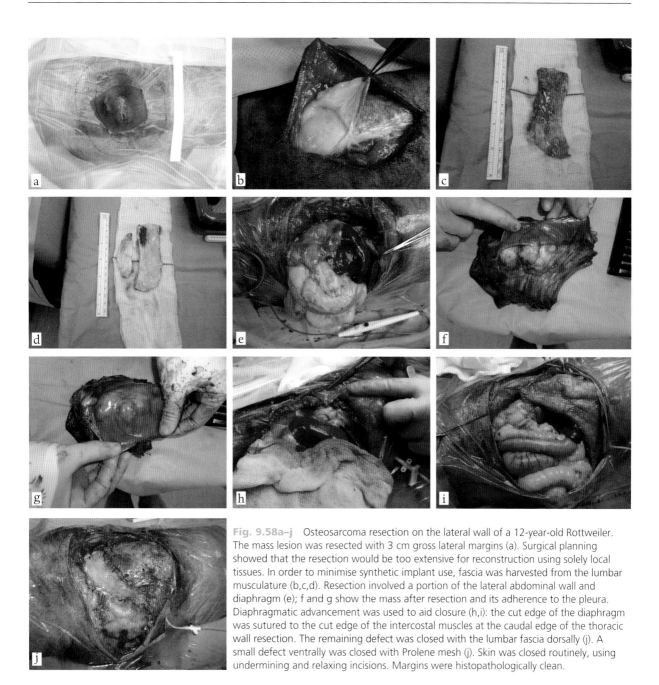

Fig. 9.58a–j Osteosarcoma resection on the lateral wall of a 12-year-old Rottweiler. The mass lesion was resected with 3 cm gross lateral margins (a). Surgical planning showed that the resection would be too extensive for reconstruction using solely local tissues. In order to minimise synthetic implant use, fascia was harvested from the lumbar musculature (b,c,d). Resection involved a portion of the lateral abdominal wall and diaphragm (e); f and g show the mass after resection and its adherence to the pleura. Diaphragmatic advancement was used to aid closure (h,i): the cut edge of the diaphragm was sutured to the cut edge of the intercostal muscles at the caudal edge of the thoracic wall resection. The remaining defect was closed with the lumbar fascia dorsally (j). A small defect ventrally was closed with Prolene mesh (j). Skin was closed routinely, using undermining and relaxing incisions. Margins were histopathologically clean.

Recommendations are to include at least one unaffected rib cranially and caudally within the *en bloc* excision (Hunt, 2012). Local anaesthetic techniques are strongly recommended. Appropriate diathermy is mandatory, and the author uses a harmonic scalpel as standard for such resections. The intercostal arteries caudal to the rib and the internal thoracic vasculature dorsal to the sternum should be ligated. Occasionally, lung lobectomy is also required if the mass lesion is adherent to the lung (Fig. 9.56). The tissue resected *en bloc* is submitted in its entirety for histopathological analysis, following appropriate inking of margins (Bowlt et al., 2013).

Before closure of the thoracic cavity, gloves and the entire surgical kit are replaced in order to minimise contamination following tumour excision. The thoracic wall is closed to create integrity of the pleural space, establish negative pressure and ensure sufficient rigidity to restore the thoracic 'bellows' (Hunt, 2012). The thoracic cavity defect does not need to be completely rigid, and large defects (usually approximately four ribs) can be closed readily with local tissue. Other options for closure include diaphragmatic advancement, latissimus dorsi muscle flap, omentalisation and use of prosthetics (native or synthetic, e.g. Prolene; Figs. 9.57a–g, 9.58a–j).

Postoperative care following thoracic wall reconstruction involves frequent monitoring of vital parameters, generous multimodal analgesia, antibiosis as appropriate, regular thoracic drainage, oxygen supplementation and nutritional support. Potential complications include haemorrhage, infection, wound-related complications, pneumothorax, pyothorax, pleural effusion, atelectasis, hypoventilation and hypothermia. Appropriate facilities and expertise for post-operative care must be provided before commencing surgery, and referral is recommended.

Prognosis

Prognosis for neoplasia of the thoracic wall depends on the tumour type. Osteosarcoma and haemangiosarcoma are most likely to metastasise, regardless of local control provided (Hunt, 2012). In 39 dogs undergoing curative intent surgery for thoracic wall neoplasms, median survival was 290 days for osteogenic osteosarcoma and was not reached for chondrosarcoma (Liptak et al., 2008).

References

Abelson, A.L, McCobb, E.C., Shaw, S., Armitage-Chan, E., Wetmore, L.A., Karas, A.Z. and Blaze, C. (2009) Use of wound soaker catheters for the administration of local anesthetic for post-operative analgesia: 56 cases. *Veterinary Anaesthesia and Analgesia* 36, 597–602.

Ackerman, N., Burk, R., Hahn, A.W. and Hayes H.M. (1978) Patient ductus arteriosus in the dog: a retrospective study of radiographic, epidemiologic, and clinical findings. *American Journal of Veterinary Research* 39, 1805-1810.

Allman, D.A., Radlinsky, M.G., Ralph, A.G. and Rawlings, C.A. (2010) Thoracoscopic thoracic duct ligation and thoracoscopic pericardectomy for treatment of chylothorax in dogs. *Veterinary Surgery* 39, 21–27.

Arora, M. (2001) Reversed patient ductus arteriosus in a dog. *Canadian Veterinary Journal* 42, 471-472.

Au, J.J., Weisman, D.L., Stefanacci, J.D. and Palmisano, M.P. (2006) Use of computed tomography for evaluation of lung lesions associated with spontaneous pneumothorax in dogs: 12 cases (1999–2002). *Journal of the American Veterinary Medical Association* 228, 733–737.

Ave, V., Parent, C. and Seiler, G. (2004) Acute lung injury and acute respiratory distress syndrome in cats: 65 cases (1993–2003). *Journal of Veterinary Emergency and Critical Care* 14, 5.

Bergstrom, A., Dimopoulou, M. and Eldh, M. (2016) Reduction of surgical complications in dogs and cats by the use of surgical safety checklist *Veterinary Surgery* 45, 571-576.

Booth, H.W., Howe, L.M., Boothe, D.M., Reynolds, L.A. and Carpenter, M. (2010) Evaluation of outcomes in dogs treated for pyothorax: 46 cases (1983–2001). *Journal of the American Veterinary Medical Association* 236, 657–663.

Bowlt, K.L., Murphy, S. and Stewart, J. (2013) Practical hints and tips for oncological surgery. *Companion Animal* 18, 277–283.

Brisson, B.A., Reggiti, F. and Biensle, D. (2006) Portal site metastasis of invasive mesothelioma after diagnostic thoracoscopy in a dog. *Journal of the American Veterinary Medical Association* 229, 980–983.

Brissot, H. (2016) Bronchial and pulmonary surgery. In: Hamaide, D. and Griffon, A. (eds) *Complications in Small Animal Surgery*. John Wiley and Sons, Ames, Iowa, pp. 305–312.

Brockman, D.J. (2016) Patent ductus arteriosus. In: Hamaide, D. and Griffon, A. (eds) *Complications in Small Animal Surgery*. John Wiley and Sons, Ames, Iowa, pp. 338–342.

Brugarolas, A. and Takita, H. (1973) Regeneration of the lung in the dog. *Journal of Thoracic and Cardiovascular Surgery* 65, 187–190.

Buchanan, J.W. (1968) Thoracic surgery in the dog and cat. 3. Patient ductus arteriosus and persistent right aortic arch surgery in dogs. *Journal of Small Animal Practice* 9, 409–428.

Buchanan, J.W. (1999) Prevalence of cardiovascular disorders. In: Fox, P.R., Sisson, D. and Moïse, N.S. (eds) *Textbook of Canine and Feline Cardiology*, 2nd edn. Saunders, Philadephia, Pennsylvania, pp. 457–470.

Buchanan, J.W. and Patterson, D.F. (2003) Etiology of patent ductus arteriosus in dogs. *Journal of Veterinary Internal Medicine* 17, 167–171.

Burton, C.A. and White R.N. (1996) Review of the technique and complications of median sternotomy in the dog and cat. *Journal of Small Animal Practice* 37, 516–522.

Cahalane, A.K. and Flanders, J.A. (2012) Use of pleural access ports for treatment of recurrent pneumothorax in two dogs. *Journal of the American Veterinary Medical Association* 241, 467–471.

Campbell, V.L. and King, LG. (2000) Pulmonary function, ventilator management, and outcome of dogs with thoracic trauma and pulmonary contusions: 10 cases (1994–1998). *Journal of the American Veterinary Medical Association* 217, 1505–1509.

Carter, J.E., Chanoit, G. and Kata, C. (2011) Anaphylactoid reaction in a heartworm-infected dog undergoing lung lobectomy. *Journal of the American Veterinary Medical Association* 238, 1301–1304.

Coceani, F. and Baragatti, B. (2012) Mechanisms for ductus arteriosus closure. *Seminars in Perinatology* 26, 92–97.

Corti, L.B., Merkley, D. and Nelson, O.L. (2000) Retrospective evaluation of occlusion of patent ductus arteriosus with hemoclips in 20 dogs. *Journal of the American Animal Hospital Association* 36, 548–551.

Cote, E. and Ettinger, S.J. (2001) Long-term clinical management of right-to-left ("reversed") patent ductus arteriosus in 3 dogs. *Journal of Veterinary Internal Medicine* 15, 39-42.

Crowe, D.T. (1983) Thoracic drainage. In: Bojrab, M.J. (ed.) *Current Techniques in Small Animal Surgery*. Lea and Febiger, Philadelphia, Pennsylvania, pp. 287–292.

Davis, K.M., Roe, S.C., Mathews, K.G. and Mente, P.L. (2006) Median sternotomy closure in dogs: a mechanical comparison of technique stability. *Veterinary Surgery* 35, 271–277.

De Lorenzi, D., Bertoncello, D. and Drigo, M.J. (2009) Bronchial abnormalities found in a consecutive series of 40 brachycephalic dogs. *Journal of the American Veterinary Medical Association* 235, 836–840.

Demetriou, J.L., Foale, R.D., Ladlow, J., McGrotty, Y., Faulkner, J. and Kirby, B.M. (2002) Canine and feline pyothorax: a retrospective study of 50 cases in the UK and Ireland. *Journal of Small Animal Practice* 43, 388–394.

Den Toom, M.L., Meiling, A.E., Thomas, R.E., Leegwater,

P.A. and Heuven, H.C. (2016) Epidemiology, presentation and population genetics of patent ductus arteriosus (PDA) in the Dutch Stabyhoun dog. *BMC Veterinary Research* 12, 105–108.

Dupre, G., Corlouer, J.P. and Bouvy, B. (2001) Thoracoscopic pericardectomy performed without pulmonary exclusion in 9 dogs. *Veterinary Surgery* 30, 21–27.

Ellison, G.W. (1980) Vascular ring anomalies in the dog and cat. *Compendium on Continuing Education for the Practising Veterinarian* 2, 693–697.

Eyster, G.E., Eyster, J.T., Cords, G.B. and Johnston, J. (1976) Patent ductus arteriosus in the dog: characteristics of occurrence and results of surgery in one hundred consecutive cases. *Journal of the American Veterinary Medical Association* 168, 435–438.

Faella, H.J. and Hijazi, Z.M. (2000) Closure of the patent ductus arteriosus with the Amplatzer PDA device: Immediate results of the international clinical trial. *Catheterisation and Cardiovascular Intervention* 51, 50–54.

Fossum, T.W., Birchard, S.J. and Jacobs, R.M. (1986) Chylothorax in 34 dogs. *Journal of the American Veterinary Medical Association* 188, 1315–1318.

Fossum, T.W., Forrester, S.D., Swenson, C.L., Miller, M.W., Cohen, N.D., Boothe, H.W. and Birchard, S.J. (1991) Chylothorax in cats: 37 cases (1969–1989). *Journal of the American Veterinary Medical Association* 198, 672–678.

Fossum, T.W., Mertens, M.M., Miller, M.W., Peacock, J.T., Saunders, A., Gordon, S., Pahl, G., Makarski, L.A., Bahr, A. and Hobson, P.H. (2004) Thoracic duct ligation and pericardectomy for treatment of idiopathic chylothorax. *Journal of Veterinary Internal Medicine* 18, 307–310.

Gasson, J. (2011) Reducing surgical complications using a safety checklist. *Veterinary Record* 169, 503.

Gawande, A. (2009). *The Checklist Manifesto: How to Get Things Right.* Henry Holt and Company, LLC, New York.

Gines, J.A., Friend, E.J., Vives, M.A., Browne, W.J., Tarlton, J.F. and Chanoit, G. (2011) Mechanical comparison of median sternotomy closure in dogs using polydioxanone and wire sutures. *Journal of Small Animal Practice* 52, 582–586.

Gordon, S.G. and Miller, M.W. (2005) Transarterial coil embolization for canine patent ductus arteriosus occlusion. *Clinical Techniques in Small Animal Practice* 20, 196–202.

Hodges, C.C., Fossum, T.W. and Evering, W. (1993) Evaluation of thoracic duct healing after experimental laceration and transection. *Veterinary Surgery* 22, 431–435.

House, E.W. and Ederstrom, H.E. (1968) Anatomical changes with age in the heart and ductus arteriosus in the dog after birth. *The Anatomical Record* 160, 289–295.

Hunt, G.B. (2012) Thoracic wall. In: Tobias, S.A. and Johnston, K.M. (eds) *Veterinary Surgery: Small Animal.* Elsevier Saunders, St.Louis, Missouri, pp. 1769–1780.

Isakow, K., Fowler, D. and Walsh, P. (2000) Video-assisted thoracoscopic division of the ligamentum arteriosum in two dogs with persistent right aortic arch. *Journal of the American Veterinary Medical Association* 217, 1333–1336.

Jackson, J., Richter, K.P. and Launer, D.P. (1999) Thoracoscopic partial pericardectomy in 13 dogs. *Journal of Veterinary Internal Medicine* 13, 529–533.

Johnston, M.S. and Martin, M.W.S. (2007) Successful medical treatment of 15 dogs with pyothorax. *Journal of Small Animal Practice* 48, 12–16.

Jones, C.L. and Buchanan, J.W. (1981) Patent ductus arteriosus: anatomy and surgery in a cat. *Journal of the American Veterinary Medical Association* 179, 364–366.

Kellum, H.B. and Stepien, R.L. (2007) Sildenafil citrate therapy in 22 dogs with pulmonary hypertension. *Journal of Veterinary Internal Medicine* 21, 1258–1264.

Kim, M., Lee, H., Lee, M., Choi, M., Kim, J., Chang, D., Choi, M. and Yoon, J. (2011) Ultrasound-guided mesenteric lymph node iohexol injection for thoracic duct computed tomographic lymphography in cats. *Veterinary Radiology and Ultrasound* 52, 302–305.

Kolata, R.J. (1981) Management of thoracic trauma. *Veterinary Clinics of North America* 11, 103–106.

Kraje, B.J., Kraje, A.C., Rohnach, B.W., Anderson, K.A., Marks, S.L. and Macintire, D.K. (2000) Intra-thoracic and concurrent orthopaedic injury associated with traumatic rib fracture in cats: 75 cases (1980–1998). *Journal of the American Veterinary Medical Association* 216, 51–54.

Krebs, I.A., Lindsley, S., Shaver, S. and MacPhail, C. (2014) Short- and long-term outcome of dogs following surgical correction of a persistent right aortic arch. *Journal of the American Animal Hospital Association* 50, 181–186.

Kudnig, S.T., Monnet, E. and Riquelme, M. (2006) Effect of positive end-expiratory pressure on oxygen delivery during one-lung ventilation for thoracoscopy in normal dogs. *Veterinary Surgery* 35, 534–542.

Kyles, A.E. (2003) Esophagus. In: Slatter, D.G (ed.) *Textbook of Small Animal Surgery.* Elsevier Saunders, Philadephia, Pennsylvania, pp. 573–592.

Kyles, A.E. and Huck, J.L. (2012) Esophagus. In: Tobias, S.A. and Johnston, K.M. (eds.) *Veterinary Surgery: Small Animal.* Elsevier Saunders, St.Louis, Missouri, pp. 1677–1699.

LaRue, S.M., Withrow, S.J. and Wykes, P.M. (1987) Lung resection using surgical staples in dogs and cats. *Veterinary Surgery* 16, 238–240.

Liptak, J.M., Monnet, E. and Dernell, W.S. (2004) Pneumonectomy: four case studies and a comparative review. *Journal of Small Animal Practice* 45, 441–447.

Liptak, J.M., Kamstock, D.A., Dernell, W.S., Monteith, G.J., Rizzo, S.A. and Withrow, S.J. (2008) Oncologic outcome after curative-intent treatment in 39 dogs with primary chest wall tumors (1992–2005). *Veterinary Surgery* 37, 488–496.

Lisciandro, G.R., Lagutchik, M.S., Mann, K.A., Voges, A.K., Fosgate, G.T., Tiller, E.G., Cabano, N.R., Bauer, L.D. and Book, B.P. (2008) Evaluation of a thoracic focused assessment with sonography for trauma (TFAST) protocol to detect pneumothorax and concurrent thoracic injury in 145 traumatized dogs. *Journal of Veterinary Emergency and Critical Care* 18, 258–269.

MacPhail, C.M., Monnet, E. and Twedt, D.C. (2001) Thoracoscopic correction of persistent right aortic arch in a dog. *Journal of the American Animal Hospital Association* 37, 577–581.

Marques, A.I., Tattersall, J. and Shaw, D.J. (2009) Retrospective analysis of the relationship between time of thoracostomy drain removal and discharge time. *Journal of Small Animal Practice* 50, 162–166.

Meakin, L.B., Salonen, L.K., Baines, S.J., Brockman, D.J., Gregory, S.P., Halfacree, Z.J., Lipscomb, V.J. and Lee, K.C. (2013) Prevalence, outcome and risk factors for postoperative pyothorax in 232 dogs undergoing thoracic surgery. *Journal of Small Animal Practice* 54, 313–317.

Merbl, Y., Kelmer, E., Shipov, A., Golani, Y., Segev, G., Yudelevitch, S. and Klainbart, S. (2010) Resolution of persistent pneumothorax by use of blood pleurodesis in a dog after surgical correction of a diaphragmatic hernia. *Journal of the American Veterinary Medical Association* 237, 299–303.

Meyhew, P.D. and Friedberg, J.S. (2008) Video-assisted thoracoscopic resection of noninvasive thymomas using one-lung ventilation in two dogs. *Veterinary Surgery* 37, 756–762.

Miller, M., Stepien, R., Meurs, K. and Boswood, A. (2005) Echocardiographic assessment of patent ductus arteriosus after occlusion. *Proceedings of the 12th ACVIM Forum* 12, 305 (abstr.).

Millward, I.R., Kirberger, R.M. and Thompson, P.N. (2011) Comparative popliteal and mesenteric computed tomography lymphangiography of the canine thoracic duct. *Veterinary Radiology and Ultrasound* 52, 295–301.

Monnet, E. (2018a) Lungs. In Johnston, K.M. and Tobias, S.A. (eds) *Veterinary Surgery: Small Animal*. Elsevier Saunders, St. Louis, Missouri, pp. 1983–2000.

Monnet, E. (2018b) Pericardial surgery. In Johnston, K.M. and Tobias, S.A. (eds) *Veterinary Surgery: Small Animal*. Elsevier Saunders, St. Louis, Missouri, pp. 2084–2092.

Mooney, E.T., Rozanski, E.A., King, R.G. and Sharp, C.R. (2012) Spontaneous pneumothorax in 35 cats (2001–2010). *Journal of Feline Medicine and Surgery* 14, 384–391.

Moores, A. (2016a) Complications after intercostal and sternal thoracotomy. In: Hamaide, D. and Griffon, A. (eds) *Complications in Small Animal Surgery*. John Wiley and Sons, Ames, Iowa, pp. 294-299.

Moores, A. (2016b) Thoracostomy and thoracocentesis. In: Hamaide, D. and Griffon, A. (eds) *Complications in Small Animal Surgery*. John Wiley and Sons, Ames, Iowa, pp. 284–293.

Murphy, K.A. and Brisson, B.A. (2006) Evaluation of lung lobe torsion in pugs: 7 cases (1991–2004). *Journal of the American Veterinary Medical Association* 228, 86–90.

Neath, P.J., Brockman, D.J. and King, L.G. (2000) Lung lobe torsion in dogs: 22 cases (1981–1999). *Journal of the American Veterinary Medical Association* 217, 1041–1044.

Oswald, G.P. and Orton, E.C. (1993) Patent ductus arteriosus and pulmonary hypertension in related Pembroke Welsh corgi dogs. *Journal of the American Veterinary Medical Association* 202, 761–764.

Patterson, D.F., Pyle, R.L., Buchanan, J.W., Trautvetter, E. and Abt, D.A. (1971) Hereditary patent ductus arteriosus and its sequelae in the dog. *Circulation Research* 29, 1–13.

Pelosi and Orton, E.C. (2018) Cardiac surgery. In Tobias, S.A. and Johnston, K.M. (eds) *Veterinary Surgery: Small Animal*. Elsevier Saunders, St.Louis, Missouri, pp. 2049–2083.

Pelsue, D.H., Monnet, E., Gaynor, J.S., Powers, B.E., Halling, K., Parker, D. and Golden, A. (2002) Closure of median sternotomy in dogs: Suture versus wire. *Journal of the American Animal Hospital Association* 38, 569–576.

Plesman, R., Johnson, M., Rurak, S., Ambrose, B. and Shmon, C. (2011) Thoracoscopic correction of a congenital persistent right aortic arch in a young cat. *Canadian Veterinary Journal* 52, 1123–1128.

Puerto, D.A., Brockman, D.J., Lindquist, C. and Drobatz, K. (2002) Surgical and nonsurgical management of and selected risk factors for spontaneous pneumothorax in dogs: 64 cases (1986–1999). *Journal of the American Veterinary Medical Association* 220, 1670–1674.

Radlinsky, M.G., Mason, D.E. and Biller, D.S. (2002) Thoracoscopic visualisation and ligation of the thoracic duct in dogs. *Veterinary Surgery* 31, 138–146.

Reichle, J.K. and Wisner, E.R. (2000) Non-cardiac thoracic ultrasound in 75 feline and canine patients. *Veterinary Radiology and Ultrasound* 41, 154–162.

Ringwald, R.J. and Birchard, S.J. (1989) Complications of median sternotomy in the dog and literature review. *Journal of the American Animal Hospital Association* 25, 430–434.

Rooney, M.B. and Monnet, E. (2002) Medical and surgical treatment of pyothorax in dogs: 26 cases (1991–2001). *Journal of the American Veterinary Medical Association* 221, 86–92.

Rooney, M.B., Mehl, M. and Monnet, E. (2004) Intercostal thoracotomy closure: transcostal sutures as a less painful alternative to circumferential suture placement. *Veterinary Surgery* 33, 209–211.

Scheepens, E.T.F., Peeters, M.E., L'Eplattenier, H.F. and Kirpensteijn, J. (2006) Thoracic bite trauma in dogs: a comparison of clinical and radiological parameters with surgical results. *Journal of Small Animal Practice* 47, 721–726.

Schrope, D.P. (2015) Prevalence of congenital heart disease in 76,301 mixed-breed dogs and 57,025 mixed-breed cats. *Journal of Veterinary Cardiology* 17, 192–202.

Scurtu, S., Pestean, S., Lacatus, R., Lascu, M. and Mircean, M. (2016) Reverse PDA – less common type of patent ductus arteriosus – case report. *Bulletin of UASVM Veterinary Medicine* 73, 351–355.

Shultz, R.M., Peters, J. and Zwingenberger, A. (2009) Radiography, computed tomography and virtual bronchoscopy in four dogs and two cats with lung lobe torsion. *Journal of Small Animal Practice* 50, 360–363.

Sigrist, N.E., Doherr, M.G. and Spreng, D.E. (2004) Clinical findings and diagnostic value of post-traumatic thoracic radiographs in dogs and cats with blunt trauma. *Journal of Veterinary Emergency and Critical Care* 14, 259–268.

Simpson, S.A., Syring, R. and Otto, C.M. (2009) Severe blunt trauma in dogs: 235 cases (1997–2003). *Journal of Veterinary Emergency and Critical Care* 19, 588–602.

Snaps F.R., McEntee, K., Saunders, J.H. and Dondelinger, R.F. (1995) Treatment of patent ductus arteriosus by placement of intravascular coils in a pup. *Journal of the American Veterinary Medical Association* 207, 724–725.

Stanley, B.J., Luis-Fuentes, V. and Darke, P.G. (2003) Comparison of the incidence of residual shunting between two surgical techniques used for ligation of patent ductus arteriosus in the dog. *Veterinary Surgery* 32, 231–237.

Tattersall, J.A. and Welsh, E. (2006) Factors influencing the short-term outcome following thoracic surgery in 98 dogs. *Journal of Small Animal Practice* 47, 715–720.

Thompson, M.S., Cohn, L.A. and Jordan, R.C. (1999) Use of rutin for medical management of idiopathic chylothorax in four cats. *Journal of the American Veterinary Medical Association* 215, 346–348.

Tivers, M. (2011) Reducing surgical complications. *Veterinary Record* 169, 334-335.

Tivers, M. (2015) Reducing error and improving patient safety. *Veterinary Record* 177, 436-437.

Tobias, K.M., Darrow, B.G. and Radlinsky, M.G. (2012) Thoracic cavity. In: Tobias, S.A. and Johnston, K.M. (eds) *Veterinary Surgery: Small Animal*. Elsevier Saunders, St.Louis, Missouri, pp. 2019–2049.

Tobias, K.M., Darrow, B.G. and Radlinsky, M.G. (2018) Thoracic cavity. In: Tobias, S.A. and Johnston, K.M. (eds) *Veterinary Surgery: Small Animal*. Elsevier Saunders, St.Louis, Missouri, pp. 2019–2048.

Tronc, F., Gregoire, J., Leblanc, P. and Deslauriers, J. (1999) Physiologic consequences of pneumonectomy. Consequences on the pulmonary function. *Chest Surgery Clinics of North America* 9, 459–473.

Valtolina, C. and Adamantos, S. (2009) Evaluation of small-bore wire-guided chest drains for management of pleural space disease. *Journal of Small Animal Practice* 50, 290–297.

Van Israel, N., French, A.T., Wooton, P.R. and Wilson, N. (2001) Hemolysis associated with patent ductus arteriosus coil embolization in a dog. *Journal of Veterinary Internal Medicine* 15, 153–156.

Waddell, L.S., Brady, C.A. and Drobatz, K.J. (2002) Risk factors, prognostic indicators and outcome of pyothorax in cats: 80 cases (1986–1999). *Journal of the American Veterinary Medical Association* 221, 819–824.

Walker, A.L., Jang, S.S., Dwight, B.A. and Hirsh, C. (2000) Bacteria associated with pyothorax of dogs and cats: 98 cases (1989–1998). *Journal of the American Veterinary Medical Association* 216, 359–363.

Yoon, J., Feeney, D.A., Cronk, D.E., Anderson, K.L. and Seigler, L.E. (2004). Computed tomographic evaluation of canine and feline mediastinal masses in 14 patients. *Veterinary Radiology and Ultrasound* 45, 542–546.

Zitz, J., Birchard, S.J., Couto, G.C., Samii, V.F., Weisbrode, S.E. and Young, G.S. (2008) Results of excision of thymoma in cats and dogs: 20 cases (1984–2005) *Journal of the American Veterinary Medical Association* 232, 1186–1192.

Case 9.1

History and presentation

A 5-year-old female neutered terrier presented as an emergency in the early hours of the morning for assessment following being attacked by a dog. There is no other significant history.

On presentation, the dog was in lateral recumbency and was panting. Physical examination showed:

- Mucous membranes are pale pink.
- Capillary refill time is 1 second.
- Heart rate and pulse rate are synchronous; heart rate 140 bpm; pulse quality is good; no cardiac arrhythmias or murmurs.
- Dressing covering the thoracic cavity.
- Thoracic auscultation is difficult because the dog is stressed and panting.
- Abdominal palpation is painful cranially.
- Neurological examination is within normal limits.
- Orthopaedic examination is within normal limits.

Problem list

- recumbency
- unknown chest injury – difficult to examine further
- painful cranial abdomen
- history of a dog fight.

Plan

- emergency blood panel: PCV/TS, urea, creatinine, lactate, electrolytes, blood gas analysis
- oxygen supplementation
- appropriate analgesia (opioid)
- thoracic imaging and assessment of any thoracic/abdominal trauma
- abdominal imaging
- intravenous access and fluid therapy.

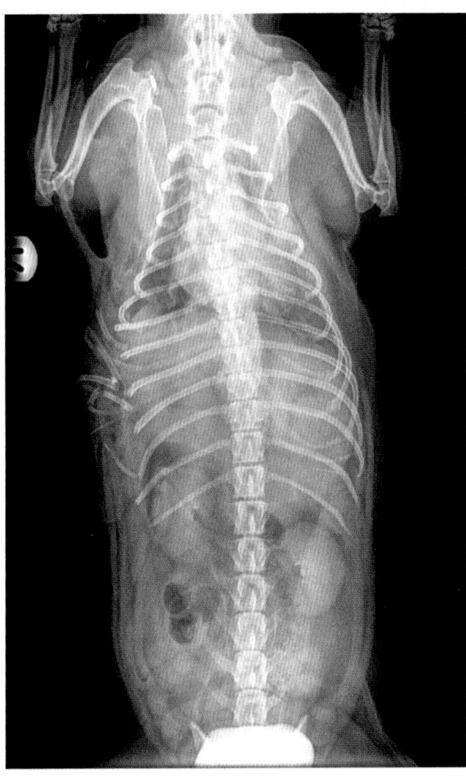

Fig. 9.59 Ventrodorsal radiograph showing pulmonary contusions and multiple rib fractures.

Investigation

Blood results were all normal. Intravenous methadone was provided. Full-body radiography was performed (Figs. 9.59, 9.60). Findings were consistent with pulmonary contusions (particularly the right caudal lobe) and multiple rib fractures. Intravenous urography was performed, which confirmed the absence of urinary tract damage.

No abdominal pathology was identifiable and the diaphragm appeared intact.

The dressing was removed from the thorax and the left side was noted to be normal. The right thoracic wall suffered from several wounds (Fig. 9.61), the largest of which communicated with the thoracic cavity when digitally explored.

Therefore, exploratory thoracotomy was performed. A skin incision was made in the region of the 7th–8th intercostal region. The regional musculature was severely damaged. Two rib fracture fragments were removed (Figs. 9.62, 9.63).

The gross appearance of the remainder of the lung lobe was consistent with diffuse contusion. A partial right caudal lung lobectomy was performed using staples. No leakage was identified after flooding the thorax with saline. The remainder of the lung lobes appeared grossly normal. The diaphragm was intact. A small-bore thoracostomy drain was placed. The intercostal musculature and ribs were repaired using 2-0 PDS in a circumcostal basket-weave formation. The overlying musculature was closed with simple interrupted sutures using 2-0 PDS. The fat and intradermal layers were closed with simple continuous sutures using 3-0 Monocryl. Skin staples were applied.

Bacteriology swabs were procured from the wounds. The wounds were flushed, active suction drains (x2) placed, and closed with 3-0 Monocryl and skin staples.

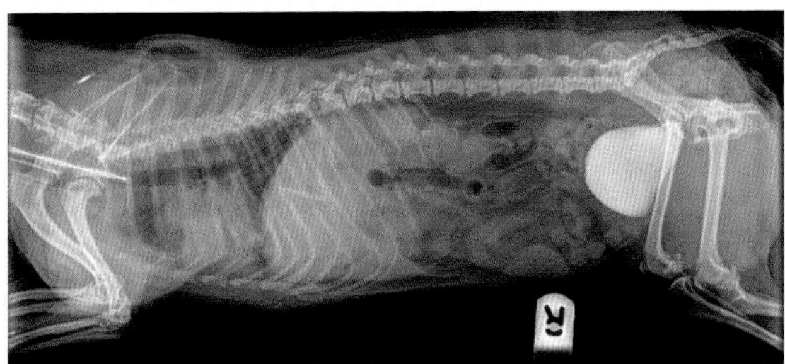

Fig. 9.60 Lateral radiograph showing pulmonary contusions and multiple rib fractures.

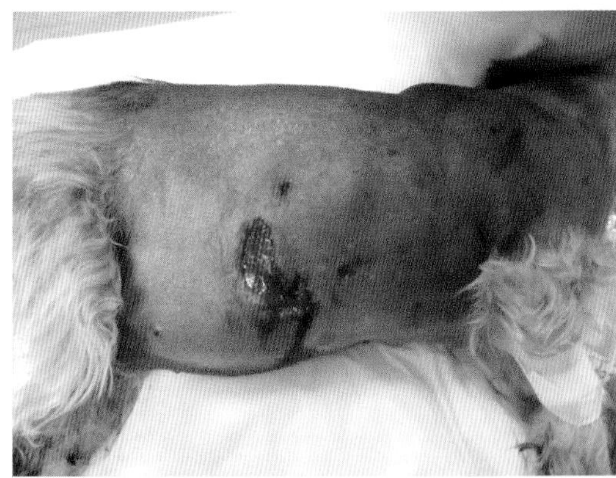

Fig. 9.61 Several wounds on the right lateral chest.

Postoperative care

- Pain scores were documented every 2 hours and methadone (0.2 mg/kg IV) provided as required. A ketamine and lidocaine infusion was administered for 24 hours. Meloxicam was administered daily.
- Intravenous crystalloids were provided at maintenance rate (2 ml/kg/h) until the patient was eating unaided (24 hours postoperatively).
- The thoracostomy drains were ordered to be aseptically evacuated every 4 hours. The drains were removed 24 hours postoperatively when air production was nil. Repeat thoracic radiographs 24 hours after thoracostomy drain removal were within normal limits.
- The active suction drains were evacuated aseptically every 4 hours and removed after 72 hours when fluid production decreased to <1 ml/kg/24 h.

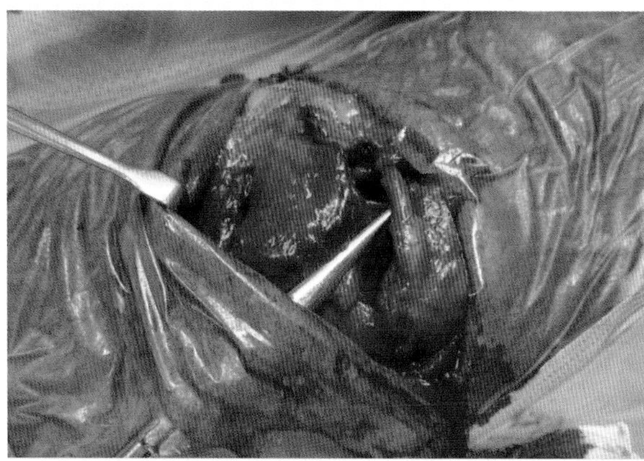

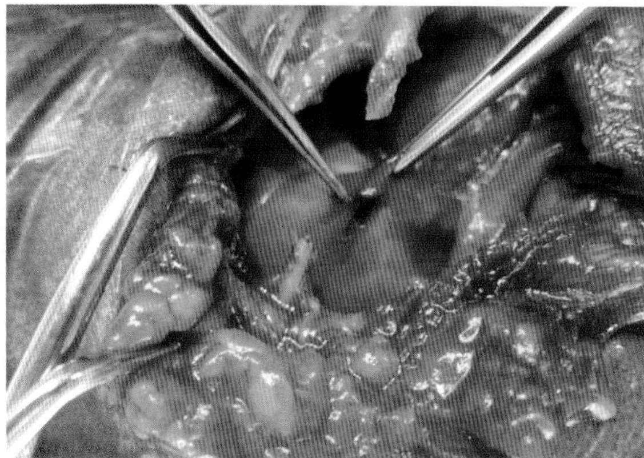

Figs. 9.62, 9.63 The right caudal lung lobe was impaled on a dorsal rib fragment, creating a hole in the lung parenchyma.

- Antibiotics (clavulanic amoxycillin) were provided intra-operatively and postoperatively for seven days.
- Upon recovery and ambulation, the patient was noted to have a 4/10 right hindlimb lameness and moderate volume of soft tissue swelling associated with this limb. There was a grade 2/3 medial patellar luxation and the swelling and luxation may explain the lameness, but we should also consider that there is an underlying orthopaedic trauma that was yet to be diagnosed. The survey radiographs did not identify any obvious fractures. The lameness resolved after 3 days.
- The patient was discharged 4 days postoperatively with oral meloxicam and clavulanic amoxicillin, with instructions for strict room rest and short-lead walks for toileting purposes only. The buster collar and protective vest were to remain in place for a further week in order to prevent interference with the wound.
- A large seroma developed postoperatively following discharge, but the dog remained bright. Antibiotics were continued until the seroma resolved (two weeks) and regular application of hot packs was recommended. The dog recovered uneventfully.

Case 9.2

History and presentation

A 9-year-old male neutered Rottweiler presented as an emergency for assessment of a three-day history of increased respiratory effort and rate, and exercise intolerance. There is no other significant history.

On presentation, he is quiet, but alert and responsive. Physical examination shows:

- Mucous membranes are pale pink.
- Capillary refill time is 1 second.
- Heart rate and pulse rate are synchronous; heart rate 100 bpm; pulse quality is good; no cardiac arrhythmias or murmurs. Dull heart sounds.
- Respiratory rate is 60 pm and lung sounds are dulled bilaterally.
- Abdominal palpation is normal.
- Neurological examination is within normal limits.
- Orthopaedic examination is within normal limits.

Problem list

- increased respiratory rate and effort
- exercise intolerance
- tachypnoea
- dull heart and lung sounds bilaterally.

Plan

- emergency blood panel: PCV/TS, urea, creatinine, lactate, electrolytes, blood gas analysis
- oxygen supplementation
- thoracic imaging
- thoracocentesis (for both stabilisation and diagnostic purposes).

Investigation

Emergency blood panel results were generally within normal limits.

Mask oxygenation was provided.

Thoracic CT showed a large-volume pneumothorax. Bilateral small-bore thoracostomy tubes were placed and the pneumothorax evacuated. Two litres of air were removed. CT was repeated and showed bilateral mild pneumothorax, with a multifocal alveolar pattern in the caudal part of the left cranial, right caudal and accessory lung lobes compatible with atelectasia. It was not possible to rule out neoplasia or other lesions, but these were considered less likely. A bulla was identified in the dorsal aspect of the left cranial lung lobe. Additionally, multi-cavitary lesions were identified. One was 20 mm in diameter in the ventromedial aspect of the left caudal lung lobe and another was 25 mm in diameter localised in the medioventral aspect of the left cranial lung lobe. Intermittent thoracic drainage was planned for overnight, but large volumes of air were produced (2–3 litres every 30 minutes), so continuous suction was utilised.

The following day the patient was taken to surgery, with median sternotomy preferred because of concerns about multiple lung lobe lesions visualised on CT.

An 8 mm pulmonary bulla was noted on the dorsal aspect of the left cranial lung lobe and was resected using a TA stapler (Figs. 9.64, 9.65). The lobectomy site was submerged in warm saline and no air leakage or haemorrhage was observed. The rest of the lung lobes were examined systematically (submerged in warm saline). No air leakage or parenchymal abnormality, except for atelectasis, was found. The lobectomy site was re-examined for any leakage or haemorrhage prior to closure of the sternotomy.

The sternotomy was apposed with USP 7 stainless steel suture in a cruciate pattern. The pectoral muscles were apposed with continuous Monocryl 2-0 suture prior to placement of a wound infusion catheter. Continuous Monocryl 3-0 subcutaneous and intradermal sutures were placed. Skin glue was applied. The thoracic cavity was drained via the previously placed thoracic drains prior to general anaesthesia recovery.

Postoperative care

- Pain scores were documented every 2 hours and methadone (0.2 mg/kg IV) provided as required. A ketamine infusion was administered for 24 hours. Meloxicam was administered daily.
- Intravenous crystalloids were provided at maintenance rates (2 ml/kg/h) until the patient was eating unaided (24 hours postoperatively).
- The thoracostomy drains were ordered to be aseptically evacuated every 4 hours. The drains were removed 24 hours postoperatively when air production was nil.
- Antibiotics (clavulanic amoxycillin) were provided intra-operatively and postoperatively for 5 days.
- Unfortunately, as is often the case following sternotomy, there was a reasonable quantity of serosanguinous fluid oozing from the wound and the dog remained hospitalised with the site dressed until this resolved. Bacterial culture of the wound fluid did not yield any growth.
- Repeat thoracic radiographs 24 hours after thoracostomy drain removal were within normal limits.
- The patient was discharged 5 days postoperatively with oral meloxicam and instructions for strict room rest, and short-lead walks for toileting purposes only. The buster collar and protective vest were to remain in place for a further week in order to prevent interference with the wound.
- Repeat thoracic radiographs one week after thoracostomy drain removal were within normal limits.
- The patient recovered uneventfully.

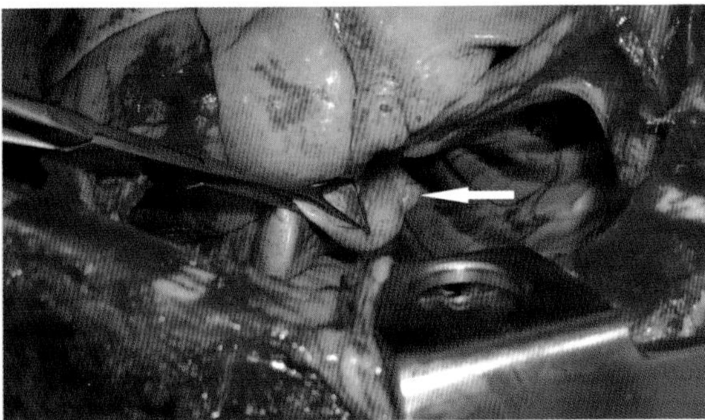

Fig. 9.64 Left cranial lung lobe retracted caudoventrally with Duval lung forceps, showing the pulmonary bleb on the dorsal aspect (white arrow).

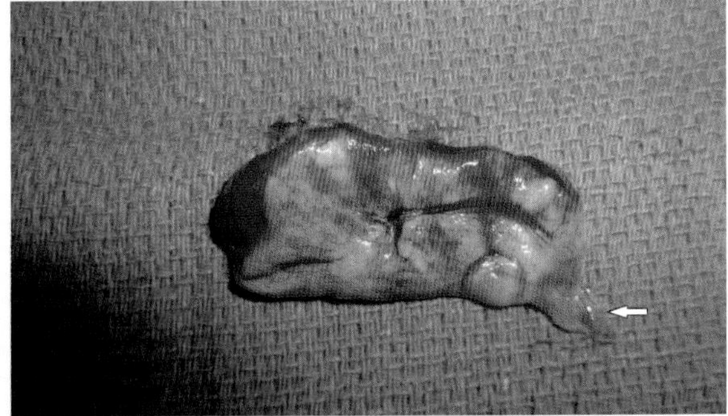

Fig. 9.65 Partially excised left cranial lung lobe with pulmonary bleb (white arrow).

10 Surgical oncology

Pieter Nelissen

Chapter summary

10.1 Principles of surgical oncology

Key points

- Surgical treatment remains an important aspect of the management of cancer.
- Malignant tumours in young animals tend to have a more aggressive biological behaviour compared to older animals.
- Clinical staging is important for malignant cancers.
- Normal tissue must be protected from tumour cells during tumour dissection.
- The timing of adjunctive therapies is an important consideration when planning curative or cytoreductive surgery.
- Re-evaluations should be individually assessed according to the tumour type, grade and stage.

In oncology it is important to consider early on in the treatment which options there are and to rely on a multimodality approach from the onset.

Veterinary oncology is a rapidly changing and constantly evolving discipline involving the use of multiple diagnostic and therapeutic modalities to achieve the most optimal outcome. Surgical treatment remains an important aspect of the management of cancer. Surgery cures more cancer than any other single modality. However, the optimal treatment for most cancer patients often involves several adjuvant treatment modalities (Gilson and Stone, 1990; Soderstrom and Gilson, 1995). Therapeutic goals (curative intent, cytoreduction or palliation) should be discussed and established with the owners before surgery is initiated. To maximise the success of treatment, each case should be strategically assessed before initiating treatment. This planning should always include a thorough discussion regarding preoperative tests, stage of the cancer, all possible treatment options, costs, postoperative care, function, cosmesis and prognosis. The goal of this planning and discussion is to provide the owners with enough information to help them make an informed choice regarding the optimal treatment for their pet.

10.1.1 *Signalment*

The patient's age, breed, gender and body score are important factors in the determination of appropriate treatment recommendations. Advanced age is not a disease and this also is not a negative prognostic indicator. However, in geriatric patients, co-morbidities such as renal impairment, hepatic disease, osteoarthritis or heart disease may limit or change specific treatment recommendations (Gilson and Stone, 1990; Soderstrom and Gilson, 1995). Age can sometimes provide prognostic information. Malignant tumours in young animals tend to have a more aggressive biological behaviour compared to older animals (Morrison, 2002) (Fig. 10.1a,b).

Certain neoplastic processes are more common in a particular gender or breed, and the oncologist should always bear this in mind. The patient's weight and body score can also play an important role. Obese and overweight patients, or patients in poor body condition, may not be able to function effectively, they

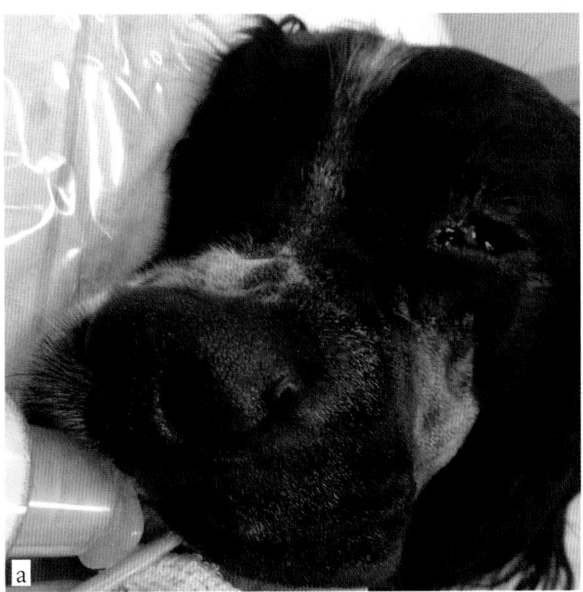

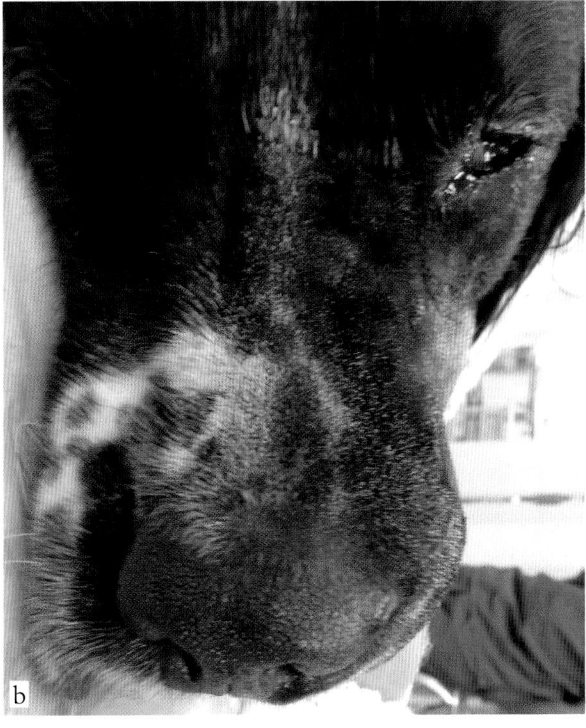

Fig. 10.1a,b Two-year-old English springer spaniel with high-grade soft tissue sarcoma over the rostral aspect of the nasal bone and maxilla.

may be more debilitated after major surgery or they may be more prone to major complications following surgery.

Handy hints

Cancer can occur in any breed at any age. Do not forget that cancer can be seen in young dogs and cats.

10.1.2 Staging

The tumour type, histological grade and clinical stage (TNM) should ideally be determined before surgery to plan optimal therapy and provide the owner with a realistic prognosis (Table 10.1). Information can be obtained from physical examination, assessment of the mass, complete blood count, biochemistry, urinalysis, thoracic and abdominal radiographs, abdominal ultrasound, cytology (FNA), biopsy of the mass and lymph nodes and advanced imaging modalities. Whilst there is still debate as to the timing of some of these diagnostic tests (before or after biopsy), for many patients a thorough screening will unmask any underlying pathology that may alter the further decision-making process (Erhart and Culp, 2012).

A thorough evaluation of the patient begins with a comprehensive physical exam and a minimum database, which includes a complete blood count and chemistry panel. The scope of the diagnostic work-up for staging purposes is dependent upon the known behaviour of the individual tumour type.

Evaluation of local disease starts with the physical exam to determine the size, appearance and mobility or fixation of the primary tumour to adjacent tissues. If the neoplasia is internal, imaging via ultrasound, radiography, computed tomography (CT) or MRI may be necessary for assessment of local extent of disease.

Regional tumour assessment involves evaluation of associated lymph nodes. Documentation of metastases to lymph nodes cannot reliably be made by palpation for size and other physical parameters, but requires cytology or histopathology. Because lymph node drainage can be highly variable, sampling of multiple nodes may be necessary. If a lymph node aspirate is non-diagnostic or if the lymph node cannot be accessed for aspiration, it is a candidate for excisional biopsy.

Distant metastasis refers to spread of cancer beyond regional lymph nodes to distant organs. Complete staging can vary depending on the particular tumour type, but distant metastasis may be revealed by a thorough physical examination, abdominal ultrasound (Fig. 10.2), abdominal and three-view thoracic radiography (Fig. 10.3), nuclear scintigraphy, CT (Fig. 10.4a–c), positron emission tomography-CT or MRI.

Table 10.1 WHO: TNM staging of tumours.

In the TNM system
T refers to the size and extent of the main (primary) tumour
N refers to the number of nearby lymph nodes that have cancer
M refers to whether the cancer has metastasised
There will be numbers after each letter that give more details about the cancer: for example, T3N1M0
Primary tumour (T)
TX: Main tumour cannot be measured
T0: Main tumour cannot be found
T1, T2, T3, T4: Size and/or extent of the primary tumour. The higher the number after the T, the larger the tumour or the more it has grown into nearby tissues
Regional lymph nodes (N)
NX: Cancer in nearby lymph nodes cannot be measured
N0: There is no cancer in nearby lymph nodes
N1, N2, N3: Refer to the number and location of lymph nodes that contain cancer. The higher the number after N, the more lymph nodes contain cancer
Distant metastasis (M)
MX: Metastasis cannot be measured
M0: Cancer has not spread to other parts of the body
M1: Cancer has spread to other parts of the body

Handy hints

When taking radiographs for staging (distant metastasis screening), always perform fully inflated three-view thoracic radiographs.

10.1.3 Surgical planning

Appropriate planning and adherence to principle of surgical oncology should address the following questions (Withrow, 2001a):

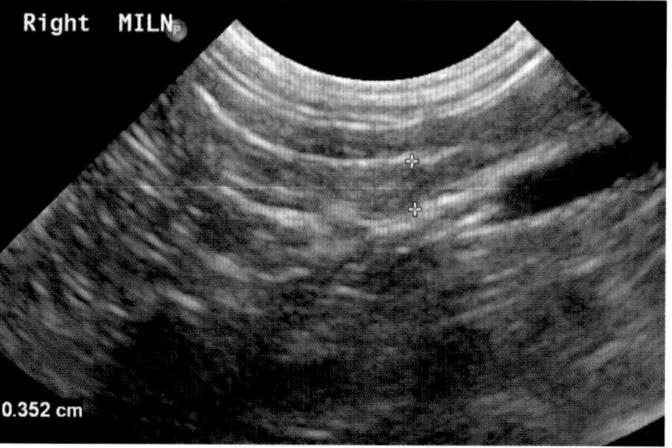

Fig. 10.2 Staging of an anal sac adenocarcinoma involved ultrasound of the abdomen, and an enlarged medial iliac lymph node was identified on the right side (the side on which there was a 2 cm nodule in the anal sac). Fine needle aspiration confirmed metastatic disease.

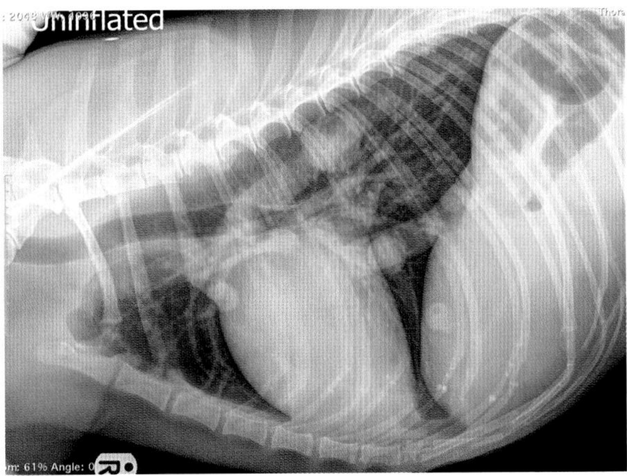

Fig. 10.3 A 10.5-year-old terrier was seen for a 'rapidly' growing mass in the ventral cervical region. Ultrasound of the mass was performed and a mass-like lesion was identified in the left thyroid gland. Thoracic radiographs revealed multiple large metastatic masses throughout the lung parenchyma.

1. What are the type and stage of the tumour?
2. Do the biopsy results correlate with the clinical presentation?
3. What is the biological behaviour of the tumour?
4. Is surgery indicated and what is the proper surgical approach?
5. What are the alternatives and adjuncts to surgery?
6. What are the owner's expectations and are these reasonable?

There are five different surgical goals with cancer: prevention, diagnosis, cure, palliation and combination therapy (Withrow, 2001b).

Preventative surgery

Forms of preventative surgery include: early ovariohysterectomy to reduce the incidence of cancers of the ovary, uterus and mammary glands; and castration to prevent Sertoli cell tumours in cryptorchid dogs and perianal adenoma (Gilson and Stone, 1990; Soderstrom and Gilson, 1995).

Diagnostic surgery: biopsy

The ideal biopsy technique should safely and simply provide an adequate sample of tissue that will consistently provide an accurate diagnosis (Soderstrom and Gilson, 1995).

Fine needle aspiration

Fine needle aspiration (FNA) is often the most minimally invasive technique for obtaining information about the mass before surgery. The accuracy of fine needle aspirates depends on many factors including: tumour type, tumour location and amount of inflammation or necrosis (Erhart and Culp, 2012). Imaging can increase the chance of obtaining a diagnostic sample. Aspirates of cutaneous and subcutaneous lesions can be obtained in most patients without sedation and with minimal discomfort (Fig. 10.5a–c). The goal of FNA is to differentiate between inflammation and neoplasia and, if the latter, to establish whether the mass is benign or malignant (Erhart and Culp, 2012). The overall purpose is to guide the staging diagnostics and surgical dose. Fine needle aspiration of internal organs can be performed, but image-guided techniques should be used when obtaining tissue from masses within a body cavity. As with most techniques, FNA is not entirely without risk: in certain cases, bleeding, fluid leakage or seeding can be problematic. However, FNA remains an effective, inexpensive and valuable tool in preoperative planning (Withrow, 2001a).

Step by step: fine needle aspiration of lymph node/mass

The following describes the equipment required and procedure.

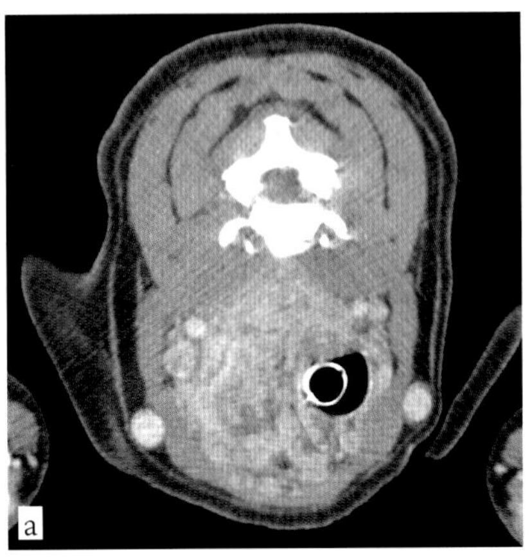

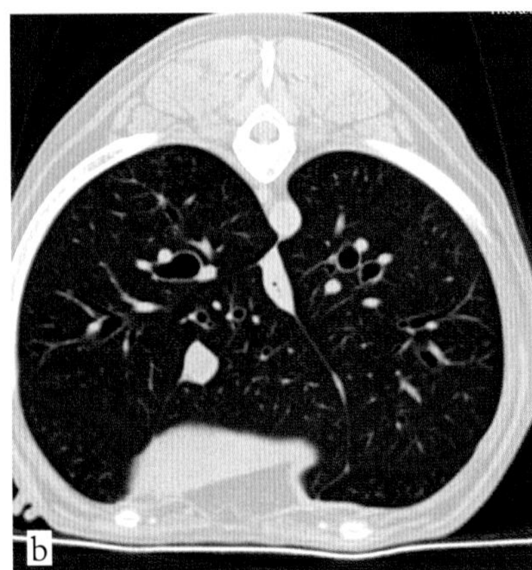

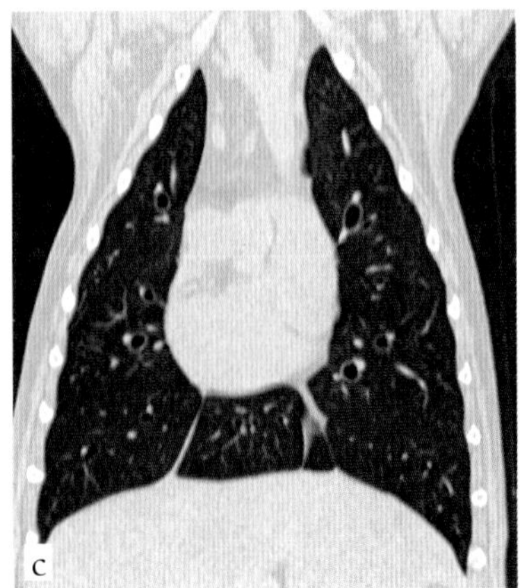

Fig. 10.4a–c A 7-year-old Labrador was seen for further investigations of dyspnoea, inappetence and a rapidly growing mass in the cervical region. A large soft tissue mass was identified rostrally (a). Several small nodules are seen in the thoracic cavity, highly consistent with metastasis (b,c).

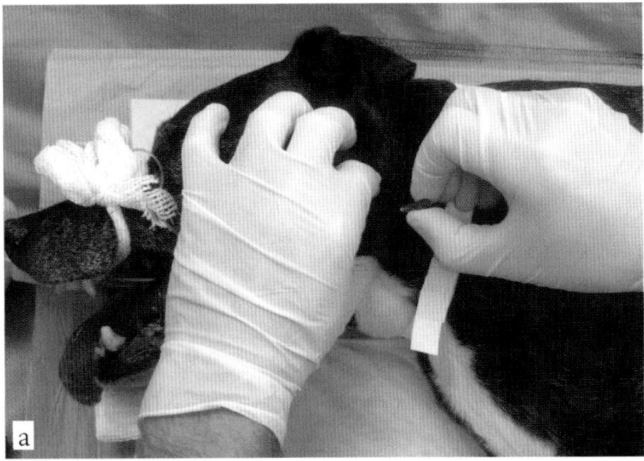

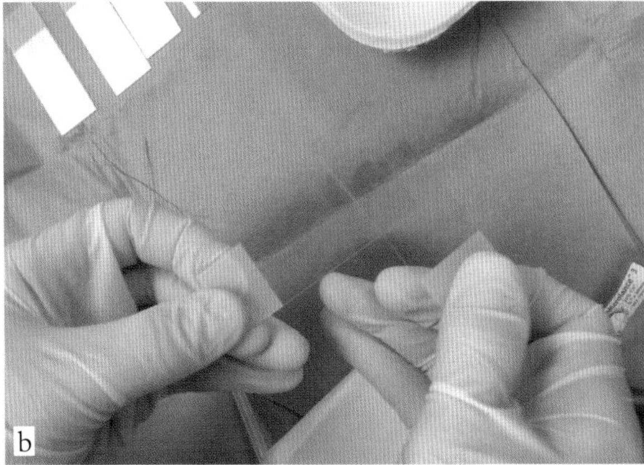

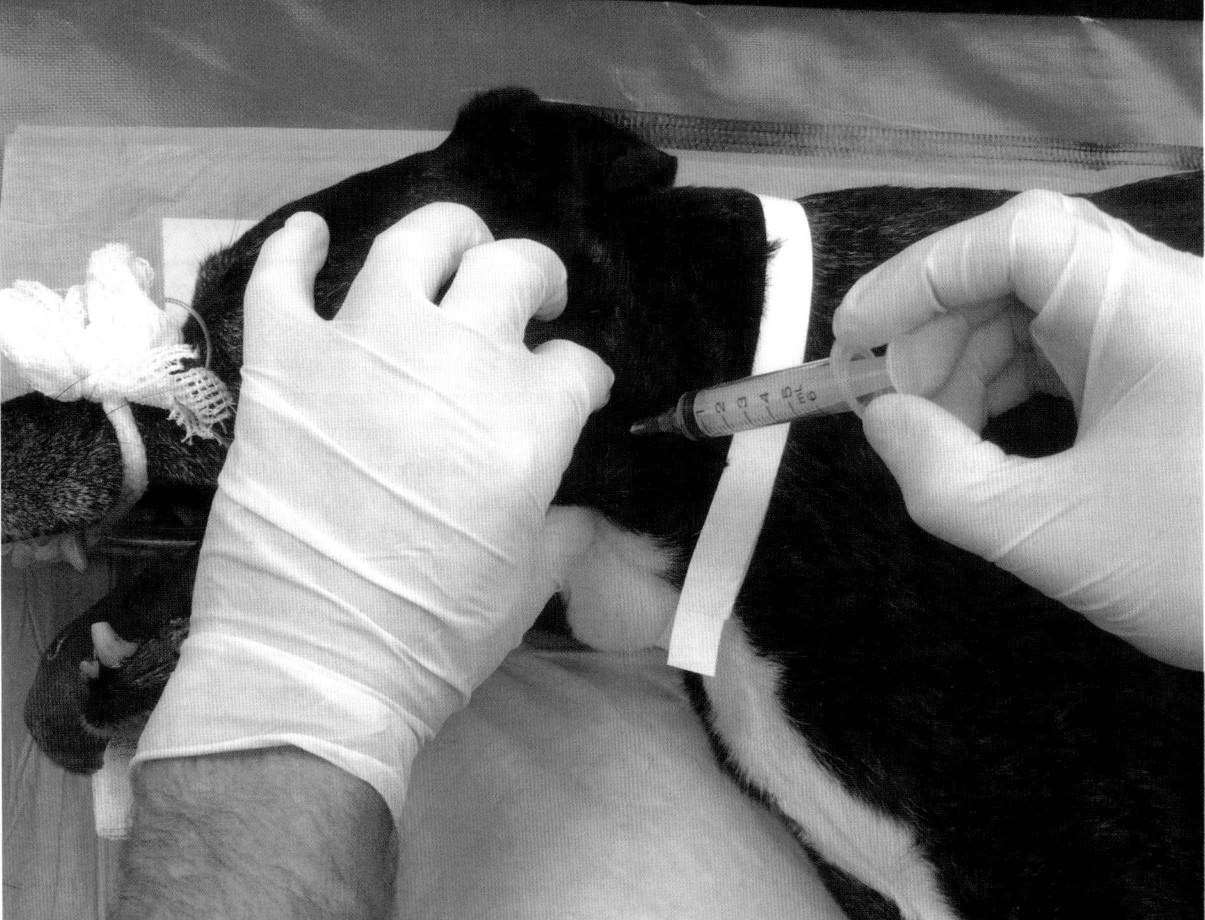

Fig. 10.5a–c Fine needle aspiration of lymph node/mass.

- 21–23-gauge needles.
- 2.5 or 5.0 ml syringe.
- Glass microscopic slides.
- Clip and/or aseptically prepare the area.
- Stabilise the mass or lymph node with one hand.
- Insert the needle into the mass (Fig. 10.5a)
- Redirect the needle several times.
- Remove the needle and aspirate air into the syringe before attaching the syringe to the needle.
- Expel the air and contents of needle onto a glass slide (Fig. 10.5b).
- Alternatively, cells can be withdrawn from the mass by aspiration with a syringe (Fig. 10.5c).

Handy hints

Fine needle aspiration cytology can be very rewarding for most cancers. Be aware that mesenchymal tumours do not shed cells readily. You can perform multiple fine needle aspirations or aspirations with large-gauge needles for mesenchymal tumours.

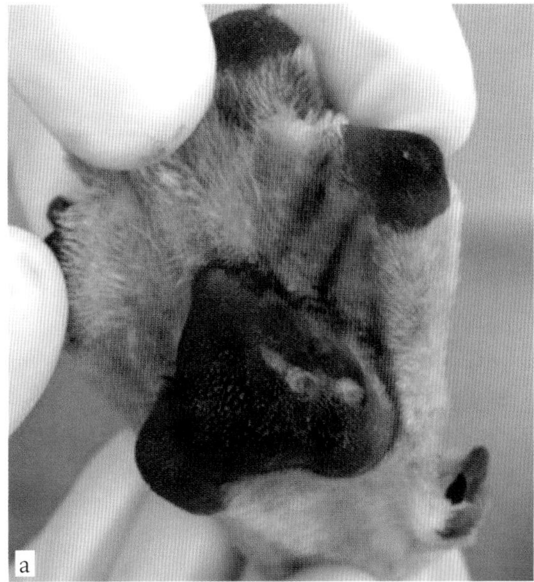

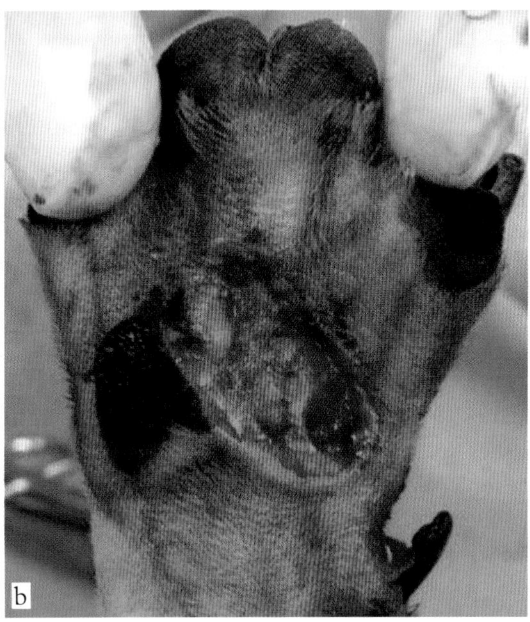

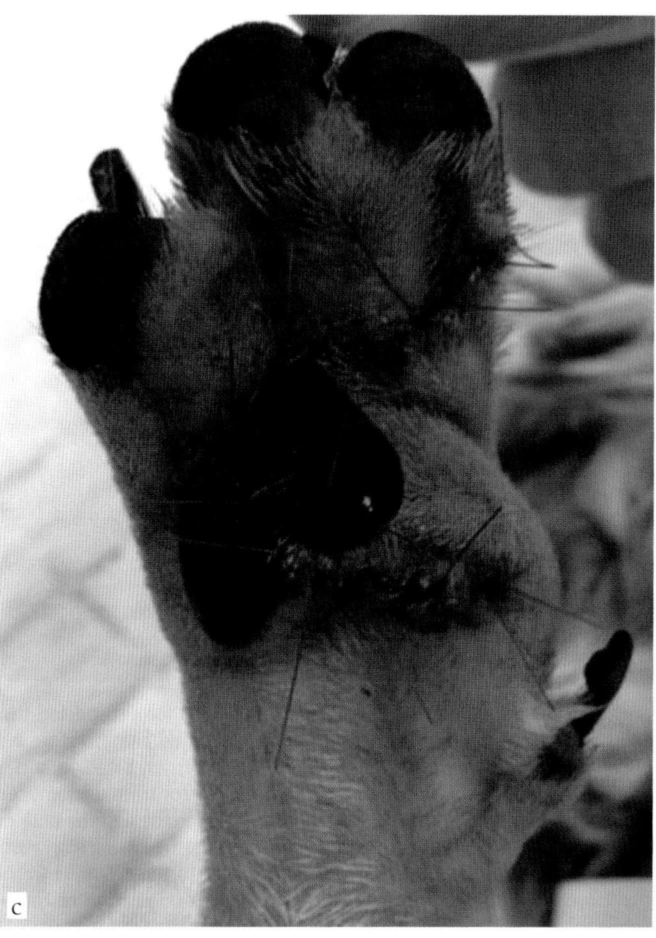

Fig. 10.10a–c A dog with a malignant melanoma on its paw pad had excisional biopsy performed by a local referring veterinary surgeon. Histopathological examination of the biopsy confirmed incomplete surgical margins.

Curative intent surgery (definitive surgery)

The first attempt at complete excision will always give the best results with locally aggressive or malignant tumours (Liptak, 2009). If a biopsy has been performed previously, then the chances of complete excision are reduced unless the biopsy was well planned (Soderstrom and Gilson, 1995). Tumours recurring after initial surgery are often more locally invasive due to altered vascularity and local immune responses, and the destruction of normal tissue planes in the initial surgery will make subsequent surgeries more difficult. Surgical planning depends on knowledge of tumour type, clinical stage and expected biological behaviour (Gilson and Stone, 1990). There are four levels of aggressiveness (doses) for surgical resection depending on location of the surgical margin. Enneking (Enneking et al., 1980; Fig. 10.11) first proposed these categories for musculoskeletal tumours, but they have since gained wide acceptance for all solid tumours (Gilson and Stone, 1990; Soderstrom and Gilson., 1995). The most common mistake in surgical oncology is to use too low a surgical dose, particularly from fear of being unable to close the resultant defect.

Wide and radical resections

Only wide and radical resections are considered curative intent surgeries aimed at resecting macroscopic and microscopic disease, including biopsy tracts, thus preventing local tumour recurrence and improving overall survival times. Wide or radical surgical resection is recommended to manage most solid tumours. For wide and radical resection of tumours, a margin of normal-appearing tissue should be excised *en bloc* with the gross tumour to eradicate any microscopic

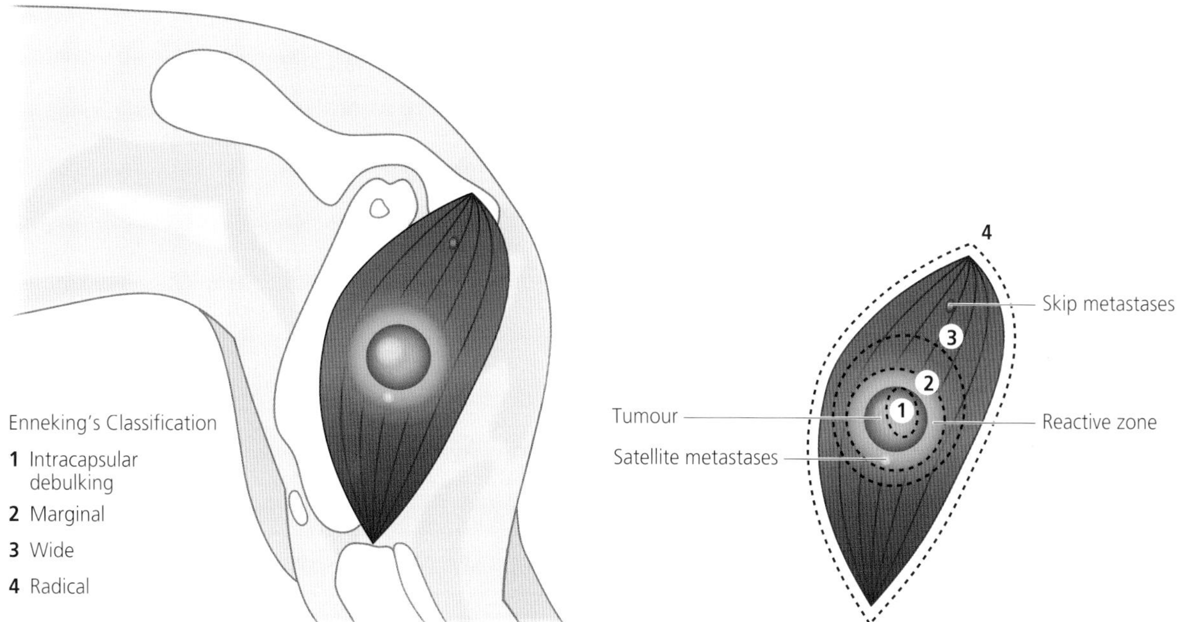

Fig. 10.11 Enneking classification for solid tumours. A tumour is seen in the biceps femoris muscle belly of a dog. The tumour is surrounded by a pseudo-capsule, which in turn is surrounded by a reactive zone. Within this reactive zone we occasionally encounter satellite tumours. Skip metastases some distance away from the primary tumour are rarely encountered (or rarely diagnosed) in small animal patients (adapted from Farese et al., 2018). *Illustrator: Elaine Leggett*

extension of the tumour (Fig. 10.12a–c). Radical resection is defined as the removal of a body part. This is occasionally required for complete excision of a tumour, such as splenectomy for splenic haemangiosarcoma (Fig. 10.13a,b), limb amputation for appendicular osteosarcoma and rib resection for a thoracic wall sarcoma (Fig. 10.14a–d).

Palliative surgery (marginal excision)

Palliative surgery is designed to improve the quality of life where the type or extent of disease prevents curative surgery. Examples of palliative surgery include removal of ulcerated mammary adenocarcinoma in a patient with asymptomatic pulmonary metastasis, splenectomy for haemangiosarcoma, limb amputation for osteosarcoma and gastrojejunostomy for duodenal obstruction. The patient gain should always outweigh the potential risk of surgery. Heroic surgery may not be indicated and the question we have to ask ourselves is: 'When do we give up?'

Marginal resection is defined as the incomplete excision of a tumour with residual microscopic disease.

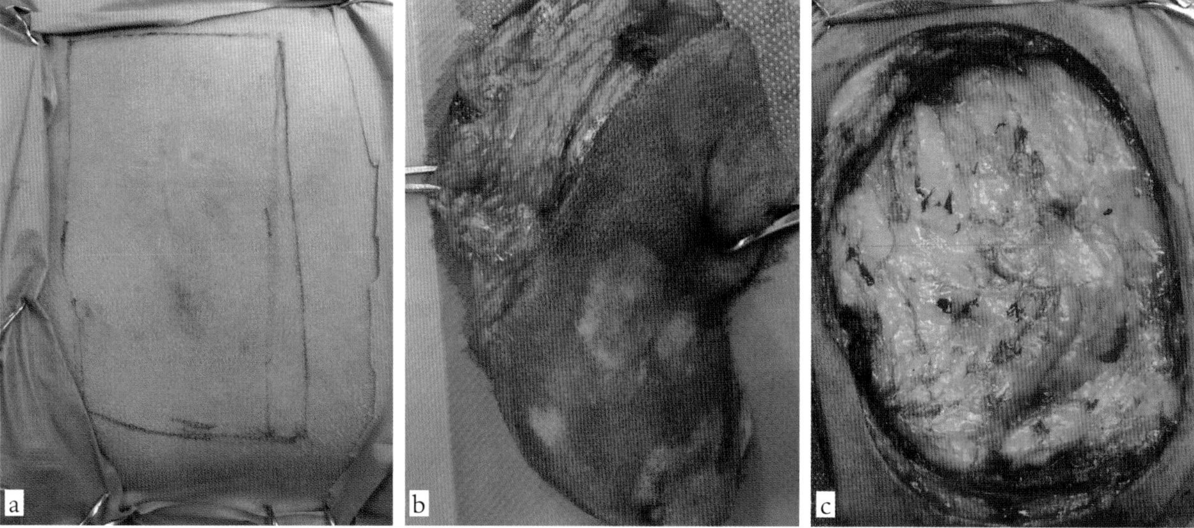

Fig. 10.12a–c Wide resection of a soft tissue sarcoma. a. A 10-year-old Labrador seen for surgical resection of an incompletely removed intermediate-grade soft tissue sarcoma on the left lateral flank. b. Complete tumour resected with lateral and deep margins, including fascial planes and muscles. c. Resulting defect after removal of tumour.

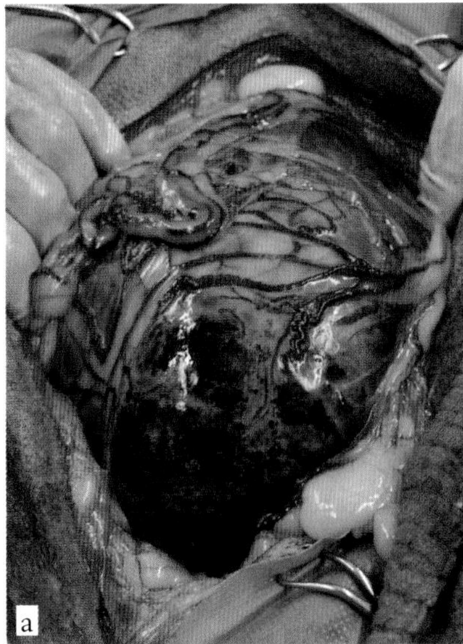

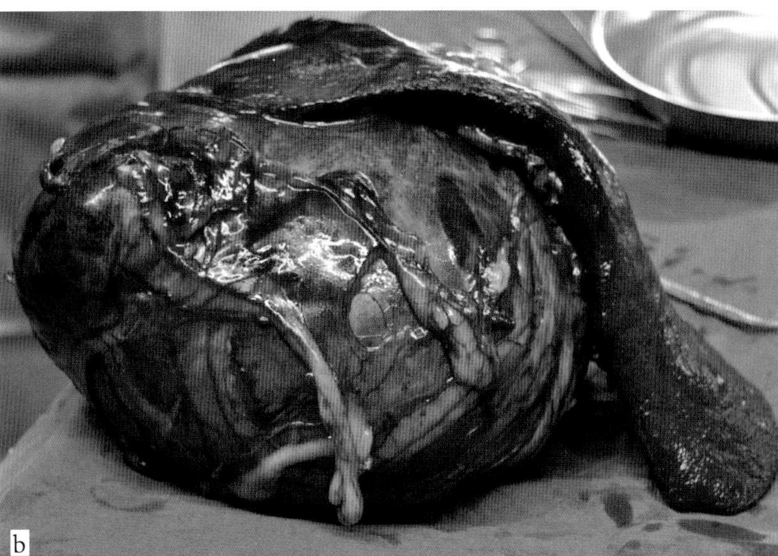

Fig. 10.13a,b Splenectomy as a form of radical oncologic resection. a. A 10-year-old Labrador with no clinical history was presented for an acute onset of weakness. No previous history of weakness had been reported. Clinical examination was fairly unremarkable except for an enlargement of the cranial abdomen. Palpation was resented by the patient. Ultrasound showed a huge cavitary lesion arising from the tail of the spleen, with no free fluid present. b. Histology of this mass revealed a large area of the splenic parenchyma characterised by loss of the normal architecture and replacement by haemorrhage and multifocal to coalescing areas of necrosis and fibrin deposition. There was moderate infiltration of haemosiderin-laden macrophages, mild accumulation of extracellular haematoidin and moderate extramedullary haematopoiesis at the periphery. There were also several areas of fibro-endothelial proliferation and, in these areas, the endothelial cells were slightly plumped, but no overt atypia or mitotic activity was seen. Further examination of different areas of the spleen revealed that the endothelial proliferation showed greater nuclear pleomorphism and more obvious bulging into the vascular lumens lined by the endothelial cells. A few mitoses (3 in 5 HPFs) were also seen. Spleen (final diagnosis): haemangiosarcoma with haemorrhage, necrosis and extramedullary haematopoiesis.

This highlights the need for multiple sections in multiple areas of the spleen when there is huge discrepancy in the organ and when there is a great suspicion of malignancy.

Marginal resection can be either planned or unplanned. Planned marginal resection is used when the tumour type is known based on preoperative biopsy. It is a useful limb-sparing technique for mast cell tumours (MCTs) and soft tissue sarcomas (STSs) of the distal extremities when combined with postoperative radiation therapy (Fig. 10.15a–c). Unplanned marginal resections occur when excisional biopsies performed without prior knowledge of tumour type result in incomplete excision. Unplanned marginal resections should be avoided by conducting appropriate preoperative biopsy, clinical staging and surgical planning.

Cytoreductive surgery

Cytoreductive surgery is the incomplete removal of a tumour, and is rarely an acceptable or indicated form of sole therapy because tumours that are incompletely excised will usually recur in a short period of time. It is a practical consideration prior to cryosurgery, and may increase the efficacy of chemotherapy or radiotherapy.

Debulking surgery (intra-lesional/ intra-capsular)

Debulking surgery is defined as the incomplete resection of a tumour with residual gross disease (Fig. 10.16). Debulking surgery is rarely an acceptable treatment for neoplastic diseases because tumour regrowth is usually rapid, and the presence of a macroscopic tumour burden makes adjunctive treatments less effective. This method is acceptable only for benign conditions.

10.1.4 Surgical technique

Following skin and subcutaneous incisions, protective drapes/swabs should be placed on skin edges to prevent tumour seeding (Fig. 10.17a–c). Normal tissue must be protected from tumour cells. Tumours are considered an infective nidus and hence careful handling is required to prevent exfoliation of tumour cells and local recurrence (Gilson and Stone, 1990; Soderstrom and Gilson, 1995). The tumour is isolated with a laparotomy sponge and, if required, manipulated with stay sutures or tissue forceps. Haemostasis, with prompt electrocoagulation or ligation of arterial, venous and lymphatic vessels, is important to prevent the release of tumour emboli into the circulation (especially for tumours with a good vascular supply, such as splenic and lung tumours) and to minimise the risk of postoperative complications. Wound lavage may dilute residual exfoliated tumour cells and decrease the risk of local tumour recurrence,

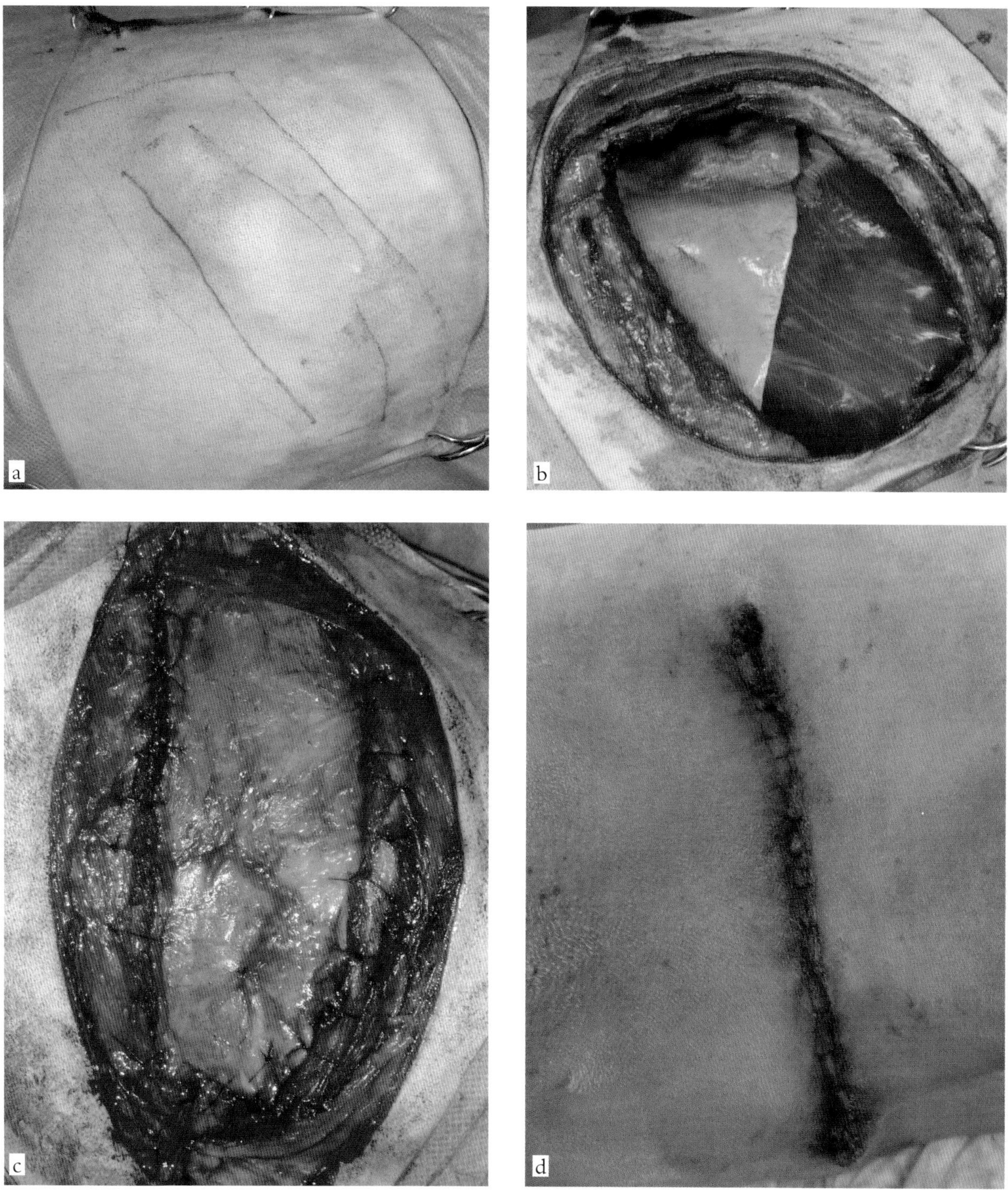

Fig. 10.14a–d Radical thoracic wall resection for a chrondrosarcoma. a. A 5-year-old Labrador was seen for a swelling on the mid- to caudal lateral thorax. The referring veterinary surgeon had taken a biopsy, which returned as a chondrosarcoma. Thoracic CT showed involvement of ribs 9 and 10. b–d. A thoracotomy with resection of four ribs (8–11) was performed with full-thickness *en bloc* resection of all layers and tissues.

or it may disseminate exfoliated cells throughout a lavaged cavity (Birchard, 1995; Soderstrom and Gilson, 1995). Drains should not be used in oncological surgery because they further disrupt deep and lateral tissue planes distant to the surgical field. Gloves, drapes and instruments should be changed after excision of the tumour (Erhart, 1998). Primary wound closure is preferred if possible, but 'it is better to leave a wound partly open with no cancer than to close the wound with residual cancer'. The aggressiveness of surgery should not be compromised by the ease of wound closure. It is preferable to avoid reconstructive surgery such as subdermal random flaps, axial pattern flaps and skin grafts at the time of initial tumour resection without knowledge of completeness of surgical resection (Gilson and Stone, 1990; Soderstrom and Gilson, 1995).

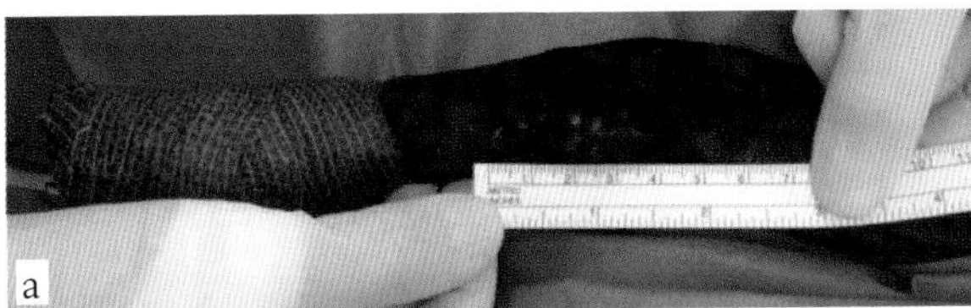

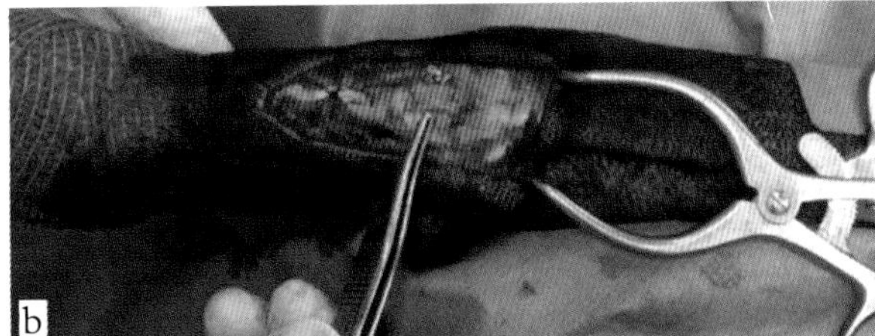

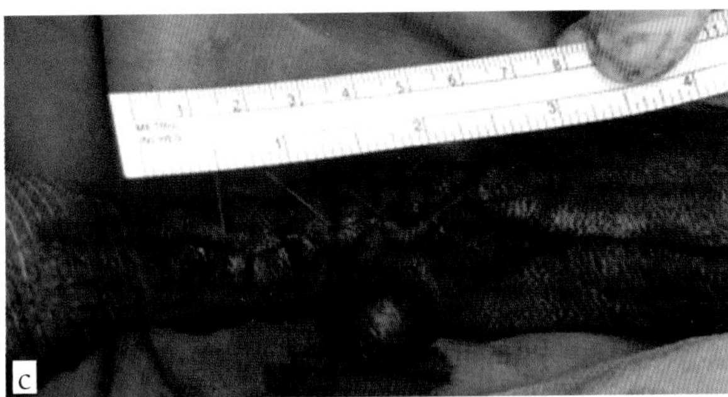

Fig. 10.15a–c Planned marginal excision before radiation therapy. Planned marginal resection for known tumour types is based on preoperative biopsy. This is commonly used as a 'limb-sparing' technique for MCTs and STSs of the distal extremities when combined with follow-up postoperative radiation therapy. a. Incompletely resected high-grade soft tissue sarcoma on the medial aspect of the distal radius. Presurgical measurement of the mass/scar tissue. b. Local/marginal resection of the scar tissue/mass with deep margins and primary closure. c. Immediate postoperative view showing primary closure and measurement. Planned radiation therapy 3–4 weeks after surgery.

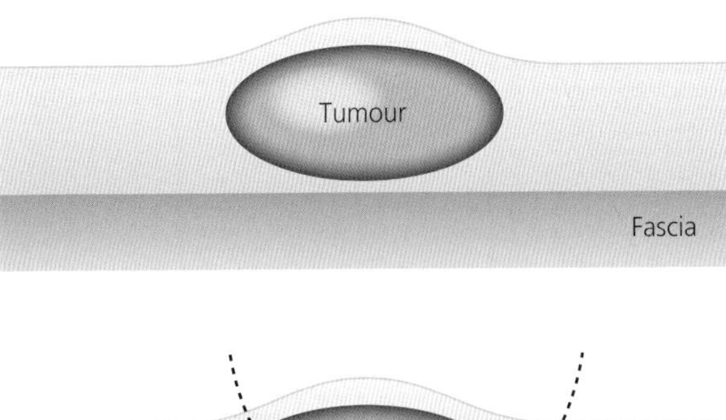

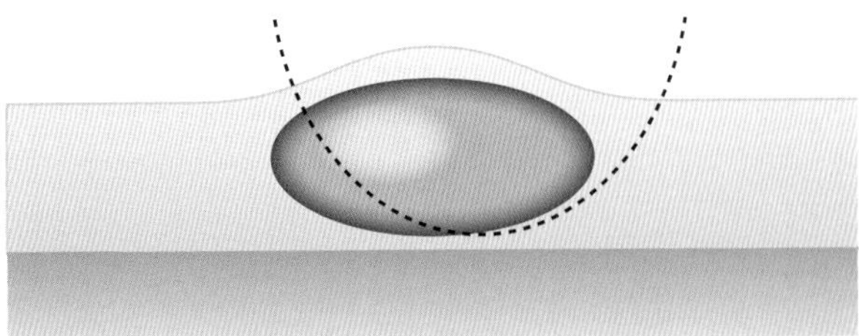

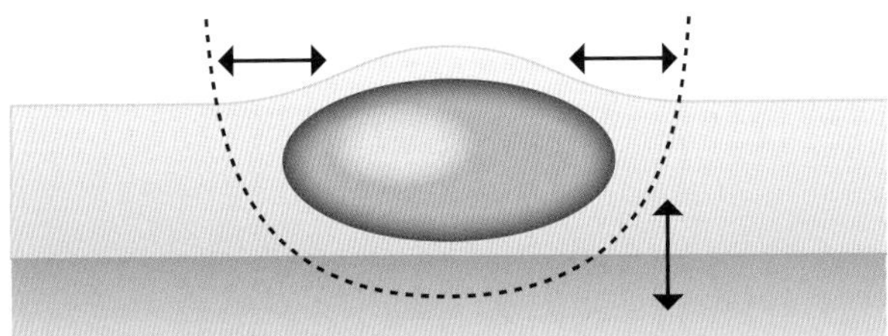

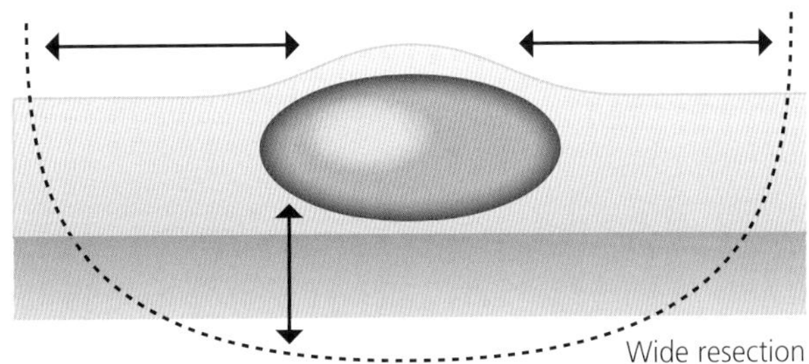

Fig. 10.16 Surgical margins. Intra-lesional resection (second from top): incomplete resection of a tumour with residual gross disease. Marginal resection (second from bottom): incomplete excision of the entire tumour with residual microscopic disease. Wide margin resection (bottom): for wide and radical resection of tumours, a margin of normal-appearing tissue should be excised *en bloc* with the gross tumour to eradicate any microscopic extension of the tumour. Generally measured laterally and along a fascial plane, as deep margins are used. *Illustrator: Elaine Leggett*

10.1.5 Histopathology and margins

The histopathological evaluation of surgical margins of an excised specimen is an essential component to appropriate care in any cancer patient. The entire resected mass should always be submitted for histopathological assessment of tumour type, grade (if appropriate) and surgical margins. This knowledge is essential so that the risk of local tumour recurrence and metastasis can be determined, further treatment can be planned if necessary and the owner can be advised of the prognosis (Gilson and Stone, 1990; Soderstrom and Gilson, 1995). Small biopsy samples should be placed in fixative immediately to prevent drying. Large tumours may need to be sliced into sections more than 1 cm thick to facilitate adequate fixation but, to maintain the ability of the pathologist to orient the sample and assess margins, the slicing should not be full-thickness through the tumour (Fig. 10.18). Tumours should be labelled and submitted to a veterinary pathologist, with a detailed history of clinical and surgical findings including anatomical location, size, shape, texture and relationship to surrounding structures. If required, a drawing of the specimen and labelling of margins may assist the pathologist in selecting the most appropriate area of the tumour to sample. Marking the tumour margins with sutures or a dye is recommended to assist in orientating the pathologist or the margins can be submitted separately (Erhart and Culp, 2012; Mann and Pace, 1993; Fig. 10.19). Pathologists do not often examine all the margins and hence clean margins should not always be interpreted as complete removal (Mann and Pace, 1993). Tumour margins define the type and magnitude of intended surgical margins. Intra-capsular margins occur with dissection through the tumour, and

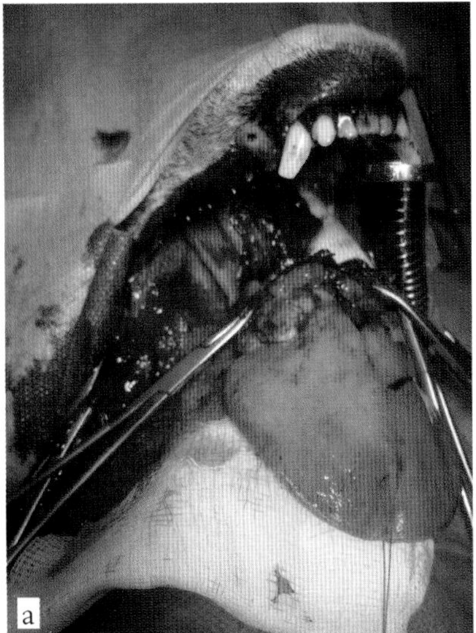

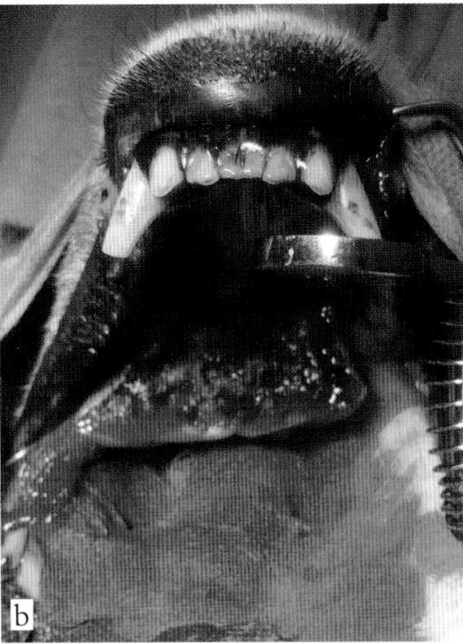

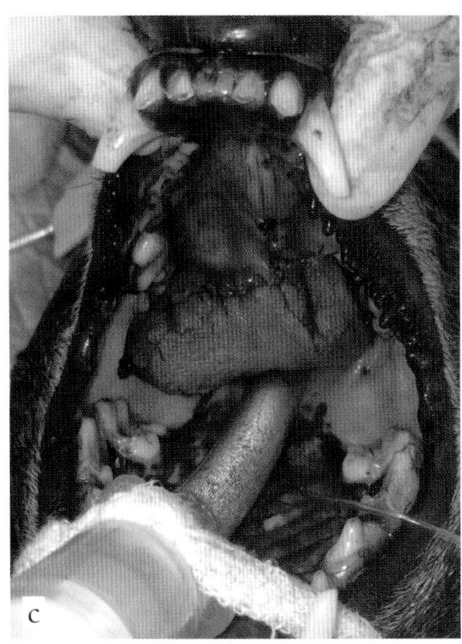

Fig. 10.17a–c Intra-operative handling of tumours – use of swabs. a. Intra-operative view during a glossectomy for resection of a squamous cell carcinoma. Protective drapes/swabs are placed on and around the edges to prevent tumour seeding. Normal tissues must be protected from tumour cells. Tumours are considered an infective nidus and hence careful handling is required to prevent exfoliation of tumour cells and local recurrence. The tumour is manipulated with stay sutures or tissue forceps. Careful haemostasis is always required. b,c. Intra-operative views of a partial distal glossectomy. The sponge protects the surrounding tissue and haemostasis has been achieved before closure of the wound.

microscopic disease always remains. Marginal excision refers to a tumour excised with a cuff of 1 cm or less of normal tissue surrounding the mass. Wide excision refers to tumours removed with 1–3 cm of normal tissue in all directions. This resection includes the pseudo-capsule and reactive zone. Dissection for a wide resection is intra-compartmental, and therefore it is distinguished from a radical excision. A radical excision is considered an excision of normal tissue greater than 3 cm or the entire anatomical compartment (i.e. amputation, splenectomy, entire muscle belly). Special focus is placed on MCT and STS when considering surgical margins, because microscopic projections of tumour cells extend out from the main tumour in the surrounding 'normal' tissues. Margins are three-dimensional, so lateral and deep margins must be considered when planning resections (Birchard, 1995; Withrow, 2001b). Lateral margins are determined by tumour type and biological behaviour. For example, lateral margins of 1 cm are recommended for benign tumours and most malignant carcinomas, whereas lateral margins of 3 cm are required for STSs. For MCTs, lateral margins are also determined by histological grade, with 2 cm lateral margins for all grade I and II (Fulcher et al., 2006; Simpson et al., 2004).

In 2013, a modified proportional margin (MPM) approach was reported (Pratschke et al., 2013), which advocates tailoring the margin to the individual tumour rather than using a blanket rule. With the MPM approach, the surgeon measures the widest diameter of the tumour and this measurement is used as the lateral margin for excision. Deep margins are determined by natural tissue barriers, as 1–3 cm-deep margins are often not possible in regions such as the extremities and trunk. Fat, subcutaneous tissue, muscle and parenchymal tissue do not provide a barrier to tumour invasion. Connective tissues, such as muscle fascia and bone, are resistant to neoplastic invasion and provide a good natural tissue barrier. Hence, deep margins should include a minimum of one fascial plane. Two fascial planes are recommended for surgical resection of vaccine-associated sarcomas. However, the true definition of a 'fascial plane' is lacking in medicine and specific guidelines remain elusive (Fasel et al., 2007). Lateral and deep margins should be greater if the tumour is invasive, recurrent or inflamed. Tumours (particularly STSs) should never be 'shelled out' because they are often surrounded by a pseudo-capsule of compressed, viable neoplastic cells and a reactive zone; these cells must also be removed completely.

Handy hints

Large tumours may need to be sliced into sections more than 1 cm thick to facilitate adequate fixation; however, the slicing should not be full-thickness through the tumour in order to maintain the ability of the pathologist to orient the sample and assess margins. Marking the tumour margins with sutures or a dye is recommended to assist in orientating the pathologist.

Handy hints

The narrowest margin after surgical excision dictates your overall surgical margin. The deep margin will always be the narrowest margin.

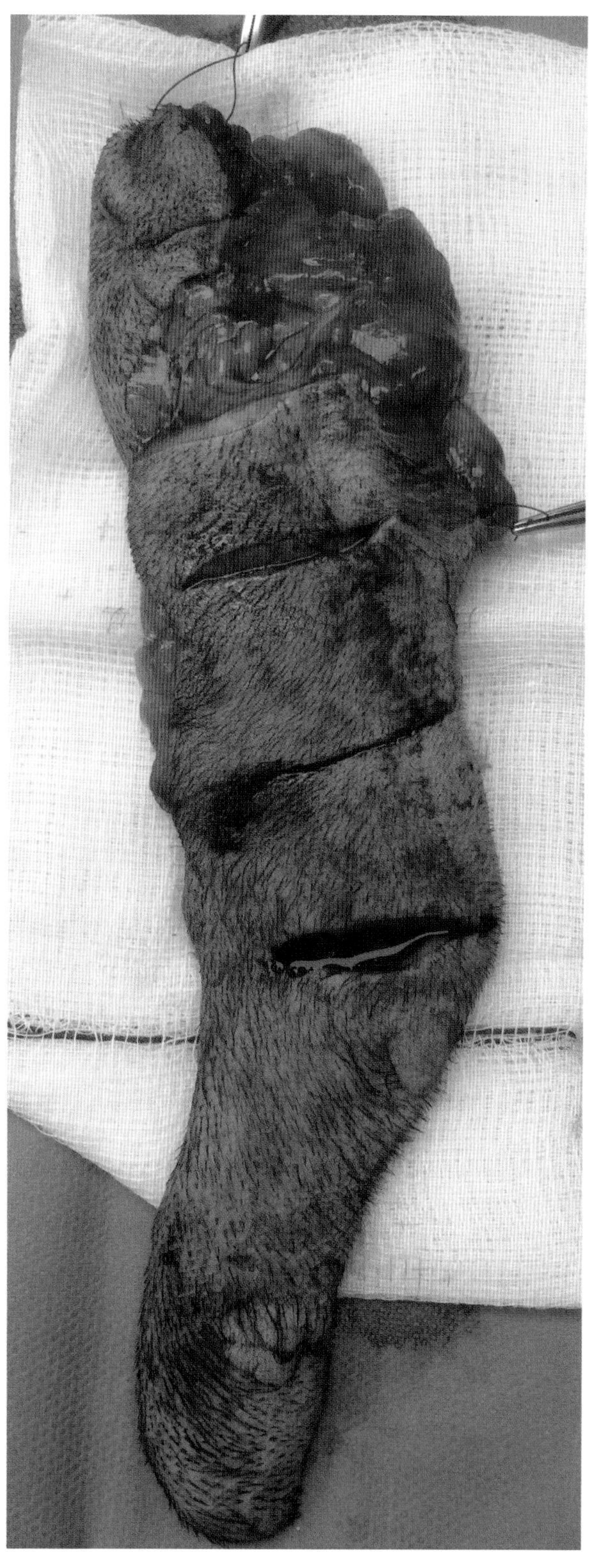

Fig. 10.18 A mammary adenocarcinoma after resection, including margins, is sliced so that the formalin can penetrate more deeply into the tissues and better fixate the tissues, allowing for faster processing. There are sutures at the cranial and medial margins.

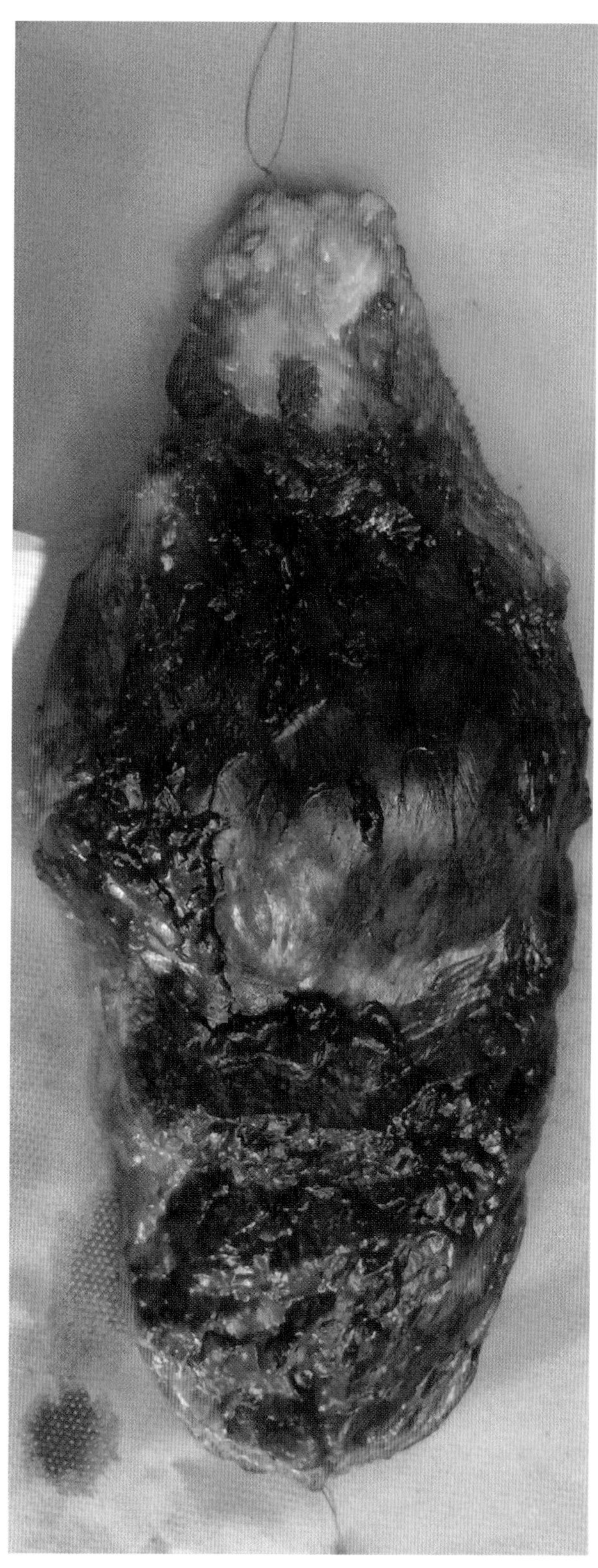

Fig. 10.19 Removal of a soft tissue sarcoma with 3 cm margins and with at least two deep fascial planes. There are sutures on the dorsal and ventral aspects of the tumour (cranial simple interrupted, caudal cruciate) to aid in orientation. The deep margin is coloured with dark ink (best not to use yellow, purple or red as these are difficult to distinguish from normal tissue colours once fixated).

10.1.6 Multimodal therapy

Nowadays it is commonplace to select multimodal therapy over a single treatment option, as this approach maximises benefits and minimises side effects (Gilson and Stone, 1990; Soderstrom and Gilson, 1995). The time to discuss the potential need for neoadjuvant or adjuvant therapy in a cancer patient is before any surgical intervention (Erhart and Culp, 2012). Even if complete excision is not possible, surgery can be effectively planned as part of a multimodal approach in combination with radiation therapy or chemotherapy. Cytoreductive surgery removes drug- and radiation-resistant tumour cells, circulating immune complexes and tumour-associated immunosuppressants (Withrow, 2001b). The timing of adjunctive therapies is an important consideration when planning curative or cyto-reductive surgery. Neoadjuvant therapy, which is administered prior to surgery, has some potential benefits but its disadvantages depend on the agent or modality being used and its adverse effects. Radiation therapy may be indicated prior to surgery and is theoretically more effective in the neoadjuvant setting, because the vascular supply of the tumour is not disturbed and hence tumour cells are better oxygenated and more radiosensitive (McChesney et al., 1995; McEntee, 1995). The risk of dissemination of tumour cells at surgery is reduced and tumour size may be decreased. Radiotherapy should be administered three weeks prior to surgery to allow the acute side effects of radiation to subside, and to minimise the delay in wound healing (McChesney et al., 1995). Adjuvant chemotherapy should be administered after the animal has recovered from surgery and wound healing has advanced to the remodelling stage. Adjuvant chemotherapy is recommended for tumours with a high metastatic risk and presumptive disseminated microscopic tumour burden (e.g. canine haemangiosarcoma, appendicular osteosarcoma, oral melanoma; McEntee, 1995). Adjuvant radiation therapy is recommended for residual microscopic disease in surgical wounds (e.g. incompletely resected canine MCT or STS; feline vaccine-associated sarcoma; McChesney, 1995).

10.1.7 Postoperative management

In the immediate postoperative period, cats and dogs should be monitored for anaesthetic and surgical complications specific to the procedure performed. The type, route and duration of analgesia are determined by the aggressiveness of the surgical procedure and response to therapy and may involve local anaesthesia, NSAIDs, opioids (partial agonists or antagonists) or N-methyl-D-aspartate (NMDA) antagonists (Liptak, 2009). Cancer has an enormous impact on the nutritional status of the patient, and so it is vital that feeding these patients pre- and postoperatively is a priority.

Postoperative management should include assessment of the wound healing process, a return to normal physiological function and checking for tumour recurrence and metastasis. This may be performed with any of the diagnostic tests previously mentioned. Re-evaluations should be individually assessed according to the tumour type, grade and stage (Gilson and Stone, 1990).

10.2 Skin and subcutaneous tumours

10.2.1 General principles

In the dog, 25–30% of all neoplasms arise in the skin. Seventy per cent of skin masses are benign and 30% are malignant (Ryan et al., 2012). The mean age at presentation is 8.3 years (Pakhrin et al., 2007). The majority of masses are located on the trunk (30%), head and neck (20%) and extremities (19%; Ryan et al., 2012). In the cat, cutaneous neoplasia accounts for 10% of all neoplasms (Miller et al., 1991). Four types are more prevalent: basal cell tumour, mast cell tumour, squamous cell carcinoma and fibrosarcoma.

Cutaneous tumours involve the skin or subcutaneous tissues. These tumours are broadly classified as epithelial, adnexal, mesenchymal, round cell or melanocytic.

- Epithelial: basal cell tumour, papilloma, squamous cell carcinoma and nail bed tumours.
- Adnexal: sebaceous gland adenoma / adenocarcinoma, ceruminous gland adenoma, apocrine gland adenocarcinoma of the anal sac, sweat gland tumours, tricho-epithelioma, pilomatrixoma, Meibomian gland adenoma.
- Mesenchymal: soft tissue sarcoma.
- Round cell: mast cell tumours, histiocytomas, melanocytic nevi, plasmocytoma and lymphoma.
- Melanocytic: benign cutaneous melanocytic nevi, malignant melanoma.

10.2.2 General approach to diagnosis and staging of cutaneous tumours

Information should include duration of presence of the mass and the rate of growth, as well as any change in appearance and growth rate. Details of concurrent disease or other tumours are important, as these could include signs of paraneoplastic disease and may affect prognosis and treatment decisions. The tumour type, histological grade and clinical stage should ideally be determined before surgical intervention. The anatomical location and measurements (in all directions) should be recorded. Cutaneous masses need to be carefully palpated to determine consistency and fixation to the underlying tissues. All skin and subcutaneous masses should be needle aspirated before surgical intervention.

A pre-treatment biopsy is indicated in the following instances (Withrow, 2001a):

- If the tumour type will alter the type of treatment.
- If the histological grade of the tumour will alter the extent, surgical dose or treatment.
- If the tumour location limits the reconstructive options.
- If the tumour type and grade affect the owner's willingness to pursue treatment based on prognosis.

Clinical staging is indicated for malignant or highly infiltrative cancers. Clinical staging includes:

- Local tumour: palpation, measurement, radiography, ultrasound, CT, MRI, cytology, histopathology.
- Regional lymph node: palpation (size, firmness, adherence), cytology, histopathology. Lymph node size is not predictive of neoplasia (Williams and Packer, 2003).
- Distant metastases: three-view thoracic radiography, abdominal ultrasound, CT, MRI, cytology.

10.2.3 Mast cell tumour (MCT)

Key points

- MCTs can vary from completely benign to some of the most malignant cancers.
- They can occur anywhere in the body.
- There is a growing number of subcutaneous MCTs being diagnosed; these generally are not classified following Patnaik or Kiupel.
- Surgery is generally considered to be the treatment of choice for localised and non-metastatic MCT.
- Radiation therapy is the primary choice for residual post-surgical microscopic disease.

MCTs are the most common malignant cutaneous tumour in the dog (London and Seguin, 2003; London and Thamm, 2013) and the second most common cutaneous tumour in the cat (Miller et al., 1991). MCTs can arise from the dermal and subcutaneous tissues. They are round cell tumours with characteristic cytoplasmic granules that contain histamine, heparin, proteases, chemotactic factors and cytokines. MCTs

Table 10.2 Clinical stages of MCT (from London and Seguin, 2003).

Clinical stage	Description
0	Single tumour, incompletely excised from dermis
I	Single tumour, confined to dermis without involvement of regional lymph nodes
II	Single tumour, confined to dermis with regional lymph node involvement
III	Multiple dermal tumour or large infiltrative tumour with or without regional lymph node involvement
IV (A,B)	Any tumour with distant metastases (blood or bone marrow)

Subtype A: no systemic signs of disease. B: signs of systemic disease.

are of varying histological appearance and biological behaviour. Dogs are generally middle aged (>5 years) and breeds reported to have a high incidence of MCT include boxers, Boston terriers, golden retrievers, Labrador retrievers, beagles and schnauzers (Murphy et al., 2004; Peters, 1969). Sixty-five to 80% of MCTs are solitary; 50–60% of MCTs occur on the trunk, with 25% on the limbs. All MCTs are locally aggressive and infiltrative. Low- to intermediate-grade MCTs have a lower metastatic potential than high-grade (Ryan et al., 2012; Table 10.2). Ninety per cent of MCTs will be diagnosed on cytology of an FNA. The typical path of metastatic spread is initially to the regional lymph nodes and then to spleen, liver or bone marrow; cutaneous MCTs rarely metastasise to the lungs. Staging should include local tumour FNA, regional lymph node aspirates and abdominal ultrasound. The routine aspiration of 'normal liver and spleen' is controversial and is currently not recommended.

Treatment

Surgery

Surgery is generally considered to be the treatment of choice for MCTs that are localised and non-metastatic. Perioperative complications may be encountered due to the release of vasoactive substances secondary to tumour manipulation. Perioperative treatment with an H1 blocker (e.g. chlorphenamine) or H2 blocker (e.g. ranitidine) is advised in tumours that will be surgically manipulated, or those that show evidence of degranulation or melaena and haemoptysis associated with gastrointestinal ulceration. Non-steroidal anti-inflammatory drugs (NSAIDs) should be avoided in patients with GI signs. Epinephrine should be available for patients in the case of an anaphylactic reaction.

Neoadjuvant prednisolone treatment may facilitate resection when tumour resection is not immediately feasible due to tumour location or size. Reduction in volume of 80% was seen in 70% of patients where neoadjuvant prednisolone was used (Stanclift and Gilson, 2008).

Several studies have investigated excisional margins, and found that margins of 2 cm laterally and one fascial plane in depth are sufficient for intermediate- and low-grade tumours that are less than 4 cm in diameter (Fulcher et al., 2006; Seguin et al., 2001; Simpson et al., 2004). A single study looked at intermediate- and low-grade MCTs and found no recurrence where tumours were excised with a 1 cm lateral margin and 4 mm in depth (Schultheiss et al., 2011). High-grade MCTs should always be excised with a lateral margin of at least 3 cm and one deep fascial plane. Where the margins of the tumour are unclear, advanced imaging may be useful to determine tumour extent, particularly the deep margins, but it is important to appreciate that in high-grade MCT the risk of local recurrence and metastasis is high, so multimodal therapy should be pursued (Thamm and Vail, 2007). Where low- or intermediate-grade MCTs are completely resected with wide margins and no evidence of metastasis is found, further treatment is generally not indicated, although monitoring is required. Owners should be warned that even after apparent complete surgical excision, local recurrence may occur in up to 23% of intermediate-grade MCTs (Fulcher et al., 2006; Schultheiss et al., 2011; Seguin et al., 2001; Simpson et al. 2004). Where incomplete margins have been demonstrated following excision of low- or intermediate-grade MCT, local recurrence is not guaranteed. Decision making in such a situation is not straightforward, and current recommendations for such cases include:

- monitoring the site
- follow-up radiation therapy
- *en bloc* excision of the scar with appropriate gross margins (2 cm laterally and one fascial plane deep).

If the MCT is high-grade and completely excised, chemotherapy should be pursued; if excision is incomplete, chemotherapy with revision surgery or radiation therapy is the gold standard (Thamm and Vail, 2007).

Options for distal extremity MCT are dictated by tumour grade. For low- and intermediate-grade MCTs, a combination of marginal surgical resection with planned external-beam radiation is a rational treatment option (Frimberger et al., 1997; LaDue et al., 1998; Michels et al., 2002; Welle et al., 2008). Only for grade III MCT is amputation considered.

Handy hints

The margins in MCT surgery are still being questioned and debated, but there generally is no consensus for a 3 cm margin. Mast cell tumours on the limbs most often are currently treated with local marginal resection, primary closure and planned follow-up radiation therapy.

Radiation therapy

Radiation therapy is the primary choice for residual post-surgical microscopic disease. Radiation therapy can be part of multimodal therapy either as adjunctive therapy after incomplete surgery, where local/regional nodal metastases are present, or as part of a planned marginal resection followed by adjuvant radiation therapy. Radiation has also been used as a palliative modality and results in an improved quality of life, but is unlikely to improve survival time significantly. Toxicity from radiation therapy is minimal, with the most common acute effects being dry desquamation and alopecia and the most common late-radiation effects being alopecia and leukotrichia. No severe adverse events are observed. In patients with MCT in the distal limbs, where achieving clean, deep margins is not possible because the tumour is wrapping around tendon, there is little to be gained in attempting to achieve clean lateral margins and the surgeon should aim for the removal of all gross disease and achieve simple primary closure (Frimberger et al., 1997; LaDue et al., 1998). The surgeon should collaborate closely with the radiotherapist and take numerous pre-, intra- and postoperative photographs to ensure there is not a geographical miss when radiation therapy is performed. Radiation offers a 3-year control rate of >90% after incomplete excision of low- and intermediate-grade MCTs (Frimberger et al., 1997; LaDue et al., 1998; Poirier et al., 2006). Disease-free intervals of >40 months can be expected in dogs with low- or intermediate-grade MCT with regional lymph node metastases treated by surgery and radiation (Chaffin and Thrall, 2002).

Chemotherapy

Chemotherapy is useful in several situations for the management of MCT:

- As a neoadjunctive to reduce tumour burden prior to complete surgical excision or radiation (such as prednisolone and vinblastin).
- Where systemic therapy is required, such as in high-grade tumours or where metastasis has been documented or is likely.
- Where microscopic disease is present and further surgery or radiation is not possible.

First-line chemotherapeutic protocols may comprise vinblastine and prednisolone, with second-line therapies including lomustine, but variations are common. In dogs with intermediate- or high-grade MCT after surgical excision and with or without radiation therapy, prednisolone and vinblastine will increase the patient's life expectancy by up to 3 years, which is a significant improvement compared with dogs undergoing only surgical resection of high-grade MCT and of whom only 6–27% are alive after one year (Welle et al., 2008). Chemotherapy needs to be discussed before and after surgical management, as vinblastine is severely irritant when injected perivascularly and can also cause myelosuppression and gastrointestinal toxicity. Lomustine can cause severe myelosuppression and hepatic toxicity.

Tyrosine kinase inhibitors

One of the most recent significant developments in the treatment of canine MCT is the use of KIT receptor tyrosine kinase inhibitors (TKIs). In the dog, 20–30% of MCTs express a mutated form of KIT. Small-molecule tyrosine kinase inhibitors, including masitinib and toceranib, have shown efficacy against certain MCTs. Such molecules competitively block the extracellular domains of receptor tyrosine kinases, which then prevents the activation and phosphorylation of the intracellular domains responsible for cell proliferation, differentiation and survival, and angiogenesis and metastasis. Toceranib is licensed for use in recurrent, non-resectable intermediate- or high-grade MCT, while masitinib is licensed for use in non-resectable intermediate- or high-grade MCT with demonstrable c-KIT mutations. In one study assessing masitinib in non-metastatic recurrent or non-resectable intermediate- or high-grade MCT, masitinib increased the overall time to progression from 75 to 118–253 days, with minimal side effects (Hahn et al., 2008, 2010).

Prognosis

Histopathological grading of an MCT is the most important single prognostic factor (Patnaik et al., 1984; Thamm et al., 1999; Turrell et al., 1988). Most MCTs are diagnosed on cytopathology. If preoperative biopsies are required, these should be performed at a site such that their excision might be readily included in the subsequent treatment protocols, without the need to enlarge the surgical site or radiation field. The Patnaik (Patnaik et al., 1984) system (Table 10.3) is the most widely used for cutaneous tumours but is subjective, resulting in <64% agreement among pathologists for grades I and II MCT and 75% agreement for grade III. To reduce subjectivity, a two-tier system described by Kiupel et al. (2011) (Table 10.4) has attempted to differentiate MCTs simply into either high or low grade.

Cell proliferation markers can also predict prognosis in response to therapy in a less subjective fashion. A mitotic index >5 is prognostic for reduced survival, and >7 results in increased recurrence (Romansik et al., 2007). Increased Ki-67 (>1.8%) and AgNOR scores are both associated with increased mortality, recurrence and metastasis, independent of histological grade (Scase et al., 2006). Increased proliferating cell nuclear antigen is associated with recurrence and metastasis, but is not independent of histological grade. Mutations in the c-Kit gene are detected in 15–40% of canine MCTs and are associated with increased metastasis, local recurrence and high histological grade (Webster et al., 2004).

Multiple cutaneous MCTs occur in 9–12% of patients (Murphy et al., 2006; Thamm and Vail, 2007). Boxers and golden retrievers and older dogs are likely to present with multiple cutaneous MCTs. Dogs with multiple MCTs have a low rate of metastasis and a good prognosis following adequate excision of all MCTs (Murphy et al., 2006; Thamm and Vail, 2007).

Table 10.3 Patnaik classification system for MCT (from Patnaik et al., 1984).

Grade	Patnaik grade	Microscopic features
Well differentiated	I Low	Well-differentiated mast cells with clearly defined cytoplasmic borders and regular spherical or ovoid nuclei Granules are large, deep-staining and plentiful Cells confined to dermis and interfollicular spaces
Intermediately differentiated	II Intermediate	Cells closely packed with indistinct cytoplasmic boundaries Nuclear/cytoplasmic ratio lower than anaplastic Frequent mitotic figures More granules than anaplastic Neoplastic cells infiltrate or replace the lower dermal and subcutaneous tissues
Anaplastic/ undifferentiated	III High	Highly cellular, undifferentiated cytoplasmic boundaries Irregular size and shape of nuclei Frequent mitotic figures Low number of cytoplasmic granules Neoplastic tissue replaces the subcutaneous and deep tissues

Table 10.4 Kiupel classification system for MCT (from Kiupel et al., 2011).

Using the 2-tier system, a tumour becomes high grade if it meets any one of the following objective criteria:
≥7 mitotic figures in 10 hpf
≥3 multi-nucleated cells (multi-nucleated defined as 3 or more nuclei per cell) in 10 hpf
≥3 bizarre nuclei (highly atypical) in 10 hpf
Karyomegaly (nuclear diameter varies by at least twofold in ≥10% of mast cells)

Handy hints

For grade II MCT it is advisable to request Ki-67 immunohistochemistry to gain an idea of the biological behaviour.

10.2.4 Soft tissue sarcoma

Key points

- Soft tissue sarcomas (STSs) are a homogenous group of mesenchymal tumours with similar behaviour.
- STSs are typically firm, plump masses that have expanded under the skin.
- Many STSs are not well diagnosed by FNA because of their limited exfoliative character.
- Histological grade is the most important prognostic factor in human STS.
- The margins for soft tissue sarcomas are challenging, although most recommend wide resection with 3 cm margins.
- STS on the limb is treated as for MCT regarding local margins (as much as possible) and primary closure, followed with planned radiation therapy.
- Chemotherapy may be beneficial in cases of metastasis, incomplete resection or high-grade tumours.

Soft tissue sarcomas are tumours derived from tissues of mesenchymal origin (Bostock and Dye, 1980; Erhart, 2005; Mayer and Larue, 2005), meaning that they can arise from almost any anatomical site. In the dog, they develop most frequently in a subcutaneous location and are remarkably common, representing between 9 and 15% of all cutaneous or subcutaneous tumours (Chase et al., 2009; Dennis et al., 2011; Erhart, 2005; Mayer, 2005). STSs have conventionally been grouped together because of key features of biological behaviour that are common to all of them (Liptak and Forrest 2013).

Several biological factors common to all STSs (Liptak and Forrest, 2013) are:

- an ability to arise from any anatomical site in the body
- the propensity to appear as pseudo-encapsulated tumours with poorly defined histological margins
- a tendency to infiltrate along fascial planes
- common local recurrence after conservative excision
- metastasise via haematogenous route
- a poor response to chemotherapy and radiation therapy in cases where gross tumour is present

One concern is that unplanned resections, performed without prior diagnostic investigations that might alert to possible malignant potential, remain very common (Bray et al., 2014; Chase et al., 2009). The metastatic potential of STS is poorly described. It is generally considered they have a low to moderate metastatic rate. Metastatic rates ranging from 1.7 to 41% have been described (Bostock and Dye, 1980; Demetriou et al., 2012; Kuntz et al 1997; Stefanello et al., 2011). The metastatic potential of STS has been associated with a higher histological grade and mitotic count (Dennis et al., 2011). Tumours metastasise most commonly to the lungs, while regional lymph nodes are a relatively rare site of metastasis (Kuntz et al., 1997).

Little is known about the pathogenetic cause of STS in the dog and cat. Changes in genetic make-up, chronic trauma, foreign bodies, vaccinations, parasites and radiation have been associated with STS in both species. P53 mutations and MDM2 gene amplification were observed in a subgroup of canine soft tissue sarcoma; however, familial predispositions have not been reported. No sex or breed predilections have been found, although certain breeds seem to be afflicted with tumours more commonly than others (Erhart, 2005; Mayer and Larue, 2005; Liptak and Forrest, 2013).

Affected dogs tend to be middle-aged or older, with a median age at diagnosis reported to be between 10 and 11 years (Bray et al., 2014; Chase et al., 2009; Erhart, 2005; Liptak and Forrest, 2013; Stefanello et al., 2011).

Animals with an STS usually present with a subcutaneous mass (Erhart, 2005; Liptak and Forrest, 2013). Although most of these are reported to have been present for many months, some large masses may arise quickly and then maintain a stable size. STSs are generally considered to be slow growing, but it is not unusual for dogs to present with a sizeable mass that has only recently been noticed by the owner. STSs are typically firm, plump masses that have expanded under the skin and are most commonly (in up to 60% of cases) found on the limbs (Bray et al., 2014; Erhart, 2005; Liptak and Forrest, 2013). The trunk (including the tail) is involved in about 35% and the head in 5% of cases.

A clinical suspicion of STS can usually be supported with cytology, based on samples obtained by FNA

(Bray et al., 2014; Erhart, 2005; Liptak and Forrest, 2013).

Many STSs are not well diagnosed by FNA because of their limited exfoliative character, but many other tumour types can be excluded as well as some inflammatory processes. It is important to note that cytology is unable to provide details on the biological aggressiveness of the mass (i.e. tumour grade) or specific morphological criteria that may be important in assisting treatment planning (Stockhaus et al., 2003).

There are currently no diagnostic tests that can reliably predict the precise surgical margins required for a particular tumour, but there are several validated and suspected prognostic factors that have been reported (Dennis et al., 2011).

Handy hints

Fine needle aspiration of soft tissue sarcomas can be challenging and disappointing.

Adjunctive diagnostic evaluations include routine blood work, radiographs of the local tumour site for possible underlying bone infiltration, ultrasound of the tumour, radiographs of the chest for possible metastatic spread, FNA of the regional lymph node and CT or MRI techniques.

STSs pose a problem to the veterinary surgeon mainly because they tend to be locally aggressive. Complete surgical excision is often impossible because of localisation or size of the tumour. Recurrence is common after incomplete resection and is the primary reason to refer STS. Most recurrences will occur within 2 years after primary tumour removal. Recurrence is caused because STS tends to spread into deeper or surrounding tissues by invasion or extension next to natural anatomical structures. These finger-like outgrowths of the tumour are often compared to the tentacles of an octopus.

Histological grade is the most important prognostic factor in human STS, and is probably one of the most validated criteria used to predict outcome following surgery in canine patients (Bray et al., 2014; Kuntz et al., 1997). A tumour grade – low (grade I), intermediate (grade II) or high (grade III) – is assigned based on various histological criteria. Higher tumour grades are associated with more aggressive biological behaviour, which translates to higher rates of local recurrence, distant metastasis and shorter disease-free intervals (Dennis et al., 2011; Kuntz et al., 1997). Grade I tumours are the predominant form in veterinary medicine (Bray et al., 2014).

Surgery

Surgery is the treatment of choice and is only successful if large margins of normal tissue are obtained, with margins of 2–3 cm in all directions being required for curative intent surgery (Dennis et al., 2011; Dernell et al., 1998; Erhart, 2005; Kuntz et al. 1997; Liptak and Forrest, 2013). The first wide surgical resection is the best chance for a cure with the least chance of recurrence (Ryan et al., 2012). Several authors have recently challenged the requirement for wide surgical excision margins (Banks et al., 2004; Bray et al., 2014; Cavanaugh et al., 2007; Chase et al., 2009), with some studies suggesting that the extent of resection did not influence the disease-free interval or overall survival time (Bray et al., 2014; Chase et al., 2009; Stefanello et al., 2011).

If the tumour is attached to a muscle or fascial plane, this should be considered 'contaminated' and the entire anatomical boundary removed. Fat and loose connective tissues are not barriers for infiltration of the mesenchymal tumour cells. The deep margins will almost always pose a difficulty, and at least one fascial plane underneath the tumour should be removed. On extremities, surgical margins are difficult to achieve and radical resection in the absence of orthopaedic and neurological abnormalities can be an option for high-grade STS limb sparing techniques, although a more conservative approach with 'limb spare' techniques may be a better alternative for low- to intermediate-grade tumours.

Marginal excision of an STS either as a sole therapy or combined with radiation therapy may result in an excellent long-term outcome with lower morbidity compared to amputation (Demetriou et al., 2012). Histological grade is a strong predictor for recurrence of marginally excised STS. McSporran (2009) highlighted the importance of tumour grade on outcome: he reported that only 7% (3/41) of low-grade tumours recurred after marginal excision compared with 34 (14/41) and 75% (3/4) for intermediate- and high-grade tumours, respectively.

Radiation therapy

Radiotherapy can be used in either a curative or palliative manner before or after surgical tumour removal. Treatment options involve hyper-fractionated or coarsely fractionated (hypofractionated) protocols. A definitive (curative) course often involves daily treatment for several days. Radiation therapy is more effective with minimal (microscopic) disease than with more bulky disease. Radiation therapy in combination with surgery results in increased disease-free intervals. Good outcomes for curative intent radiotherapy after incomplete STS resection have been reported. Forrest et al. (2000) reported a median survival time of 2270 days for incompletely resected non-oral STS after a total dose of 42–57 Gy given in 3.0–4.2 Gy daily fractions. One recent study reported the adjuvant use of hypo-fractionated radiotherapy after planned marginal

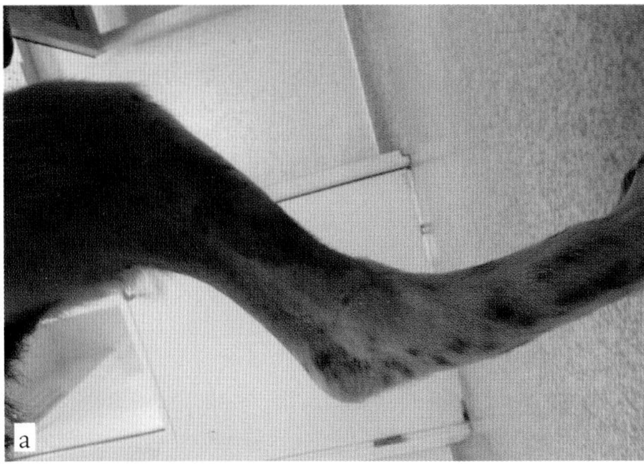

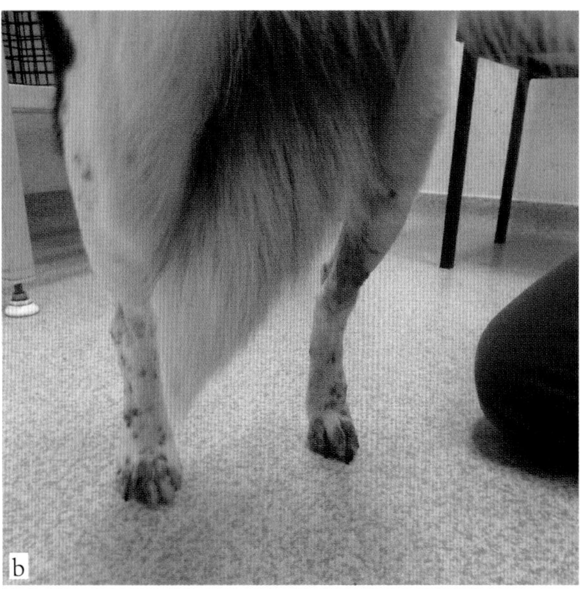

Fig. 10.20a,b Postoperative hypo-fractionated radiation therapy. A 10-year-old terrier cross had an intermediate STS resected from the medial aspect of the tibia. Only narrow margins (albeit complete) were achieved. This patient had four follow-up sessions of radiation therapy.

resection of STS (Demetriou et al., 2012). The treatment protocol consisted of four weekly doses of radiotherapy (6–9 Gy per dose) to a total treatment dose of 24–36 Gy. Local recurrences developed in 18–21% of dogs, with metastatic disease occurring in 23–25%, and follow-up periods of 240–2376 days (Fig. 10.20).

Chemotherapy

Because STSs are a heterogeneous group of tumours, it is hard to obtain sufficient data to set up solid treatment plans or protocols based on proven clinical trials. The effectiveness of chemotherapy for STS is unclear. Chemotherapy may be beneficial in cases of metastasis, incomplete resection or high-grade tumours. Multidrug chemotherapy protocols, including anthracyclines (doxorubicin, mitoxantrone), have been advocated as the most successful. Combination therapy of an anthracycline with vincristine and cyclophosphamide appeared more effective in a limited number of STSs. Scientific data supporting the efficacy of these protocols in dogs and cats are currently missing.

Metronomic cyclophosphamide chemotherapy and COX-2 inhibitors inhibit angiogenesis and suppress regulatory T cells. It has been suggested that combined therapy might elicit greater inhibition of angiogenesis and tumour growth. Piroxicam, a non-selective COX inhibitor, has been shown previously to elicit significant anti-tumour activity in dogs with transitional cell cancer. Dogs are treated with a two-drug combination consisting of orally administered low-dose cyclophosphamide (10 mg/m^2) and full-dose piroxicam (0.3 mg/kg). In a study by Elmslie et al. (2008), metronomic therapy with cyclophosphamide and piroxicam was very effective in preventing tumour recurrence in dogs with incompletely resected STS. Forty per cent of the dogs in this study developed adverse effects at some point during treatment, but in the majority the adverse effects were minor and were related primarily to gastrointestinal signs (vomiting, anorexia). Ten per cent of dogs in the current study developed haemorrhagic cystitis, a known complication of cyclophosphamide therapy in dogs.

Handy hints

Chemotherapy does not really work for STS. Only one small study looked at metronomic chemotherapy (Elmslie et al., 2008).

10.3 Oral neoplasia

Key points

- Oral tumours are common in the dog and cat.
- Biopsies of all oral tumours are recommended.
- Fifty per cent of canine oral tumours are benign.
- Histopathology can suggest whether surgery is warranted or indicated.
- Most malignant oral tumours will metastasise to the regional lymph nodes and the thoracic cavity.
- Cats do not tolerate oral surgery as well as dogs, and most cats will need a feeding tube of some sort after mandibulectomy or maxillectomy.

10.3.1 General principles

Oral tumours are common in the dog and cat, accounting for 6% of cancers in the former and 3% in the latter (Dorn and Priester, 1976; Hoyt and Withrow, 1984; Patnaik et al., 1975; Stebbings et al., 1989). The incidence of the different tumour types and their behaviour varies between dogs and cats, but surgery remains the mainstay in their treatment. However, many oropharyngeal tumours are best treated with a multimodal approach, including combinations of surgery, radiotherapy, chemotherapy and immunotherapy.

In the dog, the most frequently encountered malignant tumours of the oral cavity are malignant melanomas (31–42% of cases), squamous cell carcinomas (17–25% of cases), fibrosarcomas (7.5–25% of cases) and osteosarcomas (6–18% of cases) (Liptak, 2012). Benign odontogenic tumours are common, although their frequency is hard to estimate. In the cat, the most commonly encountered tumours are SCC (75% of cases) and FSA (7–13% of cases; Liptak and Lascelles, 2012).

Common complaints associated with oral tumours in the dog and cat include: difficulty or reluctance to eat because of oral discomfort; excessive drooling that may be blood-tinged; strong smell from the mouth; lethargy; and weight loss. Frequently there is a history of dental problems, such as loose or 'infected' teeth, which may have resulted from tumour invasion of the alveoli. Physical examination may reveal an oral mass that is visible in the mouth or palpable from the outside of the oral cavity.

The diagnostic evaluation for oral cancers is critical due to the wide ranges of cancer behaviour and therapeutic options available. If cancer is suspected, thoracic radiography/CT can be performed prior to biopsy. The most likely cancers to show positive chest radiographs at the time of diagnosis are melanoma and SCC of the caudal oral and pharyngeal areas. Most animals will require a short general anaesthetic for careful palpation, radiography/CT and biopsy. Appropriate imaging of the local site should be performed with the animal under general anaesthesia. Only when 40% or more of the bone mineral is lost will lysis be observed. However, normal radiographs do not rule out bone invasion (Liptak and Withrow, 2007). If the tumour is fixed to bone it can generally be assumed that there is at least microscopic invasion of the adjacent bone. Regional imaging will assist in determining the clinical stage of cancer and the extent of resection when surgery is indicated. Regional lymph nodes (mandibular and retropharyngeal) should be carefully palpated for enlargement or asymmetry, and these should always be aspirated. This is especially important for melanoma and caudally situated SCC. Some authors have suggested lymph node removal for staging purposes, but there is no evidence that prophylactic lymph node removal for cancer of the oral cavity improves survival rates (Herring et al., 2002; Smith, 1995). While the patient remains anesthetised, a large incisional biopsy should be taken. Oral cancers are commonly infected, inflamed or necrotic, and it is important to obtain a large specimen. Fine needle aspiration or small samples often will not be rewarding and may result in an incorrect diagnosis.

Handy hints

Normal radiographs of the oral bones do not rule out bone invasion.

Malignant melanoma

Malignant melanoma (MM) is the most prevalent canine oral cancer, but is uncommon in the cat (Fig. 10.21a–f). Oral MMs of the dog are locally aggressive, rapidly growing and frequently metastasise (50–80% of cases) to the regional lymph nodes and then to the lungs (Overley et al., 2001; Williams and Packer, 2003). MMs are amelanotic in one third of cases (Liptak and Withrow, 2007) and can therefore not be ruled out in the face of a non-pigmented oral mass. Tumours measuring <2 cm and that have not metastasised to the lymph nodes (stage I) warrant a much better prognosis than large (>4 cm) MMs or those with nodal metastasis (stage III).

Squamous cell carcinoma

Squamous cell carcinoma is the most common oral cancer in the cat, and second most common in the dog (Hoyt and Withrow, 1984; Stebbings et al., 1989). In the dog, SCCs are locally aggressive tumours that rarely metastasise. When present, underlying bone is often invaded (radiographic evidence in 77%) and needs to be resected *en bloc* with the tumour (maxillectomy, mandibulectomy). Tonsillar SCCs have a more aggressive behaviour (Liptak and Withrow, 2007). It is estimated that 90% of tonsillar SCC have already metastasised at the time of diagnosis, although overt evidence of metastatic disease is found in only 10–20% of cases at presentation (Liptak and Withrow, 2007). More generally, rostral oral SCCs (Fig. 10.22a–c) carry a much better prognosis than those situated in the caudal portion of the mouth (base of the tongue (Fig. 10.23), tonsils, pharynx; Evans and Schofer, 1988). In the cat, SCCs are more aggressive than in the dog and local recurrences are frequent after surgical excision (Bostock, 1972; Reeves et al., 1993).

Fibrosarcoma

Oral fibrosarcoma (FSA) is a malignant mesenchymal tumour with a propensity for the palate of dogs and the gingiva of cats. Achieving local tumour control is often challenging, as FSA invades bone and surrounding tissues and may be quite large before noted by the pet owner. These tumours are locally aggressive, but metastasise uncommonly (10–35% of cases) or later in the course of the disease. In the dog, there is often a

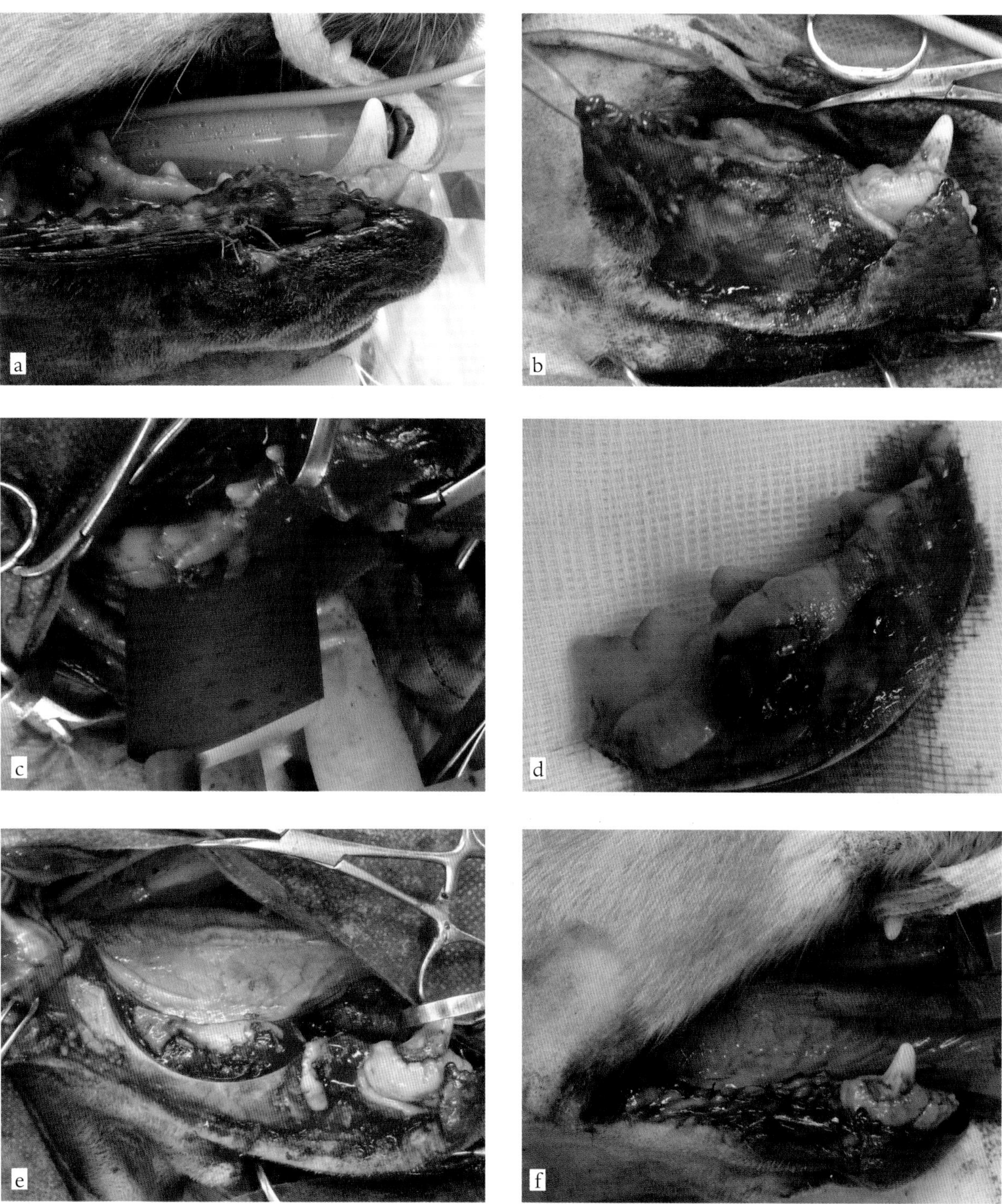

Fig. 10.21a–f Malignant melanoma. a. A 10-year-old golden retriever with a local oral MM confined to the oral mucosa, confirmed by biopsy. No lymph node or thoracic metastases were identified. b. Full-thickness resection of the skin and oral mucosa to the bone. c. A crescentic osteotomy (only locally over the tumour site) with a 30 mm TPLO saw blade. d. Resected tumour. e. Postoperative view after crescentic ostectomy. f. Postoperative view after full-thickness resection of the lip and mucosa and reconstruction.

discrepancy between the grade of the tumour, as estimated by histopathology, and its clinical behaviour (Ciekot et al., 1994). Such tumours are known as 'histologically low-grade but biologically high-grade' or 'high–low' FSAs. These tumours may appear low-grade (fibrosarcoma) or even benign (fibroma) histologically, but clinically they behave as a high-grade fibrosarcoma: they are locally aggressive and metastasise in 10–20% of cases. Therefore canine oral fibromas and FSAs *always* mandate aggressive treatment (Schwarz et al., 1991a,b). There is little information on feline oropharyngeal FSA. Where possible, aggressive surgical resection and radiotherapy is the current recommended treatment protocol.

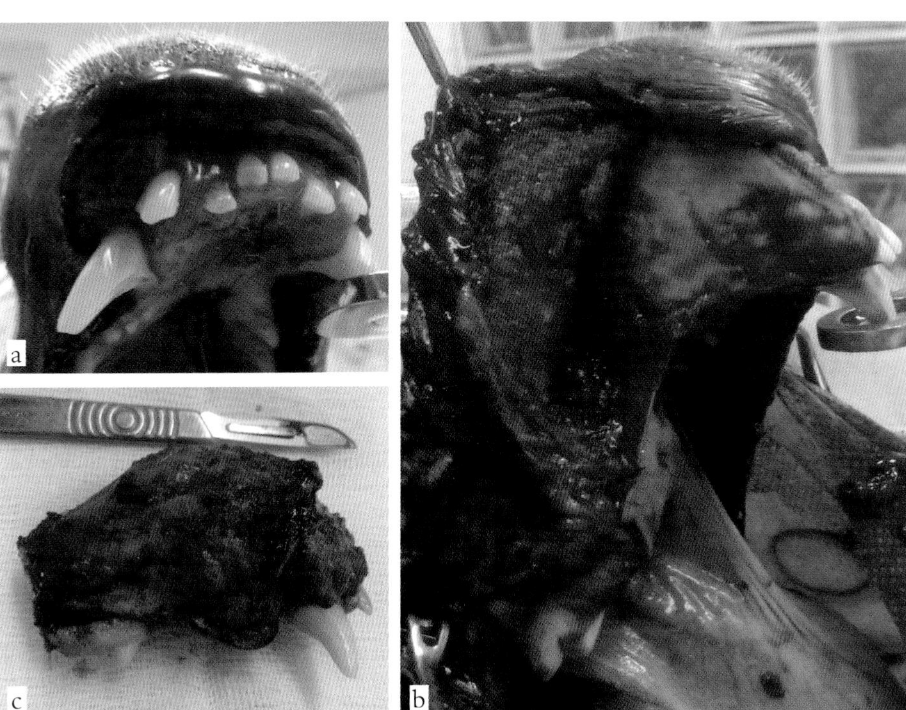

Fig. 10.22a–c Oral squamous cell carcinoma. a. An 11-year-old old crossbreed presented for bleeding from the mouth and halitosis. A rostral mandibular mass was found and biopsied by the referring veterinary surgeon. Squamous cell carcinoma was diagnosed. b. A rostral partial mandibulectomy with clear surgical margins was performed. c. Resected part of the mandible.

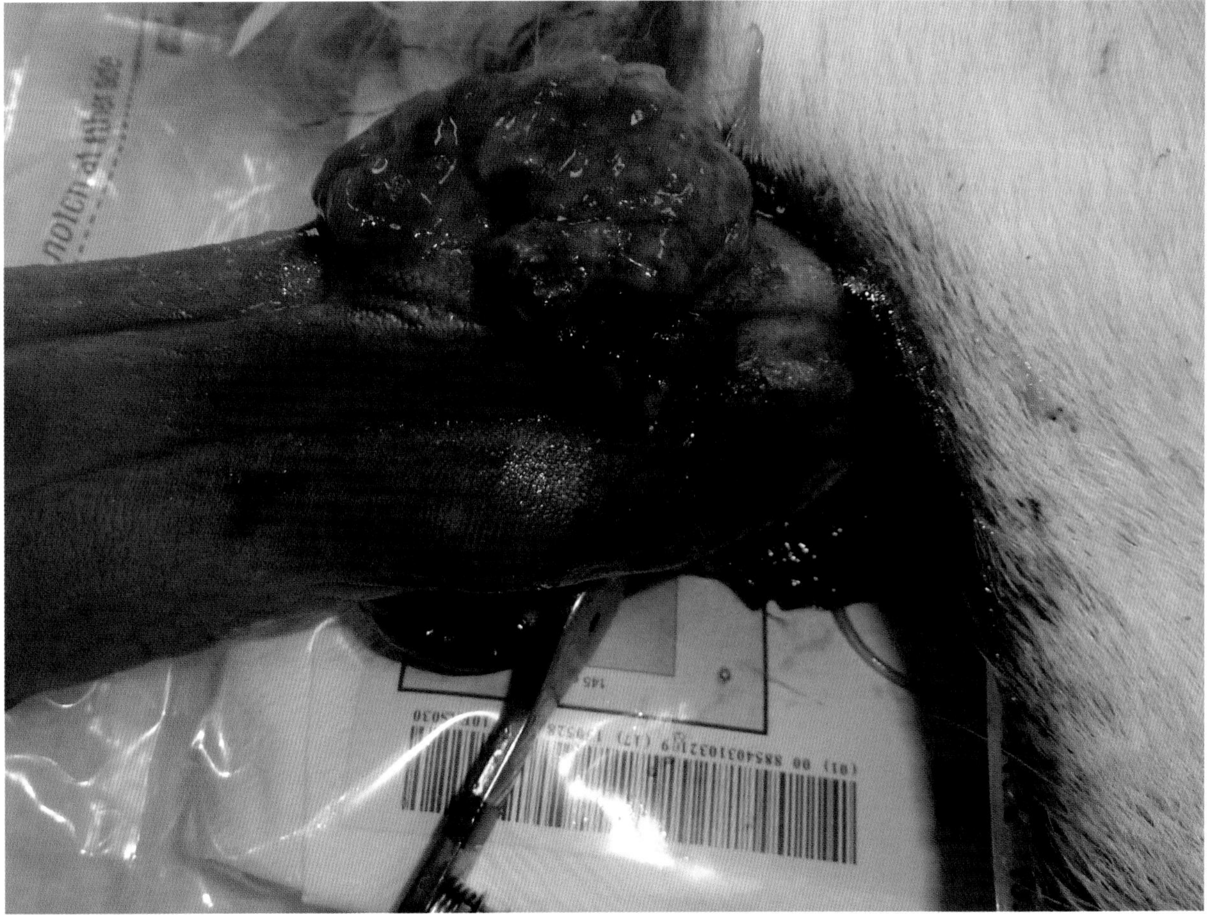

Fig. 10.23 A 12-year-old Labrador retriever was seen for halitosis, bleeding from the mouth, hypersalivation and difficulty in eating. A biopsy of the tongue revealed a squamous cell carcinoma. The mass was lateralised but caudal and, after discussion with the owner regarding palliation of the disease, a partial lateral glossectomy was performed.

Epulides and odontogenic tumours

The term epulis is a non-specific description of a localised swelling of the gingiva. Epulides are either non-neoplastic lesions (fibrous hyperplasia, fibrous epulis or fibromatous and ossifying epulis) or benign odontogenic tumours (Bjorling et al., 1987; Verstraete, 2003). Most types of epulides in the dog and cat can be resected marginally, except for ameloblastoma, amyloid-producing odontogenic tumours and feline inductive odontogenic tumours. Canine acanthomatous ameloblastoma often invades the underlying tissues and has a high recurrence rate if not widely excised (Liptak and Withrow, 2007).

Osteosarcoma

Osteosarcoma of the oropharyngeal cavity is a locally aggressive, invasive neoplasm that has a high local recurrence rate if not adequately treated, and a metastatic potential similar to osteosarcoma arising at other sites (appendicular) (Garrett et al., 2007).

10.3.2 Treatment

Treatment of oral tumours should aim to control the local disease and the potential systemic disease. Most tumours of the oral cavity that are locally invasive require wide excision for optimal local control. Therefore, in spite of major advances in other therapies (chemotherapy, radiotherapy, immunotherapy) (Bergman, 2007; Biller, 2007; Lawrence and Forrest, 2007; Mutsaers, 2007), surgery remains the mainstay in the treatment for most oral tumours. Adjuvant radiotherapy can be considered when full excision cannot be achieved because of the anatomical constraints of the area. In addition, a number of oral tumours such as MM, tonsillar SCC and OSA have a high metastatic potential, mandating systemic adjuvant treatment such as chemotherapy or immunotherapy.

Surgery

The local conditions of the oral cavity, limited availability of loose connective tissues, constant movements and bacterial burden make wound dehiscence a common complication after surgery. However, the use of proper technique limits the incidence of wound dehiscence.

Handy hints

It is recommended not to use electrocautery near the edges of the wound. Incisions using diathermy increase the risk of wound dehiscence. Where cautery is required in the depth of the wound, it is best applied with bipolar forceps to limit the effect on surrounding tissues and decrease vascular damage.

As for any other surgery, respecting tissues and their vascularisation is critical. A good knowledge of the vascular anatomy (e.g. course of the palatine arteries) facilitates resection of oral tumours as well as elevation of mucosal or mucoperiosteal flaps. Such flaps must be elevated minimally to cover the oral defect, in order to minimise vascular injury. During section of bones, the tissues must be constantly irrigated to prevent extensive thermal necrosis.

Brisk haemorrhage is commonly encountered during mandibulectomy and maxillectomy. Blood loss and hypotension have been reported as the most common intra-operative complications with such procedures (Lascelles et al., 2003; Verstraete, 2005; Wallace et al., 1992). In mandibulectomy, the mobility of the mandibles allows haemostasis after each bone section, by exposing the alveolar canal which contains the alveolar mandibular artery and vein. During maxillectomy, significant haemorrhage can be delayed by performing the bone sections in a logical order – cutting the bone that contains a large vessel last (Lascelles et al., 2003).

Closure of oral wounds is made in one or two layers, depending on the estimated risk of wound dehiscence. To reduce the risk of dehiscence, bone tunnels can be drilled to achieve increased holding power of the deeper tissues. Monofilament absorbable 3-0 to 4-0 sutures with swaged round or tapercut needles are recommended.

Handy hints

When performing surgery be aware of the biological behaviour of the tumour type and of the anatomy. You should always be prepared for a blood transfusion, as these patients can have massive haemorrhage.

Maxillectomy and mandibulectomy

Most malignant tumours and ameloblastomas invade bone, and therefore wide excision requires partial maxillectomy or mandibulectomy. Minimal 2 cm bone margins and 1 cm soft tissue margins are required for excision of mandibular and maxillary malignant tumours. Alternatively, in large dogs with small lesions of the lower dental arcade with minimal bone involvement, a more conservative excision technique preserving the ventral cortex of the mandible may be possible (Arzi and Verstraete, 2010; Murray et al., 2010). Mandibulectomy and maxillectomy can be unilateral or bilateral and rostral, lateral/segmental or caudal. Extensive mandibulectomies and maxillectomies are well tolerated in the dog (Lascelles et al., 2003; Liptak and Withrow, 2007; Schwarz, 1991a,b; Wallace et al., 1992; White, 1991). Much less information is available for the cat, but functional recovery has been reported to be much less satisfactory compared with that in the dog (Northrup et al., 2006). Patient selection is paramount in the cat, and owners must be warned about the likelihood of acute and long-term adverse postoperative effects. Owner satisfaction rates >80% after maxillectomy or mandibulectomy in dogs (Liptak and Withrow, 2007) and mandibulectomy in cats have been reported (Northrup et al., 2006).

Postoperative complications are uncommon and include incisional dehiscence, epistaxis, increased salivation, ranula formation, mandibular drift and malocclusion and difficulty in prehending food. Feeding tubes are not usually required for dogs, but are recommended for cats as eating can be difficult for 2–4 months following surgery (Northrup et al., 2006).

Radiation therapy

Radiation therapy is utilised with curative intent for small SCC or for localised tumours with incomplete margins after surgery (Blackwood and Dobson, 1996; Theon et al., 1997). Alternatively, radiation therapy can be used to downstage oral tumours prior to surgery. Response rates are best for SCC, with more moderate responses expected for FSA and MM (Blackwood and Dobson, 1996; Theon et al., 1997). For canine oral MM, coarse fractionation (once weekly) provides similar clinical responses to those with standard fractionation, and permits patients to spend more time at home.

Chemotherapy

The cause of death or euthanasia for small animal patients with oral cancer is often local disease progression rather than metastasis. For this reason, systemic chemotherapy may be less important than localised therapy for improving the clinical outcome of dogs and cats with oral cancer. In the case of canine oral MM, metastatic disease is an important cause of treatment failure but this type of cancer is relatively resistant to standard chemotherapy. Cisplatin, carboplatin and melphalan are reported to provide clinical responses in dogs with oral MM, but response rates are <30% and significant improvement in survival has not yet been demonstrated (Kitchel et al., 1994; Page et al., 1991; Rassnick et al., 2001).

10.3.3 Prognosis

For an equivalent tumour type and grade, rostral tumours are associated with a better prognosis. This is partly due to the fact that they are diagnosed earlier and are more amenable to complete excision. When complete excision can be achieved, the prognosis is better. However, some tumours such as SCC may also have a different behaviour depending on their location, with caudal tumours metastasing more often than rostral ones (Evans and Schofer, 1988; Schwarz et al., 1991 a,b). Tumour size is a clear prognostic factor in animals treated with surgery or radiotherapy. The smaller the tumour, the more likely it is to be completely excised with sufficient margins and the greater the efficacy of radiotherapy (Theon et al., 1997).

Malignant melanoma

The mean survival time (MST) without treatment is 65 days. With surgery alone, the MST is reported to be 5–17 months with 1-year survival rates of 0–35%. The prognosis is better for tumours of <2 cm in diameter (MST 511 days) compared to larger tumours (MST 164 days). With radiotherapy alone, 6–19 months progression-free survival (PFS) times have been reported (Liptak, 2009).

Squamous cell carcinoma

After surgical resection, MSTs of 3–6 months and 57–91% 1-year survival rates have been reported. Canine SCCs are very responsive to radiation therapy, and 7–28 months' PFS are reported after radiotherapy (Liptak, 2009).

In cats, surgery alone has been reported to result in MST of 2 months and in 1-year survival rates of <10% (Reeves et al., 1993). In addition, this tumour is less sensitive to radiotherapy in the cat than in the dog. However, in one study involving seven cats, a combination of surgery and radiotherapy resulted in a median survival time of 14 months (Hutson et al., 1992). Other treatment combinations of surgery, radiotherapy and/or chemotherapy have resulted in MSTs ranging from 2 to 6 months.

Fibrosarcoma

In the dog, surgery alone is associated with MSTs of 9–12 months (Fig. 10.24). Mandibulectomy resulted in 1-year survival rates of 23–50% (Theon et al., 1997; Wallace et al., 1992). Although FSAs are widely regarded as poorly responsive to radiotherapy, 26 months' PFS and 7–45 months' MST have been reported with radiotherapy (Theon et al., 1997). There is little information on feline oropharyngeal FSAs.

Osteosarcoma

After mandibulectomy, MSTs of 6–18 months and 35–71% 1-year survival rates have been reported (Heyman et al., 1992; Kosovsky et al., 1991). After maxillectomy, MSTs have been reported as 4–10 months and 1-year survival rates as 17–27%. Local recurrence is a major concern after surgery, reported in 15–44% of

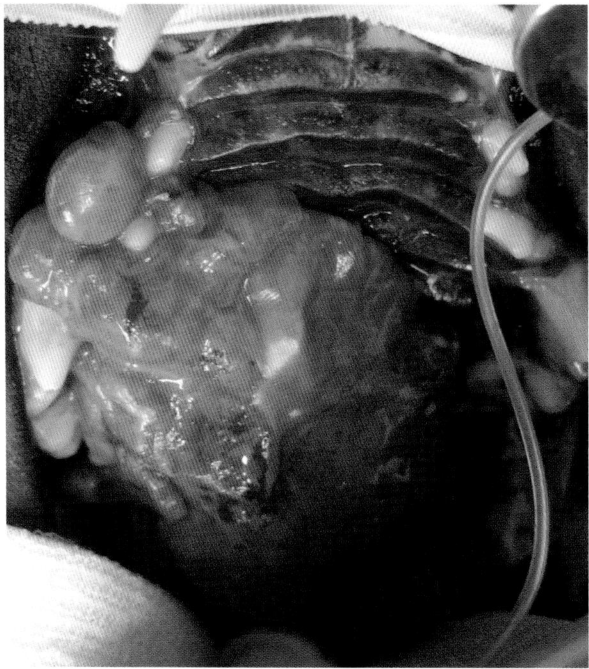

Fig. 10.24 A 13-year-old fit and healthy black Labrador retriever was presented for investigation of a large oral mass on the caudal aspect of the maxilla. A large, erosive, infiltrative mass was found invading the maxilla, zygomatic arch, orbit and palate. The mass was aspirated as oral fibrosarcoma. Local lymph nodes were negative for tumour disease and no distant metastases were found. Unfortunately, due to the extent and invasion of the disease, this tumour was deemed inoperable. Local resection and adjuvant radiation therapy was the proposed treatment plan, but this was declined by the owner.

cases after mandibulectomy and 27–100% of cases after maxillectomy. Many dogs die from failure to control local disease rather than metastatic disease. However, completely excised oral OSA is associated with a fair prognosis (MST >1500 days). On the contrary, incompletely excised oral OSA resulted in an MST of 199 days. An aggressive surgical approach is therefore warranted, especially as the combination of surgery with radiotherapy or chemotherapy has not been found to improve the outcome when oral OSA is incompletely excised (Liptak and Lascelles, 2012; Liptak and Withrow, 2007).

10.4 Gastrointestinal neoplasia

Key points

- Malignant gastric neoplasms are quite rare, but they are locally very aggressive and quickly metastasise.
- Gastric tumours generally develop in the pyloric antrum along the lesser curvature.
- Collies and German shepherds have been shown to have an increased risk for intestinal tumours, particularly adenocarcinoma to develop.
- Only immunohistochemistry can differentiate between leiomyosarcoma and gastrointestinal stromal tumour (GIST).
- Most GISTs are seen in the distal small intestine and large intestine.
- In the cat we should always think of lymphoma and MCT in GI oncology.

10.4.1 Gastric neoplasia

Gastric tumours are uncommon in the cat and dog, comprising only 1% of all malignant neoplasms in these species (Culp et al., 2012; Withrow, 2007). The most common malignant tumours in the dog are: adenocarcinoma, leiomyosarcoma and lymphoma. In the cat, lymphoma is the most common gastric tumour followed by adenocarcinoma. Other tumours reported include MCT, plasmacytoma, carcinoids and fibrosarcoma. Benign tumours include leiomyoma, fibroma and mucosal proliferations. In the dog, adenocarcinoma accounts for 42–70% and is seen in older male dogs (Fig. 10.25a–c; Swann and Holt, 2002). These tumours generally develop in the pyloric antrum along the lesser curvature. Metastatic disease is seen in 76%, with metastases to the regional lymph nodes, peritoneum, liver, spleen, lungs, adrenal glands and pancreas (Patnaik et al., 1978). Ultrasonography is a useful imaging modality combined with FNA (Beck et al., 2001; Rivers et al., 1997). Surgical treatment of gastric adenocarcinoma does not generally yield long-term survival results, because many dogs will eventually have recurrent disease or succumb to metastasis. Survival times are less than three months (Culp et al., 2012; Swann and Holt, 2002; Withrow, 2007).

10.4.2 Intestinal neoplasia

Intestinal cancer is fairly uncommon in the dog and cat (Culp et al., 2012; Patnaik et al.; 1978; Selting, 2007). Most intestinal tumours are in the large intestine (colon and rectum). Particular tumours (e.g. lymphoma) occur more commonly in the small intestine. Four general categories of tumour occur in the intestine: epithelial, smooth muscle (mesenchymal), neuroendocrine and round cell. These include adenocarcinoma, leiomyosarcoma, lymphoma, MCT, GIST, carcinoid and, rarely, plasma cell tumour or haemangiosarcoma (Selting, 2007). The most common intestinal cancer in the cat is lymphoma. Malignant tumours have the potential to spread to many areas of the body, including lymph nodes, and other organs including the liver and lungs. Benign tumours, such as polyps and adenomas, can also occur. Adenomatous polyps are found more commonly in the rectum of dogs and the small intestines in the cat. These benign tumours can be solitary or multiple. Even

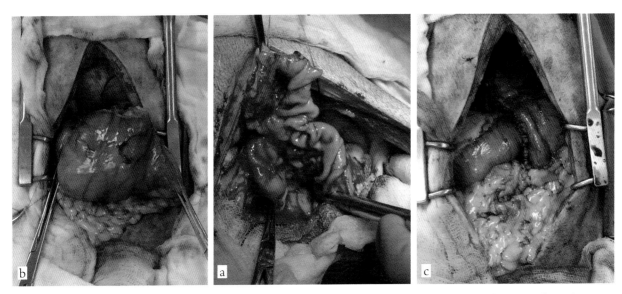

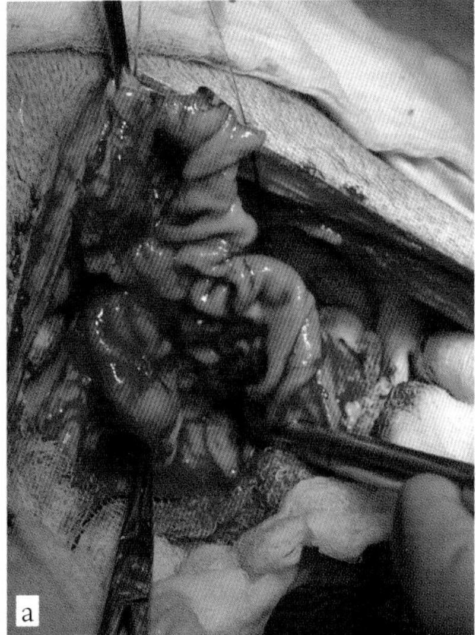

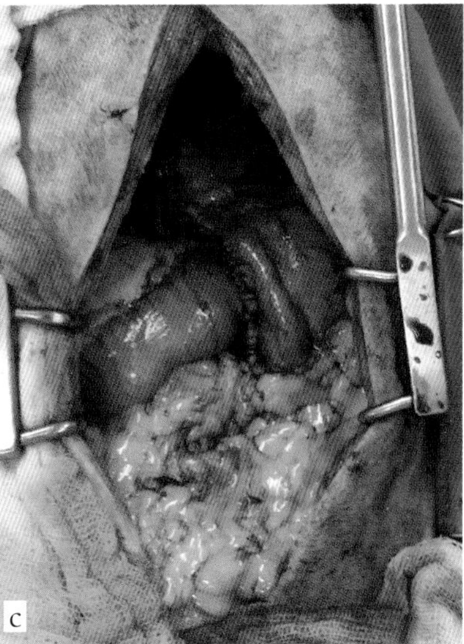

Fig. 10.25a–c Gastric adenocarcinoma. a,b. Necrosis seen in the pyloric area. c. Partial gastrectomy with clear surgical margins was performed, achieving a good medium-term outcome for this patient.

though they are benign, they can cause mechanical problems including obstruction of the intestinal tract.

The majority of animals with intestinal tumours are middle-aged to older. Some research has shown that male dogs and cats have a higher likelihood of being diagnosed with intestinal tumours. Siamese cats have a higher risk for adenocarcinoma and lymphoma, and cats with feline immunodeficiency virus (FIV) or feline leukaemia virus (FeLV) are predisposed to developing lymphoma (Selting, 2007). Certain dog breeds, such as collies and German shepherds, have been shown to have an increased risk of developing intestinal tumours, particularly adenocarcinoma (Patnaik et al., 1978).

Clinical signs usually seen with intestinal tumours include weight loss, decreased appetite, vomiting, diarrhoea and blood within the vomit or faeces. Vomiting tends to occur more commonly in tumours of the small intestine, while diarrhoea or constipation can occur in tumours of the large intestine. An abdominal mass may sometimes be palpated on physical examination. Some tumours can cause blockage (partial or complete obstruction) of the intestinal tract and require immediate medical attention. There may be an accumulation of fluid within the abdomen, causing the abdomen to appear larger than usual. Malignant tumours will cause progressive illness and weight loss, and some may have spread before a diagnosis is made.

Radiography and ultrasound (Fig. 10.26) may be useful in detecting the tumour by finding a mass in the abdomen. In order to further characterise the tumour, it is necessary to obtain a tissue or cytology sample of the tumour itself.

Fig. 10.26 Ultrasound appearance of a mid-jejunal GIST. Segment of jejunum with thickening of the outer layers and appearance of a circular mass without compression or obstruction of the lumen. The mass was extra-luminal but had infiltrated the muscularis and serosa.

Handy hints

Sometimes a needle sample can provide information, but a biopsy is often necessary to make a definitive diagnosis, especially when dealing with a carcinoma or a sarcoma.

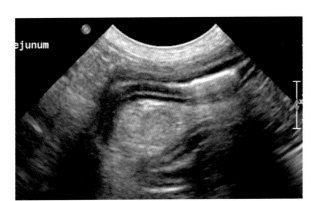

Various types of surgical sampling are available – endoscopic, laparoscopically assisted biopsies and exploratory surgery. However, endoscopic biopsies are not always diagnostic and examination of a larger tissue sample via exploratory surgery might be needed. The advantage of an exploratory surgery is that the entire tumour may be removed as part of an excisional biopsy if deemed resectable.

Treatment for most solid tumours involves surgical removal. Surgery is generally recommended if a tumour is causing obstruction of the intestinal tract or if it has resulted in perforation of the intestine. If the tumour cannot be completely removed during surgery, there is an increased risk for the intestine not healing appropriately. For cancers such as lymphoma, surgery may not be

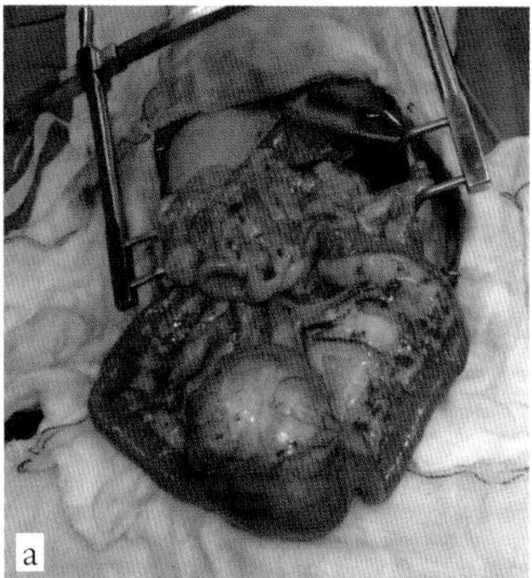

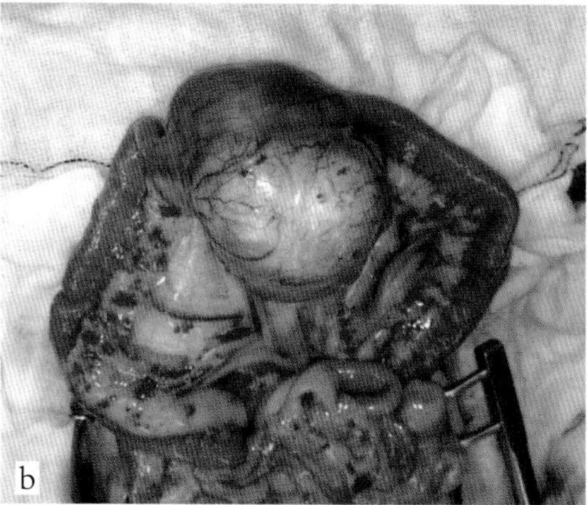

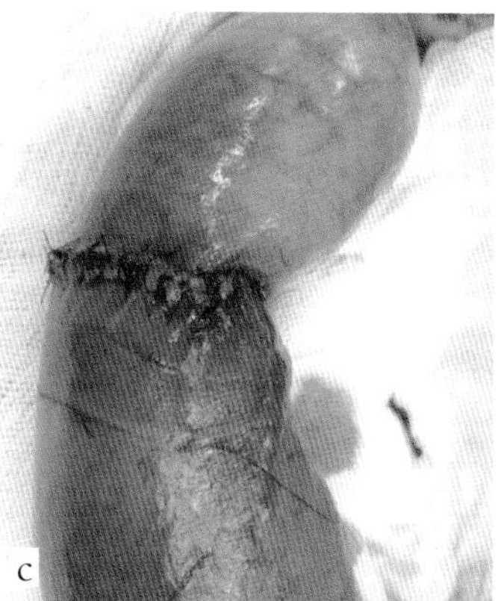

Fig. 10.27a–c A 7 Year old female Golden retriever was seen for acute vomiting and diarrhoea which was followed by inappetence and she stopped eating. The results of routine laboratory tests were unremarkable. Abdominal palpation revealed a 6 cm diameter mass in the mid abdomen. Abdominal ultrasound showed a partially obstructing inhomogeneous mass originating from the jejunum. There was at one area loss of layering of the intestine. The local lymph nodes were not enlarged. CT of the thorax did not reveal any signs of metastases. FNA of the mass was inconclusive. The mass was excised with minimum 5 cm margins and then an end to end anastomosis was performed. The histopathology returned as an enteric adenocarcinoma. The dog survived for 7 months.

recommended if the cancer involves multiple areas and a diagnosis can be obtained through FNA. Instead, this cancer is more commonly treated with chemotherapy.

The prognosis associated with intestinal tumours depends on the specific tumour type and the grade and stage of the tumour. Low-grade tumours, such as caecal GIST (Fig. 10.27a–d), may be effectively treated with surgical resection alone while patients with high-grade intestinal lymphoma have a poor long-term survival despite chemotherapy treatment. Adenocarcinoma is the most commonly treated intestinal tumour in the dog and cat. In the dog, the overall prognosis for surgically treated adenocarcinoma is 7–15 months with localised disease and 3 months with metastasised disease (Crawshaw et al., 1998; Paoloni et al., 2003). Mesenchymal neoplasms of the gastrointestinal tract have recently been divided into GIST and leiomyosarcoma (based on immunohistochemistry; Maas et al., 2007). GISTs have a higher reported rate of perforation, but they have an increased survival time. A median survival time of 37.4 months was reported for dogs with GIST versus 7.8 months for leiomyosarcoma (Russel et al., 2007). Other than for lymphoma, the effectiveness of systemic chemotherapy has not been fully evaluated in the dog and cat for many of the other primary intestinal solid tumours.

10.5 Urogenital neoplasia

10.5.1 Canine mammary tumours

Key points

- Mammary tumours are still frequently encountered in countries where ovariohysterectomy (OHE) or ovariectomy (OE) is not routinely performed.
- The presence of a mass associated with the mammary tissue warrants investigation.
- FNA cytology to differentiate benign mammary adenoma from malignant carcinoma is generally unhelpful.
- 50% of canine mammary tumours are benign.
- Inflammatory carcinomas are rare neoplasms with an extremely poor prognosis.
- OHE when mammary tumours are removed does not have a significant effect on the progression of benign and malignant disease.

Mammary tumours are the second most common tumours in the dog (second to skin tumours; Moulton, 1990). Mammary tumours are still frequently encountered in countries where OHE or OE is not routinely performed on young female dogs that are not acquired for breeding purposes. A number of studies have shown that early OHE protects female dogs from developing mammary cancer in later life. The risk of developing mammary cancer if spayed prior to the first heat is 0.05%, 8% after the first and 26% after the second, compared to intact dogs (Schneider et al., 1969). OHE after four or more cycles or >2.5 years of age has little or no protective effect on the development of malignant mammary tumours (Misdorp, 1991; Schneider et al., 1969; Sorenmo et al., 2000). It is therefore a preventable condition.

Clinical signs

The presence of a mass associated with the mammary tissue warrants investigation. The caudal mammary glands are said to be more frequently involved than the cranial glands, and tumours can present as either isolated lumps or multiples. In the case of multiple lumps, each one must be treated as an individual. Usually, these lumps are non-painful; they may appear and remain static or grow rapidly (Lana et al., 2007).

Cytology

Fine needle aspiration cytology to differentiate benign mammary adenoma from malignant carcinoma is generally unhelpful, due to mixed cell populations within mammary tumours (Allen et al., 1986).

Specific tumours

Benign mammary neoplasms

Approximately 50% of mammary tumours are benign adenomas that are curable with adequate surgery (Brodey et al., 1983; Gilbertson et al., 1983). A large percentage of mammary carcinomas are low grade and carry a fair prognosis with adequate excision.

Malignant mammary tumours

Whilst approximately 50% of canine mammary tumours are benign, between 20 and 40% are considered to be malignant and can arise from different structures within the mammary tissue (Brodey et al., 1983; Gilbertson et al., 1983).

Carcinoma

Mammary carcinoma (adenocarcinoma) is the most common malignant tumour and is variously described as solid, tubular or papillary. These can be simple (epithelium alone) or complex (epithelium and myoepithelium; Lana et al., 2007). The infiltrative characteristics of the tumour, in conjunction with the degree of invasion into local lymphatics and capillaries, is important in determining the long-term prognosis regarding local recurrence and metastatic potential. The most aggressive carcinomas have lost their identifying characteristics and are described as anaplastic or poorly differentiated tumours; the latter warrant a guarded prognosis.

The most common metastatic sites for mammary carcinomas are the draining lymph nodes, followed by the lungs. Bone, liver or brain metastases are less frequent in veterinary compared to human patients (Lana et al., 2007).

Inflammatory carcinoma

Inflammatory carcinomas (Fig. 10.28) are rare neoplasms with an extremely poor prognosis. These tumours can often be identified at the time of presentation. Typically, physical examination reveals a firmly attached mass that is painful, erythematous and warm. It may extend to involve multiple glands and cause oedema of the peripheral limb. These patients are typically in chronic disseminated intravascular coagulation (DIC).

Surgery

Important features are size and invasiveness or adherence. The treatment of choice is surgical excision with appropriate margins. No clinical trial has shown improvement in survival with radical versus local removal.

When mammary tumours are removed, OHE does not have a significant effect on the progression of malignant disease (Morris et al., 1998; Yamagami et al., 1996). One-quarter of dogs with benign mammary

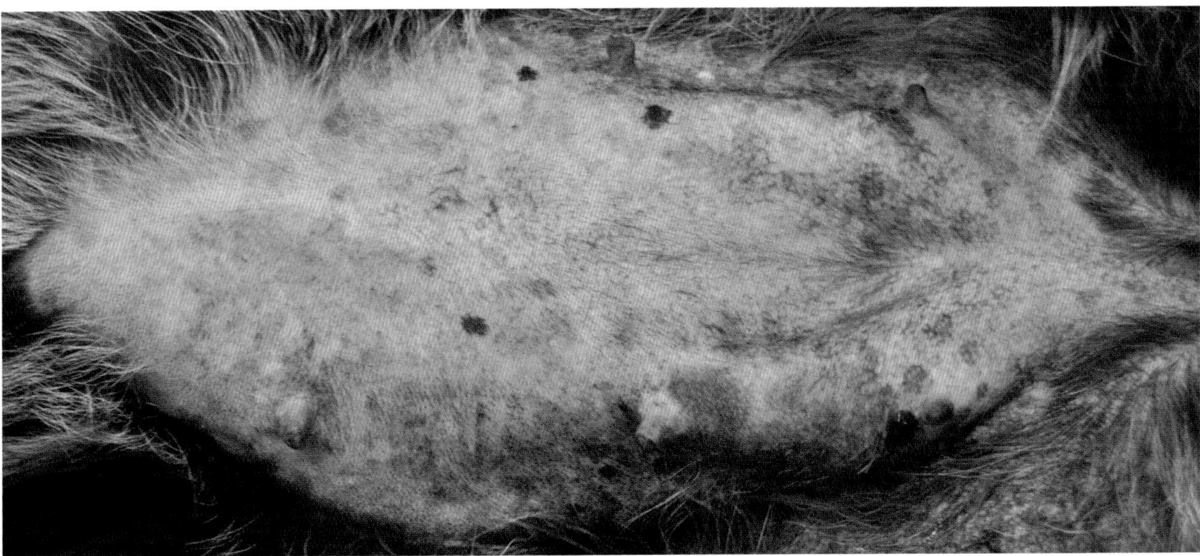

Fig. 10.28 A 13-year-old crossbreed was presented with a 2-week history of inappetance, lethargy and discomfort/pain. The referring veterinary surgeon had been treating for mastitis with antibiotics and NSAIDs. At presentation, the dog was unwell, inappetent and was extremely painful on palpation of the entire mammary chains. A biopsy was taken, which revealed an inflammatory carcinoma. The dog was euthanised 2 weeks later.

tumours developed another mammary tumour within 2 years, whether they were spayed or not (Morris et al., 1998).

Lumpectomy

Lumpectomy is performed for small nodules <0.5 cm that are firm and superficial. Incomplete margins are acceptable for benign lesions but, if malignant, re-excision to achieve clean margins is warranted.

Mammectomy

Mammectomy to remove the whole gland is used for centrally located tumours, >1 cm or with any degree of fixation to skin. Skin and abdominal wall fascia should be removed if involved. For malignant lesions, margins of 1–2 cm of grossly normal tissue are generally adequate.

Regional mastectomy

As above, with several glands removed together for ease of surgery (e.g. glands 1, 2 and 3 together or glands 4 and 5 together). The inguinal lymph node is usually removed *en bloc* with glands 4 and 5. The axillary lymph node is only removed if enlarged or cytologically positive for metastasis.

Unilateral (1–5) mastectomy

Performed to achieve multiple lumpectomies with greater ease and rapidity. It does not improve survival compared with multiple lumpectomies or mammectomies (MacEwen et al., 1985). As 50% of canine mammary tumours are benign, it is important to not perform a 'malignant' surgery for a benign disease. More surgery, if required, can be done later.

Handy hints

In the dog, there is minimal need for a bilateral (radical) mastectomy. There is usually also minimal loose skin to allow this to be achieved with clean margins. A better approach would be to do staged unilateral mastectomies, ensuring that adequate margins are achieved with each surgery.

Bilateral (radical) mastectomy

This entails considerable morbidity, time and money, and does not change survival compared to multiple mammectomies/lumpectomies.

Prognosis

The prognosis for non-invasive carcinoma is very good (Gilbertson et al., 1983). Aggressive carcinomas are seen less frequently but warrant a guarded prognosis (Kurzman and Gilbertson, 1986). Inflammatory carcinomas warrant a very poor prognosis, with a median survival time of 60 days (1–300) for all dogs (Marconato et al., 2009).

10.5.2 Tumours of the vagina and vulva

Key points

- Tumours of the vagina and vulva are seen with greater frequency than tumours of the ovary or uterus (Fig. 10.29).
- Most vaginal and vulval tumours are of mesenchymal origin.
- Surgical resection is complicated by the vascularity of the vagina and vulva, and the neovascularisation that occurs with tumour growth.
- Benign or low-grade mesenchymal lesions in the vagina or vulva have a good prognosis with surgical treatment.

Leiomyomas are typically seen in older (10–11 years) intact females and account for approximately 85% of all vaginal and vulval tumours in the dog (Kydd and Burnie, 1986; Tatcher and Bradley, 1983). Production of oestrogen is associated with growth of these tumours. The malignant variant, leiomyosarcoma, is the most common malignant tumour of the vagina and vulva. Leiomyosarcomas are locally invasive but are slow to metastasise. Other tumours reported in this region include rhabdomyosarcoma, MCT, haemangiosarcoma, squamous cell carcinoma, adenocarcinoma, epidermoid carcinoma, osteosarcoma and transmissible venereal tumours (Klein, 2007).

Clinical signs

These are usually associated with the size and position of the mass, as these tumours can be either extra- or intraluminal. Patients can present with a bulging of the perineum, prolapse of tumour from the vulva, dysuria, stranguria, haematuria, vulval bleeding or discharge, or tenesmus.

Treatment

Surgical resection is complicated by the vascularity of the vagina and vulva, and the neovascularisation that occurs with tumour growth. Blood loss during surgery can be considerable (Nelissen and White, 2012; Bilbrey et al., 1989).

Since leiomyomas, fibromas, polyps, leiomyosarcomas and most other vaginal tumours are hormone dependent, surgical excision of the vaginal tumour should be accompanied by OHE to prevent recurrence.

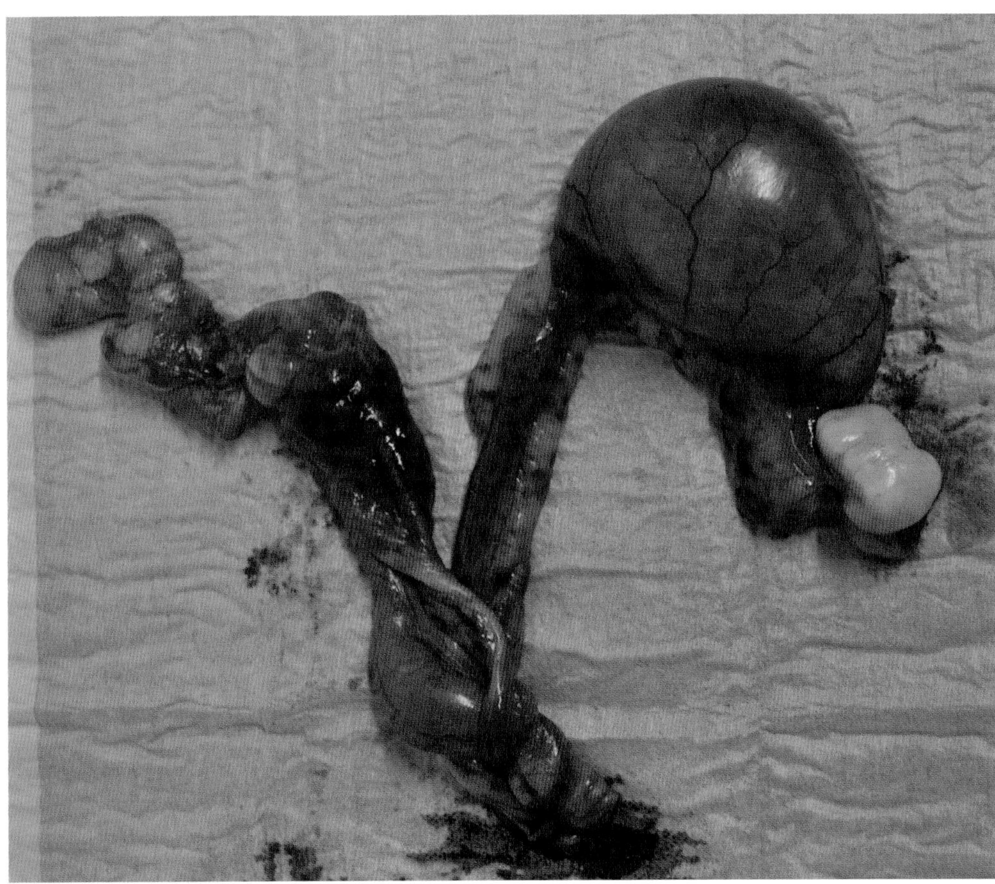

Fig. 10.29 Leiomyosarcoma of the uterus.

Step by step: vaginal tumour removal

- Retroflex the urinary bladder to gain exposure to the vagina and associated structures.
- Resect the fascial and peritoneal attachments between the vagina and the rectum within the rectogenital pouch.
- Dissect the attachment between the vagina and the urethra within the vesicogenital pouch, carefully avoiding any disruption of the craniolateral and dorsal aspect of the urethra and the periurethral tissues.
- Dissect the perivaginal tissues bluntly as far caudally as possible, ensuring that no residual vascular supply or fascial attachment remains intact.
- Assess the surgical site, ensuring that meticulous haemostasis has been achieved.
- Anchor a transfixing 0-polypropylene stay suture with a large loop through all layers of the cranial opening of the vagina; pass the loop of the suture into the vaginal lumen.
- Position the dog in sternal recumbency and perform a midline episiotomy incision.
- Identify the loop of the transfixing stay suture in the vaginal lumen and retract it caudally, withdrawing and inverting the cranial aspect of the vagina to the episiotomy site.
- Make a full-thickness circumferential incision of the vaginal wall at the junction of the vagina with the vestibule immediately cranial to the urethral orifice.
- Appose perivaginal tissues closing dead space.

Handy hints

The surgeon should obtain a packed cell volume and total protein prior to surgery, monitor for intra-operative blood loss and have an ability to provide a blood transfusion if needed.

Prognosis

The prognosis for adenocarcinoma and squamous cell carcinoma is poor, due to metastasis or local recurrence (Nelissen and White, 2012; Withrow and Susaneck, 1986), whereas benign or low-grade mesenchymal lesions have a good prognosis with treatment (Klein, 2007).

10.5.3 Tumours of the lower urinary tract

Key points

- Urinary transitional cell carcinoma (TCC) is diagnosed most frequently in both cat and dog.
- TCC is highly invasive and metastasises frequently.

- TCC is frequently located at the trigone of the bladder or in the urethra.
- Chemotherapy with piroxicam, cisplatin, doxorubicin, vinblastine, chlorambucil or mitoxantrone will generally prolong the life of affected animals.
- Obstruction is generally the main problem for patients with TCC.

Neoplasms of the ureters, bladder and urethra are uncommon in the dog and rare in the cat. The mean age of affected dogs and cats is 9 years (Knapp, 2007). In the lower urinary tract, primary neoplasms are more likely to be malignant than benign. Papillomas, leiomyomas, fibromas, neurofibromas, haemangiomas, rhabdomyomas and myxomas are found infrequently. Among primary malignant neoplasms of the lower urinary tract, transitional cell carcinomas are diagnosed most frequently in both species. Squamous cell carcinomas, adenocarcinomas, fibrosarcomas, leiomyosarcomas, rhabdomyosarcomas, haemangiosarcomas and osteosarcomas are also found (Klein et al., 1988; Knapp, 2007). Transitional cell carcinomas may be solitary or multiple papillary-like projections from the mucosa, or may develop as a diffuse infiltration of the ureter, bladder, prostate and/or urethra. Cystic transitional cell tumours are more common in certain breeds of dog, particularly Scottish terriers, have been associated with prior therapy with cyclophosphamide and may be linked to exposure to herbicides and older-generation insecticides (Knapp, 2007). Transitional cell tumours are highly invasive and metastasise frequently, most commonly to the regional lymph nodes and lungs (Knapp, 2007). Ureteral and bladder neoplasms can cause chronic obstruction to urine flow with secondary hydronephrosis. Urethral tumours are more likely to cause acute obstructive uropathy. Intractable secondary bacterial urinary tract infections are commonly associated with neoplasms of the bladder and urethra.

Clinical findings

Haematuria, dysuria, stranguria and pollakiuria are the most common signs. Animals with ureteral obstruction and unilateral hydronephrosis may show signs of abdominal pain and have a palpable, enlarged kidney. Signs of uraemia may be apparent in animals with bilateral ureteral obstruction and hydronephrosis or with urethral obstruction. The bladder wall may be thickened, and a cord-like urethra or urethral mass may be palpable rectally.

Diagnosis

History and clinical signs are highly suggestive of lower urinary tract disease in animals with tumours of the bladder or urethra. Urinalysis frequently reveals haematuria, and there may be evidence of secondary infection. Chronic, uncomplicated urinary tract infections must be differentiated from those associated with neoplasia. Neoplastic cells may be found in the sediment, particularly with transitional cell carcinomas. A cysto-urethrogram, retrograde urethrogram or ultrasonography is generally necessary to determine the location and extent of the tumour. Biopsy of the tumour is required for definitive diagnosis.

Treatment

Transitional cell carcinomas are frequently located at the trigone of the bladder or in the urethra, and may necessitate radical reconstructive surgery of the lower urinary tract. Prognosis is poor for dogs and cats with TCC even after surgery, due to recurrence and metastasis occurring rapidly. Radiation therapy and/or chemotherapy with piroxicam, cisplatin, doxorubicin, vinblastine, chlorambucil or mitoxantrone will generally prolong the life of affected animals (Bacon and Farese, 2012; Knapp, 2007). Dogs with transitional cell carcinoma, including those being treated for the tumour, are predisposed to development of bacterial urinary tract infections.

10.6 Thoracic wall neoplasia

Key points

- Rib tumours tend to occur in large-breed dogs.
- Rib tumours usually occur in the distal third of the rib adjacent to the costochondral junction.
- Intrathoracic extension and invasion of adjacent pericardium and lung lobes are relatively common (tip of the iceberg).
- Pulmonary metastasis is common with rib osteosarcoma (OSA).
- Rib OSA behaves similarly to appendicular OSA and therefore chemotherapy should be started following surgery.

Rib tumours are uncommon. OSA is the most common rib tumour, accounting for 73% of rib tumours (Martano et al., 2012). Other types of rib tumours include chondrosarcoma, fibrosarcoma and haemangiosarcoma (Martano et al., 2012). There are no breed or sex predispositions, but rib tumours tend to occur in large-breed dogs. Rib tumours usually occur in the distal third of the rib adjacent to the costochondral junction. A palpable firm and fixed mass is the most common presenting sign, although pain and dyspnoea are also reported. Radiographic changes include lysis, sclerosis or a mixture of osteolytic and osteoblastic patterns, with displacement of adjacent ribs and intrathoracic structures, such as the heart and lungs, and medial displacement of the parietal pleura resulting in an extra-pleural sign. Intrathoracic extension and invasion of adjacent pericardium and lung lobes are relatively common. CT scans are recommended to determine the location and extent of the tumour, planning of the surgical resection and clinical staging for pulmonary metastasis. Pulmonary metastasis is common, particularly with telangiectatic OSA, and up to 45% of dogs with rib OSA have metastatic disease at the time of diagnosis. Metastasis is detected in 100% of dogs with rib OSA, 53–57% with CSA, 67% with HSA and 100% with rib FSA at the time of death (Liptak, 2012; Martano et al., 2012).

Surgery

Chest wall resection is recommended for excision of rib tumours. The surgical approach is the same as a lateral intercostal thoracotomy. The caudal and cranial and dorsal and ventral margins are determined from preoperative imaging and intra-operative palpation. Caudal and cranial margins include a minimum of one intercostal space and rib, while ventral and dorsal margins should be a minimum of 3 cm from the tumour (Liptak, 2012; Liptak et al., 2008). Caudal intercostal thoracotomy should be performed first because this permits the easiest evaluation of the intrathoracic extent of the tumour (Martano et al., 2012). The ribs are then transected along the pre-planned ventral and dorsal margins with rib-cutters.

Handy hints

Caudal and cranial margins include a minimum of one intercostal space and rib, while ventral and dorsal margins should be a minimum of 3 cm from the tumour. Start with the thoracotomy caudal to the tumour, as this allows the best evaluation of the tumour extent.

Pericardectomy and lung lobectomy are required if the rib tumour is adhered to the pericardium and lung lobes, respectively. Knowledge of autogenous and prosthetic reconstruction techniques is important prior to surgery, because most resections are large and closure is not simple. Autogenous reconstruction techniques include the latissimus dorsi (Halfacree et al., 2007; Liptak, 2012) and external abdominal oblique muscles, and diaphragmatic advancement following resection of caudal rib tumours (Martano et al., 2012). Prosthetic reconstruction with non-absorbable polypropylene mesh, alone or in combination with autogenous techniques, is recommended for large defects (Liptak et al., 2008).

Chest wall resection is painful, as is the presence of the thoracostomy tube, and analgesia is mandatory to improve comfort levels, recovery time and respiratory effort. Analgesic techniques include intrapleural lidocaine and non-steroidal anti-inflammatory drugs, opioids, NMDA antagonists such as ketamine, and incisional pain-soaker catheters (Martano et al., 2012).

Adjuvant therapy

Due to the similar biological behaviour of rib and appendicular OSA, the former should be treated with rib resection and postoperative chemotherapy. The chemotherapy drugs and protocols are the same as those used for appendicular OSA. The role of chemotherapy in tumour types other than CSA is undefined (Liptak, 2012).

Prognosis

The prognosis for dogs with primary rib tumour depends on tumour type and completeness of excision (Baines et al., 2002). Local recurrence is significantly more likely following incomplete excision, and possible local recurrence significantly decreases median survival times. The MST for dogs with rib OSA is 120 days with surgery alone, and 240–290 days with surgery and adjunctive chemotherapy (Liptak, 2012). The MST is significantly longer in dogs with rib chondrosarcoma treated by surgery alone, and ranges from 1080 to 1750 days to >3820 days (Pirkey-Erhart et al., 1995). Survival times for other tumour types are based on case reports and small case series, ranging from 120–450 days for rib fibrosarcoma and 30–150 days for dogs with rib haemangiosarcoma treated with chest wall resection alone (Liptak 2012).

10.7 Feline-specific oncology

10.7.1 Feline injection site sarcoma (FISS)/vaccine-associated sarcoma (VAS)

Key points

- FISS/VAS are usually rapidly growing masses that develop at sites commonly used for injection.
- The time from last injection to tumour development can be very long.
- Excisional biopsy specimens are contraindicated due to the increased risk for tumour recurrence and decreased disease-free intervals.
- Despite extensive planning and wide or radical margins, local control is still poor with surgery alone for FISS.

Feline injection-site sarcomas primarily arise at sites of vaccination, but have also been associated with administration of injectable lufenuron, microchips and long-acting antibiotics or corticosteroids (Hendrick, 1998; Martano et al., 2011; Srivastav et al., 2012; Vaccine Associated Feline Sarcoma Task Force, 2005). FISSs have been described at locations where non-absorbable suture materials have been used. Varying lengths of latency (four weeks to ten years) between the inciting event and diagnosis of sarcoma have been reported (McEntee and Page, 2001). The diagnosis of FISS starts with signalment, with particular attention given to the injection history. FISSs are usually rapidly growing masses that develop at sites commonly used for injection; although the time from the last injection to tumour development can be very long, once the process is initiated the mass can usually reach several centimetres in diameter within a few weeks. Examination of an incisional biopsy specimen is recommended for suspected FISS. The specimen should be obtained from an easily excised site without further extension of the surgical field (Martano et al., 2011). Excisional biopsy specimens are contraindicated because of the increased risk of tumour recurrence and decreased disease-free intervals and survival times (Davidson et al., 1997; Hersey et al., 2000). Fine-needle aspiration and cytology and small, Tru-Cut biopsy specimens are not recommended as the extensive inflammation found in these tumours can lead to a misdiagnosis of granuloma (Martano et al., 2011). Surgery is an important component of treatment for FISS. As these tumours are poorly encapsulated and extend along and infiltrate fascial planes, referral and advanced imaging are recommended prior to surgery. Tumour volume on CT scans with contrast has been shown to be approximately double that of tumour volume measured with calipers on examination (McEntee and Page, 2001). This underscores the aggressive nature of FISS, as well as the importance of advanced imaging for treatment planning. An aggressive first resection offers the best chance for local control. Current treatment recommendations include surgical margins of 3–5 cm (McEntee and Page, 2001; Morrison and Starr, 2001). Median time of tumour recurrence with marginal excision is only 79 days, compared with 325–419 days following wide excision or radical surgery (Davidson et al., 1997; Hersey et al., 2000). Despite extensive planning and wide or radical margins, local control is still poor with surgery alone. Complete surgical margins are achieved in only 50% of cats with aggressive surgery, and the 1- and 2-year disease-free intervals are 35 and 9%, respectively (Davidson et al., 1997). With the high recurrence rates of surgery alone, radiation therapy is commonly used pre- or postoperatively to increase the disease-free interval of cats with FISS. The use of postoperative radiation therapy offers a median progression-free interval of 37 months. However, recurrence rates are still approximately 40% within one to two years of treatment, even with the use of pre- or postoperative radiation therapy (Cronin et al. 1998; Eckstein et al., 2009; Kobayashi et al., 2002). According to a round table convened by VAFSTF (Vaccine Associated Feline Sarcoma Task Force, 2005), even if a definitive conclusion has not been reached, a multimodal approach, combining wide surgical excision, radiation therapy (in both a neoadjuvant and adjuvant setting) and chemotherapy, is recommended.

3-2-1 biopsy

VAFSTF (Morrison and Starr, 2001; VAFSTF, 2005) recommends obtaining a biopsy specimen of a mass located at the site of a vaccine or injection based on the 3-2-1 rule:

- 3: if the mass has been present for longer than 3 months
- 2: if the mass is wider than 2 cm in diameter
- 1: if the mass increases in size after 1 month.

10.7.2 Feline mammary gland neoplasia

Key points

- 80% of mammary tumours in cats are classified as adenocarcinoma.
- Hormonal influences are involved in the development of mammary cancer in the cat.
- The treatment of choice for tumours without signs of distant metastases is radical mastectomy of the affected side, regardless of tumour size.

Mammary tumours are the third most common tumour type seen in the cat, and they account for approximately 20% of neoplastic lesions in the female cat (Misdorp et al., 1991; Morris, 2013; Simeonov and Simeonova, 2009). These tumours arise from the mammary tissue and are typically malignant (Hayes et al., 1981). Most mammary tumours in cats are classified as adenocarcinoma (Shafiee et al., 2013). Mammary neoplasia often occurs in the middle-aged to older cat, with Siamese cats being at higher risk (Lana et al., 2007; Morris, 2013).

Hormonal influences are involved in the development of mammary cancer in the cat (Morris, 2013). Several studies have found that spayed cats had a 40–60% reduced risk of developing mammary cancer

(Misdorp et al., 1991; Morris, 2013; Overley et al., 2005).

The first sign of this type of cancer may be a fluid-filled or firm lump associated with the mammary gland, or discharge originating from the nipple. These masses do not tend to be painful, but can be associated with increased grooming behaviour if discharge is present.

A biopsy of the affected tissue is needed for making a definitive diagnosis. The majority of mammary tumours in cats are malignant in nature and very likely to metastasise early in the course of the disease. The most common locations of metastasis are the local lymph nodes and lungs (Lana et al., 2007). Prior to any biopsy or treatment, palpation of the local lymph nodes and chest radiography are recommended, to look for evidence of metastasis.

Surgery can be very effective at removing the masses, but the success of surgery is hindered by the invasive nature of the disease. Due to this invasive nature of malignant masses and the tendency of these tumours to metastasise early, the treatment of choice for tumours without signs of distant metastasis is radical mastectomy of the affected side, regardless of tumour size (MacEwen et al., 1984; VanNimwegen and Kirpensteijn, 2012).

This procedure significantly reduces the chance for local regrowth of the tumour. It is important to evaluate the local draining lymph nodes during surgery due to the high risk of cancer spreading to those sites.

Since mammary cancer in the cat typically invades the lymphatic system and spreads to other locations, chemotherapy is recommended following surgery (Lana et al., 2007; MacEwen et al., 1984). Most effective protocols involve the use of doxorubicin alone or in combination with other drugs.

The average survival time for the cat with mammary cancer is variable and depends on several factors including size of the tumour, extent of surgery, grade of the tumour and whether adjuvant therapy has been received. Average survival times ranging from four months to over three years have been reported (Hayes et al., 1981; Lana et al., 2007; MacEwen et al., 1984).

Similar to the situation in women, the use of targeted therapies such as trastuzumab (a treatment that targets certain molecular and genetic defects found in cancer cells) appears to be promising for improving the outcome of treatment in mammary cancer. In veterinary medicine, there are currently two targeted therapies available, Palladia and Masivet. There are currently many research projects focused on targeted therapies.

10.7.3 Feline MCT

Key points

- Over 90% of feline cutaneous MCTs are benign, while visceral MCTs may show a more aggressive biological behaviour.
- Surgery is typically not recommended for the cat with disseminated MCT, unless the spleen is involved.

Mast cell tumours comprise about 20% of all cutaneous tumours in the cat (Miller et al., 1991; Thamm and Vail, 2007). Over 90% of cutaneous MCTs in cats are benign, while visceral MCTs may behave more aggressively (Carpenter et al., 1987). This disease is seen mostly in middle-aged cats, and Siamese cats appear to be predisposed for cutaneous MCT (Miller et al., 1991).

The actual cause of MCT is unknown. A genetic predisposition has been proposed due to the high incidence in the Siamese cat. Mutations in certain genes (such as c-KIT) have been studied extensively, although a specific cause of this mutation has not been isolated.

Cats with the visceral or disseminated form of MCT may show signs of systemic illness. They can be depressed, anorexic and show weight loss and vomiting. This visceral type is much more common in the cat in comparison to the dog (Carpenter et al., 1987).

Surgery is the treatment of choice for cats with the cutaneous form of MCT (providing there are not too many MCTs for the surgeon to remove), since most of these tumours are benign and surgical removal is likely to be curative.

Surgery is typically not recommended for cats with disseminated MCT, unless the spleen is involved. It has been shown that cats with splenic MCT usually benefit from removal of the spleen, even when there is extensive disease such as bone marrow involvement.

Relatively little is known about the effectiveness of non-surgical therapy for cutaneous MCT in the cat. Responses to certain chemotherapy medications have been reported and are typically recommended for cats with the malignant form of MCT (Thamm and Vail, 2007).

Novel therapy with small-molecular targeting drugs has shown great promise in fighting MCT in the cat. Drugs which block histamine receptors (such as cyproheptadine and famotidine) can reduce clinical signs of inflammation or stomach ulceration. Steroids are also useful for decreasing the inflammation associated with these tumours.

Many cats with the cutaneous form of MCT can do very well for years with appropriate therapy. Cats with the visceral form of MCT (spleen, intestine, liver) typically do worse than those with the skin form, although the use of combination therapies (surgery, chemotherapy and TKIs) are allowing many cats to live well over a year.

The combination of small-molecule inhibitors (e.g. Palladia and Masivet) are now being used more frequently in the cat.

10.7.4 Feline oral squamous cell carcinoma

Key points

- Squamous cell carcinoma (SCC) is the most common oral tumour in the cat.
- Surgery is the treatment of choice, but can be very difficult due to the aggressiveness and invasiveness of this tumour type.
- Surgery may be curative if the tumour is located rostrally.
- Radiation therapy or chemotherapy alone are generally ineffective in the management of most cats with oral SCC.

Squamous cell carcinoma is the most common oral tumour in the cat (Liptak, 2012; Liptak and Withrow, 2007). Oral SCC can be extremely invasive, but does not tend to metastasise very rapidly. According to research, the risk of developing oral SCC may increase significantly with the use of flea collars, high intake of canned food (especially canned tuna fish) and exposure to household tobacco smoke (Liptak, 2007). Most cats present with a mass in the mouth that may be ulcerated; they may experience increased salivation, dropping food out of the mouth when eating, facial swelling, weight loss, bad breath, pain and/or a bloody nose.

Even though SCC in the cat tends to have a low rate of metastasis, it is important to evaluate the local lymph nodes and the lungs for metastasis prior to starting any therapy. Surgery is the treatment of choice, but it can be very difficult due to the aggressiveness and invasiveness of this tumour type. If the tumour is located in the lower jaw and in the front of the mouth, it can be fairly easy to remove and most cats will have a good quality of life postoperatively. If the mass is located anywhere else in the mouth, the surgery can be much more difficult and a feeding tube might need to be placed temporarily to maintain adequate nutritional intake (Northrup et al., 2006).

Radiation therapy or chemotherapy alone is generally ineffective in the management of most cats with oral SCC. However, the combination of radiation therapy with certain types of chemotherapy can improve the response rate, quality of life and overall survival time. Local disease eventually becomes very difficult to control and is the most challenging problem with this disease. Cats with rostral mandibular SCC undergoing aggressive surgery tend to have the longest survival times. A median survival time of 3 months has been reported if oral SCC is left untreated (Liptak and Withrow, 2007).

10.7.5 Basal cell carcinoma

Basal cell carcinoma usually presents as a solitary growth that may or may not be pigmented and may occasionally ulcerate. It can occur in clusters. Basal cell tumours can be found almost anywhere in the cat, and are especially common on the face, back and upper chest areas. Most feline basal cell tumours are benign and therefore do not spread, but they still should be removed. Persian cats are predisposed to developing a malignant form of basal cell skin cancer; any bumps on a Persian should be taken seriously.

10.7.6 Squamous cell carcinoma

Squamous cell carcinoma is a malignant neoplasm arising from squamous epithelium. The skin, oral cavity and digits are the most common sites of SCC in the dog and cat (Meuten, 2002). SCCs account for 15% of skin tumours in the cat (Miller et al., 1991). Two forms of SCC *in situ* have been reported in the dog and cat: solar keratosis and multicentric SCC (MSCC) *in situ*. The lesions of solar keratosis are usually singular and range from an erythematous, scaly thickening of the skin to shallow, crusting lesions. They occur on lightly haired, non-pigmented skin and are associated with ultraviolet (UV) light exposure (Withrow and Vail, 2006). With time and continued exposure to UV light, most solar keratosis lesions can progress to SCC. MSCC, similar to Bowen's disease in the human, presents as multiple plaque-like or papillary lesions on pigmented, haired skin and is not related to UV light exposure. MSCC is rare in the cat.

Squamous cell carcinoma, also called epidermoid carcinoma, typically presents as ulcerated, crusty, weeping, necrotic, non-healing cauliflower-like or hard flat growths. They tend to show up on a cat's ear tips (Fig. 10.30a,b), lips, nose (Fig. 10.31a,b), eyelids or mouth. They can be exacerbated by exposure to sunlight, especially in white or very lightly pigmented cats with pink skin. Complete surgical excision is the treatment of choice; radiation is helpful if the masses can't be successfully removed. Plesiotherapy involves the topical application of a radiation source to the target lesion. Because topical radiation doses drop off significantly beyond a depth of 2 mm, the use of plesiotherapy is limited to superficial or incompletely excised

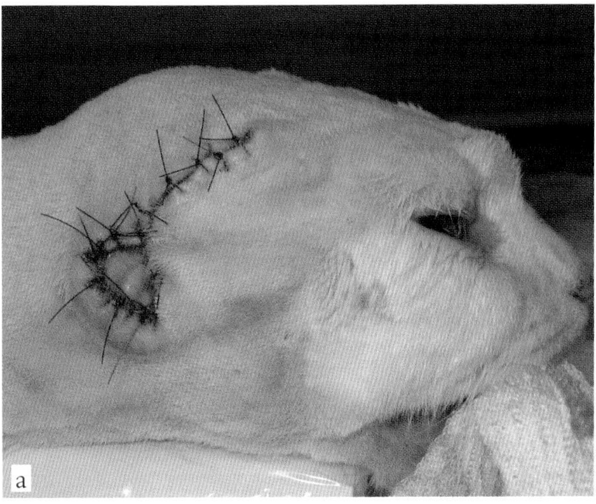

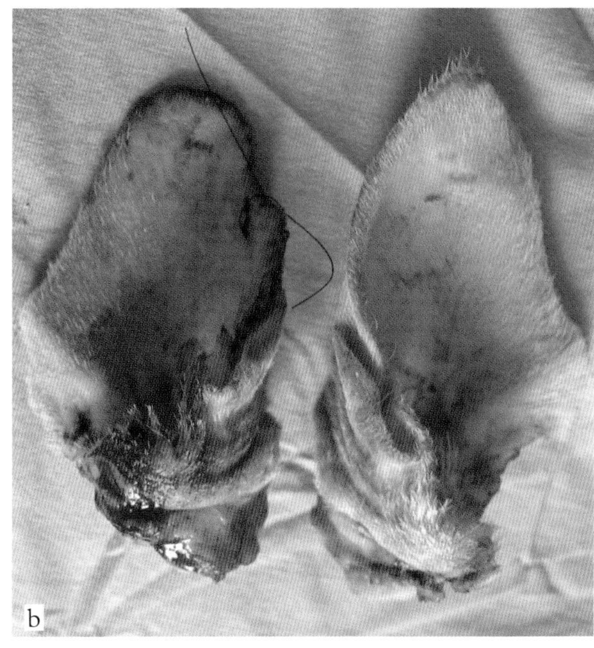

Fig. 10.30a,b 15-year-old cat with irregular changes on the tips of both pinnae. Fine needle aspiration confirmed SCC. Bilateral complete pinnectomy was performed.

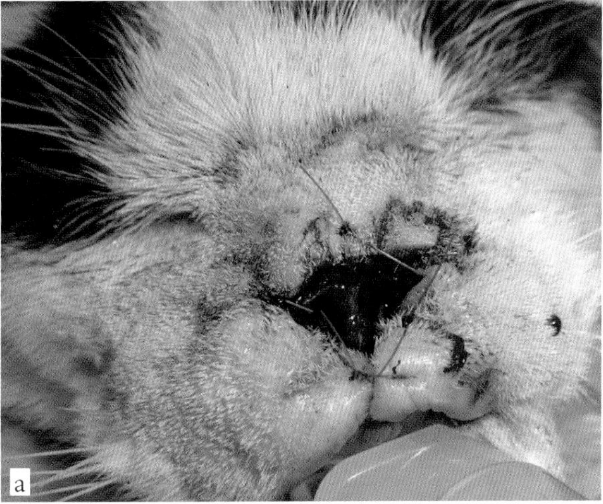

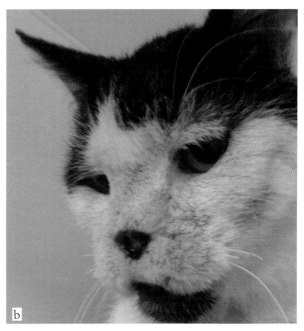

Fig. 10.31a,b 13-year-old cat with a nasal SCC. A total nasal planum resection was performed.

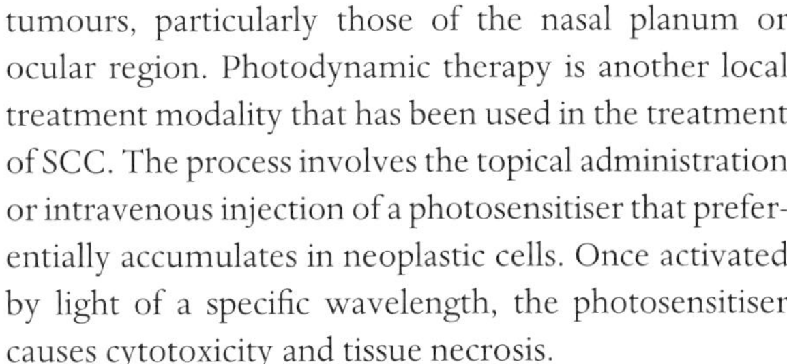

tumours, particularly those of the nasal planum or ocular region. Photodynamic therapy is another local treatment modality that has been used in the treatment of SCC. The process involves the topical administration or intravenous injection of a photosensitiser that preferentially accumulates in neoplastic cells. Once activated by light of a specific wavelength, the photosensitiser causes cytotoxicity and tissue necrosis.

References

Allen, S.W., Prasse, K.W. and Mahaffey, E.A. (1986) Cytologic differentiation of benign from malignant canine mammary tumours. *Veterinary Pathology* 40, 326–331.

Arzi, B. and Verstraete, F.J. (2010) Mandibular rim excision in seven dogs. *Veterinary Surgery* 39, 226–231.

Bacon, N.J. and Farese, J.P. (2012) Urinary tract. In: Knudig S.T. and Seguin B. (eds) *Veterinary Surgical Oncology*. Wiley-Blackwell, Chichester, UK, pp. 365–383.

Baines, S.J., Lewis, S. and White, R.A. (2002) Primary thoracic wall tumours of mesenchymal origin in dogs. A retrospective study of 46 cases. *Veterinary Record* 150, 335-339.

Banks, T., Straw, R.C., Thomson, M. and Powers, B. (2004) Soft tissue sarcomas in dogs: a study correlating optimal surgical margin with tumour grade. *Australian Veterinary Practitioner* 34, 158–163.

Beck, C., Slocombe, R.F., O'Neill, T. and Holloway, S.A. (2001) The use of ultrasound in the investigation of gastric carcinoma in a dog. *Australian Veterinary Journal*. 79, 332–334.

injection-site sarcomas in cats. *Journal of the American Veterinary Medical Association* 241, 595–602.

Stanclift, R.M. and Gilson, S.D. (2008) Evaluation of neoadjuvant prednisolone administration and surgical excision in the treatment of cutaneous mast cell tumours in dogs. *Journal of the American Veterinary Medical Association* 232, 53–62.

Stebbings, K.E., Morse, C.C. and Goldschmidt, M.H. (1989) Feline oral neoplasia: a ten year survey. *Veterinary Pathology* 26, 121–128.

Stefanello, D., Avallone, G. and Ferrari, R. (2011) Canine cutaneous perivascular wall tumours at first presentation: clinical behaviour and prognostic factors in 55 cases. *Journal of Veterinary Internal Medicine* 25, 1398–1405.

Stockhaus, C., Schoon, H. and Grevel, V. (2003) The value of cytology in the diagnosis of soft tissue sarcoma in the dog and cat. *Tierarztliche Praxis Ausgabe Kleintiere Heimtiere* 31, 148–155.

Swann, H.M. and Holt, D.E. (2002) Canine gastric adenocarcinoma and leiomyosarcoma: a retrospective study of 21 cases and literature review. *Journal of the American Animal Hospital Association* 38, 157–164.

Tatcher, C. and Bradley, R.I. (1983) Vulvar and vaginal tumours in the dog: a retrospective study. *Journal of the American Veterinary Medical Association* 183, 690–692.

Thamm, D.H. and Vail, D.M. (2007) Mast cell tumours. In: Withrow, S.J. and Vail, D.M. (eds) *Small Animal Clinical Oncology*. Saunders-Elsevier, St Louis, Missouri, pp. 402–424.

Thamm, D.H., Mauldin, E.A. and Vail, D.M. (1999) Prednisolone and vinblastin chemotherapy for canine mast cell tumour – 41 cases (1992–1997). *Journal of Veterinary Internal Medicine* 13, 491–497.

Theon, A.P., Rodriguez, C. and Griffey, S. (1997) Analysis of prognostic factors and patterns of failure in dogs with periodontal tumours treated with megavoltage irradiation. *Journal of the American Veterinary Medical Association* 210, 785–788.

Turrell, J.M., Kitchell, L.M., Miller, L.M. and Theon, A. (1988) Prognostic factors for radiation treatment of mast cell tumours in 85 dogs. *Journal of the American Veterinary Medical Association* 8, 936–940.

Vaccine-Associated Feline Sarcoma Task Force (2005) Roundtable discussion. The current understanding and management of vaccine-associated sarcomas in cats. *Journal of the American Veterinary Medical Association* 226, 1821–1842.

VanNimwegen, S. and Kirpensteijn, J. (2012) Specific disorders – neoplastic skin disorders. In: Tobias, K.M. and Johnston, S.A. (eds) *Veterinary Surgery: Small Animal*. Elsevier Saunders, St. Louis, Missouri, pp. 1303–1339.

Verstraete, J.M. (2003) Oral pathology. In: Slatter, D. (ed.) *Textbook of Small Animal Surgery*. Saunders, Philadelphia, Pennsylvania, pp. 2638–2651.

Verstraete, F.J. (2005) Mandibulectomy and maxillectomy. *Veterinary Clinics of North America: Small Animal Practice* 35, 1009–1039.

Wallace, J., Matthiesen, D.T. and Patnaik, A.K. (1992) Hemimaxillectomy for the treatment of oral tumours in 69 dogs. *Veterinary Surgery* 21, 337–341.

Webster, J.D., Kiupel, M. and Kaneene, J.B. (2004) The use of KIT and tryptase expression patterns as prognostic tools for canine cutaneous mast cell tumours. *Veterinary Pathology* 41, 371–377.

Welle, M.M., Rohrer-Bley, C. and Howard, J. (2008) Canine mast cell tumours: a review of the pathogenesis, clinical features, pathology and treatment. *Veterinary Dermatology* 19, 321–339.

White, R.A. (1991) Mandibulectomy and maxillectomy in the dog: long term survival in 100 cases. *Journal of Small Animal Practice* 32, 69–74.

Williams, L.E. and Packer, R.A. (2003) Association between lymph node size and metastasis in dogs with oral malignant melanoma. *Journal of the American Veterinary Medical Association* 222, 1234–1236.

Withrow, S.J. (2001a) Surgical oncology. In: Withrow, S.J. and MacEwan, E.G. (eds) *Small Animal Clinical Oncology*. Saunders, Philadelphia, Pennsylvania, pp. 70–76.

Withrow, S.J. (2001b) Biopsy principles. In: Withrow, S.J. and MacEwan, E.G. (eds) *Small Animal Clinical Oncology*. Saunders, Philadelphia, Pennsylvania, pp. 63–69.

Withrow, S.J. (2007) Gastric cancer. In: Withrow, S.J. and Vail, D.M. (eds) *Small Animal Clinical Oncology*. Saunders, Philadelphia, Pennsylvania, pp. 480–483.

Withrow, S.J. and Susaneck, S.J. (1986) Tumours of the canine female reproductive tract. In: Morrow, D.A. (ed.) *Current Therapy in Theriogenology*. Saunders, Philadelphia, Pennsylvania, pp. 356–372.

Withrow, S.J. and Vail, D.M. (2006) *Small Animal Clinical Oncology*, 4th edn. Saunders, Philadelphia, Pennsylvania.

Yamagami, T., Kobayashi, T. and Takahashi, K. (1996) Influence of ovariectomy at the time of mastectomy on the prognosis for canine malignant mammary tumours. *Journal of Small Animal Practice* 37, 462–464.

Case 10.1 Mast cell tumour

An 8-year-old black Labrador was presented with an acute, fast-growing non-ulcerative mass on the lateral aspect of the left pararectal fossa, lateral to the tail and overlying the ischium. The dog clinically had no other symptoms.

A fine needle aspirate was taken and this revealed mast cells.

Routine haematology and biochemistry revealed no significant abnormalities. Abdominal ultrasound was performed and no enlarged regional lymph node enlargement was found. The liver appeared normal. The spleen had several hypo-echogenic nodules. The remainder of the abdominal organs were normal.

Needle aspirates of the spleen were obtained. No increased numbers in mast cells were found, and the cytology of the spleen was consistent with extramedullary haematopoiesis. No other abnormalities were detected and, in light of the position of the mass and the cytological diagnosis of a mast cell tumour, surgery was advised.

At surgery a wide resection was performed (Figs. 10.32–10.36). Lateral margins of 2–3 cm were allowed, and one to two deep fascial planes or muscle planes were resected.

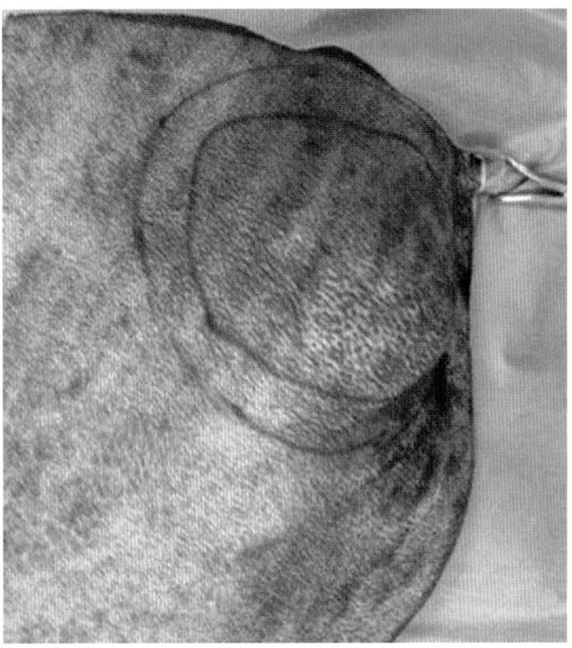

Fig. 10.32 A skin marker was used to plan surgical resection of the mass.

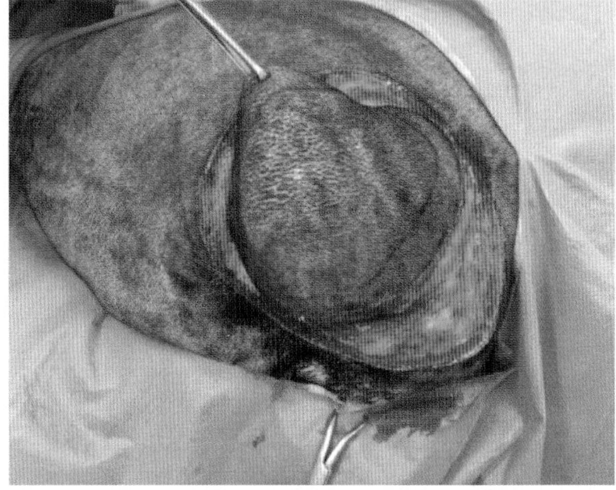

Fig. 10.33 Full-thickness skin incision allowing 3 cm lateral margins.

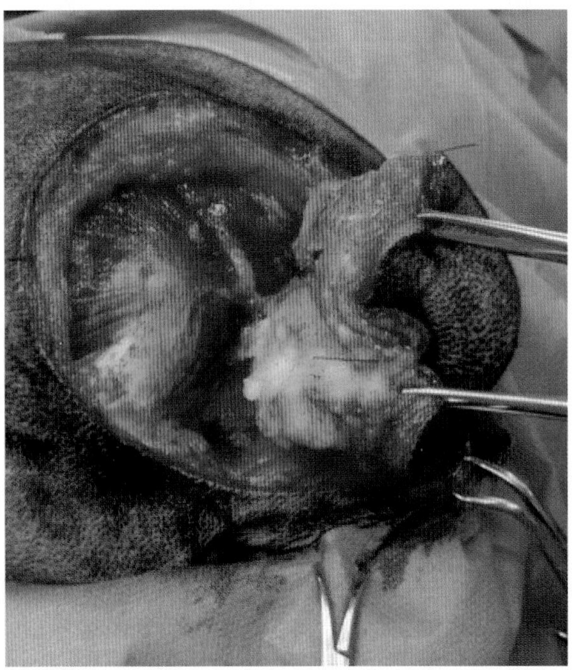

Fig. 10.34 Tumour resection including one fascial plane.

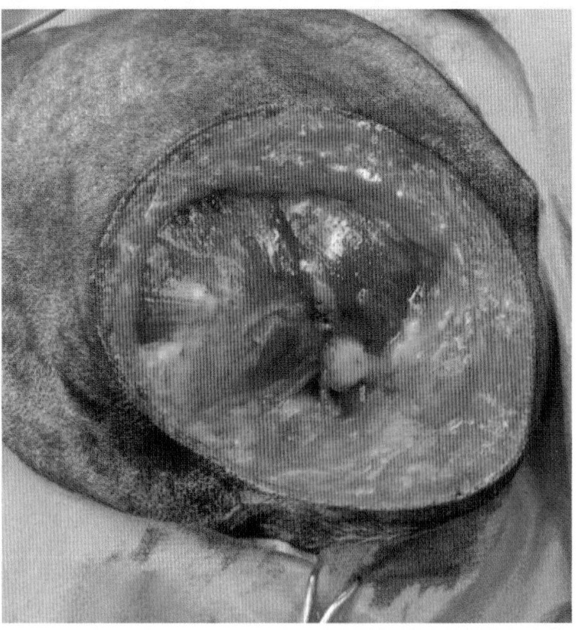

Fig. 10.35 Defect after tumour resection.

Histology of the mass returned as follows.

MICROSCOPIC FINDINGS: Haired skin (4 sections): expanding the subcutis there is a well-demarcated, unencapsulated nodule that is composed of round cells arranged in sheets, supported by abundant fibrous stroma. Neoplastic cells are round, with distinct cell margins and abundant cytoplasm containing numerous granules, and the nucleus is round, vesicular, with finely stippled chromatin and indistinct nucleolus. Anisocytosis and anisokaryosis are moderate. The mitotic rate is <1 per 10 HPFs. Numerous eosinophils are present throughout. The mass is completely excised with good lateral margins (>10 mm) and deep margin (10 mm). DIAGNOSIS: Haired skin: cutaneous mast cell tumour, intermediate grade Patnaik/low grade Kiupel. COMMENT: This is a well-differentiated mast cell tumour. Complete excision is achieved and there is no indication of satellite spread in the sections examined.

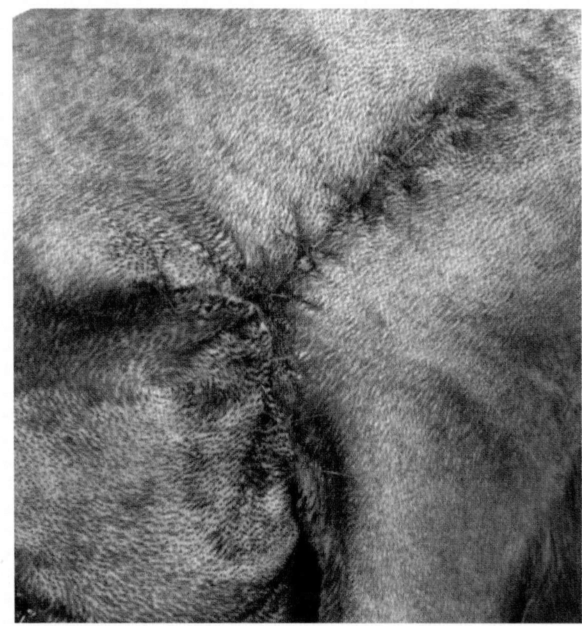

Fig. 10.36 Closure of the defect in a triangular shape.

Case 10.2 Soft tissue sarcoma

Presentation: a 2-year-old golden Labrador. Clinical examination revealed a soft tissue mass on the left lateral aspect of the maxilla, bordering the nasal planum rostrally and extending over the nasal bone laterally caudal to the eye (Fig. 10.37).

Cytology: The cellularity is very low and the preservation is poor, most of the cells being disrupted and lysed. There are only low numbers of small drops of specimen. The background contains a small amount of blood. Low numbers of lysed mesenchymal cells are found. These show variable to moderate anisokaryosis. The nuclei are oval, occasionally folded and the chromatin is finely stippled. Multiple small, round and poorly distinct nucleoli are seen. The cytoplasm, when present, is light basophilic and has ill-defined margins. Interpretation: Poorly representative sample – mesenchymal proliferation.

Surgery: a left lateral and intra-oral approach to the nasal bone and maxilla was made. The tumour was resected with 0.5–1 cm margins in all directions (Figs. 10.38–10.40).

Histopathology: present within the subcutaneous tissues of these sections of haired skin, and to deep margins, is a locally infiltrative, densely cellular, multi-nodular neoplastic mass. Neoplastic cells are arranged in short interlacing streams and bundles and storiform patterns supported by small amounts of collagenous stroma. Individual neoplastic

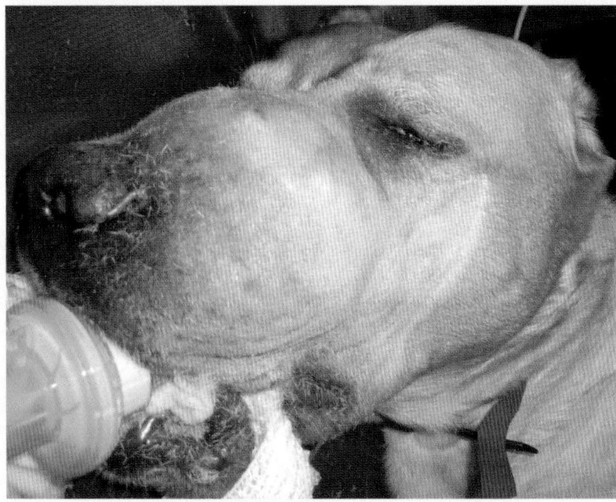

Fig. 10.37 A 2-year-old Labrador presented with a swelling over the left nasal and maxillary bone.

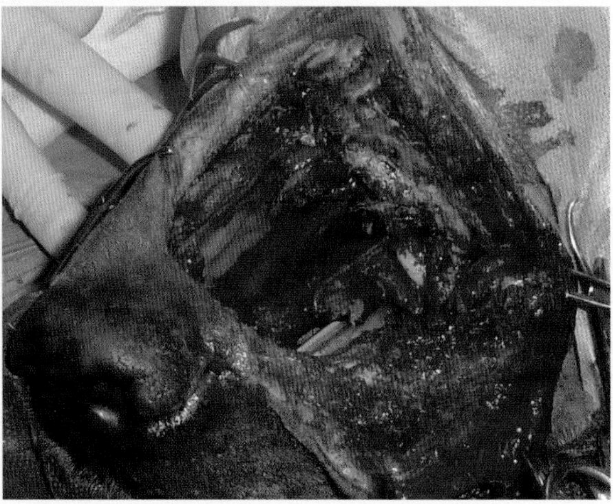

Fig. 10.38 Intra-operative view: resection of tumour, nasal bone and maxilla.

cells are spindle-shaped, contain moderate amounts of eosinophilic cytoplasm and have indistinct cell borders. Nuclei are oval to elongated oval and contain lightly stippled chromatin with 1–2 small nucleoli. Mitoses are 32 per 10 high-power field. Scattered apoptotic neoplastic cells are present and occasional areas of necrosis are present within the mass presenting <10% of the total tissue area. Histological diagnosis: soft tissue sarcoma, high-grade, mass on left side of nose. This mass represents a soft tissue sarcoma that is most likely of fibroblast or nerve sheath origin.

Follow up: This patient had four fractions of radiation therapy 4 weeks after surgery, and this was followed with metronomic chemotherapy.

Outcome: unfortunately there was recurrence of the mass within 6 months following surgery, and the patient was euthanised.

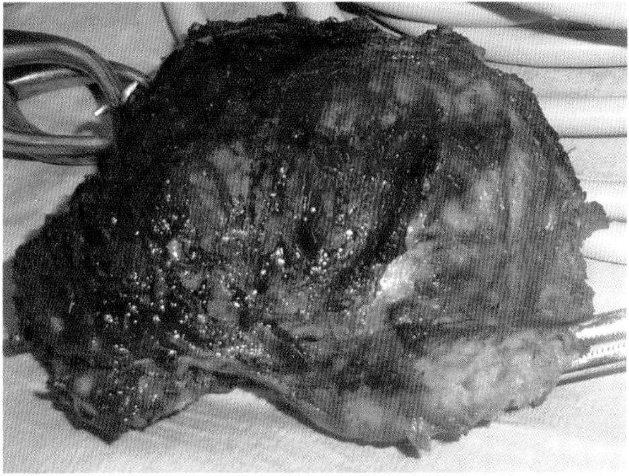

Fig. 10.39 Complete tumour resection (with clear surgical margins).

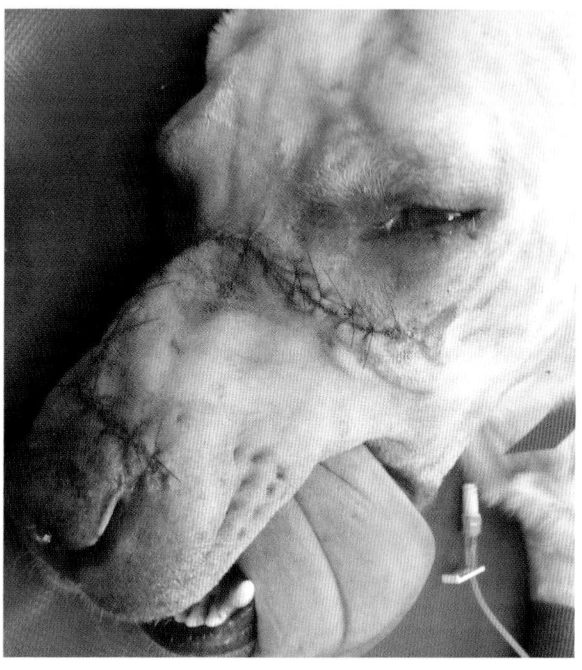

Fig. 10.40 Immediate postoperative view after resection of nasal bone and maxilla.

Case 10.3 Radiation therapy following planned surgical resection of soft tissue sarcoma on the leg

An 11-year-old lurcher was seen after three surgical attempts over the past year had been made to resect a low-grade soft tissue sarcoma (STS) (Fig. 10.41).

Each time the mass had been marginally resected.

At presentation the patient was in excellent condition.

Routine haematology and biochemistry were unremarkable except for mildly elevated urea.

Thoracic radiographs were unremarkable, with no signs of metastases.

It was discussed that a wide surgical resection would not be able to be performed and that the tumour would only be marginally resected, followed by radiation therapy (Figs. 10.42, 10.43).

Six months following surgery and radiation therapy, there were no signs of complications or recurrence.

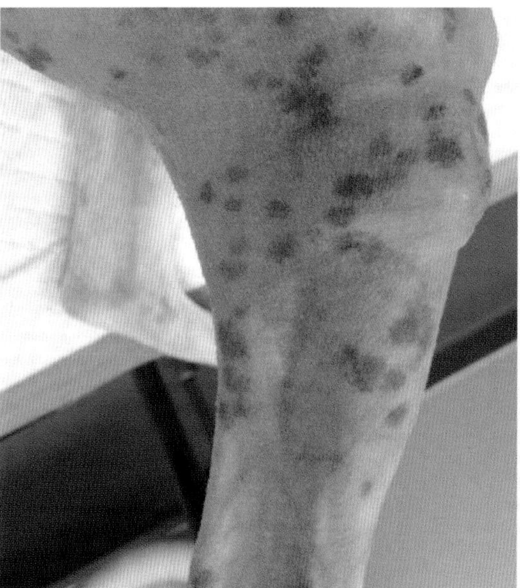

Fig. 10.41 Mass on the lateral aspect of the stifle, progressing cranially and dorsoventrally. The mass was not well defined and was very infiltrative and not mobile.

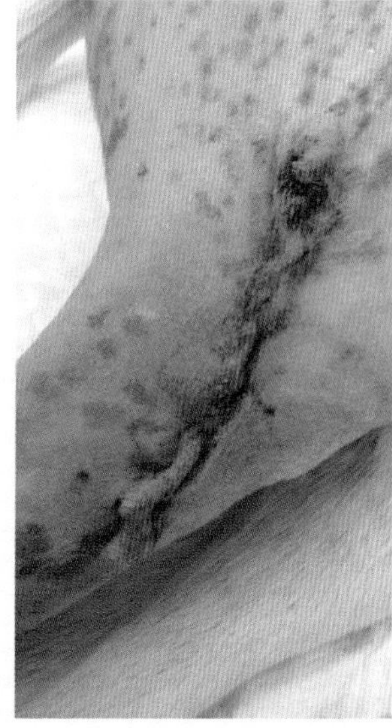

Fig. 10.42 Postoperative image. Lateral narrow margins, but deep resection to and including fascial planes.

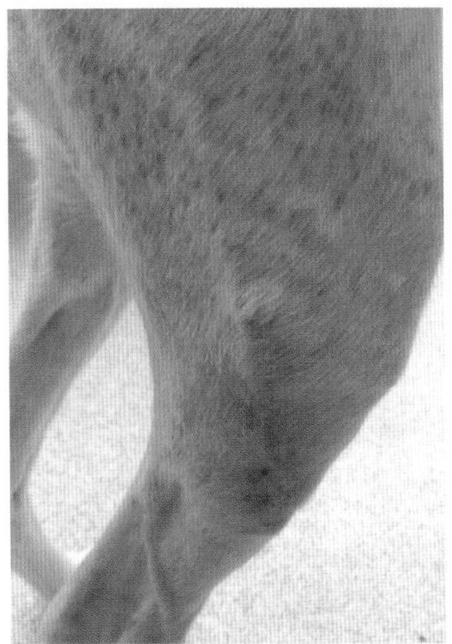

On the extremities, surgical margins are difficult to achieve and radical resection in the absence of orthopaedic and neurologic abnormalities can be an option for high-grade STS; however, a more conservative approach with limb sparing techniques may be a better alternative for low- to intermediate-grade tumours. Marginal excision of an STS, either as a sole therapy or combined with radiation therapy, may result in an excellent long-term outcome with lower morbidity compared to amputation.

Fig. 10.43 Three weeks postoperatively. At this time there were no signs of recurrence, swelling or problems with wound healing, and the patient was seen for four fractions of radiation therapy.

Case 10.4 Oral tumour

A 4-year-old, very happy, lively and healthy setter was seen for acute swelling of the lower mandible. A biopsy had been taken and this returned as a low-grade fibrosarcoma.

At presentation the patient had halitosis. There was a mild swelling lateral to the mandible caudal to the canine.

A CT scan of the head and thorax was performed (Figs. 10.44–10.46). Thoracic CT showed no signs of metastases. The regional lymph nodes were not enlarged.

Cytology (FNA) of the mandibular lymph nodes showed no signs of neoplastic cells, but in the right mandibular lymph node a reactive process was found.

CT of the mandible showed a soft tissue attenuating mass from the canine laterally to the PM2 caudally with no bony invasion.

A rostral mandibulectomy from I1 to include PM4 was performed. The labial mucosa was used to reconstruct the defect and a part of the skin had to be resected, as the lip was too large after a large part of the mandible was resected (Figs. 10.47–10.50).

Histopathology returned as:

MICROSCOPIC FINDINGS: 1) right mandible (12 sections). In the transverse section (1A) through the mandible there is an infiltrative spindle cell neoplasm that dissects through muscle and soft tissue. Neoplastic cells are spindle shaped,

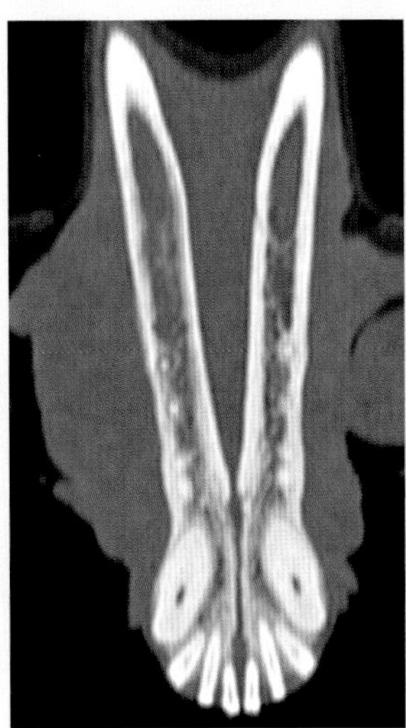

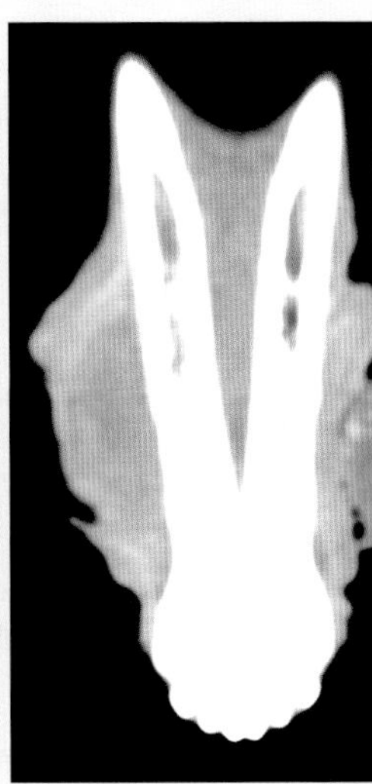

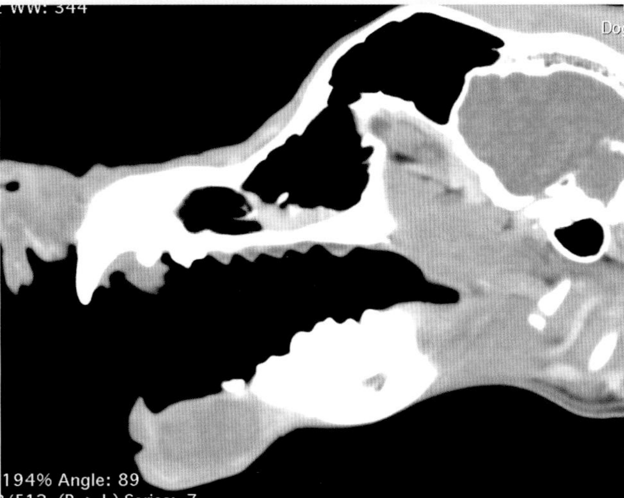

Figs. 10.44–10.46 CT of the mandible showing a soft tissue-attenuating mass (arrows) from the canine laterally to PM2 caudally with no bony invasion.

with indistinct cell margins and scant eosinophilic cytoplasm, oval nucleus with finely stippled chromatin and variably distinct nucleolus. Anisocytosis and anisokaryosis are moderate. The mitotic rate averages 1 per one high power field. In one section (1H) there is a marked inflammatory infiltrate in the mucosa, composed of neutrophils; bacterial colonies are visible on the mucosal surface which is also ulcerated. Margins: 1A yellow margin not infiltrated. 1B no evidence of neoplasia; blue margin not infiltrated. 1C no evidence of neoplasia; blue margin not infiltrated. 1D no evidence of neoplasia; blue and yellow margin not infiltrated. 1E no evidence of neoplasia; red margin not infiltrated. 1F no evidence of neoplasia; orange margin not infiltrated. 1G no evidence of neoplasia; orange margin not infiltrated. 1H no evidence of neoplasia; yellow margin not infiltrated. 1I no evidence of neoplasia; yellow and blue margin not infiltrated.

This patient made a very quick and uneventful recovery (Fig. 10.51).

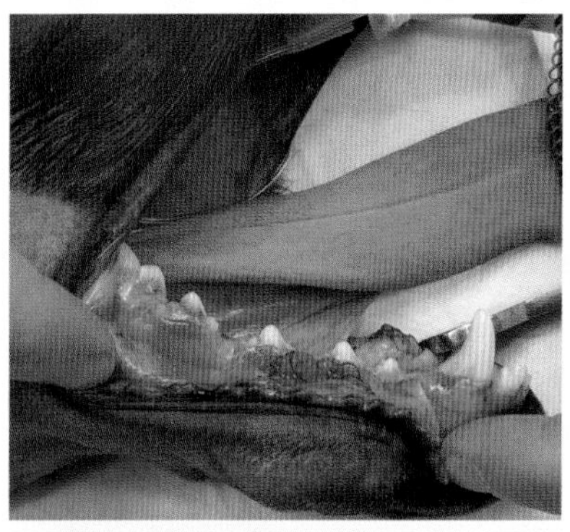

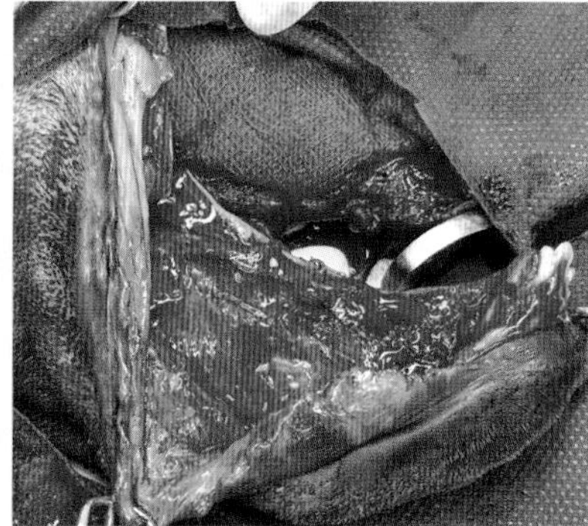

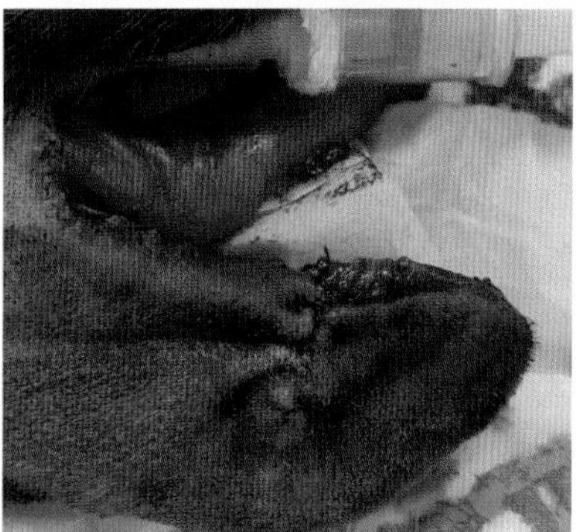

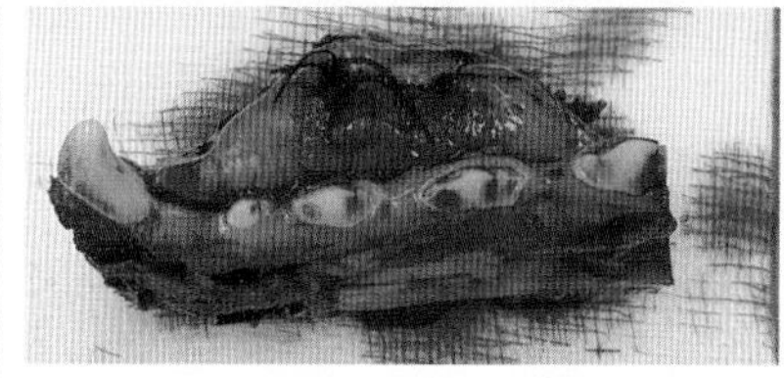

Figs. 10.47–10.50 A rostral mandibulectomy from I1 to and including PM4 was performed. The labial mucosa was used to reconstruct the defect, and part of the skin had to be resected as the lip was too large after a large part of the mandible was resected.

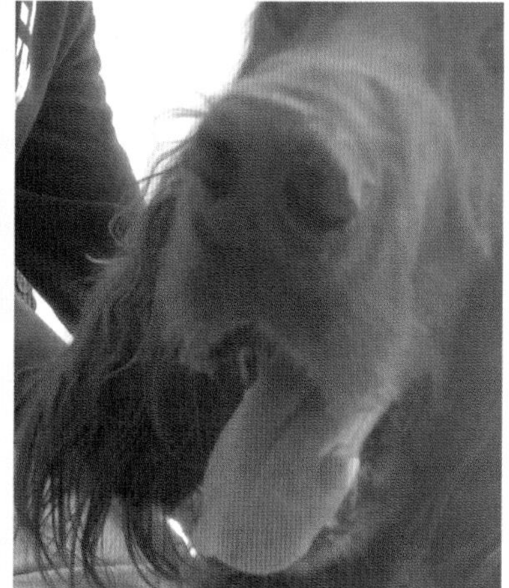

Fig. 10.51 The patient made a very quick and uneventful recovery.

Case 10.5 Mammary carcinoma

A 10-year-old terrier crossbreed was presented for further management of a mammary carcinoma in the fifth mammary gland. The dog was fit and healthy, with no abnormalities on physical examination. The results of routine haematology were unremarkable apart from slight neutrophilia. The referring veterinary surgeon had previously performed a lumpectomy to remove a small mammary nodule. The histopathology returned as a complex mammary adenocarcinoma with incomplete margins.

Ultrasound was performed and this showed no signs of increased intra-abdominal lymph nodes, but the inguinal lymph node was slightly enlarged. Needle aspiration of this lymph node revealed only a reactive process.

A regional mastectomy including the 3rd–5th mammary complex was planned (Figs. 10.52, 10.53). It is easiest to start any caudal mastectomy at the caudal border, with a V-shaped incision, to immediately locate the external pudendal artery and vein that then further lead to the mammarius and caudal superficial epigastrics (Fig. 10.54). It is also easy to then find the inguinal canal and remove the inguinal lymph node(s).

The remainder of the mammary gland can then easily be resected (this will lead to less bleeding; Fig. 10.55) and only the connection of the mammary tissue at the cranial aspect needs to be then further ligated or cauterised.

The resulting defect can then be closed in multiple layers (Fig. 10.56).

Histopathological examination of the entire specimen returned as:

Mammary gland: The largest nodule is composed of an infiltrative neoplastic proliferation of squamous epithelial cells effacing the mammary gland, ulcerating the epidermis and surrounded by severe inflammation (predominantly macrophages and neutrophils). Neoplastic cells are arranged in cords and trabeculae and are polygonal in shape, with abundant eosinophilic fibrillar cytoplasm and large round nuclei with finely stippled chromatin and indistinct nucleoli. These cells show moderate anisocytosis and anisokaryosis. The mitotic count is 12 in 10 HPFs. This neoplasm does not extend to the margins of the sample.

Three other nodules are identified in this sample. These are well demarcated and composed of a mixture of slightly atypical epithelial and myoepithelial cells. In two of them there are also foci of cartilaginous metaplasia. These three neoplasms do not extend to the margins.

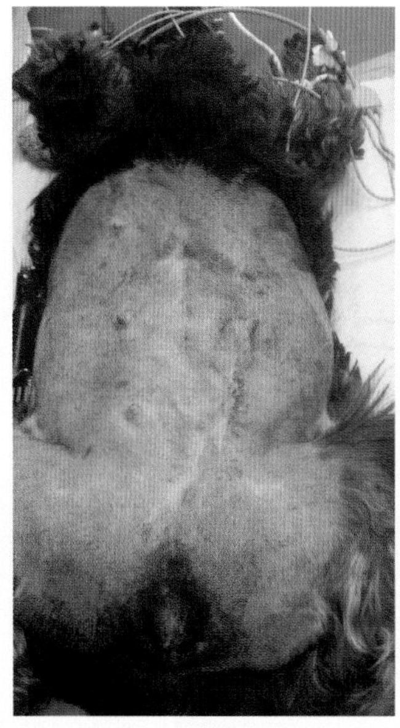
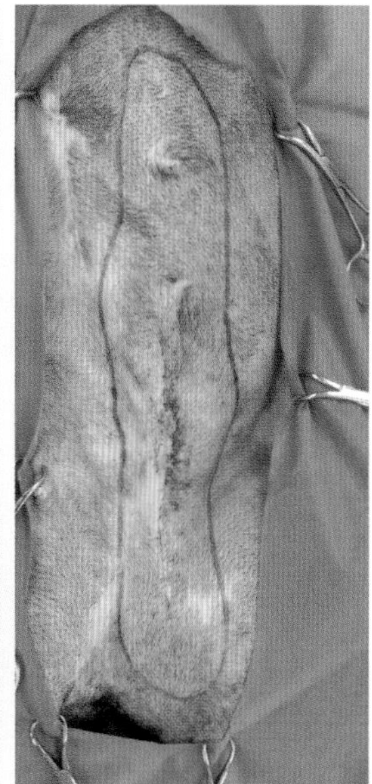

Figs. 10.52–10.53 A regional mastectomy was planned, to include the 3rd–5th mammary complex.

Medial iliac lymph node: Cortical lymphoid follicles are expanded with prominent germinal centres. Medullary sinuses are congested and paracortical areas are moderately hyperplastic.

Between 4–5 left mammary: in this sample there is a well-demarcated mammary nodule that is similar to the three well-demarcated nodules identified in the other mammary sample.

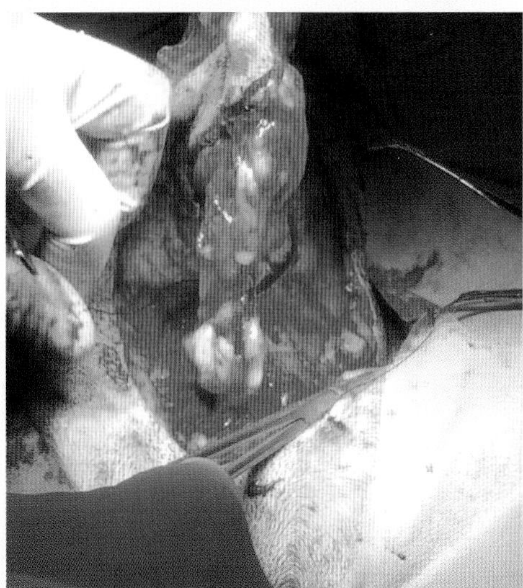

Fig. 10.54 Caudal mastectomy, starting at the caudal border with a V-shaped incision, to immediately locate the external pudendal artery.

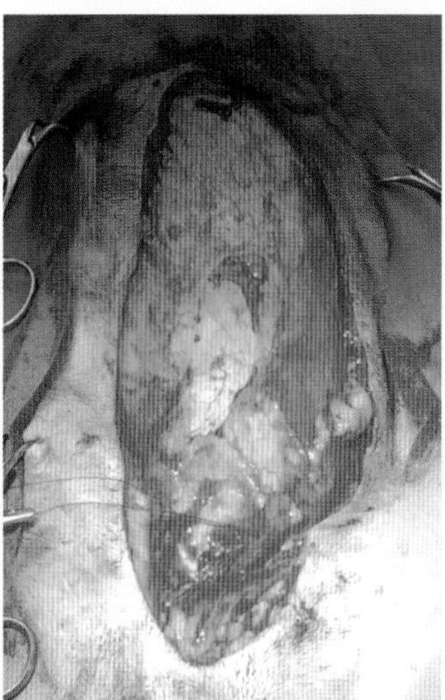

Fig. 10.55 Resection of the remainder of the mammary gland.

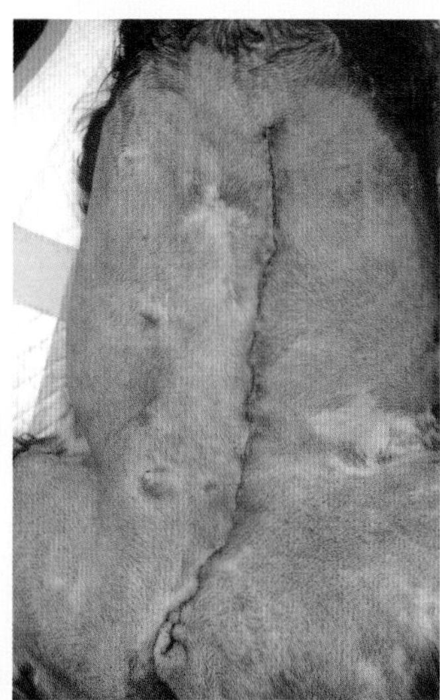

Fig. 10.56 The resulting defect was then closed in multiple layers.

Case 10.6 Vaginal tumour

A 7-year-old golden retriever was presented for a swelling in the perineal area. The patient had previously been neutered at the age of 3 years. Recently there had been vaginal discharge and also, just before the referral, the patient was having difficulty passing faeces.

Clinical examination revealed a large mass in the ventral perineum (Fig. 10.57). Vaginal palpation revealed a thickening in the vaginal wall. Abdominal palpation revealed a large caudal mass in the area of the bladder. The results of routine histology and biochemistry revealed no specific abnormalities.

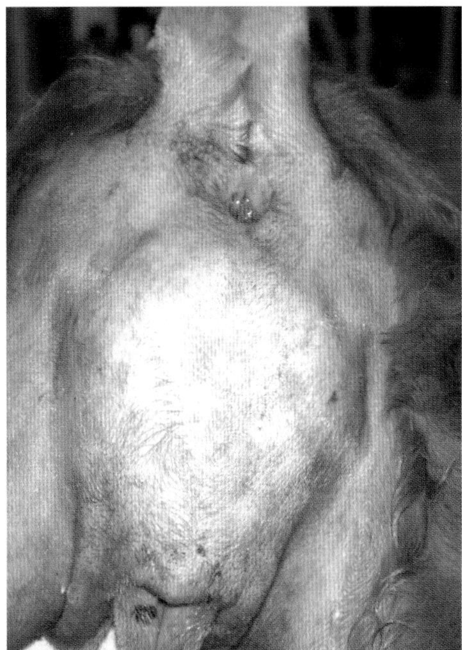

Fig. 10.57 Clinical examination revealed a large mass in the ventral perineum.

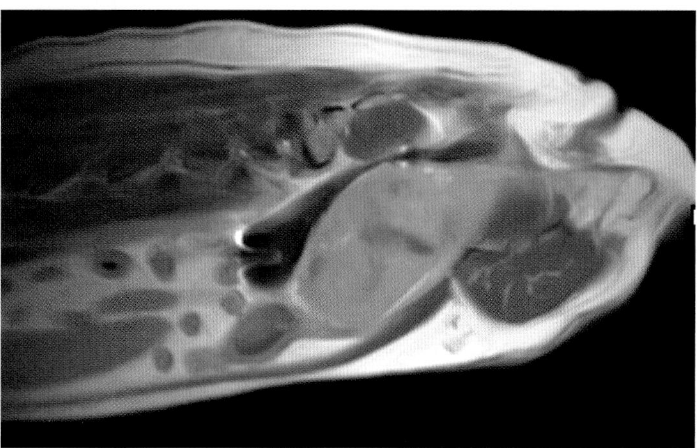

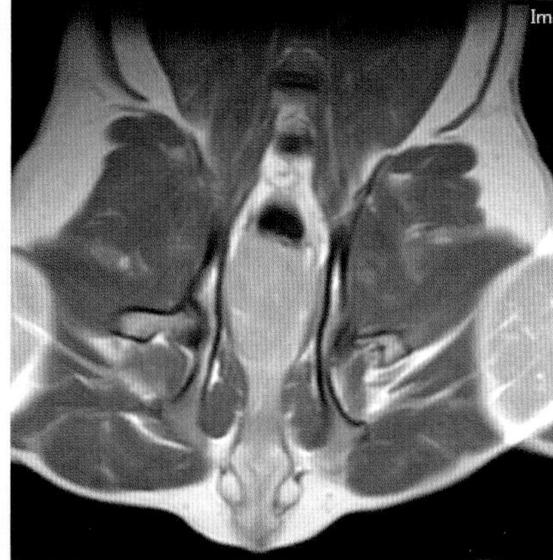

Figs. 10.58, 10.59 Abdominal CT showing a large mass in the caudal abdomen emanating from the vagina.

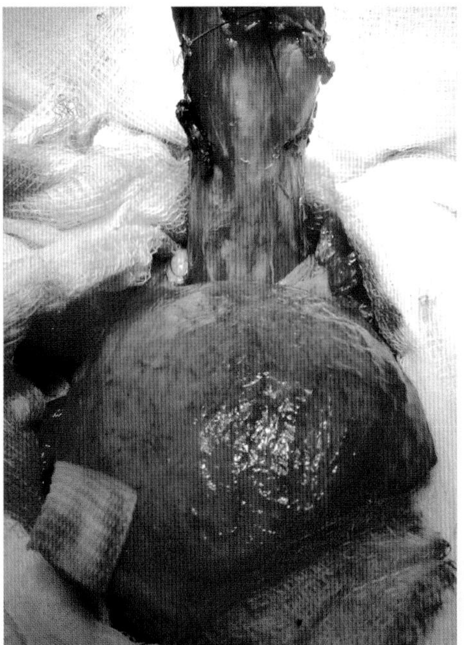

Fig. 10.60 Vagina bluntly dissected from its pelvic retroperitoneal fascial attachments between the paired levator ani.

Abdominal CT was performed, and this showed a large mass in the caudal abdomen emanating from the vagina (Fig. 10.58, 10.59).

At surgery: the dog was initially positioned in dorsal recumbency and a ventral midline coeliotomy was made. The bladder was retroflexed to gain exposure to the vagina and associated structures. The fascial and peritoneal attachments between the vagina and the rectum within the rectogenital pouch were resected using a combination of blunt and sharp dissection. Similarly, the attachment between the vagina and the urethra within the vesico-genital pouch was carefully dissected avoiding any disruption of the craniolateral and dorsal aspect of the urethra and the peri-urethral tissues. Care was taken to identify and preserve the integrity of the ureters and the urethral innervation. Excessive dissecting at the level of the bladder trigone, the level of the ureters and the dorsal surface of the urethra was avoided to prevent damage to the nerve supply of the bladder and the urethra (pelvic and pudendal nerves).The cranial and caudal branches of the vaginal artery and vein were ligated or coagulated using the vessel-sealing device. The perivaginal tissues were subsequently bluntly dissected

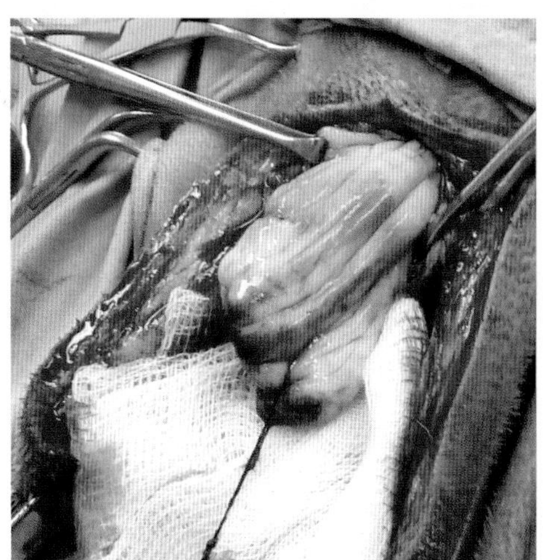

Fig. 10.61 Residual vascular supply to the cranial vagina ligated or coagulated.

as far caudally as possible, ensuring that no residual vascular supply or fascial attachment remained intact. A transfixing stay suture with a large loop was anchored through all layers of the cranial opening of the vagina; the loop of the suture was passed into the vaginal lumen. The dog was then positioned in sternal recumbency.

Alternatively both procedures can be performed with the dog in dorsal recumbency and with the legs pulled forward; this will allow access to the perineum without the need to change the patient's position.

Vaginal procedure: A midline episiotomy incision was made. The loop of the transfixing stay suture was identified in the vaginal lumen and retracted caudally, withdrawing and inverting the cranial vagina to the episiotomy site. A full-thickness circumferential incision of the vaginal wall was made at the junction of the vagina with the vestibule immediately cranial to the urethral orifice. The vagina was bluntly dissected from its pelvic retroperitoneal fascial attachments between the paired levator ani muscles (Fig. 10.60), progressing cranially until completely freed. Residual vascular supply to the cranial vagina was ligated or coagulated as previously described (Fig. 10.61). Care was taken to identify the urethral papilla during this procedure to ensure that it was not included in the closure.

Case 10.7 Rib soft tissue sarcoma

A 9-year-old pug was seen for a swelling over the caudal thorax. Fine needle aspiration by the referring vet was indicative of a soft tissue sarcoma. At presentation the dog was fit and healthy with no obvious abnormalities. A CT scan was performed, and this showed the mass to be originating from the 11th rib. There was marked lysis of the rib and swelling of the surrounding tissue.

At surgery the skin and full-thickness tissue around the mass were resected. The 10th–12th ribs were resected.

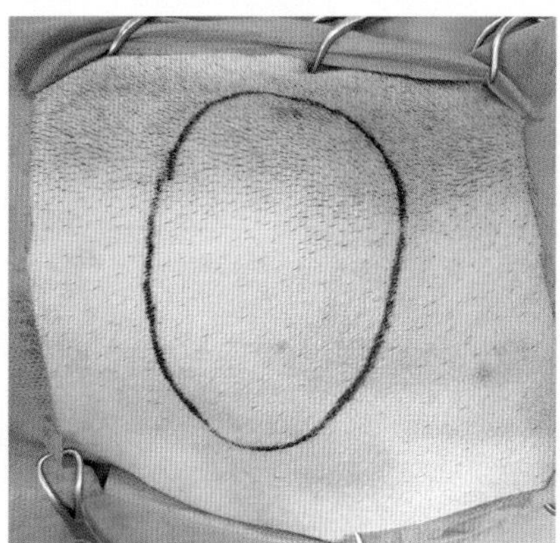

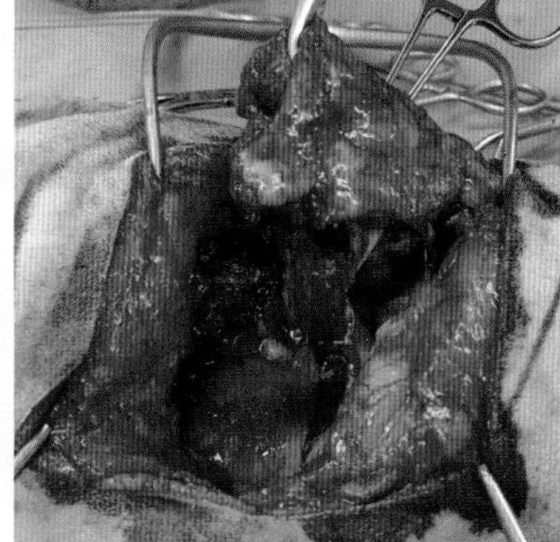

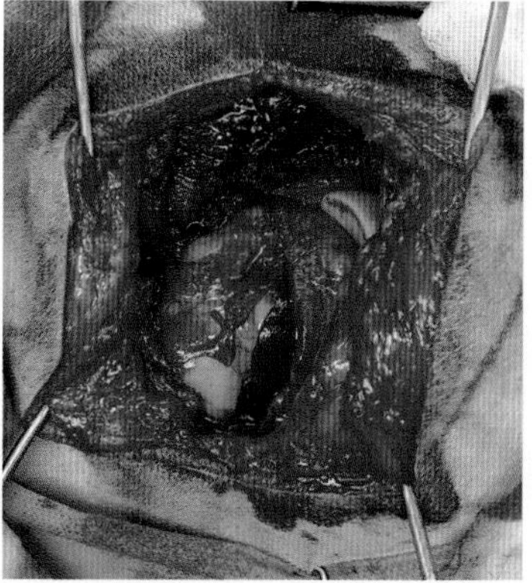

Figs 10.62–10.64 Resection of sarcoma.

The mass seemed to be attached to the diaphragm, and these tissues were resected together with the mass (Figs. 10.62–10.64).

The diaphragm was then cranially transposed and attached to the 9th rib. Wound closure was by primary apposition. No mesh was necessary: the abdominal musculature allowed primary closure of the wound and the skin was apposed.

Histopathology returned as: Thorax (four sections). In one sample there is a portion of a densely cellular mass. The mass is composed of neoplastic cells which are arranged in interlacing streams set in a fine to moderate fibrous connective tissue stroma. Individual neoplastic cells are ovoid to spindled with scant pale eosinophilic cytoplasm and indistinct borders. Nuclei are ovoid with coarse chromatin and small nucleoli. There is mild to moderate anisokaryosis and anisocytosis. Mitoses are 17 per 10 high power fields. The other sections comprise fibrous and adipose connective tissue, with in a few areas more cellular fibrous tissue in which loose streams of plump spindled cells are apparent which resemble those described above. This tissue is poorly demarcated. The margins are free of tumour cells.

Histological diagnosis: soft tissue sarcoma, intermediate grade, mass from thorax.

Case 10.8 Vaccine-associated soft tissue sarcoma

A 13-year-old cat was seen for management of a swelling left dorsolateral to the scapula (Fig. 10.65). A fine needle aspiration of the mass had been inconclusive. The cat had mild azotaemia on routine biochemistry. The mass was fixed but slightly mobile around the fixed points. The mass was about 6 cm in diameter.

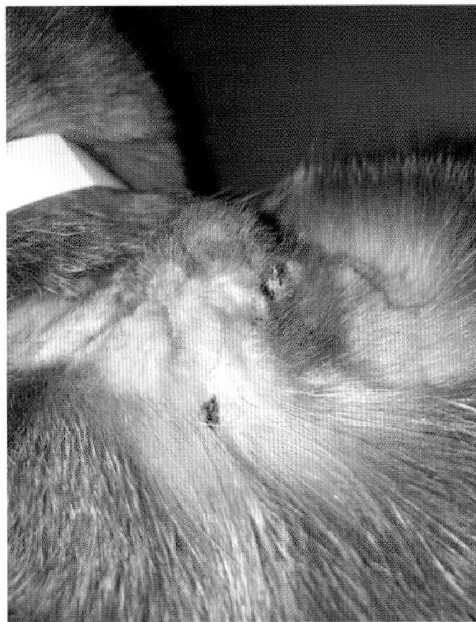

Fig. 10.65 Swelling dorsolatersal to scapula.

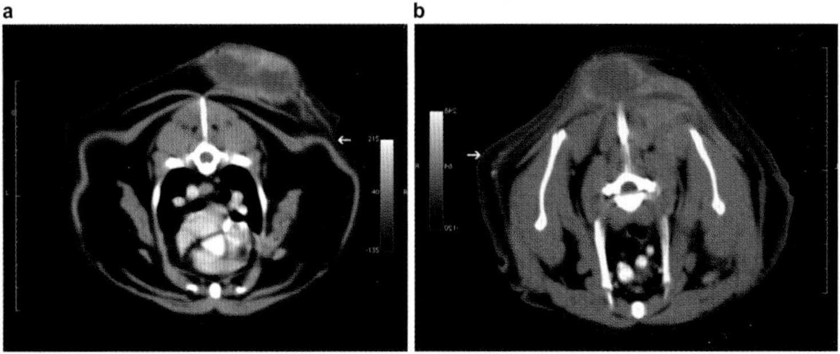

Fig. 10.66 CT highlighting a subcutaneous mass dorsal to the scapula on the left side.

CT of the mass (Fig. 10.66) showed a delineated mass in the subcutaneous tissues just dorsal to the scapula on the left side, and dorsal to the interscapular muscles and the omotransversarius. The mass, however, had medially and laterally further extensions into the subcutaneous tissues. There was an appearance of boundary between the capsule of the mass and the fascial planes.

Index